The New

Manual of Interventional Cardiology

Edited by

Mark Freed, M.D.
Cindy Grines, M.D.
Robert D. Safian, M.D.

Division of Cardiology
William Beaumont Hospital
Royal Oak, Michigan

1996

Physicians' Press
Birmingham, Michigan

DEDICATION

—We are who we are because of those who teach us and those who love us:

To my mentors, Phil Needleman, Jim Goldstein, Sarafino Garella, Burton Sobel, and William O'Neill, for leading by example; and to my family, Mom, Dad, Ralph, Susie, Paulie, Steve, Boomer, and my adorable little nephew, the Mutchie, who make the coldest, darkest days warm and sunny.

Mark Freed

"...we must have the steadfastness to see every enterprise through."
— JFK

To my wife, Maureen, who hoped I would have more free time as an editor than as an interventional cardiologist; and to my sons, Ryan and Luke, who keep me focused on the important aspects of life.

Rob Safian

To Jessica, Derek, John and Doug, for helping me remember the important things in life.

Cindy Grines

PREFACE

For the last 3 years, the Manual of Interventional Cardiology has been the most practical and popular reference in the field. Now, the Cardiology Division of William Beaumont Hospital, recognized as world's leaders in complex coronary intervention and the investigation of new technologies, proudly presents the much awaited Second Edition.

In addition to complete and extensive revisions of 30 previous chapters on simple & complex intervention, intraprocedural complications, and new devices, Second Edition features include:

- **Special Emphasis on Stents:** Among the topics reviewed in this 60-page chapter include: who, when, and how to stent; use of adjunctive imaging modalities and pharmacotherapy; and lesion-specific techniques. Almost 300 literature references are included.

- **Eight New Chapters:** Revascularization based on patient characteristics (the elderly, diabetics, renal failure patients...), radial approach to coronary intervention, intravascular ultrasound, local drug delivery & more...

- **Interventional Survey:** 27 leading interventionalists from 7 countries respond to more than 100 questions about patient triage, technical pearls & pitfalls, clinical follow-up and more...

- **Up-to-the-Minute Data:** Our unique publication process brings you the most current information available — literature references _≤ 1 week old_ at the time of book release _compared to 18-24 months old_ for most other interventional texts!

- **The "Bottom Line":** This 50-page "book-within-a-book" provides concise summaries of clinically important information from each chapter — a perfect review for the busy clinician!

We hope you enjoy reading _THE NEW_ Manual of Interventional Cardiology and find it of great practical value.

Mark Freed, M.D.
Cindy Grines, M.D.
Robert D. Safian, M.D.

ACKNOWLEDGEMENTS

To accomplish the tremendous task of presenting the data contained in this Manual, a small, dedicated team of professionals was assembled. This team focused their energy and discipline for many weeks into designing, illustrating, formatting, revising and typing the many chapters that make up this text. As editors, we wish to publicly recognize the abilities and talents of this small clerical team. We sincerely thank them, and wish to acknowledge:

Monica Crowder: As project coordinator, Ms. Crowder has played an important role in every aspect of production — from library research to design & formatting. Her committment to and enthusiasm for this project over the last year has been unsurpassed. Ms. Crowder created all the wonderfully readable tables and algorithms in the Manual.

Dianna Frye: As principal typist, Ms. Frye spent many, many hours typing the many, many revisions that went into creating the Manual. Her skillful work and indefatigable work ethic were essential to the succeessful completion of the Manual.

Steven Kronenberg — Imprint Graphic Design: Figures and cover design.

Phyllis McKinney: Typing and revisions: Chapter 5.

The Library Staff of William Beaumont Hospital: Patricia Benjamin, Nancy Bulgarelli, Ellen Carey, Jill Davidson, Kevin Davison, Joan Emahiser, Jean Gilbert, Wendy Janes, Shanan Kribs, Glen Nelson, Laurie Traks, and Jane West, for the many hours spent gathering literature references for the Manual.

We would also like to thank:
The Companies who helped us gather information on their products: Eli Lilly & Co., Centocor, Guidant (ACS, DVI), Boston Scientific (CVIS, Heart Technology, Meditech, SciMed), Johnson & Johnson Interventional Systems, Cordis, InterVentional Technologies, Cook, Spectranetics, Cardiometrics, USCI, Schneider, Medtronic, Merit Medical, Target Therapeutics, Namic, and Braun.

John Arnos Sr., for giving us the strength (Canon 586/133mHz, 1.2 gigabyte hard-drive, 28.8 baud modem) to complete this project on time.

Anne Johnson, Bob Fish, and the Staff at Quebecor Printing for their printing expertise and for helping us meet a deadline.

Mark Freed, M.D.
Cindy Grines, M.D.
Robert D. Safian, M.D.

NOTICE

The explosive growth of new equipment and drug therapy has resulted in the rapid evolution and acceptance of practice patterns often based on retrospective nonrandomized data and personal experience. Their ultimate role will require close inspection of prospective randomized trials. The clinical recommendations set forth in this book are those of the authors; they are offered as *general guidelines only and are not to be construed as absolute indications*. In addition, not all medications have been accepted by the U.S. Food and Drug Administration (USFDA) for usages described in this manual. The use of any drug should be preceded by a careful review of the package insert, which provides indications and dosages as approved by the USFDA. The reader is advised to consult the package insert before using any therapeutic agent. The authors and publisher disclaim responsibility for adverse effects resulting from omissions or undetected errors.

LIST OF CONTRIBUTORS

Katherine Abbo, MD
Director, Karen Yonts Cardiac
Awareness Center
St. Lukes Hospital
Milwakee, WI

Steven L. Almany, MD
Division of Cardiology
William Beaumont Hospital
Royal Oak, MI

Steven C. Ajluni, MD
Division of Cardiology
William Beaumont Hospital
Royal Oak, MI

Brian Annex, MD
Assistant Professor of Medicine
Duke University
Durham, NC

Phillip J. Bendick, PhD
Director, Vascular Laboratory
Director, Surgical Research
William Beaumont Hospital
Royal Oak, MI

Alan Bennett, R.C.V.T.
Division of Cardiology
William Beaumont Hospital
Royal Oak, MI

Terry T. Bowers, MD
Division of Cardiology
William Beaumont Hospital
Royal Oak, MI

Anthony C. De Franco, MD
Department of Cardiology
The Cleveland Clinic Foundation
Cleveland, OH

Daniel Diffin, MD
Staff Interventional Radiologist
Wilford Hall Medical Center
Lackland AFB
San Antonio TX

Mark Dooris, MBBS
Divison of Cardiology
Royal Brisbane Hospital
Queensland, Australia

Neal Eigler, MD
Co-Director, Cardiovascular Interventional
Center
Cedars-Sinai Medical Center
Associate Professor of Medicine
UCLA School of Medicine
Los Angles, CA

Kathleen A. Fasing, B.S., R.C.V.T.
Division of Cardiology
William Beaumont Hospital
Royal Oak, MI

Mark Freed, MD
Division of Cardiology
William Beaumont Hospital
Royal Oak, MI

Harold Z. Friedman, MD
Division of Cardiology
William Beaumont Hospital
Royal Oak, MI

Barry S. George, MD
Department of Cardiology
Riverside Methodist Hospital
Columbus, OH

Cindy L. Grines, MD
Director, Cardiac Catheterization Laboratory
William Beaumont Hospital
Royal Oak, MI

Joel K. Kahn, MD
Division of Cardiology
William Beaumont Hospital
Royal Oak, MI

Krishna Kandarpa, MD, PhD
Associate Professor of Radiology
Harvard Medical School
Co-Director, Cardiovascular & Interventional
Radiology
Brigham and Women's Hospital
Boston, MA

Barry M. Kaplan, MD
Division of Cardiology
William Beaumont Hospital
Royal Oak, MI

Kevin L. Kelco, B.S.
Division of Cardiology
William Beaumont Hospital
Royal Oak, MI

Sandeep Khurana, MD
Division of Cardiology
William Beaumont Hospital
Royal Oak, MI

James Kinn, MD
Division of Cardiology
William Beaumont Hospital
Royal Oak, MI

Patrick T. Koller, MD
Division of Cardiology
St. Paul Heart Clinic
St. Paul, MN

Frank Litvack, MD
Co-Director, Cardiovascular Interventional
Center
Cedars-Sinai Medical Center
Associate Professor of Medicine
UCLA School of Medicine
Los Angles, CA

Raymond G. McKay, MD
Director, Cardiac Laboratory
Hartford Hospital
Clinical Professor of Medicine
University of Connecticut
Hartford, CT

Mauro Moscucci, MD
Assistant Professor of Medicine
University of Michigan Medical Center
Ann Arbor, MI

David W.M. Muller, MBBS
Director, Interventional Cardiology
Associate Professor Medicine
University of Michigan Medical Center
Ann Arbor, MI

Steven E. Nissen, MD
Vice Chairman, Department of Cardiology
Director, Clinical Cardiology
The Cleveland Clinic Foundation
Cleveland, OH

William W. O'Neill, MD
Director, Divison of Cardiology
William Beaumont Hospital
Royal Oak, MI

Ashish Parikh, MD
Division of Cardiology
Cedars-Sinai Medical Center
Los Angles, CA

Gregory Pavlides, MD
Director, Cardiac Cathaterization Laboratory
Onassis Cardiac Surgery Center
Athens, Greece

Mark Reisman, MD
Director, Cardiovascular Research
Swedish Medical Center
Seattle, WA

Robert D. Safian, MD
Director, Interventional Cardiology
William Beaumont Hospital
Royal Oak, MI

Marc P. Sakwa, MD
Division of Cardiovascular Surgery
William Beaumont Hospital
Royal Oak, MI

Francis L. Shannon, MD
Division of Cardiovascular Surgery
William Beaumont Hospital
Royal Oak, MI

Gregory Stone, MD
Chariman, Cardiovascular Services
EL Camino Hospital
Mountain View, CA

Gerald C. Timmis, MD
Director, Cardiovascular Research
William Beaumont Hospital
Royal Oak, MI

E. Murat Tuzcu, MD
Associate Professor of Medicine
Ohio State University
Department of Cardiology
The Cleveland Clinic Foundation
Cleveland, OH

TABLE OF CONTENTS

SIMPLE & COMPLEX ANGIOPLASTY
1. PTCA EQUIPMENT AND TECHNIQUE 1
2. BRACHIAL AND RADIAL APPROACH 63
3. SINGLE-VESSEL & MULTIVESSEL ANGIOPLASTY 73
4. HIGH-RISK INTERVENTION 95
5. PTCA IN UNSTABLE ISCHEMIC SYNDROMES 105
6. LV DYSFUNCTION 155
7. PATIENT CHARACTERISTICS 175

CORONARY INTERVENTION BY LESION MORPHOLOGY AND LOCATION
8. OVERVIEW OF INTERVENTIONAL DEVICES 195
9. INTRACORONARY THROMBUS 209
10. BIFURCATION LESIONS 233
11. TORTUOSITY AND ANGULATION 247
12. CALCIFIED LESIONS 255
13. ECCENTRIC LESIONS 267
14. OSTIAL LESIONS 273
15. LONG LESIONS 285
16. CHRONIC TOTAL OCCLUSIONS 297
17. CORONARY ARTERY BYPASS GRAFTS 325
18. PTCA EXOTICA 351

COMPLICATIONS
19. CORONARY ARTERY SPASM 361
20. DISSECTION AND ACUTE CLOSURE 369
21. NO-REFLOW 399
22. PERFORATION 405
23. EMERGENCY BYPASS SURGERY 413
24. RESTENOSIS 425
25. MEDICAL & PERIPHERAL COMPLICATIONS 441

NEW INTERVENTIONAL DEVICES
26. CORONARY STENTS 461
27. ROTABLATOR 521
28. DIRECTIONAL CORONARY ATHERECTOMY 537
29. TRANSLUMINAL EXTRACTION CATHETER 563
30. EXCIMER LASER CORONARY ANGIOPLASTY 573
31. INTRAVASCULAR ULTRASOUND 583
32. CORONARY ANGIOSCOPY 603
33. DOPPLER BLOOD FLOW 611

Table of Contents

MISCELLANEOUS TOPICS

34. ADJUNCTIVE PHARMACOTHERAPY 625
35. LOCAL DRUG DELIVERY 645
36. PERIPHERAL AND VISCERAL INTERVENTION 661
37. BALLOON VALVULOPLASTY 689
38. SPECIAL CONSIDERATIONS FOR CATH LAB PERSONNEL 715
39. INTERVENTIONAL SURVEY 731
40. THE BOTTOM LINE 761

EXPANDED TABLE OF CONTENTS

Chapter 1. PTCA EQUIPMENT AND TECHNIQUE
PREPROCEDURAL PREPARATION 1
EQUIPMENT & TECHNIQUE 6
POSTPROCEDURAL CONSIDERATIONS 33
QUICK REFERENCE: PTCA EQUIPMENT 35

Chapter 2. BRACHIAL AND RADIAL APPROACH
PROCEDURAL OVERVIEW 63
SPECIAL INDICATIONS FOR BRACHIAL AND RADIAL TECHNIQUES 67
INTERVENTIONAL CONSIDERATIONS 68
COMPLICATIONS 69

Chapter 3. SINGLE-VESSEL & MULTIVESSEL ANGIOPLASTY
MULTIVESSEL PTCA IN PATIENTS WITH PRESERVED LV FUNCTION
    Randomized Trials 73
    Nonrandomized Trials 80
MULTIVESSEL PTCA IN PATIENTS WITH LV DYSFUNCTION 83
REVASCULARIZATION STRATEGY 85
    Complete vs. Incomplete Revascularization 85
    Approach to Moderate Stenoses 86
    Order of Dilatation 86
    Staging 88
SPECIAL SUBSET OF MULTIVESSEL DISEASE 91

Chapter 4. HIGH-RISK INTERVENTION
RISK STRATIFICATION 95
RISK REDUCTION 96
LEFT MAIN DISEASE 101

Chapter 5. PTCA IN UNSTABLE ISCHEMIC SYNDROMES
ACUTE MI
  PRIMARY (DIRECT) PTCA 105
    Non-Randomized Observational Series 106
    Thrombolytic-Ineligible Patients 108
    Cardiogenic Shock 110
    Thrombolytic-Eligible Patients 110
    Recommendations 115
  RESCUE (SALVAGE) PTCA FOR FAILED THROMBOLYSIS 115
    Observational Series 115
    Randomized Trials 117
    Recommendations 118
  IMMEDIATE PTCA—SUCCESSFUL THROMBOLYSIS, ASYMPTOMATIC 118
    Randomized Trials 118
    Limitations of Studies 118

Table of Contents

    Recommendations 118
  DELAYED PTCA—SUCCESSFUL THROMBOLYSIS, ASYMPTOMATIC 120
    Randomized Trials 120
    Limitations of Studies 120
    Recommendations 121
  DELAYED PTCA—OCCLUDED VESSEL, ASYMPTOMATIC 121
    Observational Trials 121
    Randomized Trials 122
    Recommendations 122
  PTCA FOR POST MI ISCHEMIA 122
    Randomized trials 122
    Recommendations 122
UNSTABLE ANGINA 123
  PATHOPHYSIOLOGY 123
  SUCCESS AND COMPLICATIONS 124
  MEDICAL THERAPY VS. PTCA VS. CABG 126
    Medical Therapy vs. CABG 126
    Medical Therapy vs. PTCA 126
    PTCA vs. CABG 127
DEFICIENCIES OF PTCA 127
  REPERFUSION ARRHYTHMIAS 127
  BLEEDING COMPLICATIONS 129
  ISCHEMIC COMPLICATIONS 130
DEVICES AND DRUGS FOR MI AND UNSTABLE ANGINA 131
  INTRAAORTIC BALLOON PUMP 131
  DIRECTIONAL CORONARY ATHERECTOMY 131
  TEC ATHERECTOMY 132
  ROTABLATOR ATHERECTOMY 133
  STENTS 133
  LASER 134
  THERMAL BALLOON ANGIOPLASTY 136
  LOCAL DRUG DELIVERY 136
  OTHER NEW DEVICES 137
  SYSTEMIC DRUGS 137
    Antiplatelet Agents 137
      Aspirin 137
      Ticlopidine 137
      Glycoprotein IIb/IIIa Receptor Antagonist 137
    Heparin 138
    Direct Thrombin Inhibitors 140
    Thrombolytics 141
    Contrast Agents 142
  EMERGENCY CABG 142
CLINICAL APPROACH TO THE ACUTE PATIENT 143
TECHNICAL STRATEGY FOR ACUTE ISCHEMIC SYNDROMES 143

Chapter 6. LV DYSFUNCTION

BACKGROUND 155
SYSTEMIC SUPPORT. 160
    IABP 160
    CPS 161
    Ventricular Assist Devices 165
    Left Atrial-Femoral Bypass 166
REGIONAL MYOCARDIAL SUPPORT. 167
    Autoperfusion Catheters 167
    Active Coronary Hemoperfusion 168
    Perfluorochemicals 168
    Coronary Sinus Retroperfusion 168
    Pharmacotherapy 169

Chapter 7. PATIENT CHARACTERISTICS

YOUNG PATIENTS (Age < 40 years) 175
ELDERLY PATIENTS (Age 65-75 years) 176
ELDERLY PATIENTS (Age ≥ 80 years) 179
FEMALE PATIENTS. 182
AFRICAN-AMERICANS 183
DIABETICS 185
CHRONIC DIALYSIS PATIENTS 186
CARDIAC TRANSPLANT PATIENTS 188
SILENT ISCHEMIA 189

Chapter 8. OVERVIEW OF INTERVENTIONAL DEVICES

LIMITATIONS OF INTERVENTIONAL DEVICES 195
    Failure to Cross a Chronic Total Occlusion with a Guidewire 195
    Failure to Cross a Lesion with a Device 195
    Failure to Dilate or Deploy a Device 195
    Dissection/Abrupt Closure 195
    Recurrent Ischemia and Restenosis 198
IMPORTANT CONSIDERATIONS IN EVALUATING INTERVENTIONAL DEVICES 198
    Procedural Success 198
    Assessment of Lumen Enlargement 199
    Relationship Between Immediate Lumen Enlargement and Late Outcome 199
    Cost 201
    Complications 202
IMPORTANT CONSIDERATIONS IN USING INTERVENTIONAL DEVICES 202
    Facilitated Lumen Enlargement 202
    Lesion-Specific Approach to Coronary Intervention 203
    Adjunctive Imaging Techniques 204
    Adjunctive Pharmacotherapy 204
NEW INVESTIGATIONAL DEVICES 204
    Hydrolyzer 205
    AngioJet 205

Therapeutic Ultrasound 206
Radiofrequency/Thermal Angioplasty Devices 206
Vibrational Angioplasty 207
Cutting Balloon Angioplasty 207
Pullback Atherectomy Catheter 208
Rotary Atherectomy System 208
Low-Speed Rotational Angioplasty Catheter System (ROTACS) 210
Excimer Laser Guidewire 210

Chapter 9. INTRACORONARY THROMBUS

DEFINITION 209
PATHOPHYSIOLOGY 209
PTCA AND THROMBOTIC LESIONS 210
NEW DEVICES AND THROMBOTIC LESIONS 210
INVESTIGATIONAL TECHNIQUES 220
PHARMACOLOGIC THERAPY OF PRE-EXISTING THROMBUS 222
    Heparin and Aspirin 222
    Thrombolytic Therapy 222
    Novel Antiplatelet and Antithrombin Drugs 224
    Local Drug Delivery 224
POST-PTCA THROMBUS 224
STENT THROMBOSIS 224

Chapter 10. BIFURCATION LESIONS

DESCRIPTION 233
APPROACH TO BIFURCATION LESIONS 233
    Need for Sidebranch Protection 233
    PTCA Techniques 235
PROCEDURAL RESULTS 240

Chapter 11. TORTUOSITY AND ANGULATION

TORTUOSITY 247
    Definition 247
    Procedural Outcome 247
    Technical Considerations and Approach 248
ANGULATED LESIONS 251
    PTCA 251
    New Interventional Devices 251
    Approach 252

Chapter 12. CALCIFIED LESIONS

LIMITATIONS OF ANGIOGRAPHY 255
PTCA 256
NEW INTERVENTIONAL DEVICES 257
TECHNICAL STRATEGY 261

Chapter 13. ECCENTRIC LESIONS

LIMITATIONS OF ANGIOGRAPHY 267
DEFINITIONS 267
BALLOON ANGIOPLASTY 267
NEW INTERVENTIONAL DEVICES 267
TECHNICAL STRATEGY 270

Chapter 14. OSTIAL LESIONS

DEFINITIONS 273
RESULTS 273
    PTCA 274
    New Devices 274
TECHNICAL CONSIDERATIONS 275
    Balloon Angioplasty 275
    New Devices 275
CASE SELECTION: LESION-SPECIFIC, MULTI-DEVICE THERAPY 277

Chapter 15. LONG LESIONS

BALLOON ANGIOPLASTY 285
NEW INTERVENTIONAL DEVICES 287
APPROACH TO LONG LESIONS 292

Chapter 16. CHRONIC TOTAL OCCLUSIONS

CORONARY ARTERY OCCLUSION 297
    Pathophysiology 297
    Indications and Benefits 298
    PTCA 298
    Equipment Selection and PTCA Technique 307
    New Devices 313
SAPHENOUS VEIN GRAFT OCCLUSION 316
    Pathology 316
    PTCA Results 316
    New Devices 316
    Prolonged Intragraft Thrombolysis 316

Chapter 17. CORONARY ARTERY BYPASS GRAFTS

TREATMENT OPTIONS FOR VEIN GRAFT DISEASE 325
    Repeat CABG 325
    PTCA 325
    New Interventional Devices 330
APPROACH TO THE PATIENT WITH PREVIOUS BYPASS SURGERY 336
    Graft Age 336
    Lesion Location 336
        Proximal and Aorto-ostial Lesions 336
        Lesions in the Body of the Graft 337

Distal Anastomotic Lesions 337
Lesion Morphology 337
Vein Grafts > 3 mm Diameter 337
Vein Grafts < 3 mm Diameter 337
Degenerated Grafts and Chronic Total Occlusions 337
Acute Myocardial Infarction 338
INTERNAL MAMMARY ARTERY INTERVENTION 339
GASTROEPIPLOIC ARTERY 341
APPROACH TO PTCA OF NATIVE VESSELS VIA BYPASS GRAFTS 341

Chapter 18. PTCA EXOTICA

LARGE VESSEL CORONARY ANGIOPLASTY 351
RETROGRADE NATIVE VESSEL ANGIOPLASTY 351
INABILITY TO REACH LESION THROUGH A BYPASS GRAFT 352
GUIDEWIRE TECHNIQUES 352
GUIDING CATHETER TECHNIQUES 353
PERCUTANEOUS REMOVAL OF EMBOLIZED FRAGMENTS 354
EMBOLIZATION OF CORONARY FISTULAS 354
ENTRAPPED GUIDEWIRE REMOVAL 355
ENTRAPPED BALLOON REMOVAL 355

Chapter 19. CORONARY ARTERY SPASM

PATHOPHYSIOLOGY 361
PTCA 361
NEW DEVICES 362
MANAGEMENT 362
PREVENTION 364
PTCA FOR VARIANT ANGINA 364

Chapter 20. DISSECTION AND ACUTE CLOSURE

CLASSIFICATION OF ACUTE CLOSURE 369
INCIDENCE AND TIMING OF ACUTE CLOSURE 369
CAUSES OF ACUTE CLOSURE 370
Dissection 370
Classification 371
Incidence 371
Pathophysiology 372
Risk Factors for Dissection 373
Prognosis After Dissection 373
RISK FACTORS FOR ACUTE CLOSURE 376
PREVENTION OF ACUTE CLOSURE 376
Antiplatelet Agents 376
Anticoagulants 381
IABP 382
PTCA Technique 382
RECOGNITION OF ACUTE CLOSURE 383

MANAGEMENT OF ACUTE CLOSURE 383
OTHER MANAGEMENT ISSUES 389
    Non-Flow-Limiting Dissection 389
    Primary Thrombotic Acute Closure 390
PROGNOSIS 391

Chapter 21. NO-REFLOW
DEFINITION 399
ETIOLOGY 399
INCIDENCE 399
CLINICAL MANIFESTATIONS AND PROGNOSIS 399
PROPHYLAXIS 400
MANAGEMENT 400

Chapter 22. PERFORATION
INCIDENCE AND CLASSIFICATION 405
MECHANISMS AND RISK FACTORS 405
OUTCOME 406
PREVENTION 407
MANAGEMENT 408

Chapter 23. EMERGENCY BYPASS SURGERY
INTRODUCTION 413
INCIDENCE 414
INDICATIONS FOR EMERGENCY CABG 416
CONTRAINDICATIONS TO EMERGENCY SURGERY 417
PREPARATION FOR EMERGENCY SURGERY 417
SURGICAL TECHNIQUES 418
RESULTS 420

Chapter 24. RESTENOSIS
DEFINITION 425
MECHANISMS 429
TIME COURSE 430
PREDICTORS 430
PREVENTION 431
DETECTION 433
MANAGEMENT 434
RECOMMENDATIONS 434
FUTURE DIRECTIONS 435

Chapter 25. MEDICAL & PERIPHERAL COMPLICATIONS
RENAL INSUFFICIENCY 441
    Etiology 441
    Prevention 441

Table of Contents

Management 443
CONTRAST REACTIONS 444
   Types of Contrast Agents 444
   Adverse Dye Reactions 444
   Recommendations 446
   Prevention 446
   Treatment 447
PERIPHERAL VASCULAR COMPLICATIONS 448
   AV Fistula 448
   Pseudoaneurysm 449
   Thrombotic Occlusion 450
   Arterial Perforation 450
   Dissection 451
   Retroperitoneal Hemmorrhage 451
   Atheroembolization 452
   Bleeding Complications 453
   Vascular Closure Devices 453
INFECTION 455
   Clinical Manifestations 456
   Etiology and Treatment 456
NEUROLOGIC COMPLICATIONS 457

Chapter 26. CORONARY STENTS

STENT DESIGNS 461
   Self-Expanding Stents 461
   Balloon-Expandable Stents 462
STENT CHARACTERISTICS 465
TECHNIQUE OF STENT PLACEMENT 466
   Self-Expanding Stents 466
   Balloon-Expandable Stents 467
   Radial Artery Technique 474
INDICATION FOR STENTS 474
   Definite Indications 474
   Probable Indications 477
   Possible Indications 485
   Contraindications 487
SPECIFIC CLINICAL SITUATIONS 491
   Acute MI 491
   Unstable Angina 491
   Single Patent Vessel 491
   Unprotected Left Main 492
   Sealing Perforations and Pseudoaneurysms 492
   Women 492
ADJUNCTIVE THERAPY 493
   Conventional Anticoagulation Regimen 493
   Low-Intensity Anticoagulation Regimen 493
   Intravascular Ultrasound (IVUS) 495

Doppler Flow 503
COMPLICATIONS 503
    Stent Thrombosis 503
    Ischemic Complications 505
    Bleeding and Vascular Injury 505
    Stent Embolization 505
    Sidebranch Occlusion 505
    Perforation 506
OTHER ISSUES 506
    Cost 506
    Future Directions 506

Chapter 27. ROTABLATOR

DESCRIPTION 521
PHYSICAL PRINCIPLES AND DESIGN CHARACTERISTICS 522
IMPACT OF HIGH-SPEED ROTATIONAL ABLATION 522
ROTABLATOR PROCEDURE 524
RESULTS 526
    Results 526
    Complications 527
    Restenosis 529
    Impact of Lesion Morphology on Results 532
CLINICAL TRIALS 532

Chapter 28. DIRECTIONAL CORONARY ATHERECTOMY (DCA)

DESCRIPTION 537
DCA EQUIPMENT 537
DCA TECHNIQUE 541
MECHANISM OF LUMEN ENLARGEMENT 543
PROCEDURAL RESULTS 543
    Immediate Angiographic Results 543
    Angiographic Complications 546
    Clinical Complications 548
    Restenosis and Late Outcome 550
SPECIAL CONSIDERATIONS 552
    Deep Tissue Resection 552
    Unstable Angina 553
    Acute MI 553
    Elderly 553
LESION-SPECIFIC APPLICATIONS 554
TISSUE ANALYSIS 556

Chapter 29. TRANSLUMINAL EXTRACTION CATHETER (TEC)

DESCRIPTION 563
EQUIPMENT 563
TECHNIQUE 564
MECHANISM OF ACTION 567

Table of Contents

RESULTS 567
    Native Coronary Arteries.. 567
    Saphenous Vein Grafts.. 568
SPECIAL CONSIDERATIONS. 569
    Acute Ischemic Syndromes 569
    Thrombus 570
    Saphenous Vein Bypass Grafts 570
    Ostial Lesions 570
    Contraindications 570
FUTURE DIRECTIONS 570

Chapter 30. EXCIMER LASER CORONARY ANGIOPLASTY

BACKGROUND 573
EQUIPMENT 573
CLINICAL RESULTS 575
    Laser Wire for Total Occlusions 576
    Complications 578
    New Techniques to Improve Results 578
RECOMMENDATIONS AND CASE SELECTION 578
TECHNICAL DETAILS 579

Chapter 31. INTRAVASCULAR ULTRASOUND

LIMITATIONS OF ANGIOGRAPHY 583
IVUS EQUIPMENT 583
IMAGE INTERPRETATION 586
ADVANTAGES OF IVUS 587
DISADVANTAGES OF IVUS 589
TECHNIQUE 590
DIAGNOSTIC APPLICATIONS OF IVUS 591
    Angiographically Unrecognized Disease 591
    Lesions of Uncertain Severity 591
    Cardiac Allograft Vasculopathy 592
INTERVENTIONAL APPLICATION OF IVUS 592
    Characterize Plaque for Device Selection 592
    Mechanism of Lumen Enlargement 595
    Precise Quantitative Measurements 596
    Guidance of Directional Atherectomy 597
    Coronary Stent Deployment 598
    Characterize Dissection After Intervention 599
COMPARISON OF IVUS, ANGIOSCOPY, AND DOPPLER FLOW 599
NEW INTRAVASCULAR IMAGING DEVICES 599

Chapter 32. CORONARY ANGIOSCOPY

INDICATIONS 603
LIMITATIONS OF ANGIOSCOPY 606
COMPLICATIONS 606

Chapter 33. DOPPLER BLOOD FLOW

INTRODUCTION 611
APPROACH TO DOPPLER BLOOD FLOW 611
APPLICATIONS 615
   Clinical Applications 615
   Interventional Applications 617

Chapter 34. ADJUNCTIVE PHARMACOTHERAPY

ANALGESIA AND SEDATION 625
CONTRAST REACTIONS 625
   PROPHYLAXIS AGAINST CONTRAST REACTIONS 625
   TREATMENT OF CONTRAST REACTIONS 626
PREVENTION OF ABRUPT CLOSURE 626
   ANTIPLATELET THERAPY 626
      Aspirin 626
      Ticlopidine 629
      Dipyridamole 629
      IIb/IIIa Receptor Antagonists 630
   ANTITHROMBOTIC AGENTS 634
      Heparin 634
      Low Molecular Weight Heparin 638
      Hirudin and Derivatives 638
      Other Antithrombin Agents 638
   FIBRINOLYTICS 639
   DEXTRAN 639
PREVENTING ISCHEMIA DURING ANGIOPLASTY 640
TREATMENT OF PERIPROCEDURAL HYPOTENSION 640

Chapter 35. LOCAL DRUG DELIVERY

OVERVIEW 645
MECHANISMS OF INTRAMURAL DRUG DELIVERY 645
PHARMACOKINETIC CONSIDERATIONS 645
CATHETER-BASED LOCAL DRUG DELIVERY TECHNIQUES 646
   The Double-Balloon Catheter 646
   The Wolinsky Perforated Balloon Catheter 647
   The Microporous Balloon Catheter 649
   The Transport Catheter 649
   The Hydrogel-Coated Balloon 649
   The Dispatch Catheter 651
   The Channel Balloon 652
   The Infusasleeve 653
   The Iontophoresis Catheter 654
DRUG DELIVERY CATHETERS APPROVED FOR CLINICAL USE 655
CONCLUSIONS 657

Chapter 36. PERIPHERAL AND VISCERAL INTERVENTION

PATHOPHYSIOLOGY 661
DIAGNOSIS AND PATIENT EVALUATION 662
PERCUTANEOUS ANGIOPLASTY TECHNIQUES 666
RESULTS OF PTA 674
    Renal Artery PTA 674
    Aortoiliac PTA 674
    Iliofemoral PTA 674
    Femoropopliteal PTA 676
    Infrapopliteal PTA 676
    Cerebral PTA 676
COMPLICATIONS OF PTA 676
NEW DIRECTIONS 677
    Intravascular Stents 677
    Peripheral Intra-Arterial thrombolysis (PIAT) 678
    Atherectomy 681
    Laser Ablation Techniques 681

Chapter 37. BALLOON VALVULOPLASTY

PERCUTANEOUS BALLOON MITRAL VALVULOPLASTY (PBMV) 689
    Mechanism of Mitral Valvuloplasty 689
    Preprocedural Evaluation 689
    Technique 689
    Results 694
PERCUTANEOUS BALLOON AORTIC VALVULOPLASTY (PBAV) 699
    Mechanism of Aortic Valvuloplasty 700
    Preprocedural Evaluation 700
    Technique 700
    Results 701

Chapter 38. SPECIAL CONSIDERATIONS FOR CATH LAB PERSONNEL

PRE-PROCEDURAL CONSIDERATIONS 715
INTRAPROCEDURAL CONSIDERATIONS 719
NEW DEVICES 722
POSTPROCEDURAL CONSIDERATIONS 725

Chapter 39. INTERVENTIONAL SURVEY 731

Chapter 40. THE BOTTOM LINE 761

1 CORONARY INTERVENTION: PREPARATION, EQUIPMENT & TECHNIQUE

Robert D. Safian, M.D.
Mark Freed, M.D.

PREPROCEDURAL PREPARATION

Percutaneous transluminal coronary angioplasty (PTCA) has enjoyed explosive growth and popularity since first introduced by Andreas Gruentzig in 1977. Although initially restricted to patients with single, discrete, concentric, and noncalcified stenoses, patients with unstable ischemic syndromes, multivessel disease, left ventricular dysfunction and acute MI are now routinely submitted for percutaneous revascularization with balloons and other intracoronary devices. Through improvements in PTCA hardware, adjunctive pharmacotherapy, and new interventional technologies, yesterday's "complex" procedure is today's "simple" case. Simple angioplasty, therefore, is a relative term and refers to procedures that can be performed with high success and a low complications. It is only through meticulous attention to patient selection, procedural technique and early recognition of complications that "simple" angioplasty can be performed.

A. **EVALUATION OF THE PATIENT PRIOR TO PERCUTANEOUS INTERVENTION.** The medical history, physical examination, and laboratory data are used to identify conditions which require preprocedural pharmacotherapy, technical modification, or postponement of the procedure (Table 1.1).

1. **History.** Cardiac history should be ascertained including previous myocardial infarction, coronary artery bypass grafting (CABG), congestive heart failure, arrhythmias, valvular heart disease, and complications during previous cardiac catheterization or percutaneous intervention. Additional history should identify active infection, peripheral or cerebrovascular disease, renal insufficiency, chronic obstructive pulmonary disease (COPD), hypertension, diabetes and pregnancy. Hepatic dysfunction, bleeding tendencies, and relative or absolute contraindications to thrombolytic therapy (e.g. gastrointestinal or urinary tract bleeding, recent major surgery or stroke) should also be identified. Obtaining a history of allergic reactions to x-ray dye, iodine, aspirin and other routine medications is essential; a history of eczema, asthma and hay fever should be documented as well, since these are associated with increased risk of contrast reactions.

2. **Physical Examination.** The physical exam is directed toward estimating the patient's volume status (peripheral edema, jugular venous distension, pulmonary rales), presence and severity of valvular heart disease, left ventricular dysfunction, and degree of compensation. Focal neurologic deficits, vascular bruits, peripheral pulses, and evidence of COPD should also be recorded.

3. **Laboratory Studies.** A complete blood and platelet count, electrolyte panel, BUN, creatinine, and PT/PTT are standard laboratory evaluations prior to PTCA. A 12-lead electrocardiogram should be obtained before and after intervention. A chest x-ray is recommended if there is an abnormality

Table 1.1. Medical Conditions Requiring Postponement of Elective Intervention

Allergy

- · Contrast
- · Aspirin

Cardiovascular

- · Congestive Heart Failure, decompensated
- · Severe Hypertension
- · Uncontrolled arrhythmias
- - AV block (Type II 2° or 3°)

Pulmonary Disease, decompensated

Diabetes, poorly controlled

Electrolyte abnormalities
- · K+ <3.3 or >6.0 mEq/L
- · Na+ <125 or > 155 mEq/L

Gastrointestinal

- · Acute hepatitis
- · Active GI bleeding

Hematologic

- · Platelet count <50,000/ul
- · Leukocytosis, unexplained
- · Hemoglobin <10 gm/dl, acute
- · Prothrombin time >16 seconds

Neurologic

- · Neurologic deficit, unexplained or progressive
- · Cerebral hemorrhage, recent

Renal

- · Renal insufficiency, unexplained or progressive

Systemic

- · Bacterial infection
- · Unexplained Fever

on examination of the lungs or any change in cardiopulmonary disease. Thyroid function tests and drug levels (e.g. digoxin, theophylline, antiarrhythmics) are ordered as appropriate. A blood type and screen for antibodies should be obtained in the event urgent transfusion or CABG is needed. For patients with peripheral vascular disease, noninvasive studies will help determine the severity of disease and the likelihood of being an able to use an intra-aortic balloon pump (IABP) or percutaneous cardiopulmonary bypass (CPS) should they be required. Review of previous angiograms, cardiac catheterization records, and operative reports is essential to help determine procedural risk, technical approach (femoral or brachial), dilatation strategy, equipment selection and the likelihood of adverse reactions to contrast agents and other medications.

B.   THERAPEUTIC MEASURES
1.   Routine Pre-PTCA Medications (Table 1.2)

2. **Aspirin Allergy.** Aspirin has been shown to reduce the incidence of acute occlusion following PTCA by 50-75% and is considered essential therapy prior to non-emergent interventions; at our institution, aspirin (160-325mg po) is administered at least 1 day prior to elective PTCA. Occasional patients have an aspirin allergy; the likelihood of effective desensitization depends on the nature of the previous allergic reaction (bronchospasm, rhinosinusitis, urticaria and angioedema, anaphylaxis).

Table 1.2. Preprocedural Medication Orders

Routine pre-PTCA orders:	• NPO after midnight except medications (may have clear liquid breakfast if PTCA is late in the day). • Aspirin 325mg p.o. started at least 1 day prior to the procedure. • Nitrates and/or calcium channel antagonist • Void on call to the cath lab • Sedative/anxiolytic on call to the lab
Diabetics:	• Give ½ usual A.M. insulin dose on the day of the procedure. IV fluids should contain dextrose. If possible, PTCA should be performed early in the day.
Coumadin patients:	• Stop Coumadin 4-6 days prior to the procedure. If necessary, the patient is hospitalized and receives IV heparin while Coumadin is held.
Renal insufficiency:	• The patient must be well hydrated prior to the procedure. IV crystalloids are usually administered for 6-12 hrs (100-150ml/hr) in hospitalized patients. • Supplemental diuretics may be necessary when ventricular dysfunction is present. • Mannitol (12.5-25 grams IV over 30 min) is given 1-2 hrs prior to procedure in those with moderate renal insufficiency (serum creatinine >2.5-3.0 mg/dl) and diabetic nephropathy.
Dye allergy:	• Premedication regimens vary and none are completely protective. • Our approach is to give prednisone 60mg., diphenhydramine 50 mg and cimetidine 300mg the afternoon and evening before, and the morning of the procedure. Hydrocortisone (100mg IV) and diphenhydramine (25-50mg IV) are given just prior to PTCA.
Aspirin-allergy:	• Elective PTCA is deferred; attempt to desensitize the patient (Section B2). • For a history of aspirin-induced anaphylaxis, we empirically administer ticlopidine (250 mg QD, started at least 72 hours before PTCA).

a. **Aspirin-Induced Asthma and Rhinosinusitis**

1. **Features.** Over 10% of adults with asthma and 30% of those with asthma and rhinosinusitis develop aspirin sensitivity. Reactions range from exacerbations of nasal congestion, chest tightness, and sneezing to life-threatening bronchospasm and anaphylaxis. Aspirin sensitivity can develop at any time in susceptible individuals; the absence of a prior adverse reaction does not predict continued tolerance. Most aspirin-allergic patients have nasal polyps (>80%), eosinophils and mast cells on nasal smear (>90% and >50%, respectively), and abnormal sinus radiographs (>90%) ranging from mild mucoperiosteal thickening to complete opacification.

2. **Desensitization.** Scripps Clinic and Research Foundation developed an aspirin desensitization protocol that has proven to be very safe and effective. Desensitization involves the oral administration of progressively larger doses of aspirin at specified time intervals (Table 1.3), and results in a refractory period during which aspirin can be safely

Table 1.3. Aspirin Desensitization Protocol at Scripps Clinic

1. Inclusion criteria: Asthma in remission, baseline $FEV_{1.0}$ >1.5 L and >70% of predicted value.

2. Preprocedural medication: Patient may continue steroids and methylxanthines but must stop antihistamines, cromolyn, and inhaled bronchodilators.

3. Oral aspirin challenge:* Progressively larger doses are administered until a positive reaction occurs (fall in $FEV_{1.0}$ >20% from baseline or marked nasal congestion and rhinorrhea) or 650mg is tolerated.[+] If a positive reaction develops, the same dose is re-administered once the $FEV_{1.0}$ has returned to baseline and symptoms have completely resolved.

	Day 1	Day 2	Day 3
8 AM	Placebo	3-30mg	150mg
11 AM	Placebo	60mg	325mg
2 PM	Placebo	100mg	650mg

4. Monitoring: $FEV_{1.0}$ and symptoms hourly.

5. Treatment of a positive reaction: For bronchospasm, administer aerosolized bronchodilator (albuterol 2.5mg in 3cc normal saline) every 10 minutes until asthma is controlled. Treat nasal congestion with Afrin (2 sprays intranasally) and Vasacon A (2 drops each eye), repeated every 30 minutes as necessary.

* Regimens vary (e.g. may give aspirin every 2 hrs to complete sequence in one day, although 2-day sequence provides a greater safety margin).
+ For those suspected of being highly sensitive, the initial dose should be 3mg.

administered. This desensitization period can be maintained indefinitely as long as aspirin therapy is not interrupted (325 mg every 48 hours or 80 mg QD). If aspirin has not been given for two or more days, repeat desensitization may be necessary. Patients with aspirin allergies who require desensitization should be referred to a center experienced in this technique.

b. **Aspirin-Induced Cutaneous Reactions.** Despite the success of desensitizing the aspirin-sensitive patient with asthma and rhinosinusitis, desensitization of individuals with aspirin-induced angioedema and/or urticaria remains problematic. These patients should not undergo desensitization. Fortunately, a previous cutaneous reaction to aspirin does not place the individual at increased risk of anaphylaxis upon re-administration of drug. If PTCA is required, aspirin is dosed in routine fashion. H1 and H2 antagonists can usually control cutaneous symptoms during the periprocedural period.

c. **Anaphylaxis.** Desensitization has not been attempted in individuals who have had an anaphylactic reaction to aspirin; re-administration of aspirin is contraindicated. If PTCA is required, we empirically administer other agents (see next section).

d. **Alternative Antiplatelet Agents (Chapter 34).** There are isolated case reports of the use of other antiplatelet agents such as low-molecular weight Dextran, sulfinpyrazone, and dipyridamole in aspirin-allergic patients. There insufficient data with these drugs to recommend their use in such patients. Other more potent platelet inhibitors, such as ticlopidine and clopidogrel, have demonstrated value in unstable angina and unstable cerebral ischemia, and may have value in patients with aspirin-allergy; pretreatment for 2-4 days prior to intervention is recommended to achieve optimal platelet inhibition. ReoPro (Centocor, Eli Lilly), a platelet glycoprotein IIb/IIIa receptor antagonist, has recently been shown to reduce ischemic complications following high-risk (EPIC and CAPTURE trials) and elective coronary interventions (EPILOG trial) (Chapter 34); its role in the aspirin-allergic patient has not been defined but is theoretically appealing. Investigational oral platelet receptor antagonists may be useful in the future.

C. **INFORMED CONSENT.** It is the obligation of the interventionalist to discuss the risks and benefits of intervention, bypass surgery, and medical therapy with the patient, family, and referring physician.; the likelihood of immediate success, complications (including emergency bypass surgery) and restenosis should be explained. In general, the risks of percutaneous intervention include death (1%), non-fatal myocardial infarction (4%), and emergency bypass surgery (2-3%); however, the presence of certain clinical and angiographic characteristics may increase the risk of adverse outcomes (Table 1.4). Additional complications include stroke (<0.5%), vascular injury (2-5%), infection, blood transfusion (2-8%), contrast-induced nephrotoxicity, allergic reactions, and systemic atheroembolization. Restenosis occurs in approximately 30% of patients and repeat revascularization is necessary in 20%.

Table 1.4. Clinical and Angiographic Factors Associated with Increased Risk of Complications and/or Decreased Rate of Success During PTCA

Clinical:	Angiographic:
Advanced Age	Multivessel/multilesional disease
Aortic stenosis	Left main or equivalent
Pulmonary hypertension	Single patent vessel
Ejection fraction < 40%, particularly with CHF	Lesion Characteristics:
Diabetes mellitus	Long
Female gender	Bend point ($\geq 45°$)
Hypotension	Bifurcation
Severe hypertension	Thrombus
Previous MI	Eccentric
Previous CABG	Irregular contour
Peripheral vascular disease	Proximal vessel tortuosity
Unstable angina	Calcification
Acute MI	Chronic total occlusion
Multiple PVCs	Ostial location
	Diffuse disease
	Degenerated vein graft

EQUIPMENT AND TECHNIQUE

A. PROCEDURAL OVERVIEW

1. **Intraprocedural Medication.** At the time of intervention, a narcotic and benzodiazipine are usually employed for analgesia and sedation. A continuous infusion of nitroglycerin (30-100mcg/min) may be used to attenuate ischemia and vasospasm. Some operators favor administration of a intracoronary calcium antagonists (verapamil 100-500 mcg), particularly prior to Rotablator or in clinical situations in which no-reflow is anticipated. Routine infusion of low-molecular weight dextran has fallen out of favor; there are no studies demonstrating efficacy in patients with ischemic heart disease, and potential complications (volume overload, anaphylaxis) outweigh its theoretical benefits. Heparin is universally employed during all interventional procedures (IV bolus: 150 units/kg); activated clotting time (ACT) > 300 seconds is recommended before advancing PTCA hardware into the coronary artery. Patients who have been receiving continuous heparin prior to the procedure may manifest drug resistance; a higher dose of heparin may be needed in these patients to achieve a therapeutic ACT. Supplemental heparin as a continuous drip (10 u/kg/hr) or boluses (1000-5000 units) is administered as necessary to maintain the ACT > 300 seconds. When an ACT machine is unavailable, supplemental heparin is given automatically.

2. **Vascular Access**
   a. **Femoral Approach.** To obtain vascular access, the femoral artery with the strongest pulse is identified followed by administration of a local anesthetic (10-20cc of 2% lidocaine). If pulses in both groins are equal, the femoral artery with the stronger peripheral pulse is chosen. If the femoral artery has been punctured within the last week, the contralateral artery is used for access. Synthetic grafts older than one month may be used for vascular access; sequential dilatation with progressively larger introducers may be necessary before the sheath can be inserted. Access is obtained by percutaneous puncture of the anterior wall of the common femoral artery using a beveled hollow needle via a modified Seldinger technique (Figure 1.1). It is important to access the common femoral artery since sheath placement in the superficial or profunda femoral arteries increases the risk of vascular injury, particularly when using 9F-11F sheaths. Anatomic landmarks can be used to identify the site for arterial access (Figure 1.2) and is especially useful in obese patients. Femoral venous access is recommended to serve as a port for saline, medications, pacemaker, and pulmonary artery catheter as necessary. In "simple" cases, some operators do not obtain central venous access. The brachial and radial approaches are discussed in Chapter 2.

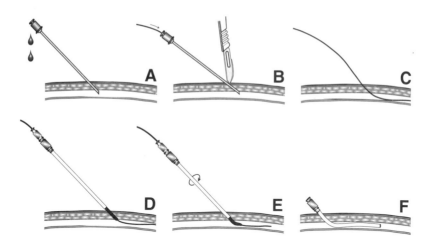

Figure 1.1 Vascular Access: Single-Wall Technique

Once blood flow is obtained through the needle (A), a 0.035-0.038" guidewire is threaded into the vessel (B) followed by needle removal (C). An arterial sheath and dilator are then tracked over the wire (D,E) into the femoral artery followed by removal of both guidewire and dilator (F). The sheath is then aspirated and connected to a pressure transducer which displays continuous systemic pressure.

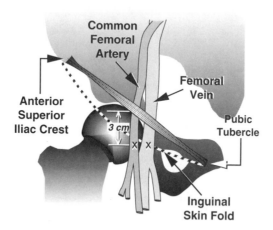

Figure 1.2   Landmarks for Vascular Access

Arterial access should be obtained 2-3cm below the inguinal ligament directly over the pulse. The inguinal ligament runs between the anterior superior iliac spine and the pubic tubercle; the inguinal skinfold may be a misleading landmark and should not be used in determining the site of access.

    b.   **Brachial and Radial Approaches (Chapter 2).**

3.   **Pacemaker Insertion.** While some operators insert a prophylactic temporary transvenous pacemaker prior to all interventions, we reserve prophylactic pacing for patients with pre-existing high-grade conduction abnormalities or those at increased risk for its development. These cases include degenerated vein grafts or thrombus-associated lesions in large RCA or left circumflex arteries, or Rotablator atherectomy of the RCA.

4.   **Equipment Setup.** A guiding catheter of appropriate size and configuration is advanced around the aortic arch. Once in the ascending aorta, the wire is removed, the catheter is connected to a manifold assembly and Y-adapter, and flushed. The manifold is connected to a pressure transducer, which continuously records blood pressure (Figure 1.3). The guide is maneuvered until it engages the coronary ostium; baseline angiograms are taken in orthogonal views to best demonstrate the lesion and serve as a "guide" during manipulations of guidewires and interventional devices. Common angiographic views are listed in Figure 1.4.

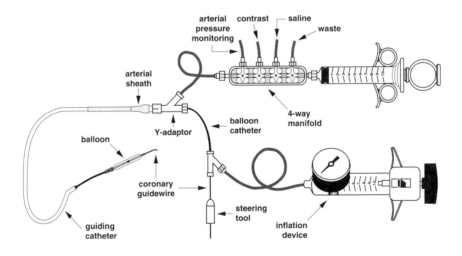

Figure 1.3   Basic Angioplasty Equipment and Setup

5.   **Balloon Sizing.** The diameter of the final balloon is chosen to achieve a balloon/artery ratio of 1:1 (e.g., if the diameter of an atheroma-free segment adjacent to the lesion is 2.5mm, a 2.5mm balloon catheter is used). The reference diameter is estimated by comparing the target vessel to the guiding catheter (e.g., 7F guide = 2.3mm, 8F = 2.7mm, 9F = 3.0mm, 10F = 3.3mm, 11F = 3.6mm). Although visual estimates of reference diameter are less accurate than digital techniques, they are the simplest and most popular method. Balloon size should be judged carefully; undersizing

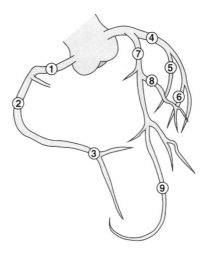

Figure 1.4 Frequently Used Angiographic Views

RCA	LCX	LAD
1) Proximal RCA: • 30° LAO, 30° caudal • 20° RAO, 20° caudal • 90° LAO, 20° caudal	**4)** Proximal LCX: • 30° RAO, 30° caudal • 30° LAO, 30° caudal	**7)** Proximal LAD: • 20° LAO, 20° cranial • 30° RAO, 30° caudal • 50° LAO, 30° caudal
2) Mid-RCA: • 30° LAO • 20° RAO • 90° LAO	**5)** Obtuse Marginal: • 20° RAO, 20° caudal • 50° LAO, 30° caudal	8) Mid-LAD: • 50° LAO, 30° cranial • 60° RAO, 20° cranial • 90° LAO • 50° LAO, 30°caudal
3) Distal RCA: • 30° LAO, 30° cranial • 90° LAO	**6)** Distal LCX: • 30° RAO, 30° caudal • 30° LAO, 30° cranial	9) Distal LAD • 20° RAO, 20° caudal • 40° LAO • 20° LAO, 20° cranial

(balloon/artery ratio <0.9) frequently results in significant residual stenosis and oversizing (balloon/artery ratio ≥ 1.2) increases the risk of emergency bypass surgery and myocardial infarction.[3]

6. **Guidewire Shaping.** Selection of the guidewire is based on coronary anatomy, lesion morphology, and operator preference. The guidewire is shaped to accommodate the morphology of the target vessel; this is easily accomplished by gentle manipulation of the wire between thumb and index finger, or by rolling the guidewire tip over the guidewire introducer. In general, the length of the distal bend should approximate the diameter of the vessel since a small distal bend limits steerability and a large bend increases the risk of wire prolapse. A double bend is very useful when steering into a steeply angled vessel (Figure 1.5).

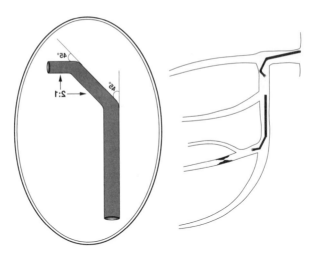

Figure 1.5 Double Bend Guidewire

The proximal bend allows the operator to steer the wire from the Left Main into the Circumflex artery. Once in the Circumflex, the smaller distal bend allows entry into the marginal branch.

7. **Purging Air from the System.** The guidewire and balloon are inserted through the O-ring of the Y-adapter into the guiding catheter. Air must be purged from the system by injecting saline from the manifold through the guiding catheter with the O-ring open and directed upward. Once a continuous stream of flush is observed, the O-ring is closed. The balloon catheter and guidewire are then advanced to the guiding catheter tip. Standard angioplasty equipment and set-up are demonstrated in Figure 1.3.

8. **Crossing the Lesion with the Guidewire.** To reduce the risk of intraprocedural vasospasm, intracoronary nitroglycerin (100-200 mcg) is recommended just prior to guidewire advancement. The guidewire is steered into the distal vessel to provide support for balloon catheter advancement, and should pass smoothly through the stenosis. If buckling occurs, the wire should be retracted and re-advanced rather than forcefully prolapsed beyond the lesion since forceful manipulation increases the risk of acute vessel closure.

9. **Balloon Dilatation.** With the guidewire fixed in place, the balloon is advanced into the target lesion. After confirming proper balloon position using contrast injections, the balloon is gradually inflated using an inflation device filled with a 50:50 mixture of contrast and saline. The inflation pressure is increased until the lesion no longer indents the balloon or the rated burst pressure has been reached. Inflation times usually last 1-2 minutes, but range from 15 seconds to several minutes depending on the patient's tolerance and the responsive of the lesion. With the balloon inflated, the patient is questioned regarding chest pain and a 12-lead EKG is obtained; these may prove useful in diagnosing abrupt closure after the patient leaves the angioplasty suite.

10. **Evaluation of Acute Angiographic Outcome.** Following each inflation, the balloon is retracted into the guiding catheter leaving the guidewire across the lesion. Cineangiograms are performed in orthogonal views to assess vessel patency and residual stenosis. Each cineangiogram must be systematically and carefully evaluated for residual stenosis, thrombus, coronary artery dissection, side branch occlusion, distal embolization, spasm, perforation, and no-reflow. If the patient is clinically stable and a good angiographic outcome has been obtained (<30% residual stenosis, normal flow, lack of high-grade dissection or thrombus), all PTCA hardware is removed and final films are taken. If a suboptimal angiographic result is obtained, a variety of technical approaches may be beneficial (Figure 1.6).

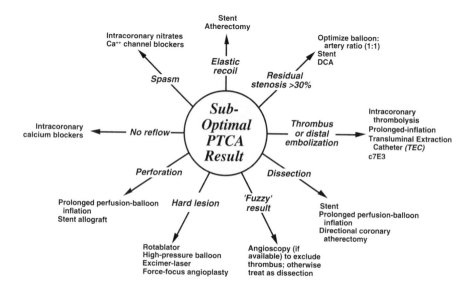

Figure 1.6 Suboptimal Angiographic Outcome Following PTCA: Causes and Management

B. EQUIPMENT SELECTION

1. **Vascular Sheaths.** Arterial sheaths commonly used for interventional procedures are 6F-8F in diameter; larger sheaths are required for atherectomy (9F-11F), valvuloplasty (12F), and percutaneous cardiopulmonary bypass (18-22F). Long sheaths (23cm) may be useful in straightening out tortuous femoral and iliac arteries, facilitating guiding catheter support and torque-control.

2. **Guiding Catheter Selection (Tables 1.5 [p. 36-39], 1.6 [p. 40-42], Figure 1.7).** The enormous variety of guiding catheters has improved the technique of coronary intervention. Many companies now manufacture guiding catheters from 6-10FR, and each guide has its own unique design and construction. For a given size guiding catheter, the internal diameter is either a standard lumen, large lumen, or giant lumen (Table 1.7). The internal diameter of the guide is an important

Table 1.7. Standard, Large-Lumen, and Giant-Lumen Guiding Catheters

FR	Standard	Large	Giant
6	≤ 0.061	0.062 - 0.065	≥ 0.066*
7	≤ 0.071	0.072 - 0.075	≥ 0.076
8	≤ 0.079	0.080 - 0.085	≥ 0.086
9	≤ 0.089	0.090 - 0.095	≥ 0.096
10	≤ 0.099	0.100 - 0.107	≥ 0.108

* Not available

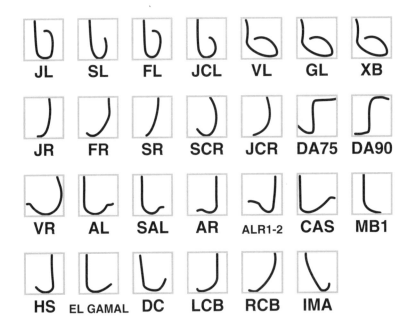

Figure 1.7 Guiding Catheter Configurations

consideration in the use of new devices and complex angioplasty (Table 1.8). Some manufactures design guides to perform passively; these guides are relatively stiff and should not be "deep-throated" or actively manipulated once the ostium is engaged). In contrast, active guides are softer and more flexible and are designed to be actively manipulated once the ostium is engaged. Most guiding catheters consist of 3-layer construction: a stainless steel or Kevlar braid, which determines stiffness and flexibility; an outer protective "jacket" (usually polyurethane or Nylon), which provides a polished, smooth surface that resists abrasion and thrombosis; and an inner coating or liner (usually PTFE or silicone), which provides a lubricious surface for passing guides and interventional devices (Figure 1.8). Important guiding catheter characteristics include the ability to provide stable coaxial alignment between catheter tip and coronary ostium, kink-free torque

Table 1.8. **Interventional Techniques and Minimum Recommended Guiding Catheter Internal Diameter**

Technique	Internal Diameter (inch)
PTCA	
Simple	0.060
Kissing balloon *	0.086
Perfusion	0.070
Stents	
GRS 2.0 mm, 2.5 mm	0.077
GRS 3.0 mm	0.080
GRS 3.5 mm, 4.0 mm	0.086
PSS	0.086
Rotablator Burr	
1.25 mm,1.5 mm	0.076
1.75 mm	0.084
2.0 mm, 2.15 mm	0.092
2.25 mm, 2.38 mm, 2.5 mm	0.107
ELCA Probe	
1.4 mm	0.084
1.8 mm	0.084
2.0 mm	0.092
DCA Atherocath	
5F	0.105
6F	0.105
7F,7FG	0.105
TEC Catheter	
5.5F, 6F	0.092
6.5F, 7.0F	0.100
7.5F	0.107
IVUS	0.076
ANGIOSCOPY	0.077

Abbreviations: GRS = Gianturo-Roubin stent; ELCA = excimer laser coronary angioplasty catethers; DCA = directional coronary atherectomy catheters (AtheroCath); TEC = transluminal extraction catheters; IVUS = intravascular ultrasound; F = French Size

*　　Virtually all low-profile 0.014-inch compatible systems and fixed wire devices can be used. To determine kissing balloon and guiding catheter combinations: Add balloon profiles for each balloon plus 0.010" for clearance; the total must be less than the guide ID.

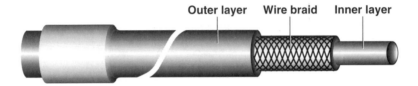

Figure 1.8 Guiding Catheter Construction

The outer layer consists of either polyurethane or polyethylene which provides overall stiffness. The middle layer is composed of a wire matrix allowing for torque generation. The inner layer is composed of a Teflon coating to allow smooth passage of the balloon dilatation catheter.

control, and sufficient back-up support for PTCA hardware. A properly selected guide should also provide reliable pressure monitoring and adequate contrast delivery. Advantages of larger guides include better opacification, support, and pressure monitoring; disadvantages include an increased risk of ostial trauma and vascular complications, and kinking of the catheter shaft. In comparison to catheters used for coronary arteriography, guiding catheters have a stiffer shaft, larger internal diameter, a shorter and more angulated tip (110° verses 90°), and re-enforced construction (3 vs 2 layers) (Figure 1.8). As shown in Tables 1.9, 1.10, and Figure 1.9, guiding catheter selection is based on aortic root width, coronary ostial origin (e.g. high, anterior), and ostial orientation (superior, horizontal, inferior).

a.   **Left Anterior Descending Coronary Artery (LAD) PTCA (Figure 1.9, Table 1.10).** The LAD normally arises in an anterior and superior position. A JL4 guide is the catheter of choice in the vast majority of cases. If the ostium of the left main is high or the aortic root is small, a JL 3.5 catheter may be preferred. Once in the left main, gentle counter-clockwise rotation of the guiding catheter will frequently direct it anteriorly. An out-of-plane femoral guiding catheter (30° anterior orientation) is available, though rarely needed. If the left main is short, a short-tip guide may be used to prevent inadvertent obstruction of the circumflex artery. Coaxial alignment between the catheter tip and left main is best confirmed in the LAO (50°)-Caudal (30°) view or in the shallow RAO (5°)-Caudal (20°) view.

b.   **Left Circumflex (LCX) PTCA (Figure 1.9, Table 1.10).** LCX angioplasty is often associated with difficulties in guidewire passage and balloon tracking due to the inherent tortuosity of this vessel. Stable coaxial alignment may be facilitated by gentle clockwise rotation of a JL4 guiding catheter once engaged in the left main. A JL5 may be of benefit in a dilated aortic root or when the tip of a JL4 points anteriorly. An Amplatz left guiding catheter should be considered for a sharply angulated or inferiorly positioned circumflex ostium. Amplatz catheters can also be extremely useful in providing additional back-up support for balloon advancement when proximal vessel tortuosity, chronic total occlusion, or a distal target lesion is present. If the Amplatz guide becomes deeply engaged, it should be partially withdrawn over an extended balloon to prevent guide-induced injury. Amplatz catheters must be carefully disengaged from the coronary artery; simple withdrawal from the vessel in a manner similar to Judkins guide can cause the tip to advance farther into the vessel. To disengage an Amplatz catheter, it is first advanced slightly to prolapse the tip out of the artery and then rotated away from the ostium prior to withdrawal. In addition to JL5 and Amplatz left guides, out-of-plane (30° posterior orientation) guiding catheters are available. The guiding catheter configuration that offers the best support for PTCA in the left coronary artery is the Voda-left guide; unlike the Amplatz and Judkins curves, which derive their support from the left Sinus of Valsalva, the Voda derives its support from the opposite wall of the aorta.

c.   **Right Coronary Artery (RCA) PTCA (Figures 1.9, 1.10, Table 1.10).** The right coronary artery is more difficult to engage than the left coronary artery, and frequently results in a dampened arterial pressure tracing. For horizontally oriented RCAs and most proximal lesions in gently superior or inferior orientations, a JR4 guiding catheter will usually suffice. However, when additional back-up support is needed a left Amplatz guide or hockey-stick are generally required. For marked superior orientations ("Shepherd's Crook"), a left Amplatz, Hockey-stick, internal mammary, El Gamal, Voda-right, or double-loop Arani catheter (75°) provide better coaxial alignment than a standard Judkin's catheter (Figure 1.10). Although double-loop Arani catheters provide excellent back-up, they are often very difficult to engage; a Voda-right guide provides similar back-up and is much easier to engage the ostium. Like the left Voda, the right Voda and double-loop Arani derive support from the opposite wall of the aorta rather than the Sinus of Valsalva. For marked inferior orientations, a Multipurpose or Amplatz catheter (left or right) are preferred for better coaxial alignment and backup.

d.   **Saphenous Vein Graft PTCA (Chapter 17) (Table 1.10).** Saphenous vein bypass grafts to the RCA usually arise from the anterior wall of the aorta several centimeters above the aortic root, and are best approached with a Judkins right, Multipurpose, or Amplatz (left or right) guiding catheter. Grafts to the LAD and left circumflex are usually positioned above and lateral to RCA grafts, and may require an EL Gamal, left coronary bypass, Hockey stick, right Judkins, or Amplatz guiding catheters.

e.   **Internal Mammary Artery PTCA (Chapter 17).** Internal mammary guiding catheters are used most frequently for internal mammary artery intervention.

f.   **"Dampening" of the Arterial Pressure Tracing (Figure 1.11).** Occasionally, guiding catheter engagement obstructs coronary flow, causing an immediate fall in diastolic pressure ("ventricularization") or a fall in both systolic and diastolic pressure ("dampened" pressure). Although most commonly due to the presence of a diseased ostium, ventricularization and dampening may be caused by coronary spasm, non-coaxial alignment of the guide and vessel wall, or mismatch between the vessel diameter and the diameter of the guide; in these instances, forceful contrast injections increase the risk of coronary dissection and must be

Table 1.9. Guiding Catheters Configurations

Guiding Catheter	Description	Recommended Use
JL	Judkins left	Most left coronary artery interventions
FL	Femoral left	Most left coronary artery interventions
JCL	Judkins "C" left	Same relationship of tip to shaft as JL, but more gentle transition; DCA of left coronary artery; may also be used for biliary stents, Rotablator
VL	Voda left	Back-up support from opposite wall of aorta; excellent for difficult anatomy (tortuous; angulated; calcified; total occlusion; etc) in left coronary artery
VLHT	Voda left, high takeoff	Back-up support from opposite wall of aorta; excellent for difficult anatomy (tortuous; angulated; calcified; total occlusion; etc) in left coronary artery with high takeoff
XB	Extra-backup	Back-up support from opposite wall of aorta; excellent for difficult anatomy (tortuous; angulated; calcified; total occlusion; etc) in left coronary artery
GL	Geometric left	Back-up support from opposite wall of aorta; excellent for difficult anatomy (tortuous; angulated; calcified; total occlusion; etc) in left coronary artery
AL	Amplatz left	Versatile configuration; particularly useful for Shephard Crook RCA, high-anterior RCA, tough anatomy in left coronary artery (especially LCx), virtually all vein grafts
JR	Judkins right	Most RCA interventions; also useful for many interventions on vein grafts to the left coronary artery; may not provide coaxial alignment for vein grafts to the RCA
FR	Femoral right	Most RCA interventions; also useful for many interventions on vein grafts to the left coronary artery; may not provide coaxial alignment for vein grafts to the RCA
NR	No-torque right	Most RCA interventions; minimal catheter manipulation
SCR	Shephard Crook right	Shephard Crook RCA; may be useful for vein grafts to the left coronary artery with vertical upward origin
SHR	Shani right	Shephard Crook RCA; may be useful for vein grafts to the left coronary artery with vertical upward origin
JCR	Judkin's "C" right	DCA of RCA and vein grafts to the left coronary artery with horizontal or slightly inferior origin; also used for biliary stents
DA 75,90	Double-loop Arani (75°, 90°)	Excellent back-up support for difficult anatomy in RCA or Shephard Crook; difficult catheters to manipulate

Guiding Catheter	Description	Recommended Use
VR	Voda right	Excellent back-up support for difficult anatomy in RCA, Shephard Crook RCA, or vein grafts to the left coronary artery with vertical upward origin
VRSC	Voda right, Shephard Crook	Excellent back-up support for difficult anatomy in RCA, Shephard Crook RCA, or vein grafts to the left coronary artery with vertical upward origin
AR	Amplatz right	Useful for interventions in RCA or vein grafts to RCA with inferior origin
ALR 1-2	Amplatz left-right (modified Amplatz)	Similar to AL and AR; slightly longer reach than AR, and shorter reach than AL
MP	Multipurpose	Useful for RCA or vein grafts to RCA with inferior origin; also useful for many vein grafts to the left coronary artery with gentle inferior or horizontal origin
SON	Sones	Useful for RCA or vein grafts to RCA with inferior origin; also useful for many vein grafts to the left coronary artery with gentle inferior or horizontal origin
HS	Hockey-Stick	Good guiding catheter for horizontal or gentle superior origin of RCA or vein grafts to left coronary artery
Champ	Champ	Good guiding catheter for horizontal or gentle superior origin of RCA or vein grafts to left coronary artery
ELG	EL Gamal bypass	Good guiding catheter for horizontal or gentle superior origin of RCA or vein grafts to left coronary artery
LCB	Left coronary bypass	Similar to JR and HS; useful for vein grafts to left coronary artery with horizontal or slightly superior origin
RCB	Right coronary bypass	Useful for vein grafts to the left coronary artery with horizontal origin; may not provide coaxial alignment with vein grafts to the RCA with inferior origin
IMA	Internal mammary	Target lesions in LIMA, RIMA, or native vessel beyond anastamosis
CAS	Castillo	Left Amplatz type of confirguration; intended use from brachial approach (similar to Simmons).
DC	Doctor's choice	Multipurpose catheter for RCA or left coronary artery; extra backup from opposite wall of aorta

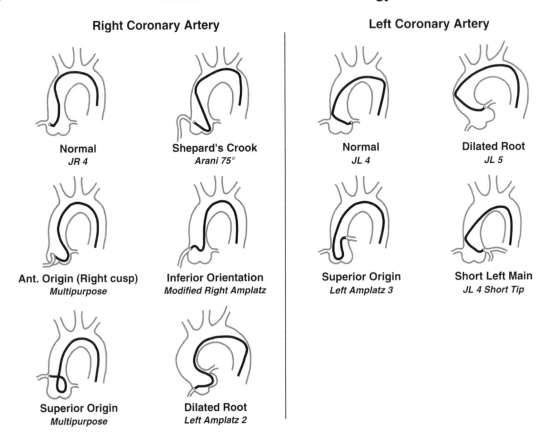

Right Coronary Artery | Left Coronary Artery

Normal
JR 4

Shepard's Crook
Arani 75°

Normal
JL 4

Dilated Root
JL 5

Ant. Origin (Right cusp)
Multipurpose

Inferior Orientation
Modified Right Amplatz

Superior Origin
Left Amplatz 3

Short Left Main
JL 4 Short Tip

Superior Origin
Multipurpose

Dilated Root
Left Amplatz 2

Figure 1.9   Guide Catheter Selection Based on Anatomic Variations in Aortic Root Width and Coronary Artery Orientation

avoided. When dampening is due to the presence of a small coronary artery or an ostial obstruction, the guiding catheter should be replaced with a sidehole catheter; sideholes allow passive entry of aortic blood into the guiding catheter and coronary artery. If a sidehole catheter is not available, sideholes can be created with a sidehole cutter or the beveled end of the vascular access needle. Potential problems with sidehole catheters include suboptimal opacification (contrast escapes through the sideholes); decreased back-up support due to weakness of the catheter shaft; and kinking at the sideholes, particularly in giant lumen guides. When sidehole guides are used for ostial lesions, the presence of sideholes will permit passive perfusion, but does not decrease the chance of guiding catheter injury to the vessel ostium.

Table 1.10. Guiding Catheter Selection

Target Vessel	Configuration	Guiding Catheters
RCA	**Aortic root:**	
	Normal	JR4, AL1, AR1
	Dilated	JR≥5, AL ≥ 2, AR ≥ 2
	Narrow	JR 3, AL ≤ 0.75
	Orientation *	
	Normal	JR,AL,AR,
	Anterior Superior	AL,HS,MP,HS,
	Inferior	MP,AR,JR
	Shephard Crook	AL,SCR,VR,VRSC,DA,ELG, SHR, Champ
	Horizontal	JR,HS
LCA	**Aortic root:**	
	Normal	JL4,AL2,VL4,GL4
	Dilated	JL≥5; AL≥2; VL≥4,GL≥ 4
	Narrow	JL3.5,VL3.5,GL3.5
	Orientation *	
	Normal Anterior	JL,AL,VL,GL
	Posterior	AL,VL,GL
	Superior	JL,VL,GL
	Supraselect	
	LAD	JL3.5,JL (anterior)
	LCx	JL4.5,AL,JL (posterior)
SVG→RCA	**Orientation***	
	Inferior	MP,AL,AR,JR
	Horizontal	JR,AL,MP
SVG→LCA	**Orientation***	
	Horizontal	JR,HS,MP,AL,RCB,AR
	Superior	HS,ELG,LCB,MP,SCR, Champ,SHR

* Size of curve depends on the diameter of the aortic root; see Table 1.9 and Figure 1.8 for description of guiding catheters.

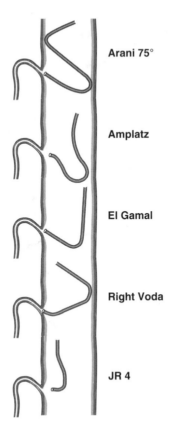

Arani 75°

Amplatz

El Gamal

Right Voda

JR 4

Figure 1.10 Guide Catheter Selection for Shepards' Crook RCA

Note suboptimal alignment with JR4 catheter compared to Arani 75°, Amplatz, El Gamal, and Right Voda guides.

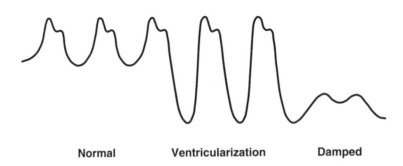

Normal   Ventricularization   Damped

Figure 1.11   Arterial Pressure Tracings Recorded from Guiding Catheter

3. **Guidewires**

    a. **Composition.** Guidewires consist of 3 basic components, including a central core or shaft (usually stainless steel or nitinol); a distal flexible spring coil (usually platinum or tungsten); and a lubricious coating (silicone, PTFE, or other hydrophilic coating) (Figures 1.12, 1.13). Although virtually all guidewires can be used for most coronary interventions, guidewire construction does influence performance, particularly in difficult anatomy such as severe tortuosity and/or angulation (Table 1.11, p. 43-47) (Chapter 11). In general, single-core constructions provide a smoother transition, enhanced torque response, and less prolapse compared to dual-core constructions. Guidewires with nitinol cores are virtually kink-resistant, which those with stainless steel cores are more susceptible to kinking.

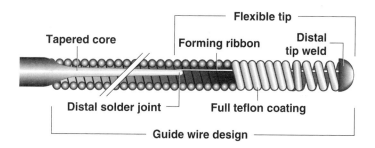

Figure 1.12   Guidewire Construction

    b. **Characteristics.** Features to consider when choosing a guidewire include its torque-control, steerability, visibility, flexibility, and support for balloon catheter advancement. Unfortunately, the perfect angioplasty guidewire does not exist: Wires with increased flexibility have decreased steerability; those with increased torque-control have decreased flexibility. Coronary guidewires are available in 0.010, 0.012, 0.014, 0.016, 0.017, and 0.018" diameters. Larger wires (0.016"-0.018") have increased steerability, result in greater straightening of tortuous coronary segments, and provide more support for balloon catheter advancement; balloon catheter selection, however, is more limited. Guidewire tips come with either a preformed "J" or are straight and require shaping. Most guidewires have radiopaque tips (usually platinum) in short (2-3 cm) and long (25-40 cm) lengths. Although there are no differences in performance per se, each has its own advantages and disadvantages: Long radiopaque tips are readily visible in the guiding catheter and target vessel — kinks or loops

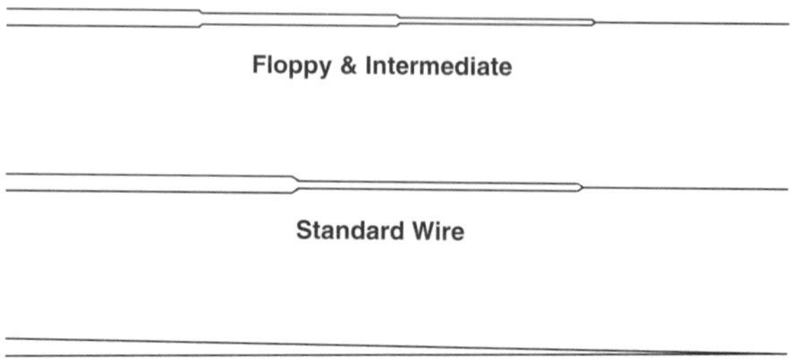

Floppy & Intermediate

Standard Wire

Tapered Core

Figure 1.13　Guidewire Core Construction

in the wire and the exact path of the wire in the coronary vasculature are readily apparent at all times; however, the radiopacity of the guidewire frequently inhibits assessment of fine details of lumen morphology, such as intraluminal filling defects, haziness, or dissection, particularly in small vessels. In addition, most on-line digital QCA programs are unable quantitate lumen diameter if such radiopaque wires are in place. Because of these limitations, guidewires with long radiopaque tips are not routinely recommended during coronary stent implantation.

c.　**Exchange-Length and Extension Wires.** Exchange-length wires are available in 270, 300, and 400 cm lengths. As shown in Table 1.12, many conventional length guidewires can be extended using special extension wires.

d.　**Specialty Wires**
　　1.　**Magnum Wire** (Schneider). The Magnum wire, which is available in 0.014, 0.018, 0.021 inch diameters, consists of a stainless steel core; a flexible, gold-plated tungsten spring; and a 1mm olive-shaped tip. Its principal use has been in recanalizing chronic total occlusions (Chapter 16).

Table 1.12.　Extension Wires

Company	Name	Length (cm)	Compatible Guidewire (inch)
ACS	DOC	145	0.014, 0.018
ACS	DOC-Tite	145	0.010
Cordis	Cinch-3	145	0.012, 0.014, 0.018
USCI	Linx-EZ	145	0.012, 0.014, 0.016
Schneider	DOC/EXT	130	0.014, 0.018

2. **Glidewire**. The angled 0.016 and 0.018" Glidewires consist of a kink-resistant nitinol core, which is coated with a low-friction hydrophilic polymer to facilitate smooth passage through high-grade obstructions and total occlusions. Disadvantages include poor steerability and the inability to extend the wire beyond 180 cm; poor visualization has been aided by the addition of a 2-mm gold tip. Other nitinol guidewires with either tungsten (Jagwire, Boston Scientific) or platinum (Roadrunner, Cook) spring tips have exceptional steerability, flexibility, kink resistance, and radiopacity.

4. **Balloon Dilatation Catheters.** Angioplasty balloon catheters are arbitrarily classified into three different categories: Over-the-wire (OTW) systems; single-operator-exchange (SOE) or monorail systems; and fixed-wire systems (formerly called "balloon-on-a-wire") (Table 1.13). In addition, several specialty balloons have unique "niche" applications (Figure 1.14, Tables 1.14 [p.48-51] and 1.15 [p. 52-57]).

a. **Classification of Balloon Catheters**

1. **Over-the-Wire (OTW) Systems.** In the United States, the majority of operators use OTW systems that accommodate either 0.014 or 0.018" guidewires. The availability of many ultra-low profile balloons have led most manufacturers to eliminate or markedly curtail the production of balloons that accommodate 0.010" guidewires. Although the standard usable length of most balloons is 135cm, longer shaft balloons (145,150 cm) are available and may be useful for dilating target lesions in distal vessels, particularly beyond bypass graft anastomoses.

   The two techniques of guidewire manipulation with OTW balloons are the "thru-wire" and "bare-wire" techniques — both are equally acceptable. In the thru-wire technique, the operator advances the guidewire-loaded balloon into the O-ring and through the guiding catheter. Just proximal to the vessel ostium, the operator advances the guidewire across the lesion, and after confirming proper position, the balloon is tracked into the lesion. If the operator has difficulty crossing the lesion with the guidewire, the balloon catheter can be advanced into the target vessel to provide additional support and enhance torque control. If the lesion still cannot be crossed, the balloon catheter can be left in the target vessel to function as a transport catheter — the operator can fashion a different curve on the guidewire or use a new guidewire as necessary. The bare-wire technique involves advancing the guidewire into the O-ring, through the guiding catheter, and across the lesion *without* the balloon. This technique may allow better visualization during contrast injections, but does not permit use of the balloon to enhance support or facilitate exchanges. If a bare-wire technique is employed with over-the-wire balloons, the operator must also use an exchange-length or extendable wire, a Trapper, or a magnetic device (Table 1.16).

2. **Single-Operator Exchange (SOE) Systems.** Outside the United States, SOE systems, also commonly referred to as "monorail" or "rapid-exchange" balloons, comprise the overwhelming majority of balloon catheter sales. SOE balloons are modified over-the-

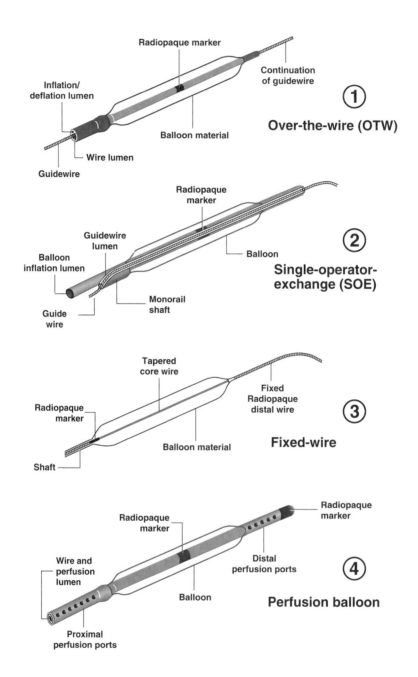

Figure 1.14   Balloon Dilatation Catheter Designs

Table 1.16. Exchange Devices

Company	Name	Description
SciMed	Trapper	Unique device with small inflatable balloon that traps the guidewire inside the guiding catheter, allows easy rapid exchange with over-the-wire balloons and non-exchange length guidewires.
SciMed	Magnet	Adjustable flip cover to secure wire; rapid exchange of Sceptor and Choice guidewires.
Baxter	Relay	Unique device for exchanging guiding catheters; 282 cm-long monorail catheter (4.1F) is placed in the distal vessel; provides a platform for exchanging vascular sheaths and guiding catheters, without giving up guidewire position.

wire balloons — only the distal portion of the balloon catheter tracks coaxially over the guidewire; the remaining portion of the catheter shaft does not have a guidewire thru-lumen. Compared to over-the-wire balloons, SOE balloons have a somewhat lower profile and are well-suited for single operator use. Standard-length (175 cm) guidewires are recommended using a bare-wire technique; exchange-length guidewires are not necessary. Disadvantages of SOE balloons include less pushability and trackability; inability to reshape or exchange the guidewire without a transport catheter; and inability to use the balloon catheter for additional guidewire back-up support while crossing a difficult lesion.

3. **Fixed-Wire Systems.** Formerly referred to as "balloon-on-a-wire" systems, these devices do not permit independent movement of the guidewire and balloon. Although fixed-wire devices have always had the lowest profile of all balloon catheters, a significant limitation is the inability to exchange balloons or guidewires without having to recross the lesion. The important role of PTCA as an adjunct to virtually all laser, atherectomy, and stent devices (which themselves require a movable guidewire), and the availability of ultra-low-profile over-the-wire systems, has substantially reduced the need for fixed-wire devices. Nevertheless, fixed-wire balloons are occasionally useful in tortuous vessels or highly angulated stenosis when other over-the-wire or single-operator exchange balloons have failed (Chapter 11).

4. **Specialty Balloons.** There are a variety of "specialty" balloons that can be used for specific "niche" indications (as well as for routine PTCA). The most common specialty balloon is the perfusion balloon catheter, which is available as an over-the-wire or single-operator-exchange balloon. Multiple sideholes in the catheter shaft proximal and distal to the balloon permit passive flow of arterial blood to the distal myocardial bed during balloon inflation (perfusion rates are 30-60 cc/min); these balloons are particularity useful in patients who are unable to tolerate conventional balloon inflations (due to severe angina or hemodynamic dysfunction) or in situations where prolonged inflations (>5 minutes) are used to manage suboptimal PTCA results (dissection, abrupt closure, elastic recoil, residual thrombus). In general, perfusion balloons have larger profiles than their over-the-

wire or single-operator-exchange counterparts, and trackability in tortuous anatomy is inferior to non-perfusion balloon catheters. Because of their perfusion capabilities, these catheters may also be used as bail-out devices during triage of patients to emergency CABG after failed PTCA. Other specialty balloons are also available: The tapered balloon, which tapers by 0.5 mm from the distal-to-proximal ends of a 25-mm balloon, has been used successfully for tapering vessels (Chapter 15). The Focus balloon (Cardiovascular Dynamics, Santa Clara, CA) is an interesting and potentially useful balloon for adjunctive PTCA before and after stenting (Chapter 26). The balloon is 20-mm long, and consists of a central PE segment (10 mm) and two PET segments on each end (5 mm each); during high-pressure inflations (>12 ATM), the central PE segment is 0.2-0.5 mm larger than the PET segments on either end. The "Cutting balloon" (InterVentional Technologies, San Diego, CA) contains 3-4 longitudinal microtomes that incise plaque and create controlled, localized dissection during balloon inflation; it is currently under investigation in a large randomized trial (Chapter 8).

b. **Characteristics of Balloon Catheters**
   1. **Balloon Material, Compliance, and Creep.** Balloon compliance, defined as the change in balloon diameter per atmosphere of inflation pressure, is an index of the stretchability of a balloon. Balloon materials can be classified as highly-compliant, moderately-compliant, and minimally-compliant: more compliant balloons are generally associated with more "creep", which refers to the tendency of a balloon to enlarge after serial inflations at the same pressure (Table 1.17). Balloon compliance ranges from 0.095mm/ATM (POC balloons) to 0.010 mm/ATM (PET balloons). Although in-vitro testing suggests that PET balloons are less compliant than POC or PE balloons, most studies have found that these differences are not clinically relevant (Chapter 20). In fact, high compliance is marketed by some manufactures as an advantage (sizing "flexibility") and by others as a disadvantage ("less predictable" balloon sizing). Concerns about balloon compliance and creep have been heightened by clinical studies suggesting that accurate balloon sizing (ideal balloon/artery ratio = 0.9-1.1) is needed to minimize the risk of dissection, abrupt closure, and major ischemic complications. Despite the recognized importance of proper balloon sizing, there are no data to suggest clear superiority of certain balloon materials: Only two retrospective studies reported different results for compliant and noncompliant balloons; one reported better results for noncompliant balloons, whereas the other reported better results for compliant balloons. In contrast, five nonrandomized studies and two prospective randomized studies (over 4000 lesions in all) failed to show any difference in angiographic results or ischemic complications (Chapter 20). Although early studies suggested that angulated lesions may respond better to noncompliant balloons, more recent data from a prospective randomized study suggested no difference in outcome for angulated lesions, lesions > 20 mm, ostial lesions, calcified lesions, or eccentric lesions. Nevertheless, noncompliant balloons are associated with higher burst pressures (see below) and are clearly useful in rigid lesions that cannot be dilated at inflation pressures < 10 ATM, and as adjuncts to stenting (Table 1.18).

Table 1.17. Balloon Material and Compliance

Company	Material	Compliance* (%)	Nominal (ATM)	RBP (ATM)
ACS	P-Flex	Low (4%)	8	12
ACS	PE-600	Medium (13%)	6	8
Cordis	Duralyn	Low (9%)	8	10
Cordis	Duralyn-ST	Low (3-4%)	12	16
Medtronic	PE	Medium (12%)	6	8
Schneider	PET	Low (4%)	10	16
Schneider	Thin PET (Thaline)	Low (4%)	5	14
Schneider	PE (Repeat)	Medium (14%)	5	9
Schneider	Nylon (PM300)	Medium 10%)	6	14
SciMed	POC-6	High (21%)	6	9
SciMed	POC-8	High (19%)	8	9
SciMed	Triad-PET	Low (4%)	6	16
SciMed	Coex	Low (5%)	3	15
SciMed	LEAP	Medium (10%)	6	14
SciMed	T4	Low (3-4%)	3	18
USCI	PET	Low (6%)	5	12

Abbreviations: RBP=rated burst pressure; ATM = atmospheres; P-Flex = polyethylene blend; POC = polyolefin copolymer; Coex = Coextruded; T4 = Triad-4 (PET); LEAP = Pebax
*   Compliance: High: >15%; Medium: 10-15%; Low: <10%

2. **Burst Pressure.** Nominal pressure, which refers to the inflation pressure required to achieve the inflated balloon diameter on the package label, usually ranges from 3-10 ATM. Burst pressure (usually reported as rated burst pressure; RBP) is defined as the pressure below which 99.9% of balloons will not rupture. RBP is an important component of product labeling (and as such is monitored by the FDA); it provides the operator with a good idea about the safe range of inflation pressures. RBP commonly ranges from 6-16 ATM. Mean burst pressure (MBP), defined as the pressure at which 50% of balloons will rupture, is higher than RBP and ranges from 10-27 ATM. Many manufacturers do not publish data about MBP because of FDA regulatory issues and concerns about balloon rupture.

3. **Profile.** There are considerable data about deflated profile (measured diameter of the

Table 1.18. High-Pressure Balloons For Stents

Company	Balloon	Material	Nominal (ATM)	RBP (ATM)	MBP (ATM)
ACS	Rx-Lifestream	PFlex	8	12	NR
ACS	OTW Lifestream	PFlex	8	12	NR
ACS	NC Bandit	T4	8	18	25
Cordis	Titan	Duralyn ST	12	16	27
CVD	Focus	PET/PE	NA	NA	NA
Schneider	Mongoose	PET	10	16	21-23
Schneider	Shortgoose 10	PET	10	16	21-23
Schneider	Shortgoose 20	PET	10	16	21-23
SciMed	Mighty	Coex	3	15	24
SciMed	NC Cobra	Triad PET	6	14	24

Abbreviations: RBP = rated burst pressure; MBP = mean burst pressure; ATM = atmospheres; NA = not available; NR = not reported by manufacturer; PFlex = polyethylene blend; PET = polyethylene terephthalate; PE = polyethylene; Coex = coextruded; T4 = Triad-4 (PET)

deflated balloon and distal catheter shaft). Although measured profile was relevant 5-10 years ago, contemporary PTCA products from virtually all manufacturers are extremely low-profile. Although measured differences in profile do exist, their clinical relevance is probably less important than differences in trackability and pushability (see below). While deflated profiles after one or more initial balloon inflations are extremely important, virtually no companies report these data. Clinical experience suggests that inadequate refolding of the balloon (i.e., "winging") is worse for PET balloons; this observation may explain the recognized difficulty recrossing lesions after a series of initial balloon inflations.

4. **Pushability and Trackability.** Unlike compliance, creep, nominal pressure, burst pressure, and profile (which can all be measured in-vitro), there are no reliable in-vitro methods for measuring "trackability" (the ease of tracking a balloon over the guidewire up to the target lesion) or "pushability" (the ability to advance the balloon across the lesion). And yet, trackability and pushability are more important to the practice of interventional cardiology than any other in-vitro measurement. The guiding catheter, guidewire, and operator experience also influence the operator's perception of trackability and pushability.

5. **Balloon Diameter and Length.** Most PTCA balloons are available in 0.5mm increments

from 2.0-4.0 mm in diameter; 1.5-mm balloons and quarter-sizes are also available from many manufacturers. Although the "standard" PTCA balloon is 20-mm in length, long balloons (30 and 40-mm) and short balloons (8, 9, 10, 15-mm) are also available; the former are particularly useful for long segments of diffuse disease, ostial lesions, and angulated lesions, whereas the latter are useful for very focal lesions and for adjunctive PTCA after stenting.

5. **Accessories (Tables 1.19, 1.20, 1.21, 1.22).** Y-adapters attach to the guiding catheter and provide a means of advancing interventional hardware and injecting contrast, while maintaining hemostatic control. Standard adapters consist of two channels (one for PTCA hardware, the other for contrast); a three-channel adapter contains three channels for bifurcation angioplasty. It is important to verify that other accessories, such as Y-adapters, guidewire introducers, and torque devices can accommodate planned devices and guidewires.

Table 1.19. Rotating Hemostatic Valves (Y-Adapters)

Company	Max ID		Tri-Adapter	Device Restrictions
	Inch	mm		
ACS	0.096	2.44	Yes	DCA
ACS	0.115	2.92	Yes	None
Braun	0.125	3.18	Yes	None
DVI	0.094	2.38	No	None
Medtronic	0.110	2.79	Yes	None
Schneider/Namic	0.113	2.87	Yes	None
Schneider/Namic	0.125	3.18	Yes	None
SciMed	0.118	2.99	Yes	None
USCI	0.125	3.18	Yes	None

Abbreviations: ID = internal diameter; DCA = directional coronary atherectomy

6. **Transport and Infusion Catheters (Tables 1.23 [p. 58-59], 1.24 [p. 60-61]).** A variety of end-hole transport catheters can be used for guidewire exchanges; sideholes are usually absent. Infusion catheters and wires are designed for selective drug infusion, but can also be used as transport catheters; most contain multiple sideholes and variable infusion lengths.

7. **Coating.** As shown in Table 1.25, there are a variety of lubricious coatings for guidewires, guiding catheters, and balloon catheters.

Table 1.20. Guidewire Introducers

Company	Maximum Guidewire (inch)	Material
ACS	0.018	Plastic or Metal
Braun	0.025	Plastic or Metal
Medtronic	0.035	Plastic
Medtronic	0.021	Metal
Schneider/Namic	0.018	Metal
SciMed	0.018	Metal
USCI	0.018	Metal

Table 1.21. Guidewire Torque Devices

Company	Name	Guidewire (inch)
ACS	Torque Device	0.009 - 0.018
Braun	LTD	< 0.022
Cook	Pin-Vise	0.014 - 0.018
Cook	Olcott Torque Device	0.014 - 0.045
Cordis	E-Z Twist	≤ 0.018
Cordis	Tweak	≤ 0.018
Meditech	Multi-Torque Vise	0.010 - 0.038
Medtronic	Torque Handle	≤ 0.018
Schneider/Namic	Torque Device	$\leq 0.010 - 0.018$
SciMed	Grip	≤ 0.018
SciMed	TD2	≤ 0.018
USCI	Steering Handle	≤ 0.018

   8.   Cost. The approximate cost of commonly used interventional hardware is shown in Table 1.26.

Table 1.22. Inflation Devices

Company	Name	Volume (cc)	Pressure (ATM)	Comments
ACS	Indeflator-Plus-20	10	20	Low-light readibility
ACS	Indeflator-20/20	20	20	Low-light readibility
DVI	LP-90	10	6	Useful for DCA
Medtronic	Everest	20	20	Low-light readibility
Merit	Monarch	20	20	Digital display, timer
Merit	Basix	20	20	Low-light readibility
Schneider/Namic	Breeze	25	22	Low-light readibility
SciMed	Classic	20	20	Low-light readibility
SciMed	Encore	20	20	Low-light readibility; lighted dial
USCI	Presto	20	20	Low-light readibility
USCI	Ideal-20	20	30	Low-light readibility
USCI	Wizard	10	20	Low-light readibility

Abbreviations: ATM = atmospheres; DCA = directional coronary atherectomy

Table 1.25. Lubricious Coatings

Company	Coating	Chemical Name	PTCA Equipment
ACS	Microglide	Silicone compound	Distal guidewire shaft and outer balloon shaft
		PTFE	Proximal guidewire shaft
Cook	SlipCoat	PTFE	Guidewires; inner lumen of guiding catheter
Cordis	Dura Glide	PTFE	Guidewires; Extensions; Inner lumen of guiding catheter
	SLX	Silicone	Inner, outer balloon shaft; balloon surface
Meditech	Glidex	Hydrophilic polymer	Guidewires
Medtronic	Enhance	Silicone	Inner balloon lumen and distal 30 cm of outer balloon shaft
		PTFE	Inner lumen of guiding catheters
Schneider	Expresscoat	Silicone heptane	Outer balloon shaft
		PTFE	Guidewires; Inner lumen of guiding catheter
SciMed	Bioslide	Hydrophilic polymer	Outer balloon shaft
	Hydroplus	Hydrophilic polymer	Outer balloon shaft
	ICE	Hydrophilic polymer	Guidewires
	Xtra	Silicone	Outer balloon shaft
USCI	Propel	Silicone	Guidewires, outer balloon shaft, vascular sheaths

Abbreviations: PTFE = teflon; SLX - silicone

Table 1.26 Cost of Interventional Hardware

Equipment	Cost ($)	Equipment	Cost ($)
Devices		**Accessories**	
PTCA balloons	300-500	Y-connector	15
DCA AtheroCath	1250	Torque tool	5
Rotablator burr	1095	Inflation device	25
ELCA catheter	1100	DCA-MDU	99
TEC cutter	925	TEC powerpack	65
PSS (coronary)	1595	TEC vacuum bottles	8
GRS (coronary)	1150	TEC-MDU	275
Biliary stent	800*		
IVUS catheter	650		
Doppler Wire	450		
Angioscope	695	**Miscellaneous**	
		Vascular sheath-short	13
		Vascular sheath-long	30
		Manifold	9
		J-wire (0.035" x 145 cm)	7
Guiding Catheters		Contrast syringe	6
		Contrast agent	
Conventional	60-80	Low osmolar (100 cc)	100
DCA	162	High osmolar (100 cc)	5
TEC	120		
Guidewires			
Conventional			
175 cm	110		
300 cm	140		
Extension	60		
Rotablator	140		
TEC	135		

Abbreviations: DCA = directional coronary atherectomy; ELCA = excimer laser coronary angioplasty; TEC = transluminal extraction catheter; PSS = Palmaz-Schatz stent; GRS = Gianturco-Roubin stent; IVUS = intravascular ultrasound; MDU = motor drive unit

*　Biliary stent alone - no delivery balloon

POSTPROCEDURAL CONSIDERATIONS

A.　　**TRIAGE AND MONITORING.** After an uncomplicated procedure, patients are observed for 12-36 hours in a skilled nursing telemetry unit. If the intervention was complicated by acute closure, severe dissection in a large vessel, or prolonged hypotension, observation in a cardiac intensive care unit is preferred. A 12-lead electrocardiogram is obtained immediately after the case and the following morning to identify silent ischemia and new conduction disturbances, and to serve as a new baseline if chest pain recurs. We routinely obtain a complete blood count and creatinine 12-24 hours post-procedure to identify potential complications.

B. **COMPLICATIONS.** Recurrent chest pain occurs in up to half of all hospitalized patients after PTCA. The decision to return to the catheterization laboratory is based on the character of the chest pain and the presence of ECG changes (particularly when compared to pre-PTCA); the triage and management of such patients is discussed in Chapter 20. Mild hypotension may occur following PTCA and is usually caused by medications (sedatives, nitrates, calcium channel blockers, beta blockers) and volume depletion (NPO status, contrast-induced diuresis); hypotension from these causes should respond promptly to saline administration. Postprocedural hypotension may also be caused by more serious conditions such as acute vessel closure, retroperitoneal bleeding, or sepsis. It is important to systematically exclude concomitant non-cardiac causes of hypotension when acute closure is present; it is not uncommon for a large retroperitoneal hemorrhage to cause hypotension and acute coronary occlusion. The recognition, diagnosis, and management of complications are reviewed in Chapter 20.

C. **POST-PTCA PHARMACOTHERAPY.** If a good final result has been obtained (<30% stenosis, normal flow; absence of dissection or thrombus), additional heparin is usually not required. However, if a suboptimal angiographic result is obtained, prolonged (18-48 hrs) post-procedural heparin may be warranted (Chapters 20, 34). Dosing is adjusted to maintain the ACT at 160-200 seconds or PTT 2.0-2.5 times control value. We empirically administer intravenous nitroglycerin (30-100 mcg/min) until the vascular sheaths have been discontinued, followed by oral or transdermal nitrates. Most interventionalists maintain patients on aspirin (160-325 mg po qd) indefinitely and long-acting nitrates for 1-6 months. The potential value of new platelet receptor antagonists is discussed in Chapter 34.

D. **SHEATH REMOVAL, AMBULATION, & PATIENT DISCHARGE.** Femoral sheaths are removed 4-6 hrs after discontinuing heparin (ACT <140 seconds or PTT < 50 seconds); if thrombolytics have been given, the fibrinogen level should be > 150 mg/dl prior to sheath removal. When uninterrupted anticoagulation is required (e.g., extensive coronary dissection with thrombus), the heparin infusion is decreased by 50% prior to sheath removal. When the ACT is 140-160 seconds, the sheaths are pulled and the site meticulously compressed until bleeding stops (usually 30-45 minutes). The use of special femoral compression and arterial closure devices is described in Chapter 25. Patients are kept recumbent in bed for a minimum of one hour for each French size of the arterial sheath (e.g., 6F = 6 hrs, 10F = 10 hrs). The evaluation and management of a new bruit, pulsatile mass, or loss of distal pulses is discussed in Chapter 25. The majority of uncomplicated PTCA patients are discharged within 24-36 hrs after the procedure; the patient is instructed to immediately report any new or recurrent symptoms; activity instructions, discharge medications, and follow-up appointment(s) are reviewed.

QUICK REFERENCE: PTCA EQUIPMENT

Table 1.5   Guiding Catheters: Size, Shape & Configuration 36-39

Table 1.6   Guiding Catheters: Technical Features 40-42

Table 1.11   Guidewires 43-47

Table 1.14   Balloon Catheters: Balloon Characteristics 48-51

Table 1.15   Balloon Catheters: Technical Features 52-57

Table 1.23   Transport Catheters 58-59

Table 1.24   Infusion Catheters 60-61

Table 1.5. Guiding Catheters for Coronary Intervention: Size, Shape, and Configuration

Name	FR	SH	Short Tip	Soft Tip	JR	JL
COOK						
LuMax-Flex, LuMax	6	Y	JL	Y	3,3.5,4,4.5,5,6	3.5,4,4.5,5
LuMax-Flex, LuMax	7	Y	JL	Y	3,3.5,4,4.5,5,6	3.5,4,4.5,5
LuMax-Flex	8	Y	JL	Y	3,3.5,4,4.5,5,6	3.5,4,4.5,5
LuMax-Flex	9	Y	JL	Y	3,3.5,4,4.5,5,6	3.5,4,4.5,5
USCI						
Super-7	7	JR,AR	JL	Y	3,3.5,4,4.5,5	3,3.5,4,4.5,5,6
Illumen-8	8	JR,AR	JL	Y	3,3.5,4,4.5,5	3,3.5,4,4.5,5,6
Illumen-8 Flexguard	8	JR,AR	JL	Y	3,3.5,4,4.5,5	3,3.5,4,4.5,5,6
Super-9	9	JR,AR	JL	Y	3,3.5,4,4.5,5	3,3.5,4,4.5,5,6
CORDIS						
Vista Petite Tip	6	Y	JR,JL,AL	Y	3.5,4,4.5,5,6	3.5,4,4.5,5,6
Vista Brite Tip	6	Y	JL	Y	3.5,4,4.5,5,6	3.5,4,4.5,5,6
Vista Brite Tip	7	Y	JL	Y	3,3.5,4,5	3.5,4,4.5,5
Brite Tip	7	Y	JR,JL,AL	Y	3,3.5,4,5,6	3.5,4,4.5,5,6
Vista Brite Tip	8	Y	JR,JL,AL	Y	3.5,4,4.5,5,6	3.5,4,4.5,5,6
Brite Tip	8	Y	JR,JL,AL	Y	3.5,4,4.5,5,6	3.5,4,4.5,5,6
Vista Brite Tip	9	Y	JR,JL,AL	Y	3.5,4,4.5,5,6	3,3.5,4,4.5,5,6
Vista Brite Tip	10	Y	JR,JL,AL	Y	3.5,4,5	3.5,4,5
MEDTRONIC						
Sherpa	6	Y	JL,JR	Y	3,3.5,4,4.5,5,6	3,3.5,4,4.5,5,6
Ascent	6	Y	JL,JR,AL	Y	3,3.5,4,4.5,5	3,3.5,4,4.5,5,6
Ascent	7	Y	JL,JR,AL	Y	3,3.5,4,4.5,5	3.5,4,4.5,5
Sherpa	7	Y	JL,JR,AL,AR	Y	3,3.5,4,4.5,5,6	3,3.5,4,4.5,5,6
Sherpa-peak flow	7	Y	JL,JR,AL,AR	Y	3,3.5,4,4.5,5,6	3,3.5,4,4.5,5,6
Sherpa	8	Y	JL,JR,AL,AR	Y	3,3.5,4,4.5,5,6	3,3.5,4,4.5,5,6
Sherpa Main	8	Y	JL,JR	Y	3,3.5,4,4.5,5	3,3.5,4,4.5,5,6
Sherpa-peak flow	8	Y	JL,JR,AL,AR	Y	3,3.5,4,4.5,5,6	3,3.5,4,4.5,5,6
Ascent	8	Y	JL,JR,AL,AR	Y	3,3.5,4,4.5,5	3,3.5,4,4.5,5,6
Sherpa 0.086	8	Y	JL,JR,AL,AR	Y	3,3.5,4,4.5,5,6	3,3.5,4,4.5,5,6
Ascent	9	Y	JL,JR,AL,AR	Y	3,3.5,4,4.5,5	3,3.5,4,4.5,5,6
Sherpa	9	Y	JL,JR,AL,AR	Y	3,3.5,4,4.5,5,6	3,3.5,4,4.5,5,6
Sherpa	10	Y	JL,JR,AL,AR	Y	3.5,4,5	3.5,4,5
Sherpa-Firm	10	Y	JL,JR,AL	Y	3.5,4	3.5,4,5
ACS						
Tourguide	6	Y	JL,AL,JR	Y	3.5,4,5,6	3.5,4,4.5,5,6
Tourguide	7	Y	JL,AR,AL,JR,DL	Y	3,3.5,4,5	3,3.5,4,4.5,5,6
Powerbase	7	Y	JL,JR,AL,AR	Y	3,3.5,4,5,6	3,3.5,4,4.5,5,6
Powerbase	8	Y	JL,JR,AL,AR	Y	3,3.5,4,5,6	3,3.5,4,4.5,5,6
Powerbase	9	Y	JL,JR,AL,AR	Y	3,3.5,4,5,6	3,3.5,4,4.5,5,6
Tourguide	8F	Y	JL,AR,AL,JR,DL	Y	3,3.5,4,5,6	3,3.5,4,4.5,5,6
Tourguide	9F	Y	JL,AR,AL,JR,DL	Y	3,3.5,4,5,6	3,3.5,4,4.5,5,6
Tourguide	10F	Y	JL,AR,DL	Y	4	3.5,4,5

Table 1.5. Guiding Catheters for Coronary Intervention: Size, Shape, and Configuration

AL	AR	Hockey	MP	IMA	Cor Bypass	Other Curves
COOK						
0.75,1,1.5,2,3,4	1,2	Y	A,B	Y	L,R	None
0.75,1,1.5,2,3,4	1,2	Y	A,B	Y	L,R	None
0.75,1,1.5,2,3,4	1,2	Y	A,B	Y	L,R	None
0.75,1,1.5,2,3,4	1,2	Y	A,B	Y	L,R	None
USCI						
1234	1,2	Y	A,B	Y	L,R	Champ
1234	1,2	Y	A,B	Y	L,R	Champ
1234	1,2	Y	A,B	Y	L,R	Champ
1234	1,2	Y	A,B	Y	L,R	Champ
CORDIS						
0.75,1,1.5,2,3	1,2	Y	A1	Y	L,R	XB;SON;DA;ELG;NR;CAS
1,1.5,2,3	1,2	Y	A1	Y	L,R	XB;SON;DA;ELG;CAS
1,1.5,2,3	1,2	Y	A1	Y	L,R	XB;DA;ELG
1,1.5,2,3	1,2	Y	A1	Y	L,R	XB;DA;ELG
0.75,1,1.2,1.5,2,3	1,2	Y	A1,B1	Y	L,R	XB;SON;DA;ELG;CAS
0.75,1,1.2,1.5,2,3	1,2	Y	A1	Y	L,R	XB;DA;ELG
0.75,1,1.5,2,3	1,2,ALR 1.2	Y	A1,B1	Y	L,R	XB;JCL;SCR;SON;DA;NR;ELG;CAS;JLGRF
1,2	NA	Y	A1	NA	L	JCL;JCR;JLGRF;JRG
MEDTRONIC						
1,1.5,2,3,4	1,2	Y	B1,B2	Y	L,R	FR;SCR;ELG
1.0,1.5,2,3,4	1,2,ALR 1-2	Y	B1,B2	Y	L,R	SCR;DC;FR;ELG
0.75,1,1.5,2,3	1,2,ALR 1-2	Y	B1,B2	Y	L,R	FL;FR;SCR;DC
0.75,1,1.2,1.5,2,3	1,2,ALR 1-2	Y	B1,B2	Y	L,R	FR;SCR;ELG;DA;DC
0.75,1,1.2,1.5,2,3	1,2,ALR 1-2	Y	B1,B2	Y	L,R	FL;FR
0.75,1,1.2,1.5,2,3	1,2,ALR 1-2	Y	B1,B2	Y	L,R	FR;SCR;DA
1,1.5,2,2.5,3	1,2	Y	B1,B2	Y	L,R	ELG;SCR
0.75,1,1.2,1.5,2,3	1,2,ALR 1-2	Y	B1,B2	Y	L,R	FR;SCR;DA
0.75,1.0,1.5,2,3,4	1,2,ALR 1-2	Y	B1,B2	Y	L,R	FL;SCR;JCL;FR;DA;JC;DC
0.75,1,1.5,2,2.5,3	1,2,ALR 1-2	Y	B1,B2	Y	L,R	FL;FR;JCR;SCR;DA;DC
0.75,1.0,1.5,2,3,4	1,2,ALR 1-2	Y	B1,B2	Y	L,R	FL;FR;JCR;SCR;DA;DC
0.75,1,1.5,2,2.5,3	1,2,ALR 1-2	Y	B1,B2	Y	L,R	JCL;FR;JCR;SCR;DA;ELG;DC
1,2	NA	Y	B1,B2	NA	L,R	JCL;ELG;DA;DC
NA	NA	Y	B1,B2	NA	L,R	JCL;JCR;DC
ACS						
0.75,1,1.5,2,3,4	1,2	Y	Y	Y	L,R	GL;SHR;DA
1,1.5,2,3	1,2	Y	Y	Y	L,R	GL;SHR;DA
0.75,1,1.5,2,3,4	1,2,3	Y	Y	Y	L,R	GL;SHR;DA
0.75,1,1.5,2,3,4	1,2,3	Y	Y	Y	L,R	GL;SHR;DA
0.75,1,1.5,2,3,4	1,2,3	Y	Y	Y	L,R	GL;SHR;DA
.75,1,1.5,2,3	1,2,3	Y	Y	Y	L,R	GL;SHR;DA;JCL;JCR
1,1.5,2,3	1,2	Y	Y	Y	L,R	GL;SHR;DA;JCL;JCR
NA	NA	Y	Y	NA	L,R	GL;SHR;DA;JCL;JCR

Table 1.5. Guiding Catheters for Coronary Intervention: Size, Shape, and Configuration

Name	FR	SH	Short Tip	Soft Tip	JR	JL
SCHNEIDER						
Pink Power	6	Y	JL,JR	Y	3.4,4,5,6	3,3.5,4,4.5,5,6
Soft tip Standard	7	Y	JL,JR	Y	3,3.5,4,5	3,3.5,4,4.5,5,6
Guidezilla	7	Y	JL,JR	Y	3.5,4,5,6	3,3.5,4,4.5,5,6
Superflow	7	JL4	JL,JR	Y	3.5,4,4.5,5	3.5,4,4.5,5
Soft tip Standard	8	Y	JL,JR	Y	3,3.5,4,4.5,5,6	3,3.5,4,4.5,5,6
Visiguide	8	Y	JL,JR	Y	3,3.5,4,4.5,5,6	3,3.5,4,4.5,5,6
Superflow	8	Y	JL,JR	Y	3.5,4,5	3.5,4,4.5,5
Guidezilla	8	Y	JL,JR	Y	3.5,4,5,6	3.5,4,4.5,5
Soft tip Standard	9	Y	JL	Y	3.5,4,5,6	3.5,4,4.5,5
Superflow	9	Y	JL,JR	Y	3.5,4,5,6	3.5,4,4.5,5
Superflow	10	Y	JL,JR	Y	3.5,4,5,6	3.5,4,4.5,5
SCIMED						
Triguide-Elite	6	N	FL 3.5,4	Y	FR 3.5,4,5	3,3.5,4,4.5,5
Triguide-Lite	7	Y	FR,FL,AR,AL	Y	FR 3.5,4,5,6	3,3.5,4,4.5,5,6
Mighty Max	7	Y	FR,FL,AR,AL	Y	FR 3.5,4,5,6	3,3.5,4,4.5,5,6
Standard	8	Y	FL	Y	FR 3.5,4,5,6	3,3.5,4,4.5,5,6
Intermediate	8	Y	FR,FL,AR,AL	Y	FR 3.5,4,5,6	3,3.5,4,4.5,5,6
Big Max	8	Y	FR,FL,AL	Y	FR 3.5,4,5	3,3.5,4,4.5,5
Triguide Plus	9	Y	FL	Y	FR 3.5,4,5	3.5,4,4.5,5
Triguide Flex	10	Y	FCR,FL	Y	NA	3,3.5,4,4.5,5
DVI						
	9.5	Y	JR	Y	4	NA
	10	Y	NA	Y	NA	3.5,4,4.5,5
	11	Y	NA	Y	NA	3.5,4,4.5,5

Abbreviations: FR = French size; SH = sideholes; Hockey = Hockey stick; MP = multipurpose; IMA = internal mammary artery catheter; Cor bypss = coronary artery bypass catheter

*   See table 1.9 and Figure 1.8 for description of all configurations

AL	AR	Hockey	MP	IMA	Cor Bypass	Other Curves

SCHNEIDER

AL	AR	Hockey	MP	IMA	Cor Bypass	Other Curves
1,1.5,2,3	1,2	Y	Y	Y	L,R	ELG;DA
1,1.5,2,3	1,2,1	Y	Y	Y	L,R	ELG;DA
1,1.5,2,3	1,2	Y	Y	Y	L,R	ELG;DA
1,2,3	1,2	Y	Y	Y	L,R	
0.75,1,1.5,2,3	1,2,3	Y	Y	Y	L,R	ELG;DA
0.75,1,1.5,2,3	1,2,3	Y	Y	Y	L,R	ELG;DA
1,1.5,2,3	1,2	Y	Y	Y	L,R	ELG
1,1.5,2,3	1,2	Y	Y	Y	L,R	ELG
1,2,3	1,2	Y	Y	Y	L,R	ELG;DA
1,1.5,2,3	1,2	Y	Y	Y	L,R	ELG
1,1.5,2,3	1,2	Y	Y	Y	L,R	ELG

SCIMED

AL	AR	Hockey	MP	IMA	Cor Bypass	Other Curves
0.75,1,2,3	1,2	Y	1,2	Y	L,R	VR;VRSC;VL;VLHT;RC;SC;BR
0.75,1,1.5,2,2.5,3	1,1.5,2,2.5	Y	1,2	Y	L,R	VR;VRSC;VL;ELG;DA;VLHT;RC;SC;BR
0.75,1,1.5,2,2.5,3	1,1.5,2.5	Y	1,2	Y	L,R	VR;VRSC;VL;VLHT;DA;BR;FCL;FCR;RC;SC
0.75,1,1.5,2,3,4	1,2	Y	1,2	Y	L,R	VR;VRSC;VL;ELG;DA;RC;SC
0.75,1,1.5,2,2.5,3	1,1.5,2,2.5	Y	1,2	Y	L,R	VR;VRSC;VL;ELG;DA;VLHT;RC;SC;BR
0.75,1,2,3	1,2	Y	1,2	Y	L,R	VR;VRSC;VL;FCR;FCL;ELG;VLHT;BR
1,2,3	1,2	Y	1,2	Y	L,R	VR;VRSC;VL;FCR;ELG;FCL;RC;SC;VLHT
1,2	NA	Y	1	N	L	VR;VRSC;VL;FCR;FCL;FRGRF;FLGRF;VLHT

DVI

AL	AR	Hockey	MP	IMA	Cor Bypass	Other Curves
NA	NA	Y	NA	NA	NA	JRGRF;JR4IF
NA	NA	NA	NA	NA	NA	JLGRF
NA	NA	NA	NA	NA	NA	JLGRF

Abbreviations: FR = French size; SH = sideholes; Hockey = Hockey stick; MP = multipurpose; IMA = internal mammary artery catheter; Cor bypss = coronary artery bypass catheter

* See table 1.9 and Figure 1.8 for description of all configurations

Table 1.6. Guiding Catheters for Coronary Intervention: Technical Features

Name	FR	ID (inch)	L (cm)	Construction	Inner Liner	Comments
COOK						
LuMax-Flex, LuMax	6	0.060	100	Nylon; stainless steel braid	PTFE	Flex = more flexible tip
LuMax-Flex, LuMax	7	0.073	100	Nylon; stainless steel braid	PTFE	Flex = more flexible tip
LuMax-Flex	8	0.086	100	Nylon; stainless steel braid	PTFE	Flex = more flexible tip
LuMax-Flex	9	0.099	100	Nylon; stainless steel braid	PTFE	Flex = more flexible tip
USCI						
Super-7	7	0.070	100	Pebax; Kevlar braid	PTFE	
Illumen-8	8	0.080	100	Pebax; Kevlar braid	PTFE	
Illumen-8 Flexguard	8	0.080	100	Pebax; Kevlar braid	PTFE	More flexible tip than Illumen-9
Super-9	9	0.092	100	Pebax; Kevlar braid	PTFE	
CORDIS						
Vista PetiteTip	6	0.062	100	Nylon blend; stainless steel braid	PTFE	Modular design; Eco Pacs available
Vista Brite Tip	6	0.064	100	Nylon blend; stainless steel braid	PTFE	Modular design; Eco Pacs available
Vista Brite Tip	7	0.074	100	Nylon blend; stainless steel braid	PTFE	Modular design; Eco Pacs available
Brite Tip	7	0.072	100	Nylon blend; stainless steel braid	PTFE	Modular design; Eco Pacs available
Vista Brite Tip	8	0.086	100	Nylon blend; stainless steel braid	PTFE	Modular design; Eco Pacs available
Brite Tip	8	0.084	100	Nylon blend; stainless steel braid	PTFE	Modular design; Eco Pacs available
Vista Brite Tip	9	0.098	100	Nylon blend; stainless steel braid	PTFE	Modular design; Eco Pacs available
Vista Brite Tip	10	0.110	100	Nylon blend; stainless steel braid	PTFE	Modular design

Name	FR	ID (inch)	L (cm)	Construction	Inner Liner	Comments
MEDTRONIC						
Sherpa	6	0.057	100	Polyurethane; stainless steel braid	PTFE	Active guide
Ascent	6	0.062	100	Pebax blend; stainless steel braid	PTFE	Passive guide
Ascent	7	0.073	100	Pebax blend; stainless steel braid	PTFE	Passive guide
Sherpa	7	0.070	100	Polyurethane; stainless steel braid	PTFE	Active guide
Sherpa-peak flow	7	0.072	100	Polyurethane; stainless steel braid	PTFE	Active guide
Sherpa	8	0.079	100	Polyurethane; stainless steel braid	PTFE	Active guide
Sherpa Maine	8	0.079	100	Polyurethane; stainless steel braid	PTFE	Active guide; 16cm flexible intermediate shaft
Sherpa-peak flow	8	0.083	100	Polyurethane; stainless steel braid	PTFE	Active guide
Ascent	8	0.086	100	Pebax blend; stainless steel braid	PTFE	Passive guide
Sherpa 0.086	8	0.086	100	Polyurethane; stainless steel braid	PTFE	Active guide
Ascent	9	0.096	100	Pebax blend; stainless steel braid	PTFE	Passive guide
Sherpa	9	0.092	100	Polyurethane; stainless steel braid	PTFE	Active guide
Sherpa	10	0.108	95	Polyurethane; stainless steel braid	PTFE	Active guide
Sherpa-Firm	10	0.108	95	Polyurethane; stainless steel braid	PTFE	Active guide
ACS						
Tourguide	6	0.064	100	Nylon; stainless steel braid	PTFE	
Tourguide	7	0.075	100	Nylon; stainless steel braid	PTFE	
Powerbase	7	0.072	100	Polyurethane; vectran braid	PTFE	
Powerbase	8	0.085	100	Polyurethane; vectran braid	PTFE	
Powerbase	9	0.092	100	Polyurethane; vectran braid	PTFE	
Tourguide	8	0.087	100	Nylon; stainless steel braid	PTFE	
Tourguide	9	0.101	100	Nylon; stainless steel braid	PTFE	
Tourguide	10	0.112	100	Nylon; stainless steel braid	PTFE	

Table 1.6. Guiding Catheters for Coronary Intervention: Technical Features

Name	FR	ID (inch)	L (cm)	Construction	Inner Liner	Comments
SCHNEIDER						
Pink Power	6	0.062	100	Urethane; stainless steel	PTFE	Active guide
Soft tip Standard	7	0.063	100	Urethane; stainless steel	PTFE	Active guide
Guidezilla	7	0.072	100	Nylon blend; stainless steel braid	PTFE	Passive guide
Superflow	7	0.072	100	Urethane; stainless steel	PTFE	Active guide
Soft tip Standard	8	0.076	100	Urethane; stainless steel	PTFE	Active guide
Visiguide	8	0.079	100	Urethane; stainless steel	PTFE	Active guide
Superflow	8	0.082	100	Urethane; stainless steel	PTFE	Active guide
Guidezilla	8	0.086	100	Nylon blend; stainless steel braid	PTFE	Passive guide
Soft tip Standard	9	0.080	100	Urethane; stainless steel	PTFE	Active guide
Superflow	9	0.092	100	Urethane; stainless steel	PTFE	Active guide
Superflow	10	0.107	100	Urethane; stainless steel	PTFE	Active guide
SCIMED						
Triguide-Elite	6	0.060	100	Trilon; Stainless steel braid	PTFE	Extra support & torque
Triguide-Lite	7	0.072	100	Trilon; Stainless steel braid	PTFE	Extra support & torque
Mighty Max	7	0.074	100	Trilon; Stainless steel braid	PTFE	Extra support & torque
Standard	8	0.080	100	Trilon; Stainless steel braid	PTFE	Extra support & torque
Intermediate	8	0.080	100	Trilon; Stainless steel braid	PTFE	More tip flexibility than 8F Standard
Big Max	8	0.086	100	Trilon; Stainless steel braid	PTFE	Extra support & torque
Triguide Plus	9	0.096	100	Trilon; Stainless steel braid	PTFE	Extra support & torque
Triguide Flex	10	0.107	100	Trilon; Stainless steel braid	PTFE	Extra support & torque
DVI						
	9.5	0.104	100	Urethane; stainless steel braid	PTFE	
	10	0.104	100	Urethane; stainless steel braid	PTFE	
	11	0.111	100	Urethane; stainless steel braid	PTFE	

Abbreviations: FR = French size; ID = internal diameter; L = length of shaft; PTFE = teflon; Eco Pacs = economy packs

Table 1.11. Guidewires for Percutaneous Coronary Intervention

Name	Diameter (inch)	Length (cm)	Extend	Coating	Construction	Materials	Comments	Opaque Tip (cm)
SCIMED/MEDITECH								
Platinum Plus	0.014;0.016; 0.018;0.025	180,300	NA	Glidex on distal platinum coils	Single core	Distal platinum coils, stainless steel core	Excellent heavy-duty wire for stent placement	1,3,5
Glidewire Gold	0.016;0.018	180	NA	Hydrophilic polymer	Single core	Nitinol shaft, gold tip (2 mm)	Preformed J; superior torque, wire movement; kink resistant	2
Jagwire	0.016	180,300	NA	Silicone shaft, hydroplus tip	Single core	Nitinol shaft, tungsten tip	Superb torque, steerability, flexibility; kink resistant	2
COOK								
Roadrunner	0.014;0.016; 0.017,0.018	180,270, 300,400	NA	PTFE	Single core	Nitinol shaft, platinum spring (3-4 cm)	Excellent flexibility and kink resistance	4
CORDIS								
Reflex-super soft	0.012;0.014; 0.014;0.018	18,300	Cinch III	DuraGlide shaft; SLX coil	Single core (tritaper); broad transition	Stainless steel core; platinum spring	Broad transition causes less prolapse,improved steerability	25
Reflex-soft	0.012;0.014; 0.014;0.018	18,300	Cinch III	DuraGlide shaft; SLX coil	Single core (tritaper);broad transition	Stainless steel core; platinum spring	Broad transition causes less prolapse,improved steerability	25
Reflex-standard	0.012;0.014; 0.014;0.018	18,300	Cinch III	DuraGlide shaft; SLX coil	Single core (tritaper);broad transition	Stainless steel core; platinum spring	Broad transition causes less prolapse,improved steerability	25
Marvel-Super Soft	0.012	18,300	Cinch III	DuraGlide shaft; SLX coil	Single core (tritaper);broad transition	Stainless steel core; platinum spring	Broad transition causes less prolapse,improved steerability	25

Table 1.11. Guidewires for Percutaneous Coronary Intervention

Name	Diameter (inch)	Length (cm)	Extend	Coating	Construction	Materials	Comments	Opaque Tip (cm)
Stabilizer-Super Soft	0.014,0.018	180,300	Cinch III	DuraGlide spray; PTFE sleeve	Single core (tritaper);broad transition	Stainless steel core; platinum spring	Broad transition causes less prolapse, improved steerability; Flex-joint bond; balanced performance	3,25
Stabilizer-Soft	0.014,0.018	180,300	Cinch III	DuraGlide spray; PTFE sleeve	Single core (tritaper);broad transition	Stainless steel core; platinum spring	Broad transition causes less prolapse, improved steerability; Flex-joint bond; balanced performance	3,25
Wizdom-Super Soft	0.014	180,300	Cinch III	DuraGlide spray; PTFE sleeve	Single core (tritaper);broad transition	Stainless steel core; platinum spring	Broad transition causes less prolapse, improved steerability; Flex-joint bond; balanced performance	3
Wizdom Soft	0.014	180,300	Cinch III	DuraGlide spray; PTFE sleeve	Single core (tritaper);broad transition	Stainless steel core; platinum spring	Broad transition causes less prolapse, improved steerability; Flex-joint bond; balanced performance	3
USCI								
Pilot wire	0.014	165	Linx	PTFE	Double core, deflectable tip	Stainless steel core; platinum spring	Routine use, acute angles, in-vivo tip shaping	2,30
LumiSilk	0.012	180	Linx	Pro/Pel	Transitionless; 2 round forming wires	Stainless steel core, gold plated spring	Exceptional 1:1 torque ; severe tortuosity	2
Phantom	0.014	180,300	Linx	Pro/Pel	Transitionless; 2 round forming wires	Stainless core and ribbons; gold plated spring	Routine use; excellent trackability	2
Silk	0.012	180,300	Linx	Pro/Pel	Transitionless; 2 round forming wires	Stainless steel core; Platinum spring	Excellent trackability	30
Hi-PerFlex	0.014,0.016	180,300	Linx	Pro/Pel	Double core with forming ribbon	Stainless steel core; Platinum spring	Excellent steerability and trackability	30
VeriFlex	0.014,0.016	180	Linx	Pro/Pel	Single core with forming ribbon	Stainless steel core; Platinum spring	Very steerable, 3 cm soft tip	30

Name	Diameter (inch)	Length (cm)	Extend	Coating	Construction	Materials	Comments	Opaque Tip (cm)
Flex	0.014,0.016	180	Linx	Pro/Pel	Single core with forming ribbon	Stainless steel core; Platinum spring	Very steerable, high support	30
Standard	0.014,0.016	180	Linx	Pro/Pel	Single core	Stainless steel core; Platinum spring	Chronic total occlusions	30
SCIMED								
Sceptor floppy	0.014	300	NA	Xtra	Unibody core	Stainless steel core; platinum spring with polymer sleeve	Straight and J-wire	3
Sceptor floppy	0.014,0.018	182	NA	Xtra	Unibody core	Stainless steel core; platinum spring with polymer sleeve	Straight and J-wire	3
Sceptor intermediate	0.014,0.018	182	NA	Xtra	Unibody core	Stainless steel core; platinum spring with polymer sleeve	Straight and J-wire	2
Sceptor standard	0.014,0.018	182	NA	Xtra	Unibody core	Stainless steel core; platinum spring with polymer sleeve	Straight and J-wire	2
Sceptor extra support	0.014	300	NA	Xtra	Unibody core	Stainless steel core; platinum spring with polymer sleeve	Straight and J-wire	3
Choice floppy	0.014	182,300	NA	ICE	Unibody core	Stainless steel core; platinum spring with polymer sleeve	Straight and J-wire	3
Choice intermediate	0.014	182,300	NA	ICE	Unibody core	Stainless steel core; platinum spring with polymer sleeve	Straight and J-wire	3
Choice standard	0.014	182,300	NA	ICE	Unibody core	Stainless steel core; platinum spring with polymer sleeve	Straight and J-wire	3
Choice PT	0.014	182,300	NA	ICE	Unibody core	Stainless steel core; platinum spring with polymer sleeve	Straight and J-wire	35
Choice extra support	0.014	182,300	NA	ICE	Unibody core	Stainless steel core; platinum spring with polymer sleeve	Straight and J-wire	3
ACS								
HI-Torque Floppy	0.014	175,300	DOC	Teflon & Microglide	Multiple tapers, shaping ribbon tip	Stainless steel core; stainlesssteel and/or platinum tip	Straight and J	2,30
	0.018	175,300	DOC				Straight and J	2
	0.010	175,300	DOC-T				Straight and J	3,30

Table 1.11. Guidewires for Percutaneous Coronary Intervention

Name	Diameter (inch)	Length (cm)	Extend	Coating	Construction	Materials	Comments	Opaque Tip (cm)
HI-Torque Floppy II	0.014 0.018 0.010	175,300 175,300 175,300	DOC DOC DOC-T	Teflon & Microglide	Multiple tapers, shaping ribbon tip	Stainless steel core; stainless steel and/or platinum tip	Straight and J Straight and J Straight and J	2,30 2 3,30
HI-Torque Traverse	0.014	175,300	DOC	Teflon & Microglide	Broad transition, tapered core to tip	Stainless steel core; stainless steel and/or platinum tip	Straight and J	3,30
HI-Torque Intermediate	0.014 0.018 0.010	175 175 175,300	DOC DOC DOC-T	Teflon & Microglide	Multiple tapers; core to tip design	Stainless steel core; stainless steel and/or platinum tip	Straight and J Straight and J Straight and J	3,30 3 2,30
HI-Torque Standard	0.014 0.018 0.010	175 175 175,300	DOC DOC DOC-T	Teflon & Microglide	Multiple tapers; core to tip design	Stainless steel core; stainless steel and/or platinum tip	Straight and J Straight and J Straight and J	2,30 2 2,30
HI-Torque Balance	0.014	175,300	DOC	Teflon & Microglide	Broad transition; shaping ribbon tip	Stainless steel proximal shaft; nitinol distal core	Straight and J; designed for tortuous anatomy; exceptional steerability	3,40
HI-Torque Extra Sport	0.014	175,300	DOC	Teflon & Microglide	Multiple tapers, core to tip design	Stainless steel core, stainless steel and/or platinum tip	Straight and J; excellent support for DCA and stents	3
HI-Torque Floppy II Extra Support	0.014 0.018	175,300 175,300	DOC DOC	Teflon & Microglide	Multiple tapers; core to tip design	Stainless steel core; stainless steel and/or platinum tip	Straight and J	2,30 2,30
HI-Torque Approach	0.010	175,300	DOC-T	Teflon & Microglide	Multiple tapers, core to tip design		Straight and J	3,30
SCHNEIDER								
C-Thru Floppy	0.014	185,300	DOC/E	PTFE	Single moveable core, flat wire design	Stainless steel core; 18-K gold plated tungsten tip	Straight and J, flatwire = less surface area for platelet aggregation	3,30
C-Thur Intermediate	0.014	185,300	DOC/E	PTFE	Single moveable core, flat wire design	Stainless steel core; 18-K gold plated tungsten tip	Straight and J, flatwire = less surface area for platelet aggregation	3,30
C-Thru Standard	0.014	185,300	DOC/E	PTFE	Single moveable core, flat wire design	Stainless steel core; 18-K gold plated tungsten tip	Straight and J, flatwire = less surface area for platelet aggregation	3,30

Name	Diameter (inch)	Length (cm)	Extend	Coating	Construction	Materials	Comments	Opaque Tip (cm)
C-Thru Finder	0.010 0.014 0.018	185,300	DOC/E	PTFE	Single moveable core, flat wire design	Stainless steel core; 18-K gold plated tungsten tip	Straight and J, flatwire = less surface area for platelet aggregation	3,30
C-Thru Flex	0.010 0.014 0.018	185,300	DOC/E	PTFE	Single moveable core, flat wire design	Stainless steel core; 18-K gold plated tungsten tip	Straight and J, flatwire = less surface area for platelet aggregation	3,30
C-Thru Forte	0.010 0.014 0.018	185,300	DOC/E	PTFE	Single moveable core, flat wire design	Stainless steel core; 18-K gold plated tungsten tip	Straight and J, flatwire = less surface area for platelet aggregation	3,30
Magnum 14	0.014	185	NA	PTFE	Single core; 1 mm olive tip	Stainless steel core; 18-K gold plated tungsten tip	Flexible tip length 30 cm; 1mm oliver tip	25
Magnum 18	0.018	185	NA	PTFE	Single core; 1 mm olive tip	Stainless steel core; 18-K gold plated tungsten tip	Flexible tip length 30 cm; 1mm oliver tip	25
Magnum 21	0.021	185	NA	PTFE	Single core; 1 mm olive tip	Stainless steel core; 18-K gold plated tungsten tip	Flexible tip length 30 cm; 1mm oliver tip	25

Abbreviations: NA = not available; PTFE = teflon; SLX = Silicone; DOC = detachable on command; Extend = type of extension

Table 1.14. Coronary Angioplasty Balloon Catheters: Balloon Characteristics

Type	Catheter Name	Balloon Length (mm)	QTR Sizes	Max GW (inch)	Balloon Material	NOM (ATM)	RBP (ATM)	MBP (ATM)
			SCIMED					
OTW	Ally 14	20	Yes	0.014	HDPE	6	10	NR
OTW	Ally 18	20	Yes	0.018	HDPE	6	10	NR
OTW	Bandit	20	Yes	0.014	LEAP	6	14	20
OTW	Bandit-Long	30	Yes	0.014	LEAP	6	14	20
OTW	Bandit-Long	40	Yes	0.014	LEAP	6	14	20
OTW	Cobra 10	20	No	0.010	POC 6	6	9	NR
OTW	Cobra 14	20	No	0.014	POC 6	6	9	NR
OTW	Cobra 18	20	No	0.018	POC 6	6	9	NR
OTW	Cobra 18-Long	30	No	0.018	POC 8	8	10	NR
OTW	Cobra 18-Long	40	No	0.018	POC 8	8	10	NR
OTW	Mighty	20	Yes	0.018	Coex	3	15	24
OTW	Mighty-Long	30	Yes	0.018	Coex	3	15	24
OTW	Mighty-Long	40	Yes	0.018	Coex	3	15	24
OTW	Mirage	20	No	0.018	POC 6	6	9	NR
OTW	MVP	20	No	0.018	POC 8	8	10	NR
OTW	NC Bandit	15	Yes	0.014	T4	6	16	24
OTW	NC Cobra	20	Yes	0.014	Triad PET	6	16	24
OTW	NC Cobra-18	20	Yes	0.018	Triad PET	6	16	24
OTW	NC Cobra-18	10	yes	0.018	Triad PET	6	16	24
OTW	NC Shadow	20	Yes	0.014	Triad PET	6	16	24
OTW	SC Shadow	20	No	0.014	POC 8	8	10	NR
OTW	Shadow	20	No	0.014	POC 6	6	9	NR
OTW	Skinny	20	No	0.014	POC 8	8	10	NR
OTW	Skinny Long	30	No	0.014	POC 8	8	10	NR
OTW	Striker	20	No	0.014	EVA	6	9	NR
OTW	Trio 14	20	No	0.014	POC 6	6	9	NR
FW	ACE 1 cm	20	No	NA	POC 6	6	9	NR
FW	ACE 2 cm	20	No	NA	POC 7	7	8	NR
FW	ACE 2 cm Flex	20	No	NA	POC 6	6	9	NR
FW	ACE Graft	20	No	NA	POC 7	7	8	NR
FW	ACE Long	40	No	NA	POC 7	7	8	NR
FW	Pivot	20	No	NA	POC 6	6	9	NR
SOE	Express Plus-II	20	Yes	0.014	POC 6	6	9	NR
SOE	Express Plus-Leap	20	Yes	0.014	LEAP	6	14	20
SOE	Express Plus-Leap	30	Yes	0.014	LEAP	6	14	20
SOE	Express Plus-Leap	40	Yes	0.014	LEAP	6	14	20
SOE	NC-Express Plus	20	Yes	0.014	Triad PET	6	16	24
RX-OTW	Synergy 14	20	Yes	0.014	HDPE	6	10	NR
RX-OTW	Synergy 14-long	30	No	0.014	HDPE	6	10	NR
RX-OTW	Synergy 14-long	40	No	0.014	HDPE	6	10	NR
RX--OTW	Synergy 18	20	Yes	0.014	HDPE	6	10	NR

Type	Catheter Name	Balloon Length (mm)	QTR Sizes	Max GW (inch)	Balloon Material	NOM (ATM)	RBP (ATM)	MBP (ATM)
RX-OTW	Synergy 18-long	30	No	0.018	HDPE	6	10	NR
RX-OTW	Synergy 18-long	40	No	0.018	HDPE	6	10	NR
				CORDIS				
OTW	Olympix	20	No	0.018	Duralyn	8	10	21
OTW	Olympix Long	30	No	0.018	Duralyn	8	10	21
OTW	Olympix Long	40	No	0.018	Duralyn	8	10	21
OTW	Olympix-II	20	No	0.018	Duralyn	8	10	21
OTW	Olympix-II Long	30	No	0.018	Duralyn	8	10	21
OTW	Olympix-II Long	40	No	0.018	Duralyn	8	10	21
OTW	Predator	20	No	0.014	Duralyn	8	10	21
OTW	Predator-Long	30	No	0.014	Duralyn	8	10	21
OTW	Predator-Long	40	No	0.014	Duralyn	8	10	21
OTW	Sleek	20	No	0.014	Duralyn	8	10	21
OTW	Sleek Long	30	No	0.014	Duralyn	8	10	21
OTW	Sleek Long	40	No	0.014	Duralyn	8	10	21
OTW	Titan-18	9	No	0.018	Duralyn-ST	12	16	27
OTW	Titan-18	18	No	0.018	Duralyn-ST	12	16	27
OTW	Trakstar-14	20	No	0.014	Duralyn	8	10	21
OTW	Trakstar-14 Long	30	No	0.014	Duralyn	8	10	21
OTW	Trakstar-14 Long	40	No	0.014	Duralyn	8	10	21
OTW	Trakstar-18	20	No	0.018	Duralyn	8	10	21
OTW	Trakstar-18 Long	30	No	0.018	Duralyn	8	10	21
OTW	Trakstar-18 Long	40	No	0.018	Duralyn	8	10	21
SOE	Europass	20	No	0.014	Duralyn	8	10	21
SOE	Europass-Long	30	No	0.014	Duralyn	8	10	21
SOE	Europass-Long	40	No	0.014	Duralyn	8	10	21
SOE	Passage	20	No	0.014	Duralyn	8	10	21
SOE	Passage-Long	30	No	0.014	Duralyn	8	10	21
SOE	Passage-Long	40	No	0.014	Duralyn	8	10	21
FW	Lightning	20	No	NA	Duralyn	8	12	23
FW	Orion	20	No	NA	Duralyn	8	12	23
				USCI				
OTW	Agil	20	Yes	0.014	PET	5	12	19
OTW	Force	20	Yes	0.018	PET	5	12	19
OTW	Force-Long	40	No	0.018	PET	5	12	19
OTW	Force-Long	30	No	0.018	PET	5	12	19
OTW	Solo	20	Yes	0.014	PET	5	12	19
OTW	Sprint	20	Yes	0.018	PET	5	12	19
OTW	Tapered	25	No	0.018	PET	5	12	19
OTW	XPRT	20	Yes	0.014	PET	5	12	19
FW	Probe III	20	No	NA	PET	5	11	18

Table 1.14. Coronary Angioplasty Balloon Catheters: Balloon Characteristics

Type	Catheter Name	Balloon Length (mm)	QTR Sizes	Max GW (inch)	Balloon Material	NOM (ATM)	RBP (ATM)	MBP (ATM)
			ACS					
OTW	Edge	20	Yes	0.014	PE 600	6	8	NR
OTW	Edge-Long	30	No	0.014	PE 600	6	8	NR
OTW	Edge-Long	40	No	0.014	PE 600	6	8	NR
OTW	Omega	20	Yes	0.010	PE 600	6	8	NR
OTW	Pinkerton	20	No	0.018	PE 600	6	8	NR
OTW	Pinkerton	10	No	0.018	PE 600	6	6	NR
OTW	Pinkerton Long	30	No	0.018	PE 600	6	8	NR
OTW	Pinkerton Long	40	No	0.018	PE 600	6	8	NR
OTW	Prism	20	Yes	0.014	PE 600	6	8	NR
OTW	Prism	15	No	0.014	PE 600	6	8	NR
OTW	Prism	10	No	0.014	PE 600	6	8	NR
OTW	Prism Long	30	Yes	0.014	PE 600	6	8	NR
OTW	Prism Long	40	Yes	0.014	PE 600	6	8	NR
FW	Slalom	20	No	NA	PE 600	6	8	NR
SOE	RX Elipse	20	Yes	0.014	PE 600	6	8	NR
SOE	RX Streak	20	Yes	0.014	PE 600	6	8	NR
SOE	RX-Elipse Long	40	No	0.014	PE 600	6	8	NR
SOE	RX-Streak Long	30	No	0.014	PE 600	6	8	NR
SOE	RX-Streak Long	40	No	0.014	PE 600	6	8	NR
Perfusion	RX Flow Track 40 (40)	20	Yes	0.018	PE 600	6	8	NR
Perfusion	RX Lifestream (40)	20	Yes	0.014	PFlex	8	12	NR
Perfusion	OTW Lifestream (40)	20	Yes	0.014	PFlex	8	12	NR
Perfusion	RX Perfusion (60)	20	Yes	0.018	PE 600	6	8	NR
Perfusion	RX Perfusion Long (55)	30	No	0.018	PE 600	6	8	NR
Perfusion	RX Perfusion Long (50)	40	No	0.018	PE 600	6	8	NR
Perfusion	Stack Perfusion (60)	20	No	0.018	PE 600	6	6	NR
Perfusion	Stack Perfusion (60)	25	No	0.018	PE 600	6	6	NR
	(Numbers in parenthesis indicate flow rates)							
			MEDTRONIC					
OTW	14 K	20	No	0.014	PE	6	8	12
OTW	14K-Long	30	No	0.014	PE	6	8	12
OTW	18K	20	No	0.018	PE	5	6	10
OTW	18K-Short	12	No	0.018	PE	5	6	10
OTW	Evergreen	20	Yes	0.014	PE	6	8	14
OTW	Evergreen	30	No	0.014	PE	6	8	14
OTW	Evergreen	40	No	0.014	PE	6	8	14
OTW	Panther	20	Yes	0.014	PE	6	8	14
OTW	Panther	40	No	0.014	PE	6	8	14
OTW	Panther	30	No	0.014	PE	6	8	14
OTW	Spirit	20	No	0.014	PE	7	10	14
OTW	Spirit	30	No	0.014	PE	7	10	14

Type	Catheter Name	Balloon Length (mm)	QTR Sizes	Max GW (inch)	Balloon Material	NOM (ATM)	RBP (ATM)	MBP (ATM)
OTW	Spirit	40	No	0.014	PE	7	10	14
SOE	Falcon	20	No	0.014	PE	6	8	14
				SCHNEIDER				
OTW	Asuka	20	Yes	0.014	Nylon	6	12	NR
OTW	Asuka-Long	30	Yes	0.014	Nylon	6	12	NR
OTW	Asuka-Long	40	Yes	0.014	Nylon	6	12	NR
OTW	Freeflight	20	Yes	0.014	Repeat (PE)	5	9	NR
OTW	Freeflight-Long	30	Yes	0.014	Repeat (PE)	5	9	NR
OTW	Freeflight-Long	40	Yes	0.014	Repeat (PE)	5	9	NR
OTW	Magnum Meier	20	No	0.021	PET	10	16	NR
OTW	Mystic MC	20	Yes	0.014	Thaline	5	12	NR
OTW	Mystic MC Long	30	Yes	0.014	Thaline	5	12	NR
OTW	Mystic MC Long	40	Yes	0.014	Thaline	5	12	NR
OTW	Takumi	20	No	0.014	Nylon	6	14	NR
SOE	Bypass Speedy**	20	No	0.018	Nylon	10	18	NR
SOE	Chubby*	20	No	0.018	Nylon	8	18	NR
SOE	Forte 30	30	Yes	0.014	PET	10	16	NR
SOE	Freehand	20	Yes	0.014	Repeat (PE)	5	9	NR
SOE	Freehand-Long	30	Yes	0.014	Repeat (PE)	5	9	NR
SOE	Freehand-Long	40	Yes	0.014	Repeat (PE)	5	9	NR
SOE	Goldie	20	No	0.014	Nylon	6	14	NR
SOE	Goldie-Long	30	No	0.014	Nylon	6	10	NR
SOE	Goldie-Long	40	No	0.014	Nylon	6	10	NR
SOE	Magna Rail	20	No	0.021	PET	10	16	NR
SOE	McRail	20	Yes	0.014	Thaline	5	12	NR
SOE	McRail-Long	30	Yes	0.014	Thaline	5	12	NR
SOE	McRail-Long	40	Yes	0.014	Thaline	5	12	NR
SOE	Mongoose	20	Yes	0.014	PET	10	16	NR
SOE	Shortgoose	10	Yes	0.014	PET	10	16	NR
SOE	Shortgoose	15	Yes	0.014	PET	10	16	NR
Perfusion	RX Speedflow Junior	20	No	0.018	Nylon	6	12	NR
Perfusion	RX Speedflow Junior	30	No	0.018	Nylon	6	12	NR
Perfusion	RX Speedflow Junior	40	No	0.018	Nylon	6	12	NR

Abbreviations: QTR = quarter sizes; Max GW = maximum guidewire; NOM = nominal pressure; RBP = rated burst pressure; MBP = mean burst pressure; ATM = atmospheres; OTW = over-the-wire; SOE = single operator exchange (Monorail); RX-OTW = rapid exchange-over-the-wire (hybrid); PET = Polyethylene terephthalate; PE = polyethylene; Pflex - polyethylene blend; LEAP = Pebax; NA = not applicable; NR = not reported by manufacturer; HDPE = high density polyethylene; POC = polyolefin copolymer; Coex - Coextruded; T4 = triad-4 (PET); EVA = ethyl vinyl acetate; FW = fixed wire
*   Available in 3.5 - 5.0 mm
**   Available in 2.0 - 6.0 mm

Table 1.15. Coronary Angioplasty Balloon Catheters: Technical Features

Type	Catheter Name	Shaft[+] (F)	Published Balloon Profiles						Usable Length (cm)	Coating
			1.5	2.0	2.5	3.0	3.5	4.0		
			SCIMED							
OTW	Ally 14	3.4/2.9	NA	0.029	0.033	0.035	0.039	0.040	135	Hydroplus
OTW	Ally 18	3.4/2.9	NA	0.032	0.035	0.039	0.041	0.044	135	Hydroplus
OTW	Bandit	2.9/2.0	0.027	0.027	0.028	0.031	0.032	0.035	135	Bioslide
OTW	Bandit-Long	3.1/2.0	NA	0.027	0.028	0.031	0.032	0.035	135	Bioslide
OTW	Bandit-Long	3.1/2.0	NA	0.027	0.028	0.031	0.032	0.035	135	Bioslide
OTW	Cobra 10	2.8/2.5	0.027	0.029	0.031	0.033	0.034	NA	135	Xtra
OTW	Cobra 14	3.0/2.7	0.030	0.031	0.033	0.037	0.039	0.042	135	Bioslide
OTW	Cobra 18	3.2/2.9	0.032	0.034	0.036	0.038	0.040	0.045	135	Bioslide
OTW	Cobra 18-Long	3.2/2.9	NA	0.033	0.037	0.040	0.042	0.046	135	Bioslide
OTW	Cobra 18-Long	3.2/2.9	NA	0.034	0.037	0.041	0.042	0.046	135	Bioslide
OTW	Mighty	2.9/2.9	NA	0.035	0.037	0.040	0.042	0.043	135	Glidecoat
OTW	Mighty-Long	2.9/3.4	NA	0.033	0.035	0.037	0.039	0.043	135	Glidecoat
OTW	Mighty-Long	2.9/3.4	NA	0.033	0.035	0.037	0.039	0.043	135	Glidecoat
OTW	Mirage	3.6/2.9	NA	0.034	0.035	0.038	0.040	0.044	135	Xtra
OTW	MVP	3.5/3.0	0.031	0.034	0.037	0.039	0.040	0.044	135	Xtra
OTW	NC Bandit	3.2/3.2	NA	NA	0.032	0.035	0.037	0.040	135	Xtra
OTW	NC Cobra	3.0/2.7	0.030	0.032	0.033	0.037	0.040	0.045	135	Xtra
OTW	NC Cobra-18	3.2/2.9	NA	0.032	0.035	0.035	0.040	0.043	135	Xtra
OTW	NC Cobra-18	3.2/2.9	NA	0.031	0.034	0.035	0.038	0.042	135	Xtra
OTW	NC Shadow	3.6/2.7	NA	0.031	0.032	0.036	0.040	0.042	135	Xtra
OTW	SC Shadow	2.7/3.6	NA	0.032	0.034	0.038	0.038	0.042	135	Xtra
OTW	Shadow	3.6/2.7	0.030	0.031	0.033	0.037	0.039	0.042	135	Xtra
OTW	Skinny	3.5/3.0	0.028	0.031	0.033	0.037	0.040	0.042	135	Xtra
OTW	Skinny Long	3.5/3.0	NA	0.031	0.034	0.038	0.040	0.044	135	Xtra
OTW	Striker	3.0/2.7	0.030	0.031	0.033	0.037	0.040	0.042	135	Xtra
OTW	Trio 14	2.6/2.0	0.030	0.031	0.033	0.037	0.039	0.042	135	Xtra
OTW	ACE 1 cm	1.8/1.8	0.020	0.022	0.030	0.032	0.036	NA	135	Bioslide
Fixed Wire	ACE 2 cm	1.8/1.8	0.020	0.022	0.030	0.032	0.036	NA	135	Xtra
Fixed Wire	ACE 2 cm Flex	1.8/1.8	0.020	0.022	0.030	0.032	0.036	NA	135	Xtra

Published Balloon Profiles

Type	Catheter Name	Shaft+ (F)	1.5	2.0	2.5	3.0	3.5	4.0	Usable Length (cm)	Coating
Fixed Wire	ACE Graft	1.8/1.8	0.020	0.022	0.030	0.032	0.036	NA	135	Xtra
Fixed Wire	ACE Long	1.8/1.8	0.022	0.024	0.032	0.035	0.039	NA	135	Xtra
Fixed Wire	Pivot	1.8/1.8	0.020	0.024	0.028	0.033	0.036	NA	135	Xtra
Fixed Wire	Express Plus-II	2.3/1.8	0.031	0.032	0.034	0.037	0.040	0.013	135	Bioslide
SOE	Express Plus-Leap	2.3/1.8	0.027	0.027	0.028	0.031	0.032	0.035	135	Bioslide
SOE	Express Plus-Leap	2.3/1.8	0.027	0.027	0.028	0.031	0.032	0.035	135	Bioslide
SOE	Express Plus-Leap	2.3/1.8	0.027	0.027	0.028	0.031	0.032	0.035	135	Bioslide
SOE	NC-Express Plus	2.3/1.8	NA	0.034	0.036	0.040	0.042	0.047	135	Bioslide
Rx-OTW	Synergy 14	2.9/2.9	Discontinued in August, 1996						135	Bioslide
Rx-OTW	Synergy 14-long	3.4/3.4	Discontinued in August, 1996						135	Hydroplus
Rx-OTW	Synergy 14-long	3.4/3.4	Discontinued in August, 1996						135	Hydroplus
Rx-OTW	Synergy 18	2.9/2.9	Discontinued in August, 1996						135	Hydroplus
Rx-OTW	Synergy 18-long	3.4/3.4	Discontinued in August, 1996						135	Hydroplus
Rx-OTW	Synergy 18-long	3.4/3.4	Discontinued in August, 1996						135	Hydroplus
CORDIS										
OTW	Olympix	3.5/3.0	NA	0.030	0.031	0.031	0.033	0.035	135	SLX
OTW	Olympix Long	3.5/3.0	NA	0.030	0.031	0.031	0.033	0.035	135	SLX
OTW	Olympix Long	3.5/3.0	NA	0.030	0.031	0.031	0.033	0.035	135	SLX
OTW	Olympix-II	3.5/3.0	NA	0.032	0.033	0.033	0.035	0.035	135,150	SLX
OTW	Olympix-II Long	3.5/3.0	NA	0.032	0.033	0.033	0.035	0.035	135,150	SLX
OTW	Olympix-II Long	3.5/3.0	NA	0.032	0.033	0.033	0.035	0.035	135,150	SLX
OTW	Predator	3.0/2.5	0.026	0.026	0.026	0.027	0.030	NA	135,150	SLX
OTW	Predator-Long	3.0/2.5	0.026	0.026	0.026	0.027	0.030	NA	135,150	SLX
OTW	Predator-Long	3.0/2.5	0.026	0.026	0.026	0.027	0.030	NA	135,150	SLX
OTW	Sleek	3.2/2.5	0.025	0.027	0.028	0.030	0.031	NA	135	SLX
OTW	Sleek Long	3.2/2.5	0.025	0.027	0.028	0.030	0.031	NA	135	SLX
OTW	Sleek Long	3.2/2.5	0.025	0.027	0.028	0.030	0.031	NA	135	SLX
OTW	Titan-18	3.9/3.3	NA	NA	NA	0.039	0.041	0.044	135	SLX
OTW	Titan-18	3.9/3.3	NA	NA	NA	0.039	0.041	0.044	135	SLX
OTW	Trakstar-14	3.2/2.5	0.029	0.029	0.029	0.031	0.032	0.032	135	SLX
OTW	Trakstar-14 Long	3.2/2.5	0.029	0.029	0.029	0.031	0.032	0.032	135	SLX

Table 1.15. Coronary Angioplasty Balloon Catheters: Technical Features

Type	Catheter Name	Shaft+ (F)	Published Balloon Profiles						Usable Length (cm)	Coating
			1.5	2.0	2.5	3.0	3.5	4.0		
OTW	Trakstar-14 Long	3.2/2.5	0.029	0.029	0.029	0.031	0.032	0.032	135	SLX
OTW	Trakstar-18	3.5/3.0	NA	0.033	0.034	0.035	0.036	0.037	135	SLX
OTW	Trakstar-14 Long	3.2/2.5	0.029	0.029	0.029	0.031	0.032	0.032	135	SLX
OTW	Trakstar-14Long	3.2/2.5	0.029	0.029	0.029	0.031	0.032	0.032	135	SLX
OTW	Trakstar-18	3.5/3.0	NA	0.033	0.034	0.035	0.036	0.037	135	SLX
OTW	Trakstar-18 Long	3.5/3.0	NA	0.033	0.034	0.035	0.036	0.037	135	SLX
OTW	Trakstar-18 Long	3.5/3.0	NA	0.033	0.034	0.035	0.036	0.037	135	SLX
SOE	Europass	3.0/2.5	0.026	0.026	0.026	0.027	0.030	NA	135	SLX
SOE	Europass-Long	3.0/2.5	0.026	0.026	0.026	0.027	0.030	NA	135	SLX
SOE	Europass-Long	3.0/2.5	0.026	0.026	0.026	0.027	0.030	NA	135	SLX
SOE	Passage	2.6/2.6	0.025	0.026	0.027	0.030	0.031	0.031	135	SLX
SOE	Passage-Long	2.6/2.6	0.025	0.026	0.027	0.030	0.031	0.031	135	SLX
SOE	Passage Long	2.6/2.6	0.025	0.026	0.027	0.030	0.031	0.031	135	SLX
Fixed Wire	Lightning	2.4/1.5	NA	0.024	0.027	0.030	0.032	NA	135	SLX
Fixed Wire	Orion	2.4/1.6	NA	0.024	0.028	0.030	0.032	NA	135	SLX
					USCI					
OTW	Agil	3.2/2.9	NA	0.029	0.030	0.031	0.034	0.037	135	Propel
OTW	Force	3.5/3.5	NA	0.031	0.033	0.034	0.036	0.036	135	Propel
OTW	Force-Long	3.5/3.5	NA	NA	0.033	0.035	0.036	NA	135	Propel
OTW	Force-Long	3.5/3.5	NA	0.032	0.033	0.035	0.036	0.037	135	Propel
OTW	Solo	3.0/3.0	0.027	0.028	0.030	0.032	0.034	0.036	135	Propel
OTW	Sprint	3.5/3.5	NA	0.032	0.033	0.034	0.036	0.036	135	Propel
OTW	Tapered	3.5/3.5	NA	NA	NA	0.033	0.034	0.036	135	Propel
OTW	XPRT	3.0/3.0	0.022	0.024	0.026	0.029	0.032	0.033	135	Propel
Fixed Wire	Probe III	1.7/1.7	NA	0.019	0.021	0.026	NA	NA	135	None
					ACS					
OTW	Edge	3.5/2.9	0.029	0.029	0.030	0.032	0.035	0.035	135	Microglide
OTW	Edge-Long	3.5/2.9	NA	0.029	0.030	0.032	0.035	0.035	135	Microglide
OTW	Edge-Long	3.5/2.9	NA	0.029	0.030	0.032	0.035	0.035	135	Microglide
OTW	Omega	2.9/2.9	0.024	0.026	0.027	0.028	0.030	0.033	135	Microglide

Published Balloon Profiles

Type	Catheter Name	Shaft+ (F)	1.5	2.0	2.5	3.0	3.5	4.0	Usable Length (cm)	Coating
OTW	Pinkerton	3.5/3.6	0.034	0.035	0.037	0.039	0.040	0.042	135	Microglide
OTW	Pinkerton	3.5/3.5	NA	0.035	0.037	0.039	0.040	0.042	135	Microglide
OTW	Pinkerton Long	3.5/3.5	NA	0.035	0.037	0.039	0.040	0.042	135	Microglide
OTW	Pinkerton Long	3.9/3.9	NA	0.035	0.037	0.039	0.040	0.042	135	Microglide
OTW	Prism	3.3/3.3	0.029	0.031	0.032	0.034	0.035	0.037	135	Microglide
OTW	Prism	3.3/3.3	NA	0.031	0.032	0.034	0.035	0.037	135	Microglide
OTW	Prism	3.3/3.3	NA	0.031	0.032	0.034	0.035	0.037	135	Microglide
OTW	Prism Long	3.3/3.3	NA	0.031	0.032	0.034	0.035	0.037	135	Microglide
OTW	Prism Long	3.3/3.3	NA	0.031	0.032	0.034	0.035	0.037	135	Microglide
Fixed Wire	Slalom	2.5/1.9	NA	0.023	0.025	0.029	NA	NA	135	Microglide
SOE	RX Elipse	2.3/2.4/3.0	0.028	0.030	0.031	0.033	0.033	0.035	135	Microglide
SOE	RX Streak	2.3/3.3	0.029	0.030	0.031	0.033	0.034	0.035	135	Microglide
SOE	RX-Elipse Long	2.3/2.4/3.0	0.028	0.030	0.032	0.033	0.033	NA	135	Microglide
SOE	RX-Streak Long	2.3/3.3	NA	0.030	0.031	0.033	0.034	0.035	135	Microglide
SOE	RX-Streak Long	2.3/3.3	NA	0.030	0.031	0.033	0.034	0.035	135	Microglide
Perfusion	RX-Flow Track 40 (40)	2.3/3.5	NA	0.048	0.049	0.050	0.051	0.052	135	Microglide
Perfusion	RX Lifestream (40)	2.3/3.3/3.5	NA	0.041	0.041	0.042	0.043	0.044	135	Microglide
Perfusion	OTW Lifestream (40)	3.5/3.3	NA	0.041	0.041	0.042	0.043	0.044	135	Microglide
Perfusion	RX Perfusion (60)	3.7/4.2	NA	0.053	0.054	0.055	0.056	0.059	135	Microglide
Perfusion	RX Perfusion Long (55)	3.7/4.2	NA	0.053	0.054	0.055	0.056	0.059	135	Microglide
Perfusion	RX Perfusion Long (50)	3.7/4.2	NA	0.053	0.054	0.055	0.056	NA	135	Microglide
Perfusion	Stack Perfusion (60)	3.9/4.5	NA	0.056	0.057	0.058	0.060	0.062	135	Microglide
Perfusion	Stack Perfusion (60)	3.9/4.5	NA	NA	0.057	0.058	0.059	0.062	135	Microglide
MEDTRONIC										
OTW	14 K	2.9/2.9	0.026	0.030	0.033	0.036	0.041	0.043	135	Enhance
OTW	14K-Long	3.1/3.1	0.025	0.028	0.032	0.034	0.036	0.040	135	Enhance
OTW	18 K	3.5/3.5	NA	0.035	0.038	0.042	0.048	NA	135	Enhance
OTW	19K-Short	3.5/3.5	NA	NA	NA	0.042	0.048	NA	135	Enhance
OTW	Evergreen	2.9/2.9	0.022	0.024	0.025	0.026	0.027	0.033	135	Enhance
OTW	Evergreen	2.9/2.9	0.021	0.023	0.025	0.028	0.029	0.032	135	Enhance
OTW	Evergreen	2.9/2.9	NA	0.024	0.025	0.028	0.029	0.032	135	Enhance

Table 1.15. Coronary Angioplasty Balloon Catheters: Technical Features

Type	Catheter Name	Shaft+ (F)	Published Balloon Profiles						Usable Length (cm)	Coating
			1.5	2.0	2.5	3.0	3.5	4.0		
OTW	Panther	2.9/2.6	0.025	0.027	0.032	0.034	0.037	0.039	135	Enhance
OTW	Panther	3.1/2.9	NA	0.027	0.031	0.034	0.037	0.041	135	Enhance
OTW	Panther	3.0/2.6	0.025	0.026	0.030	0.034	0.037	0.039	135	Enhance
OTW	Spirit	3.2/2.9	0.028	0.030	0.033	0.037	0.039	0.043	135	Enhance
OTW	Spirit	3.2/2.9	NA	0.030	0.033	0.037	0.040	0.041	135	Enhance
OTW	Spirit	3.2/2.9	NA	0.029	0.034	0.038	0.040	0.043	135	Enhance
SOE	Falcon	1.8/2.2/3.0	NA	0.025	0.028	0.031	0.034	0.037	135	Enhance
					SCHNEIDER						
OTW	Asuka	3.0/2.9	0.027	0.028	0.029	0.031	0.033	0.037	135	Expresscoat
OTW	Asuka-Long	3.0/2.9	NA	NA	0.035	0.037	0.040	NA	135	Expresscoat
OTW	Asuka-Long	3.0/2.9	NA	NA	0.035	0.037	0.040	NA	135	Expresscoat
OTW	Freeflight	3.3/2.9	0.024	0.026	0.028	0.031	0.036	0.039	135	Expresscoat
OTW	Freeflight-Long	3.3/2.9	NA	0.027	0.029	0.032	0.037	0.039	135	Expresscoat
OTW	Freeflight-Long	3.3/2.9	NA	0.026	0.029	0.032	0.037	0.039	135	Expresscoat
OTW	Magnum Meier	4.3/4.3	NA	0.038	0.039	0.040	0.041	0.042	135	Expresscoat
OTW	Mystic MC	2.9/2.9	0.026	0.027	0.030	0.030	0.033	0.034	135	Expresscoat
OTW	Mystic MC Long	3.1/2.9	NA	0.027	0.030	0.030	0.033	0.034	135	Expresscoat
OTW	Mystic MC Long	3.3/2.9	NA	0.027	0.030	0.030	0.033	0.034	135	Expresscoat
OTW	Takumi	2.8/2.7	0.027	0.027	0.029	0.029	0.033	0.035	135	Expresscoat
SOE	Bypass Speedy**	2.8/2.9	NA	0.032	0.033	0.036	0.035	0.040	160	Expresscoat
SOE	Chubby*	3.0/2.9	NA	NA	NA	0.036	0.037	0.039	135	Expresscoat
SOE	Forte 30	3.2/3.0	NA	NA	0.034	0.037	0.038	0.039	135	Expresscoat
SOE	Freehand	3.2/2.9	0.024	0.026	0.028	0.031	0.036	0.039	145	Expresscoat
SOE	Freehand-Long	3.2/2.9	NA	0.027	0.029	0.032	0.037	0.039	145	Expresscoat
SOE	Freehand-Long	3.2/2.9	NA	0.027	0.029	0.032	0.037	0.039	145	Expresscoat
SOE	Goldie	2.4/2.9	0.025	0.025	0.026	0.026	0.028	NA	135	Expresscoat
SOE	Goldie-Long	2.4/2.9	NA	NA	0.030	0.030	0.032	NA	135	Expresscoat
SOE	Goldie-Long	2.4/2.9	NA	NA	0.030	0.030	0.032	NA	135	Expresscoat
SOE	Magna Rail	3.3/3.8	NA	0.034	0.036	0.037	0.041	0.042	135	Expresscoat
SOE	McRail	2.9/2.9	0.026	0.027	0.031	0.031	0.033	0.034	135	Expresscoat
SOE	McRail-Long	2.9/2.9	NA	0.027	0.030	0.031	0.033	0.033	135	Expresscoat

Published Balloon Profiles

Type	Catheter Name	Shaft[+] (F)	1.5	2.0	2.5	3.0	3.5	4.0	Usable Length (cm)	Coating
SOE	RcRail-Long	2.9/2.9	NA	0.027	0.030	0.030	0.033	0.033	135	Expresscoat
SOE	Mongoose	3.2/3.1	0.027	0.029	0.029	0.032	0.034	0.038	135	Expresscoat
SOE	Shortgoose	3.2/3.1	NA	NA	NA	0.033	0.035	0.038	135	Expresscoat
SOE	Shortgoose	3.2/3.1	NA	NA	NA	0.032	0.036	0.036	135	Expresscoat
Perfusion	RX Speedflow Junior	2.4/2.4	NA	NA	0.050	0.050	0.052	0.054	135	Expresscoat
Perfusion	RX Speedflow Junior	2.4/2.4	NA	NA	0.050	0.050	0.052	0.054	135	Expresscoat
Perfusion	RX Speedflow Junior	2.4/2.4	NA	NA	0.050	0.050	0.052	0.054	135	Expresscoat

Abbreviations: F = French size; OTW = over-the-wire; SOE = single operator exchange; RX-OTW = rapid exchange/over-the-wire (hybrid); SLX = silicone; NA = not available by manufacturer

*   Available 3.0-5.0 mm

** Available in 2.0-6.0 mm

+   proximal/distal shaft size

Table 1.23. Transport Catheters*

Name	Shaft (F)+ Prox/Dist	ID (inch)	Length (cm)	Max GW (inch)	Tip Marker	Coating	Comments
ACS							
Coronary Infusion Catheter	2.5/2.5	0.0/21	130	0.018	Yes	None	End-hole only
BAXTER							
Relay	4.1/3.1	0.021	282	0.018	Yes	None	Facilitates guiding catheter exchanges; partial monorail design
COOK							
Infusion Catheter	3.0/3.0	0.025	135,150	0.021	Yes	None	
CORDIS							
Infusion Catheter	2.5/2.5	0.021	125	0.018	No	None	Polyethylene catheter
Transit Infusion Catheter	3.0/2.5	0.021	70,85,100, 135,150,170	0.018	Yes	Hydrophilic	Proximal braided shaft; luer-lock hub radio-opaque distal shaft (platinum coil)
Rapid Transit	3.0/2.3	0.021	70,100,150, 170	0.018	Yes	Hydrophilic	Radio-opaque distal shaft
MEDITECH							
GlideCath	5.0/5.0	0.038	100	0.038	No	Hydrophilic	
Cragg FX	3.0/3.0	0.027	145,170	0.025	Yes	Hydrophilic	

Name	Shaft (F)+ Prox/Dist	ID (inch)	Length (cm)	Max GW (inch)	Tip Marker	Coating	Comments
Buchbinder	2.0/3.0	0.016	90,130,150	0.014	Yes	Enhance	Coaxial construction, Coil shaft
Buchbinder	3.7/3.7	0.021	90,130,150	0.018	Yes	Enhance	Coaxial constructing, Coil shaft; available in tip lengths of 5mm or 25mm
SCHNEIDER							
Guidewire Exchange Catheter	4.2/4.2	0.020	144	0.018	Yes	Expresscoat	Dual lumen, peel-away, rapid exchange
SCIMED							
Ultrafuse-X	3.6/2.9	NA	135	0.018	Yes	Bioslide	Separate guidewire & infusion lumen; coaxial dual lumen
TARGET							
Fast Tracker	3.0/2.5	0.021	135,150	0.018	Yes	Hydrolene	Variable shaft stiffness
USCI							
Probing Catheter	4.0/4.0	0.023	125	0.021	Yes	None	

Abbreviations: F = French size; ID = internal diameter; Max GW = maximum guidewire; NA = not applicable; PTFE = teflon

* can also be used for drug infusion, but without sideholes (See Table 1.20)

+ shaft diameter (proximal/distal)

Table 1.24. Infusion Catheters

Name	Shaft (F)+ Prox/Dist	ID++ (inch)	Length (cm)	Max GW (inch)	Tip Marker	Distal Lumen	Comments
ACS							
Coronary Infusion Catheter	4.4/3.0	0.041/0.028	135	0.018	No	Open	36 sideholes
COOK							
Roubin Infusion Catheter	4.0/2.5	0.027/0.027	135,150	0.018	Yes	Open	4,6, or 8 cm long infusion segment; end-hole only also available
CORDIS							
Transit with sideholes	3.0/2.5	0.021/0.021	135,150,175	0.018	Yes	Open	3,6, or 12 sideholes; infusion length = 3,6,12 cm
Infusion Wire	2.6/2.6	0.024/0.024	150	0.035	Yes	Open	Removable luer-lock hub; removable stylet; platinum coil
Infusion Wire	2.9/2.9	0.027/0.027	150	0.038	Yes	Open	Removable luer-lock hub; removable stylet; platinum coil
MEDITECH							
Katzen Infusion Wire	3.0/3.0	0.035/0.035	145	0.035	No	Closed	Multiple sideholes; infusion length = 3,6,9,12 cm
Cragg Convertible Wire	3.0/3.0	0.037/0.037	145,170	0.025	Yes	Open	Polyimide sleeve with PTFE jacket
SCIMED							
Ultrafuse-4	3.6/2.9	NA/NA	140	0.018	Yes	Closed	Co-axial dual lumen; infusion length = 4 cm

Name	Shaft (F)+ Prox/Dist	ID++ (inch)	Length (cm)	Max GW (inch)	Tip Marker	Distal Lumen	Comments
TARGET							
Tracker (Softstream)	3.5/3.0	0.023/0.021	135,150	0.018	Yes	Open	Variable shaft stiffness
USCI							
Dorros Infusion Catheter	3.0/3.0	0.023/0.023	125	0.021	Yes	Open	

Abbreviations: F = French size; ID = internal diameter; Max GW = maximum guidewire; NA = not applicable; PTFE = teflon

* can also be used for drug infusion/but without sideholes (See Table 1.20)
+ shaft diameter (proximal/distal)
++ internal diameter (proximal/distal)

See Table 1.19 for transport catheters, which can also be used for infusion

2 BRACHIAL AND RADIAL APPROACH TO CORONARY INTERVENTION

Steven J. Yakubov, M.D.
Barry S. George, M.D.

Percutaneous revascularization via the brachial approach is often useful when the femoral approach is undesirable or impossible. Although similar to the femoral technique,[1-3] brachial cutdown requires considerable expertise not routinely obtained in most training programs. More recently, radial artery cannulation has been introduced for diagnostic and interventional catheterization. It shares many similarities with the femoral approach, but unlike the brachial approach, does not require cutdown techniques. Successful mastery of these alternative approaches greatly increase the range of options available to the interventionalist, and in selected cases, many increase the comfort, safety and/or efficacy of catheter-based intervention.

A. **PROCEDURAL OVERVIEW.** The selection of the access site is mostly determined by operator preference, although there are advantages and disadvantages to each technique (Table 2.1).[4] Overall, less than 3% of angioplasty procedures are performed via the brachial or radial route. However, given the important role of potent new antithrombin and antiplatelet agents, which increase the risk of bleeding complications, it is possible that brachial and radial techniques may become more widely used.

Table 2.1. Comparison of Femoral, Brachial, and Radial Catheterization for Coronary Intervention

	Femoral	Brachial	Radial
Physician Factors			
Training	Common	Uncommon	Virtually none
Experience	Extensive	Minimal	Rare
Catheter Manipulation	Easy	More difficult	More difficult
Radiation Exposure	Less	More	More
Superselective intubations	Difficult	Easy	Difficult
Complications			
Bleeding	More common	Less common	Less common
Loss of pulse	Less common	More common	More common
Transfusion	More common	Less common	Less common
Surgical repair	Uncommon	Uncommon	Uncommon
Technical Factors			
Percutaneous	Yes	Yes	Yes
Cut-down/Repair	No	Yes	No
Repeated access	Yes	Limited	Unknown
Bedrest > 8 hours	Common	Not necessary	Not necessary

1. **Cutdown Approach to Brachial Artery Access (Figure 2.1)**
    a. **Technique.** A variety of techniques have been used for brachial artery access.[3,5,6] Regardless of the approach, strict sterile technique (cap, gown, mask) is essential to limit infection. We have found the following technique to be simple and reliable:

    •   Sterilize the antecubital fossa with a povidone-iodine solution

    •   Anesthetize the area just above the elbow crease over the brachial pulse with a subdermal injection of 2% lidocaine (10-20cc).

    •   Make a horizontal incision (0.75 to 1.5 inches) over the brachial artery. If a previous cutdown has been performed within the last 5 days, the same site can be reopened; if the previous cutdown site is > 5 days old, make a new skin incision 1-1.5" above or below the previous site.

    •   Use a Wheatlaner retractor and curved hemostat to carefully perform blunt dissection and isolate the brachial artery.

    •   Identify the artery just below the bicipital aponeurosis and carefully separate other soft tissue from the artery. Extreme care should be taken to avoid the median nerve.

    •   Retract a 1-inch segment of brachial artery to the skin surface using curved or right-angle hemostats.

    •   Place cotton umbilical tapes under the artery proximally and distally for hemostatic control.

    •   With traction on the proximal tape, inject 3000 - 5000 units of dilute heparin (500 units/ml saline) into the distal brachial artery using a 22-gauge needle (or a 22-gauge angiocath after the arteriotomy is created).

    •   Create a vertical arteriotomy (3-4 mm) using a No. 11 blade. Use of a 6-8F arterial sheath and a 0.035" guidewire permits easy exchange of guiding catheters for PTCA, stent implantation, and other interventional devices.

    b. **Brachial Artery Repair (Figure 2.1)**
    •   Maintain traction on the proximal and distal umbilical tapes while removing the sheath; traction may be released slightly to ensure flow in antegrade and retrograde directions.

    •   Repair the brachial artery arteriotomy with 6-0 or 7-0 prolene using interrupted sutures placed ~ 1-2 mm apart. Meticulous attention to suture technique is necessary to achieve complete hemostasis; subdermal oozing may be managed with gentle pressure, electrocautery, topical thrombin or Gelfoam.

- Close the skin with interrupted silk sutures or an absorbable subcuticular repair.

- Gentle pressure over the arteriotomy may be necessary if oozing persists despite adequate arterial repair.

- If an adequate radial artery pulse is not obtained, consider revision of the arteriotomy ± Fogarty catheter embolectomy; liquid hematoma is manually "milked" from the antecubital fossa at this time to decrease the risk of brachial artery and/or median nerve compression.

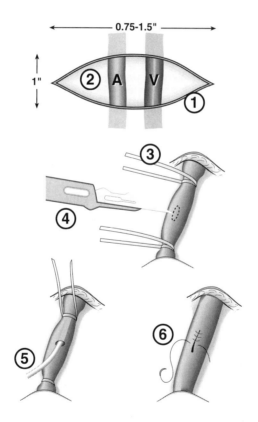

Figure 2.1   Brachial Artery Access: Cutdown Technique

1.   Horizontal incision 1 cm above antecubital crease.
2.   Blunt dissection to expose brachial artery (A) and vein (V).
3.   Tag the artery with umbilical tape; the vein with 3-0 silk.
4.   With traction on proximal tape, create arteriotomy
5.   Insert vascular sheath and catheter.
6.   Repair brachial artery with 6-0 prolene (interrupted sutures).

2. **Percutaneous Approach to Brachial Artery Access (Figure 2.2).** Local sterilization and anesthesia are identical to the cutdown technique. After careful palpation of the brachial pulse, a modified Seldinger or micropuncture technique is used to cannulate the brachial artery. Usually, a 6-8F sheath can be inserted without difficulty. It is sometimes possible to insert a 10F sheath, especially in large patients with large brachial arteries, but is considerably less likely in smaller patients and those with peripheral vascular disease or diabetes.

3. **Radial Artery Approach (Figure 2.2).** Modifications in technique continue to evolve, but the following technique is commonly employed:

   a. **Technique:**
   - Perform the Allen Test by simultaneously compressing both the radial and ulnar artery of the same hand for 30-60 seconds, followed by release of the ulnar artery. The test is considered normal (i.e., a good dual blood supply to the palm is present) when hand color returns to normal within 10 sec. after release of the ulnar artery. Although either radial artery way be used, access via the left radial artery is preferred because of better engagement of the coronary ostia.

   - Abduct the arm to about 70° and hyperextend the wrist.

   - Sterilize and anesthetize the area locally with povidone-iodine solution and a subdermal injection of 2% lidocaine.

   - Puncture the radial artery with an 18- or 22-gauge needle (micropuncture kit) at a 30-45° angle approximately 1 cm from the styloid process.

   - Once pulsatile blood return is confirmed, advance a 0.025" guidewire into the brachial artery.

   - Predilate the radial artery with a 4 or 5F dilator followed by insertion of a 6F introducing sheath over a 0.035' J-guidewire. A 23-cm sheath may be preferable to a 10-cm sheath to prevent radial artery spasm and facilitate movement of guiding catheters; intra-arterial nitroglycerin (100-200 mcg delivered through the sidearm of the sheath) may also minimize spasm. Special attention should be directed toward selection of guiding catheters to ensure coaxial alignment and adequate backup support: Amplatz and Voda curves for the left coronary artery and Amplatz and multipurpose curves for the right coronary artery may be preferred.

   b. **Sheath Removal and Hemostasis**
   - The arterial sheath can be immediately removed upon completion of most cases.

- Apply a specially-made tourniquet at the radial puncture site for at least 30 minutes; gradually release pressure until hemostasis is achieved. If this special tourniquet is not available, manual compression is adequate.

- Apply a pressure bandage and instruct the patient to restrict wrist movement for 6 hours.

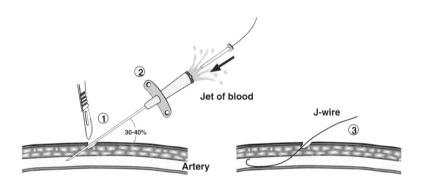

Figure 2.2   Arterial Access: Percutaneous Technique

1. Create a skin-nick inferior to the arterial pulsation.
2. Use single wall puncture to enter vessel lumen.
3. After brisk blood return is achieved, insert J-wire and sheath.

B. SPECIAL INDICATIONS FOR BRACHIAL AND RADIAL TECHNIQUES

1. **Peripheral Vascular Disease.** Femoral artery access may be difficult (morbid obesity, extensive post-operative scarring, severe peripheral vascular disease), impossible (aortic occlusion), or relatively contraindicated (coagulopathy). For these patients, the brachial cutdown technique allows an alternative approach for coronary angiography, peripheral aortography, and angioplasty. We perform all diagnostic lower extremity angiography through the brachial approach — selective iliac and renal angiography is easier and requires less contrast.

2. **Patient Preference.** Brachial and radial artery angioplasty allow immediate ambulation; this may be important in selected patients, including those with severe lumbosacral pain aggravated by prolonged bed rest.

3. **Need for Uninterrupted Anticoagulation.** Brachial artery repair allows continuous anticoagulation (with heparin or warfarin) and may be useful in decreasing length of stay in stent patients.

4. **Difficult Internal Mammary Artery Cannulation.** In some cases, selective angiography of an internal mammary artery conduit cannot be accomplished via the femoral route because of severe tortuosity of the subclavian or brachiocephalic arteries. However, selective angiography (and intervention, if necessary) can usually be performed by the ipsilateral (right Judkins or internal mammary artery catheter) or contralateral brachial artery (Simmons catheter).

5. **Severe Coronary Artery Tortuosity.** Compared to the femoral approach, the left brachial approach can more readily achieve deep guiding catheter intubation of the target vessel. This may be particularly useful when severe tortuosity of the target vessel precludes advancement of interventional hardware from the femoral approach.

C. INTERVENTIONAL CONSIDERATIONS

   1. **Guide Catheter Selection (Table 2.2)**

Table 2.2. Preferred Guiding Catheters from the Brachial Approach

Target Vessel	Preferred Guide(s)
Right Coronary Artery Right or left brachial approach	Right Judkins (especially good fit from left brachial approach) Amplatz (may have greater difficulty navigating the subclavian artery and aortic arch) Multipurpose

Left Coronary Artery*
    Right brachial approach
    Left brachial approach
	Amplatz (excellent support and maneuverability)
	Left Judkins (first choice)
	Amplatz
	Voda

Saphenous Vein Grafts Right or left brachial approach	Amplatz Multipurpose

Internal Mammary Grafts
    Ipsilateral
 	
    Contralateral
	Internal mammary (first choice)
	Right Judkins
	Simmons, Castillo

* Due to the orientation of the left subclavian artery and aortic arch, the left guide catheter should be 0.5F smaller than the typical corresponding femoral guide.

   2. **New Devices.** New device angioplasty (rotational atherectomy, directional atherectomy, and stents) can be safely and easily performed via the brachial technique, as long as the appropriate sheath can be placed in the brachial artery and arterial repair is meticulous.[7] Elective PTCA or

intracoronary stenting via the brachial approach or radial approach is particularly appealing because it can decrease length of stay, allow uninterrupted full-dose anticoagulation, minimize bed rest and immobility, and decrease the incidence of bleeding and vascular complications.[8,9,9a,9b,9c] Although insertion of an IABP via the brachial artery is feasible, it may predispose the patient to infection and vascular injury, since the catheters must remain in place for several days.

D. COMPLICATIONS

1. **Brachial Approach.** In general, the incidence of peripheral vascular complications associated with brachial cutdown and percutaneous femoral techniques are similar, including significant hematoma (1.3%), retroperitoneal hemorrhage (0.4%), false aneurysm (0.4%), vessel occlusion (0.1%), infection (0.1%), and cholesterol embolization (0.1%).[10] However, femoral vascular complications are usually associated with greater patient morbidity.[8] Compiled data from the TAMI trials show comparable success rates using brachial and femoral access sites, but complication rates were slightly lower from the brachial site.[11-14]

2. **Radial Approach.** In a study 1300 coronary interventions from the radial approach, vascular access complications occurred in 1.1% (mainly forearm or arm hematomas); only 0.15% of patients required surgery and no blood transfusions were needed.[20] In a study of 100 patients treated with elective PTCA from the radial artery, there were no major cardiac complications, blood transfusions, or vascular surgical repairs.[15] Asymptomatic radial artery occlusion has been reported in 6-10%,[15-17] although ~ 40% appear to spontaneously recanalize after 1 month. In another study, however, the incidence of stroke was 2%.[16] The ACCESS study is a prospective randomized study of PTCA with 6F catheters using the transradial, transbrachial, and transfemoral approach (Table 2.3). Preliminary analysis of the first 450 patients revealed more access-site failures and fewer bleeding complications after transradial PTCA; PTCA success and cardiac events were similar using all 3 approaches.[18] Another prospective randomized study of transradial and transfemoral PTCA with 6F catheters revealed fewer vascular complications, shorter length of stay, and lower hospital charges with transradial PTCA (Table 2.4).[19]

Table 2.3. Randomized Comparison of Transradial, Transbrachial, and Transfemoral PTCA (ACCESS)[18]

	Transradial	Transbrachial	Transfemoral
No. patients	152	146	152
Failed access (%)	7.9	3.4	0*
Major bleeding (%)	0	4.1	1.3**
PTCA success (%)	93.4	95.1	96.0
Cardiac events (%)	7.2	6.4	4.7

* p ≤ 0.001 ** p = 0.03

Table 2.4. Randomized Study of Transradial and Transfemoral PTCA[19]

	Transradial	Transfemoral
No. patients	73	95
PTCA success (%)	95	97
Emergency CABG (%)	1	0
Vascular complications (%)	0	4*
Lenth of stay (days)	2.1	2.6*
Hospital charge ($)	14,374	15,796*

Abbreviations: CABG = coronary artery bypass surgery
* $p < 0.05$

＊ ＊ ＊ ＊ ＊

REFERENCES

1. Sones FM, Shirey EK: Cine coronary arteriography. Mod Conc. Cardiovasc Dis. 31:735, 1962.
2. Judkins MP: Selective coronary arteriography: A percutaneous transfemoral technique. Radiology 89:815-824, 1967.
3. Stertzer SH: Brachial approach to transluminal coronary angioplasty. In Angioplasty. New York, McGraw-Hill, 1986, pp 260-294.
4. Yakubov SJ, George, BS: Coronary Intervention: Brachial Technique. In interventional Cardiovascular Medicine: Principles and Practice. New York, Churchill-Livingston Co., 1994, pp 451-64.
5. Huepler F: Coronary arteriography and left ventriculography: Sones technique. In Coronary Arteriography and Angioplasty. Hew York, McGraw-Hill, 1985, pp 137-181.
6. Kamada RO, Fergusson DJ, Itagaki RK: Percutaneous entry of the brachial artery for transluminal coronary angioplasty. Cathet Cardiovasc Diagn 15:132-133, 1988.
7. George BS: Brachial Technique to Intervention. In Textbook of Interventional Cardiology. Vol. 2. Philadelphia, W.B. Saunders Company, 1994, pp 549-564.
8. Kiemeneij F, Laarman, GJ. Percutaneous transradial artery approach for coronary stent implantation. Cath Cardiovasc Diagn. 30:173-178, 1993.
9. Keimeneij F, Laarman GJ, Slagboom T, Stella P. Transradial Palmaz-Schatz coronary stenting on an outpatient basis: Results of a prospective pilot study. J Invas Cardiol 7:5A-11A, 1995.
9a. Barbeau GR, Carrier G, Ferland S, Larriviere MM. Transradial approach for coronary angiography, angioplasty and stent delivery: Procedural results. Circulation 1995;92:I-196.
9b. Kiemeneij F, Laarman GJ, Slagboom T, van der Wieken R. Transradial coronary stenting in outpatients. Circulation 1995;92:I-535.
9c. Vallabhan RC, Anwar A, Bret JR, et al. Radial artery access for cardiac catheterization and coronary angioplasty. Circulation 1995;92:I-602.
10. Johnson LW, Esenta P, Giambartolomei A, et al. Peripheral vascular complications of coronary angioplasty by the femoral and brachial techniques. Cath Cardiovasc Diagn. 1994;31"165-172.
11. George BS, Candela RJ, Topol EJ, et al. The brachial approach to emergency cardiac catheterization during thrombolytic therapy for acute myocardial infarction. Cathet Cardiovasc Diagn 20(4):221-226, 1990.
12. Topol EJ, Califf RM, George BS, et al. A randomized trial of immediate vs. delayed elective angioplasty after intravenous tissue plasminogen activator in acute myocardial infarction. N. Engl J Med 317:581-588, 1987.
13. Topol EJ Califf RM, George BS, et al. Coronary arterial thrombolysis with combined infusion of recombinant tissue-type plasminogen activator and urokinase in patients with acute myocardial infarction. Circulation 77:1100-1107, 1988.
14. Topol EJ, George BS, Kereiakes DJ, et al. A randomized controlled trial of intravenous tissue plasminogen activator and early intravenous heparin in acute myocardial infarction. Circulation 79:281-286, 1989.
15. Kiemeneij, F, Laarman GJ, de Melker E. Tranradial artery coronary angioplasty. AM Heart J 1995;129:1-7.
16. Lotan C, Hasin Y, Mosseri M, Rozenman Y, et al. Transradial approach to coronary angiography and angioplasty. Am J Cardiol 76:164-167, 1995.
17. Stella P, Kiemeneij F, Laarman G, et al. Incidence and outcome of radial artery occlusion following transradial artery coronary angioplasty. Circulation 1995;92:I-225.
18. Kiemeneij F, Laarman GJ, Odekerken D, et al. Interim analysis of the ACCESS-study: A randomized comparison of transradial,-brachial and -femoral coronary angioplasty with 6-French guiding catheters. Circulation 1995;92:I-476.
19. Cubeddu MG, Arrowood ME, Mann JT. Right radial access for PTCA: A prospective study demonstrates reduced complications and hospital charges. Circulation 1995;92:I-662.
20. Fajadet J, Brunel P, Cassagneau B, et al. Transradial approach fo interventional cardiology procedures: analysis of complications. J Am Coll Cardiol 1996;March Special Issue.

3 SINGLE-VESSEL & MULTIVESSEL ANGIOPLASTY

Mark Freed, M.D.
William O'Neill, M.D.
Robert D. Safian, M.D.

SINGLE-VESSEL ANGIOPLASTY

Patients with single-vessel CAD have excellent longterm survival (mortality ~ 1% per year), but may have persistent angina, decreased functional capacity and employment status, the need for longterm medical therapy, and impaired psychological well-being. Observational and randomized studies (Table 3.1) have shed insight into relative merits of medical therapy, percutaneous revascularization, and bypass surgery (Table 3.2); decisions to triage patients are based on symptomatic status and the amount of jeopardized myocardium (Figure 3.1). The management of left main disease is discussed in Chapter 4, "High-Risk Intervention."

MULTIVESSEL ANGIOPLASTY

A. MULTIVESSEL ANGIOPLASTY IN PATIENTS WITH PRESERVED LV FUNCTION

1. **Randomized Trials.** To determine the optimal revascularization technique for patients with multivessel coronary disease, more than 4000 patients have been randomized in six PTCA vs. CABG trials (Table 3.3).

   a. **Inclusion and Exclusion Criteria (Table 3.3).** Specific entry criteria differ between each trial; most excluded patients with previous PTCA or CABG, evolving MI, left main disease, or severe non-cardiac illness. *Importantly, less than 10% of patients with symptomatic multivessel coronary disease were actually enrolled into these trials.*

   b. **Study Design and Baseline Characteristics (Tables 3.4, 3.5).** PTCA was generally confined to diameter stenoses > 50% in vessels > 1.5 mm in diameter supplying viable myocardium and causing ischemia (i.e., complete "functional" revascularization); lesions in small vessels and those supplying nonviable myocardium were generally not dilated. New device intervention was permitted only in CABRI (atherectomy and stents) and BARI (bailout stents). Internal mammary arteries were used in > 75% of CABGs but only 37% in GABI. *Importantly, most patients enrolled into these trials had 2-vessel disease and well-preserved LV function.*

Table 3.1. Treatment of Single-Vessel Disease: Acute & Longterm Outcomes

Series	Modality	N	Success(%)	In-hospital (%) D / QMI / CABG	Follow-up (%) Years	D / MI / TLR	Other ***
RITA[1] (1995)*	PTCA	456 overall	-	-	4.7	3.8 / 5.1 / 40.5	Angina at 3 yrs (17.5% vs 16.1%)
	CABG			-		3.8 / 10.8 / 9.5	
Goy[2] (1994)*	PTCA + devices	68	94	0 / 0 / 3	2.5	0++ / 11.8 / 25.7	Class 0-1+ angina (94% vs. 95%); exercise duration similar; ≥ 1 antianginal med (85% vs 43%)
	CABG-IMA	66**		1 / 0 / -		1.5++/ 3 / 3	
Mark[3] (1994)	Medicine	2919	-	-	5	6 / - / -	
	PTCA	1693		-		5 / - / -	
	CABG	339		-		7 / - / -	
Cameron[4] (1994)	PTCA	254	93	- / 3 / 3		3 / 8 / 33	Class 0-1 angina (81% vs. 90%); hospital stay (3 vs. 8.7 days)
	CABG	104		1 / - / -	5.5	7 / 2 / 1	
ACME[5,6] (1992)*	Medicine	107	-	-		1 / 3 / 1	Class 0 angina (46% vs. 63%); ↑ in exercise duration (0.5 vs. 2.1 min)
	PTCA	105	82	0 / 1 / 2	0.5	0 / 5 / 23	
	Medicine					11 / 7 / 38	Unstable angina (27% vs. 7%)
	PTCA				4+++	10 / 8 / 14	
Frierson[7] (1992)	PTCA	537	96	0.4 / 0.9 / 3	4.6	5.2 / 2.5 / 19	Asymptomatic 76%
	PTCA	295	80	-	2.9	6 / 7 / 36	Asymptomatic 74%
Henderson[8] (1991)							

Abbreviations: CABG = coronary artery bypass grafting; TLR = target lesion revascularization (i.e., PTCA or CABG); IMA = internal mammary artery

*   Randomized trial

**   6 patients assigned to CABG group actually treated by PTCA

***   Values in parentheses reflect PTCA vs. CABG (ACME values reflect Medicine vs. PTCA)

\+   Class 0 = asymptomatic, Class 1 = angina during strenuous exercise

\+\+   Cardiac death

\+\+\+   Follow-up events occuring between 6 mos. to 4 years after randomization

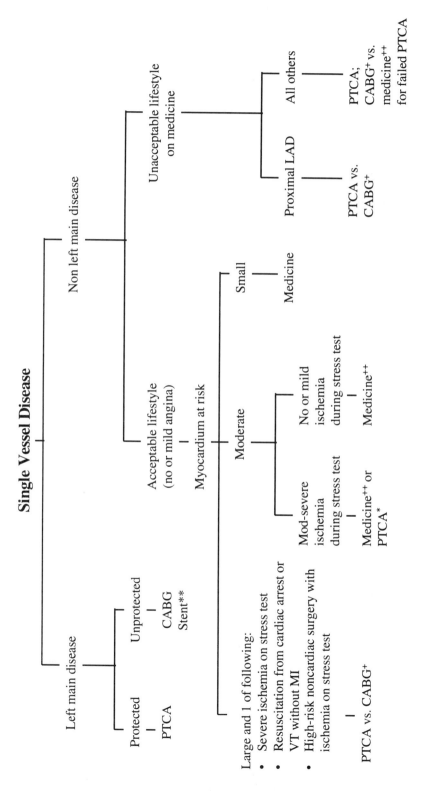

Figure 3.1. Revascularization Guidelines for Single-Vessel Coronary Disease & Chronic Stable Angina

* High-risk occupation (pilot, bus driver) favors PTCA; consider CABG for proximal LAD stenosis

** Non-surgical candidates

+ Factors tending to favor PTCA = younger age, cerebrovascular disease, severe COPD, illness limiting survival, Type A lesion, patient desires to avoid CABG and accepts 20-30% risk of repeat procedures.
Factors tending to favor CABG = severe LV dysfunction, older age, severe mitral regurgitation, diabetes, renal dialysis, complex lesion morphology, patient desires to minimize number of procedures.

++ Medicine = risk factor modification + antianginal therapy

Table 3.2. Treatment Strategies for Single Vessel Disease

Initial Treatment	Advantages
Medical therapy	**Advantages over PTCA:** • No procedural risk **Advantages over CABG:** • No procedural risk, protracted convalescence, or concern about SVG disease. • Severe progression of underlying CAD can be treated with first CABG (as opposed to repeat CABG, which is associated with lower angina-free survival)
PTCA	**Advantages over Medical Therapy:** • Less angina • Fewer antianginal meds • Better functional capacity • Better quality of life • Fewer late revascularizations **Advantages over CABG:** • Shorter and less expensive hospitalization • Shorter convalescence • Earlier functional recovery and return to work • No concern about SVG disease • Severe progression of underlying CAD can be treated with first CABG (as opposed to repeat CABG, which is associated with ↓ angina-free survival).
CABG	**Advantages over Medical Therapy:** • Less angina • Fewer antianginal meds • Better functional capacity • Better quality of life **Advantages over PTCA:** • IMA used more often when CABG is elective rather than emergent (for failed PTCA) • Less angina • Fewer antianginal meds • Fewer late revascularizations

Abbreviations: SVG = saphenous vein graft, IMA = internal mammary artery, CABG = coronary artery bypass grafting

Table 3.3. Randomized Trials of PTCA vs. CABG: Inclusion and Exclusion Criteria

Trial	N	Randomized (%)	Criteria
RITA[10]	1011	6	**Inclusion:** 1, 2, or 3-vessel disease ($\geq$ 70% stenosis); lesion supplying $\geq$ 20% of myocardium; angina or objective evidence of ischemia; equivalent revascularization by PTCA or CABG. **Exclusion:** Previous PTCA or CABG; left main disease, hemodynamically-severe valve disease; noncardiac illness threatening survival.
ERACI[11]	127	9	**Inclusion:** Multivessel disease ($\geq$ 2 vessels with $\geq$ 70% stenosis) and either significant angina despite medical therapy or a large area of myocardium at risk by exercise testing. **Exclusion:** Dilated ischemic cardiomyopathy; severe 3-vessel disease with EF $\leq$ 35%; significant left main stenosis; severe valvular or hypertrophic heart disease; evolving acute MI; noncardiac illness threatening survival.
GABI[12]	358	4	**Inclusion:** Age < 75 years; angina $\geq$ Class 2; multivessel disease ($\geq$ 2 vessels with $\geq$ 70% stenosis). **Exclusion:** Previous PTCA or CABG; total occlusion; left main stenosis $\geq$30%; > 50% of LV at risk during abrupt closure; lesion length > 2 cm; diffuse disease; coronary aneurysm, MI within 4 weeks.
CABRI[13]	1054	4.6	**Inclusion:** Age $\leq$ 76 years with multivessel disease ($\geq$ 2 vessels with $\geq$ 50% stenosis); clinical ischemia; equivalent degrees of revascularization not required. **Exclusion:** Previous PTCA or CABG; left main stenosis $\geq$ 50%; last remaining vessel; acute MI within previous 10 days; EF $\leq$ 35%; overt CHF; recent stroke; severe concomitant illness.
EAST[14]	392	7.6	**Inclusion:** Patients of any age with 2 or 3-vessel disease; angina or objective evidence of ischemia. **Exclusion:** Previous PTCA or CABG; chronic total occlusion > 8 weeks; left main stenosis $\geq$ 30%; $\geq$ 2 total occlusions; EF < 25%; MI within 5 days; noncardiac illness threatening survival.
BARI[15]	1011	7	**Inclusion:** Age > 17 and < 80; multivessel disease ($\geq$ vessels with $\geq$ 50% stenosis); and clinically severe angina (class III-IV or unstable angina; recent non-Q-MI; or class I-II angina either with severe ischemia on exercise testing; recent Q-MI; or EF < 50%), or no angina if severe ischemia on noninvasive testing and either a prior Q-MI or history of angina. **Exclusion:** Emergency revascularization; left main stenosis $\geq$ 50%; noncardiac illness that was a contraindication to PTCA or CABG or might limit survival; primary coronary spasm; severe ascending aortic calcification; need for other major surgery at same time as revascularization, known or suspected pregnancy.

CONCLUSIONS: Only a small percentage (< 25%) of patients with multivessel disease met inclusion criteria, and even fewer (< 10%) were actually randomized.

Abbreviations: MVD = multivessel disease; LV = left ventricle; EF = ejection fraction; MI = myocardial infarction

Table 3.4. Randomized Trials of PTCA vs. CABG: Study Design and Baseline Characteristics

	RITA[10]	ERACI[11]	GABI[12]	CABRI[13]	EAST[14]	BARI[15]
Patients (N)	1011	127	359	1054	392	1829
Study Design						
Planned follow-up (yrs)	10	3	1	5-10	5	10
Complete revascularization required	Yes	No	Yes	No	No	No
Total occlusion eligible	Yes	Yes	No.	Yes	No	Yes
New devices	No	No	No	Yes+	No	Yes*
IMA (%)	74	77	37	81	90	82
Baseline characteristics						
Age (yrs)	57	57	-	60	61	61
Male (%)	81	54	80	78	73	74
Previous MI (%)	43	31	47	43	41	55
Unstable angina (%)	59	53	14	15	62	65
LVEF (%)	-	61	56	63	62	57
No. diseased vessels (%)						
1	45	0	0	0	0	0
2	43	55	82	58	60	59
3	12	45	18	40	40	41

CONCLUSIONS:
- ▸ **Complete revascularization goal varied between trials.**
- ▸ **Patients with total occlusions were excluded from some trials but not others.**
- ▸ **Use of new devices and IMA grafting varied between trials.**
- ▸ **Most patients had 2-vessel disease and normal LV function.**

Abbreviations: IMA = internal mammary artery; LVEF = left ventricular ejection fraction; CABG = emergency coronary artery bypass grafting; - = not reported
+ Atherectomy or stenting
* Bailout stenting
** Complete anatomical revascularization whenever possible
- Not reported

Table 3.5. Randomized Trials of PTCA vs. CABG: PTCA Success and Revascularization Goals

Trial	PTCA success (%)	Staged PTCA (%)	PTCA Revascularization Goal
RITA[10]	87	7	Complete functional revascularization. Among patients with 2- and 3- vessel disease, attempted PTCA of all lesions occurred in 81% and 63%, respectively.
ERACI[11]	92	-	Complete functional revascularization in 89%.
GABI[12]	92	30	Complete anatomic revascularization in 86%.
CABRI[13]	91	-	Complete functional revascularization.
EAST[14]	88	40	Complete functional revascularization. Dilate lesions thought to be contributing to ischemia.
BARI[15]	88	17	Complete functional revascularization.

CONCLUSIONS:
- ▸ **PTCA success rates were high.**
- ▸ **Usual goal of PTCA: To dilate significant stenoses supplying viable myocardium; obstructions supplying nonviable myocardium or small territories were generally left untreated.**

Definitions: Complete anatomical revascularization: PTCA of all lesions regardless of viability of myocardial territory; *Complete functional revascularization:* PTCA of only those lesions thought to be causing ischemia; lesions with small territories or nonviable myocardium were rarely dilated.
* At least one lesion successully dilated
- Not reported

c. **In-hospital Outcome (Table 3.6).** In these randomized studies, PTCA success was achieved in 87-92%, with death in 1-5%, MI in 2.3-6.3%, and emergency CABG in 1.5-10.3%. Mortality rates were similar between PTCA and CABG groups, but PTCA patients had a lower rate of in-hospital MI and a shorter length of stay.

d. **Late Outcome (Table 3.7)**
　1. **Overall.** Clinical follow-up at 1-3 years revealed no difference in death, MI, or exercise capacity between groups. However, compared to CABG, PTCA patients had more recurrent angina (30-40% vs. 20-25%), a greater need for antianginal therapy (66-88% vs. 51-75%), and a 3-10 fold increase in repeat target vessel revascularization (32-54% vs. 2-13%); approximately 20% of PTCA patients required CABG during the follow-up period.

　2. **Diabetics.** Results from BARI, the largest of the randomized trials, prompted the NIH to issue a clinical alert in September 1995 regarding excess mortality in diabetics treated by multivessel PTCA; 5-year mortality was 35% in diabetics randomized to PTCA compared to 19% in CABG patients (p < 0.01). The excessive death was unrelated to periprocedural

Table 3.6. Randomized Trials of PTCA vs. CABG: In-Hospital Results

Trial	Group	Complications (%)			Other
		D	MI	CABG	
RITA[10]	PTCA	0.7	3.5	4.5	Length of stay (4 vs. 12 days)
	CABG	1.2	2.4	-	
ERACI[11]	PTCA	1.5	6.3	1.5	Stroke (1.5% vs. 3.1%)
	CABG	4.6	6.2	-	
GABI[12]	PTCA	1.1	2.3	2.8	Stroke (0% vs. 1.2%); post-op pneumonia (1.1% vs. 10.6%, <
	CABG	2.5	8.1*	-	0.001); length of stay (5 vs. 19 days); angina (18% vs. 7%, p < 0.005)
CABRI[13]	PTCA	1.3	-	3.3	-
	CABG	1.3	-	-	
EAST[14]	PTCA	1	3	10.1	Stroke (0.5% vs. 1.5%)
	CABG	1	10.3*	-	
BARI[15]	PTCA	1.2	2.1	6.3	Stroke (0.2% vs. 0.8%), respiratory failure (1% vs. 2.2%,
	CABG	1.3	4.6*	-	p < .05)

CONCLUSIONS:
▸   **In-hospital mortality similar between PTCA and CABG groups.**
▸   **In-hospital MI higher in CABG group.**
▸   **Emergency CABG for failed PTCA in 1.5-10%.**
▸   **Length of hospital stay 2-3 fold higher in CABG group.**

Abbreviations: D = death; Q-MI = Q-wave myocardial infarction; CABG = emergency coronary artery bypass grafting; - = Not reported
*   p < 0.01

      mortality, which was similar between groups (PTCA 0.6%, CABG 1.2%). CABG may be the preferred mode of revascularization for diabetics with multivessel coronary disease who meet the BARI inclusion criteria; however, these data do not reflect the improving results of multivessel angioplasty (see below) or stenting, and further studies are needed. Nevertheless, these results may have profound implications for coronary revascularization, since 20-30% of all multivessel angioplasties are performed on diabetics.

    e.   **Conclusions From the Randomized Trials (Table 3.8)**

2.   **Lessons Learned From Nonrandomized Studies of Multivessel Angioplasty**
    a.   **Ischemic Endpoints.** The Multivessel Angioplasty Prognosis Study (MAPS)[16] compared the results of multivessel PTCA in 1991 vs. 1986-87 (when many of the randomized trials enrolled patients). Despite older age and lower ejection fraction, the 1991 cohort had *higher* procedural success, *more complete* revascularization, and *better* clinical outcome than the earlier cohort (Table 3.9).[16] Another study reported continued improvement in in-hospital outcomes for

Table 3.7. Randomized Trials of PTCA vs. CABG: Late Outcome

Trial	F/U (yrs)	Modality	D / MI / TLR / ASX (%)	Other
RITA[10]	2.5	PTCA	3.1 / 6.1 / 35 / 69	See 1, below
		CABG	3.6 / 3.9 / 3.8+ / 79+	
ERACI[11]	1	PTCA	3.2 / 3.2 / 32+ / -	PTCA less expensive at 1- and 3-year follow-up
		CABG	0 / 1.8 / 3.2+/ -	
GABI[12]	3	PTCA	- / - / 37 / 60	
		CABG	- / - / 3.2+ / 80+	
	1	PTCA	2.6 / 4.5 / 44 / 71	See 2, below
		CABG	6.5 / 9.4 / 6 / 74	
CABRI[13]	1	PTCA	3.9 / 4.9 / 35.6 / 67	Need for antianginals (84% vs. 65%)
		CABG	2.7 / 3.5 / 2.1 / 75+	
EAST[14]	3	PTCA	7.1 / 14.6 / 54 / 80†	See 3, below
		CABG	6.2 / 19.6 / 13 +/ 88†+	
BARI[15]	5	Overall		See 4, below
		PTCA	14 / 8 / 54 / -	
		CABG	11 / 9 / 8 + / -	
		Diabetic++		
		PTCA	35 / - / 62 / -	
		CABG	19 / - / 8 +/ -	

CONCLUSIONS:
- **Infarct-free survival at 1-year similar; diabetics treated with PTCA had higher late mortality.***
- **PTCA resulted in more angina, antianginal therapy, and repeat revascularization (3-10 fold) compared to CABG; ~ 20% of PTCA patients required CABG at 1-3 years.**

Other results:
1. PTCA vs. CABG: Death, MI, or reintervention (38% vs. 11%+); severe angina 6% in both groups; PTCA less expensive. Pre vs. post-revascularization: 40% of those not working at baseline had returned to work at 6 months; revascularization had no effect on ejection fraction
2. PTCA vs. CABG: Death or MI (5% vs. 11%) + *, antianginals (88% vs 78%)+
3. PTCA vs. CABG: Abnormal thallium stress (9.6% vs. 5.7%); use of antianginals (66% vs. 51%) + ; costs equal; no difference in LVEF
4. PTCA vs. CABG: Infarct-free survival (79% vs. 80%); 70% of PTCA patients survived 5 years without CABG and at most one repeat PTCA procedure; severe angina present in only 3% of PTCA & CABG groups, but PTCA patients more likely to have angina of all grades

Abbreviations: ASX = asymptomatic; D = death; Q-MI = Q-wave myocardial infarction; CABG = emergency coronary artery bypass grafting; EF = ejection fraction; - = not reported
* Does not include high mortality among CABG patients during the waiting period (time between randomization and revascularization)
+ (p <0.05) ++ Patients receiving oral hypoglycemics or insulin at study entry

Table 3.8. Randomized PTCA vs. CABG Trials: Summary of Conclusions

Trial	In-hospital (%)		Late (%)				Other
	D	MI	D	MI	TLR	Angina	
RITA[10]	ND	ND	ND	ND	↑	↑	Severe angina (ND), cost (↓), exercise capacity (ND)
ERACI[11]	ND	ND	ND	ND	↑	↑	Cost (↓)
GABI[12]	ND	↓	ND	ND	↑	ND	Death or MI (↓), need for antianginals (↑)
CABRI[13]			ND	ND	↑	ND	Need for antianginals (↑)
EAST[14]	ND	↓	ND	ND	↑	↑	Abnormal thalluim (ND), need for antianginals (ND), cost (ND), exercise capacity (ND)
BARI[15]		ND	ND*	-	↑	↑	

CONCLUSIONS:

■ For patients with multivessel disease and significant ischemia who are candidates for either PTCA or CABG and meet the entry criteria for the randomized trials (i.e., no previous PTCA or CABG; well-preserved LV function; and no left main stenosis, evolving or very recent MI, or severe noncardiac illness):

   ► PTCA and CABG result in similar acute and longterm (1-5 yr) infarct-free survival. However, diabetic patients treated by PTCA have higher mortality than CABG patients.

   ► Patients treated by PTCA have more angina, require more antianginal therapy, and need more revascularization procedures in the first 1-5 years, including CABG in 20%.

   ► Patients initially treated with CABG have a longer convalescence. Longterm follow-up will determine whether more revascularization is needed after 5 years in CABG patients (i.e., to treat vein graft disease).

■ For patients with multivessel disease and either left main stenosis, single stenosis supplying > 50% of viable myocardium, severe LV dysfunction, diffusely diseased vessels, or undilatable occlusions supplying viable myocardium, CABG may be preferred over PTCA.

Abbreviations: D = death; Q-MI = in-hospital Q-wave myocardial infarction; CABG = emergency coronary artery bypass grafting: TLR = target lesion revascularization; - not reported

ND = No difference between PTCA and CABG groups

↑ Incidence higher in PTCA group

↓ Incidence lower in PTCA group

* Diabetics treated by PTCA with higher late mortality compared to those treated by CABG

Table 3.9. Nonrandomized Series of Multivessel PTCA

Series	Subset	N	Success (%)	In-Hospital (%) D / Q-MI / CABG	Follow-up Years	Event (%)	
						Death	CABG
Weintraub[32] (1995)	1-VD	7604	-	0.2 / 0.4 / 1.2	1,5,10	1 / 7 / 14	8/13/23
	2-VD	2587	-	0.8 / 0.9 / 0.2		3 / 11 / 24	11/21/42
	3-VD	592	-	1.7 / 3.0 / 3.2		5 / 10 / 30*	14/27/41+
Ellis[16] (1995)	1991	200	90	1 / 1.5 / 1	1	1991 vs. 1986-87: EFS (74% vs. 64%); CABG (8.1% vs. 13.4%); complete revascularization (35% vs. 21%); use of new devices (26% vs. 0%)	
	1986-87	400	84	1 / 2 / 5.5			
Cowley[31] (1993)		370	92	-	3	EFS (77%); asymptomatic (74%)	
LeFeuvre[33] (1993)		703	91	0 / 2.5 / 1.5	6	Death (7.1%); MI (9.2%); Class 0-1 angina (84%)	

Abbreviations: VD = vessel disease; D = death; Q-MI = Q-wave myocardial infarction; CABG = emergency coronary artery bypass grafting; EFS = event-free survival; - not reported
* 9-year + 8-year

multivessel angioplasty in 1994 compared to 1990-1991 (in-hospital MI, death, or CABG: 2% vs. 5%, p < 0.05).[17] Finally, Ellis and colleagues at the Cleveland Clinic found a 40% reduction in ischemic complications for coronary interventions performed in 1995 compared to 1993-1994 (1.7% vs. 3.0%, p = 0.004), probably related to the increased frequency of elective stenting (23% vs. 5%).[41] These improving results may have important implications for proper interpretation of the randomized PTCA vs. CABG trials, which enrolled patients 5-9 years ago.

b. **Restenosis.** Symptomatic status is not a reliable indicator of restenosis after multivessel PTCA. In one report, restenosis occurred in 55% of patients (the majority were asymptomatic), and correlated with a greater number of dilated segments.[13] Patients with asymptomatic restenosis managed medically had 6-year outcomes similar to patients *without* restenosis; these data support functional assessment of borderline lesions (50-70% stenosis) rather than routine repeat intervention based on angiographic findings alone (i.e., "oculostenotic reflex").

B. **MULTIVESSEL ANGIOPLASTY IN PATIENTS WITH LV DYSFUNCTION.** Data from the Coronary Artery Surgery Study (CASS) Registry demonstrate the powerful adverse impact of LV dysfunction on the natural history of medically-treated patients;[38] as shown in Table 3.10, patients with single-vessel disease and poor LV function had higher mortality than those with 3-vessel disease and

**Table 3.10. The Impact of LV Function and Extent of Coronary Disease on
4-Year Survival in Medically-Treated Patients[38]**

| LV function* | No. Diseased Vessels | | |
	1	2	3
Good	94	91	79
Poor	67	61	42

* Systolic contraction was assessed in 5 selected LV segments and assigned a value of 1 (normal wall motion) to 6 (dyskinetic). Systolic contraction score is the sum of all segmental values; scores of 5-11 and 17-30 represent good and poor LV function, respectively.

normal LV function. LV dysfunction has also been shown to adversely impact longterm outcome after multivessel PTCA:[18] CABG resulted in more periprocedural stroke and longer hospital study, but improved 5-year event-free survival and less angina (Table 3.11) compared to PTCA patients. Late outcome, however, was most influenced by *completeness* of revascularization, *not the mode* of revascularization; patients with complete revascularization demonstrated similar event-free survivals regardless of treatment mode. These data suggest that CABG may be preferred if PTCA cannot achieve complete revascularization, particularly in patients with diabetes, unstable angina, high-risk lesion morphology, and/or proximal LAD disease.[19,20]

Table 3.11. PTCA vs. CABG for Patients with Multivessel Disease and LV Dysfunction[18]

Event (%)	PTCA (n=100)	CABG (n=100)
In-hospital Outcome		
Complete revascularization	37	82
Death	3	5
Q-MI	2	2
Stroke	0	7
Length of stay	4.3	12.8
5-year Follow-up		
Death	33	24
Death or MI	54	24
Repeat revascularization	50	0
Class III-IV angina	11	1

C. REVASCULARIZATION STRATEGY (Figure 3.2)

1. Complete vs. Incomplete Revascularization: "To dilate or not to dilate... that is the question." The concept of complete revascularization evolved from the early surgical experience, which demonstrated improved anginal status, exercise capacity, and intermediate (5-7 year) event-free survival when all stenoses > 50% were bypassed.[21-25] The early PTCA experience seemed to corroborate the benefits of this approach.[26-28] However, patients with incomplete revascularization were at higher risk (i.e., older, worse LV function, greater comorbidity, more complex coronary disease) than those with complete revascularization. Once these differences were accounted for, many studies concluded that revascularization status had no impact on infarct-free survival (although late PTCA or CABG was required more often in patients with incomplete revascularization).[29,30] Complete revascularization can be subdivided into 2 groups: complete "anatomical" revascularization and complete "functional" revascularization (Table 3.12). The optimal revascularization strategy is unknown, but may depend on LV function:

   a. **Nondiabetics with 2- or 3-Vessel Disease and Good LV Function.** The goal of multivessel PTCA is to improve symptomatic status and functional capacity, which can be achieved by treating all culprit stenoses > 60-70% with moderate-to-large myocardial territories. Routine PTCA of stenoses that supply nonviable myocardium, or of mild stenoses (< 60%) in small vessels (subtend < 10% of LV mass), does not appear necessary to achieve a good longterm clinical outcome.[31] In the ERACI trial, there was no difference in 1-year outcome between CABG patients who had all stenosis >50% bypassed (complete "anatomic" revascularization) and PTCA patients who had only those lesions causing ischemia dilated (complete "functional" revascularization); 96% of PTCA patients were asymptomatic at follow-up. In the CABRI trial, incomplete revascularization was predictive of reintervention, but not survival or MI at one year.[40]

   b. **Nondiabetics with 3-Vessel Disease and Poor LV Function.** The goal of revascularization is to improve symptomatic status, functional capacity, and possibly prolong survival. While most patients with high-risk lesions are traiged to CABG, select patients with low-risk lesions may be considered for percutaneous revascularization. When PTCA and other devices are used, we attempt to revascularize all stenoses in vessels ≥ 1.5 mm, including chronic total occlusions supplying nonviable myocardium, since they can serve as a source of collaterals. Subset analyses of patients with LV dysfunction in the randomized PTCA vs. CABG trials will help determine optimal revascularization for this important group of patients.

   c. **Diabetics (On Insulin or an Oral Hypoglycemic) with 2- or 3-vessel Disease.** Results from the BARI trial suggest that CABG can improve longterm survival compared to multivessel PTCA and should be considered the preferred mode of revascularization. However, these data do not reflect the improving results of multivessel angioplasty and stenting. Further studies are indicated. Regardless of whether CABG or PTCA is performed, longterm mortality rates are high, emphasizing the need for aggressive risk factor modification.

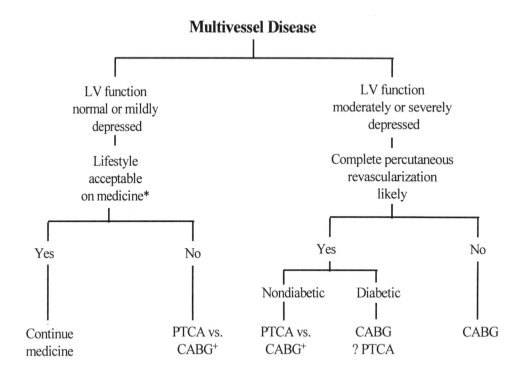

Figure 3.2. Revascularization Guidelines for Multivessel Disease & Chronic Stable Angina

* Medicine = risk factor modification + antianginal therapy
+ **Factors tending to favor PTCA** = younger age, cerebrovascular disease, severe COPD, illness limiting survival, Type A lesion morphology, patient desires to avoid CABG and accepts 20-30% risk of repeat procedures. **Factors tending to favor CABG** = older age, severe mitral regurgitation, diabetes, renal dialysis, complex lesion morphology, patient desires to minimize number of procedures.

2. **Approach to "Moderate" Stenoses.** Moderate (50-70%) stenoses may or may not be functionally significant and require treatment. Factors favoring intervention include: ischemic ECG changes, a regional wall motion abnormality, or a reversible thallium defect in the distribution of the stenosis; lesion morphology suggesting ruptured plaque or intracoronary thrombus; or coronary flow reserve < 2.0 when a Doppler wire is used (Chapter 33).

3. **Order of Dilatation.** The order in which stenoses are dilated can directly impact the safety and efficacy of multivessel PTCA. As outlined in Figure 3.3, total occlusions that supply large jeopardized areas or furnish collaterals are dilated first, followed by culprit lesion(s) that supply moderate-to-large myocardial regions. If the culprit lesion supplies little viable myocardium or

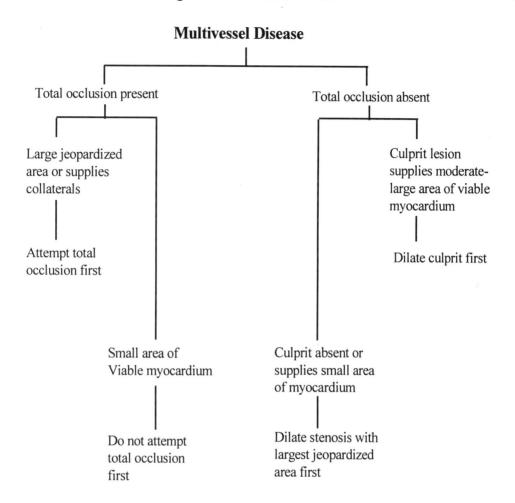

Figure 3.3. Dilatation Order for Patients Requiring Elective Multivessel PTCA

cannot be identified, we dilate the most important stenosis (largest jeopardized area) next. If two stenoses are present in vessels of equal caliber and distribution, the better collateralized vessel is dilated first. When proximal and distal stenoses are present, we attempt to dilate the distal lesion first; this allows the balloon to retain its lowest profile as it advances across the more distal lesion. If the balloon impedes flow or cannot be easily advanced across the proximal stenosis, this site is dilated first.

Table 3.12. Percutaneous Revascularization Strategies and Expected Clinical Outcome

Revascularization Strategy	Definition	Expected Clinical Outcome
Complete anatomic revascularization	Dilatation of all stenoses > 50% in vessels ≥ 1.5 mm in diameter	Similar to complete functional revascularization
Complete functional revascularization	Dilatation of only those lesions thought to be causing ischemia	Similar to complete anatomic revascularization in patients with well-preserved LV function; anatomic revascularization may be preferred in pateints with LV dysfunction.
Incomplete functional revascularization	Inability to dilate ≥ 1 lesion thought to be causing ischemia	Worse than either of the other 2 groups

4. **Staging**
    a. **Elective Intervention.** For most patients with multivessel disease, complete functional revascularization is attempted during the initial procedure. Small branches (≤ 1.5 mm) may be left untreated. When further PTCA might compromise patient comfort or safety, other stenoses are treated at a later time ("staged") (Table 3.13). A "next-day" staging strategy is useful, allowing the majority of patients to be completely revascularized during their initial hospital stay (Figure 3.4). When this approach is chosen, patients usually receive an overnight infusion of heparin (aPTT maintained at 60-70 or ACT 180-200 sec). If the original lesion looks good the next day, other stenoses may be dilated at this time. If the original result is suboptimal, the operator may elect to perform additional intervention on the original lesion, defer further percutaneous intervention for 2-4 weeks, or refer the patient for CABG.

Table 3.13. Indications for Staging

·   Thrombus prior to or immediately after PTCA

·   Severe dissection or impaired flow after intervention

·   Procedure duration > 3 hrs

·   Contrast media volume > 400 cc

·   Borderline lesions (50-70% stenosis) without objective evidence for ischemia

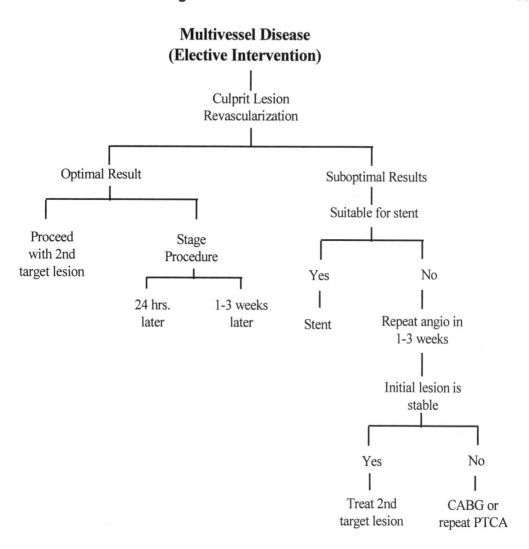

Figure 3.4. Staging of Multivessel Disease During Elective Intervention

b. **Urgent Intervention.** When PTCA is being performed for acute MI or post-infarct angina, the culprit lesion is usually dilated during the initial procedure (Chapter 5). Additional high-grade stenoses may be deferred to the next day or several weeks later, depending on symptom status and LV function (Figure 3.5).

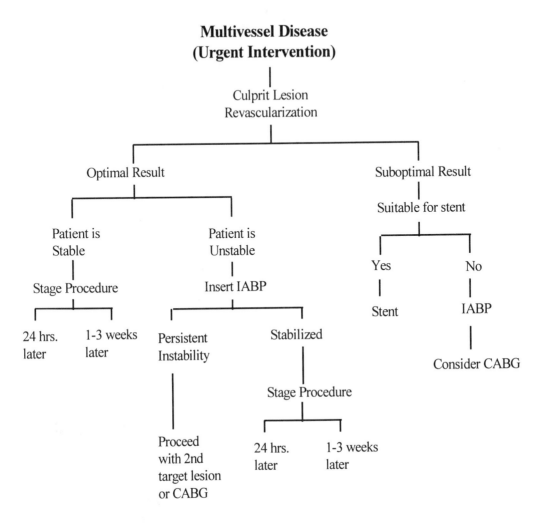

Figure 3.5. Staging of Multivessel Disease During Urgent Intervention

Abbreviations: IABP = intraaortic balloon pump; CABG = coronary artery bypass grafting

Table 3.14. PTCA of One Major Artery When the Other is Occluded

Series	Group	N	In-Hosp (%) D/Q-MI/CABG	Follow-Up (%) Mos.	Follow-Up (%) D/Q-MI/PTCA/CABG	No Angina (%)
Lafont[4+] (1993)	PTCA of LAD or RCA when the other is occluded	193	0.5 / 0.5 / 5.7	33	4.7 / 3.7 / 23.6 / 13.1	76
	PTCA of LAD & RCA	214	0.5 / 0.5 / 3.3		5.3 / 4.3 / 11.6 / 8.2	80
	CABG of LAD + RCA	194	1.5 / 1.0 / 0		8.5 / 3.7 / 1.6 / 2.1	74
DeBruyne[35] (1991)	PTCA of LAD or LCX when RCA is occluded	61	0 / 0 / 4.9	5	- / - / 25 / 5	65
Teirstein[36] (1990)	PTCA of left coronary:					
	RCA occluded	65	1.5 / - / 0	17	8 / 3 / - / 18	61
	RCA not occluded	105	0 / - / 1.5		7 / 1 / - / 9	84

Abbreviations: D = death; Q-MI = Q-wave myocardial infarction; CABG = emergency coronary artery bypass grafting; LAD = left anterior descending coronary artery; RCA = right coronary artery; LCX = left circumflex artery
+   Groups matched for number and location of stenoses, EF, age, gender and study period.
-    Not reported

D. SPECIAL SUBSET OF MULTIVESSEL DISEASE: PTCA OF ONE MAJOR ARTERY WHEN THE OTHER IS OCCLUDED. Several studies have evaluated the results of PTCA in a major artery when the other vessel is occluded.[34-36] As shown in Table 3.14, success and complications rates are acceptable. Nevertheless, many interventionalists refer such patients for bypass surgery, particularly when the occluded vessel supplies a large myocardial territory, LV function is poor, or the target lesion has high-risk morphology for PTCA (e.g., thrombus, angulation, long). These patients should understand that although PTCA may be a viable alternative to CABG, repeat revascularization (including CABG) may be required 30-40% of the time.

* * * * *

REFERENCES

1. Henderon RA, Pocock SJ, Hampton JR. Revascularization for patients with single vessel disease: Results from the randomized interventional treatment of angina (RITA) trial at 4.7 years. Circulation 1995;92:I-476.
2. Goy JJ, Eckhout E, Burnand B, et al. Coronary angioplasty versus left internal mammary artery grafting for isolated proximal left anterior descending artery stenosis. Lancet 1994;343:1149-1453.
3. Mark DB, Nelson CL, Califf RM, et al. Continuing evolution of therapy for coronary artery disease. Initial results from the era of coronary angioplasty. Circulation 1994;89:2015-2025.
4. Cameron J, Mahanonda N, Aroney C, et al. Outcome five years after percutaneous transluminal coronary angioplasty or coronary artery bypass grafting for significant narrowing limited to the left anterior descending coronary artery. Am J Cardiol 1994;74:544-549.
5. Parisi A, Folland E, Hartigan P. A comparison of angioplasty with medical therapy in the treatment of single-vessel coronary artery disease. N Engl J Med 1992;326:10-16.
6. Morris KG, Folland ED, Hartigan PM, et al. Unstable angina in late follow-up of the ACME trial. Circulation 1995;92:I-725.
7. Frierson JH, Dimas AP, Whitlow PL, Hollman JL. Angioplasty of the proximal left anterior descending coronary artery: Initial success and long-term follow-up. J Am Coll Cardiol 1992;19:745-751.
8. Henderson RA, Karani S, Dritsas A, et al. Long-term results of coronary angioplasty for single vessel, proximal left anterior descending disease. Eur Heart J 1991;12:642-47.
9. Kramer JR, Proudfit W, Loop FD, et al. Late follow-up of 781 patients undergoing PTCA or bypass surgery for an isolated obstruction in the left anterior descending coronary artery. Am Heart J 1989;118:1144-53.
10. Coronary angioplasty versus coronary artery bypass surgery: The randomized intervention treatment of angina (RITA) trial. RITA Trial Participants. Lancet 1993;341:573-80.
11. Rodriguez A, Boullon F, Perez-Balino N. Argentine randomized trial of percutaneous transluminal coronary angioplasty versus coronary artery bypass surgery in multivessel disease (ERACI): In-hospital results and 1-year follow-up. J Am Coll Cardiol 1993;22:1060-1067.
12. Hamm C, Reimers J, Ischinger T, Rupprecht H. A randomized study of coronary angioplasty compared with bypass surgery in patients with symptomatic multivessel coronary disease. N Engl J Med 1994;331(16):1037-1043.
13. First-year results of CABRI Coronary Angioplasty versus Bypass Revascularization Investigation). CABRI Trial Participants. Lancet 1995;346:1179-84.
14. King S, Lembo N, Weintraub W, Kosinski A. A randomized trial comparing coronary angioplasty with coronary bypass surgery. N Engl J Med 1994;331:1044-1150.
15. The Bypass Angioplasty Revascularization Investigation (BARI): Five-year mortality and morbidity in a randomized study comparing CABG and PTCA in patients with multivessel coronary disease. The BARI Investigators. N Engl J Med (submitted).
16. Ellis S, Cowley M, Whitlow P, et al. Prospective case-control comparison of percutaneous transluminal coronary revascularization in patients with multivessel disease treated in 1986-1987 versus 1991: Improved in-hospital and 12-month results. J Am Coll Cardiol 1995;25(5):1137-42.
17. Danchin N, Cador R, Dibon O, et al. Changes in immediate outcome of PTCA in multivessel coronary artery disease: Implications for the interpretation of randomized trials of PTCA versus CABG. Circulation 1995;92:I-475.
18. O'Keefe JH, Allan JJ, McCallister BD, McConahay DR. Angioplasty versus bypass surgery for multivessel Coronary artery disease with left ventricular ejection fraction <40%. Am J Cardiol 1993;71:897-901.
19. Ellis SG, Vandormael MG, Cowley MJ, et al. Coronary morphologic and clinical determinants of procedural outcome with angioplasty for multivessel coronary disease: Implications for patient selection. Circulation 1990;82:1193-1202.
20. Ellis SG, Cowley MK, DiSciascio G, et al. Determinants of 2-year outcome after coronary angioplasty in patients with multivessel disease on the basis of comprehensive preprocedural evaluation: Implications for patient selection. Circulation 1991;82:1905-1914.
21. LaVee J, Rath S, Hoa, et al. Does complete revascularization by the conventional method truly provide the best possible results? Analysis of results and comparison with revascularization of infarct-prone segments (systematic segmental myocardial revascularization): The Sheba Study. J Thorac Cardiovasc Surg 1986;92:279-290.
22. Schaff HV, Gersh BJ, Pluth JR, et al. Survival and functional status after coronary artery bypass grafting: Results 10

to 12 years after surgery in 500 patients. Circulation 1983;68 (Suppl II):II-200-204.

23. Lawrie GM, Morris GC, Silvers A, et al. The influence of residual disease after coronary bypass on the 5-year survival rate of 1274 men with coronary artery disease. Circulation 1982;66:717-723.

24. Jones EL, Craver JM, Guyton RA, et al. Importance of complete revascularization in performance of the coronary bypass operation. Am J Cardiol 1983;51:7-12.

25. Cukingham RA, Carey JS, Wittig JH, et al. Influence of complete coronary revascularization on relief of angina. J Thorac Cardiovasc Surg 1980;79:188-193.

26. Mabin TQA, Holmes DR, Smith HC, et al. Follow-up clinical results in patients undergoing percutaneous transluminal coronary angioplasty. Circulation 1985;71:754-760.

27. Vandormael MG, Chaitman BR, Ischinger T, Aker UT. Immediate and short-term benefit of multilesion coronary angioplasty: Influence of degree of Revascularization. J Am Coll Cardiol 1985;6:983-991.

28. Bourassa MG, Yeh W, Detre K, for the NHLBI PTCA Investigators. Five-year event rates after multivessel PTCA when complete revascularization is not possible or not intended. J Am Coll Cardiol 1994;February:223A.

29. Bell M, Bailey K, Reeder G, Lapeyre A, Holmes D. Percutaneous transluminal angioplasty in patients with multivessel coronary disease: How important is complete revascularization for cardiac event-free survival? J Am Coll Cardiol 1990;16:553-562.

30. Reeder GS, Holmes DR, Detre K, et al. Degree of revascularization in patients with multivessel coronary disease: A report from the National Heart, Lung and Blood Institute Percutaneous Transluminal Coronary Angioplasty Registry. Circulation 1988;3:638-644.

31. Cowley M, Vandermael M, Topol E, et al. Is traditionally defined complete revascularization needed for patients with multivessel disease treated by elective coronary angioplasty? J Am Coll Cardiol 1993;22:1289-1297.

32. Weintraub W, King S, Douglas J, Kosinski A. Percutaneous transluminal coronary angioplasty as a first revascularization procedure in single-, double, and triple-vessel coronary artery disease. J Am Coll Cardiol 1995;26:142-151.

33. Le Feuvre C, Bonan R, Cote Gilles, et al. Five-to-10 year outcome after multivessel percutaneous transluminal coronary angioplasty. Am J Cardiol 1993;71:1153-1158.

34. Lafont A, Dimas AP, Grigera F, Pearce G. Percutaneous transluminal coronary angioplasty of one major coronary artery when the contralateral vessel is occluded. J Am Coll Cardiol 1993;22(5):1298-1303.

35. De Bruyne B, Renkin J, Col J, Wijns W. Percutaneous transluminal coronary angioplasty of the left coronary artery in patients with chronic occlusion of the right coronary artery: Clinical and functional results. Am Heart J 1991;122:415.

36. Teirstein P. Giorgi L, Johnson W, et al. PTCA of the left coronary artery when the right coronary artery is chronically occluded. Am Heart J 1990;119:479.

37. Le Feuvre C, Bonan R, Lesperance J, et al. Predictive factors of restenosis after multivessel percutaneous transluminal coronary angioplasty. Am J Cardiol 1994;73:840-844.

38. Mock M, Ringqvist I, Fisher L, et al. Survival of medically treated patients in the Coronary Artery Surgery Study (CASS) Registry. Circulation 1982;66:562-8.

39. Hueb WA, Bellotti G, de Oliveira A, et al. The Medicine, Angioplasty or Surgery Study (MASS): A prospective, randomized trial of medical therapy, balloon angioplasty or bypass surgery for single proximal left anterior descending artery stenoses. J Am Coll Cardiol 1995;26:1600-5.

40. Breeman A, Boersma E, Deckers JW, et al. The impact of the completeness of revascularization on adverse cardiac events at 1 year follow-up in 1021 CABRI patients. J Am Coll Cardiol 1996;March Special Issue.

41. Ellis SG, Whitlow PL, Guetta V, et al. A highly significant 40% reduction in ischemic complications of percutaneous coronary intervention in 1995: Beginning of a new era? J Am Coll Cardiol 1996;March Issue.

HIGH-RISK INTERVENTION

4

Mark Freed, M.D.
William O'Neill, M.D.
Robert D. Safian, M.D.

RISK STRATIFICATION

The risk of a fatal ischemic complication after coronary intervention may vary up to 50-fold depending on clinical, procedural, and angiographic factors. This risk can be minimized by meticulous case selection, risk-factor modification, optimal technique, adjunctive imaging modalities and pharmacotherapy, and immediate recognition and management of complications. As shown in Table 4.1, the risk of procedural death can be estimated from (1) the risk of acute vessel closure, which is best judged from lesion morphology before and immediately after PTCA; and (2) the risk of a fatal outcome after acute closure, which is best judged from clinical characteristics such as age, baseline ventricular function, number of diseased vessels, and possibly gender (see Jeopardy Score, Chapter 20).

Table 4.1 Estimation of Procedural Mortality

Lesion Closure Risk*	+	Patient Mortality Risk**	∝	Procedural Risk
High		High		Highest
Low		High		High
High		Low		Intermediate
Low		Low		Low

Lesion Closure Factors::
Unstable angina
Thrombus
Multilesion/multivessel CAD
Angulation > 45-60°
Long lesion (> 20 mm)
Branch point stenosis
No aspirin
Suboptimal ACT
Balloon-to-artery ratio > 1
Residual stenosis > 30%
Dissection: long, spiral, cap

Patient Mortality Factors:
LVEF < 35%
Age > 65 years
Three-vessel or left main CAD
Recent MI
No prior CABG
Jeopardy score ≥2.5 (Chapter 20)
Female gender?

Abbreviations: ACT = activated clotting time; CABG = coronary artery bypass graft; CAD = coronary artery disease; LVEF = left ventricular ejection fraction
*   The risk of developing acute closure; estimated from the number of lesion closure factors.
**   The risk of death following acute closure; estimated from the number of patient mortality factors.

In one study,[1] at least one clinical or lesion risk factor was present in 87% and 22% of fatal PTCA outcomes, respectively, suggesting that procedural risk is more closely associated with patient characteristics than lesion morphology. The Registry Committee of the Society for Cardiac Angiography and Interventions (SCAI) identified risk factors for major in-hospital complications (death, MI, emergency CABG) among 10,622 patients undergoing angioplasty;[2] after developing a simplified predictive index based on the number of "high-risk" variables, they validated this index in a separate cohort of 5250 PTCA patients (Table 4.2).

RISK REDUCTION

Figure 4.1 summarizes important prophylactic and therapeutic measures aimed at reducing the risks of high-risk angioplasty. Most of these issues are discussed elsewhere; however, a few considerations will be detailed here.

A. PREPROCEDURAL CONSIDERATIONS
1. **Patient Referral.** Procedures involving high-risk lesions in high-risk patients are best performed at interventional centers experienced in the use of new interventional devices, IABP, and CPS. The need for an experienced operator and support staff cannot be overstated.

Table 4.2 Risk of Major Complications After PTCA[32]

Risk Class	Risk Factors[†] (N)	Patients (N)	Complications* (%)
Low	0	37,333	1.3
Moderate	1-2	5,400	2.6
High	3	326	8.6
Very high	> 3	79	23

†   Risk factors = aortic valve disease, left main PTCA, shock, acute MI < 24 hrs, Type C lesion, multivessel disease, and unstable angina

*   In-hospital death, MI (within 24 hours of the procedure), and emergency CABG.

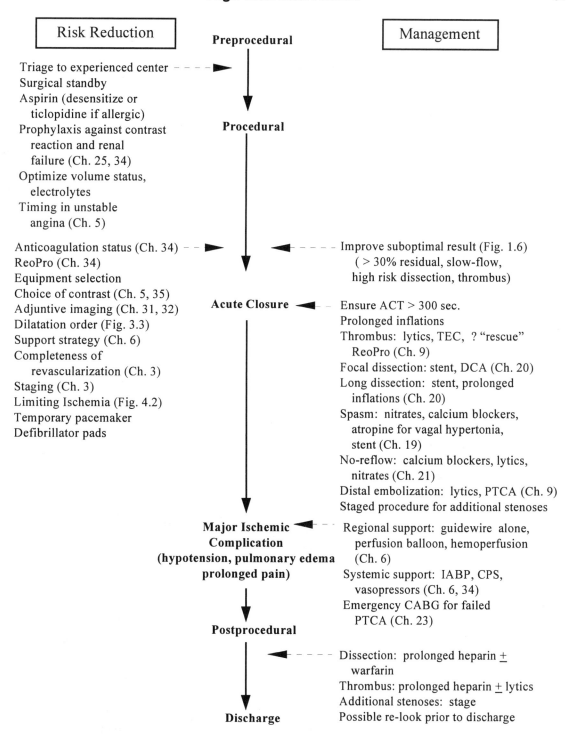

Figure 4.1. Overview of High-Risk Angioplasty: Risk Reduction and Management

2. **Optimizing Volume Status and Electrolytes.** Intravascular volume depletion exaggerates the hypotensive effects of contrast agents, nitrates and balloon-induced ischemia, and is a risk factor for adverse outcome following acute closure.[3] Aggressive administration of IV fluids (coupled with the negative inotropic effects of contrast agents and balloon-induced ischemia) can readily induce heart failure in patients with marginal LV reserve. Therefore, careful assessment of intravascular volume is mandatory during high-risk intervention; a pulmonary artery catheter is recommended in all patients with labile hemodynamic performance or heart failure. Electrolyte disturbances must also be corrected prior to PTCA in order to reduce the risk of arrhythmias during balloon inflation. Some operators withhold β-blockers the day of the procedure to ensure that compensatory mechanisms (reflex tachycardia, hypercontractility) are fully operative should they be needed to maintain systemic blood pressure and end-organ perfusion.

3. **Surgical Standby.** When high-risk angioplasty is performed, we recommend that an operating room be immediately available for the duration of the case, minimizing the time to emergency CABG, if needed.

4. **Prophylaxis Against Renal Failure.** Patients with pre-existing renal insufficiency or a history of renal dysfunction following contrast exposure must be well-hydrated prior to PTCA. In hospitalized patients, we aim to maintain urine output > 40 cc/hr with IV crystalloids (100-150 cc/hr starting 8-10 hours prior to the case); supplemental diuretics may be needed to prevent pulmonary congestion when LV dysfunction is present. Upon completion of the case, the crystalloid infusion is usually continued for an additional 8-24 hours to facilitate excretion of the contrast agent. If urine output falls below 40-60 cc/hr in patients without CHF, one or more bolus infusions of normal saline (200 cc) may be given. If urine output remains low, particularly in those with LV dysfunction or baseline renal insufficiency, supplemental use of diuretics (e.g., furosemide 20-80 mg IV over 1-2 minutes) may improve urine flow. Mannitol (12.5-25 grams IV over 30 minutes before and immediately after contrast exposure) may be of value for insulin-dependent diabetics with serum creatinines above 1.7-2.0 mg/dl,[4] although randomized data are lacking. Mannitol should be administered judiciously, if at all, to patients with severe LV dysfunction due to the risk of precipitating pulmonary edema; if given, supplemental therapy with a loop diuretic is usually required.

5. **Choice of Contrast (Chapter 25) and Prophylaxis Against Reactions (Chapter 34).**

6. **Hemodynamic Support.** A Swan-Ganz catheter is used to optimize volume status and continuously monitor pulmonary artery pressure in patients with LV dysfunction or a large area of jeopardized myocardium. A transvenous pacemaker is inserted prophylactically when a pre-existing high-grade conduction disturbance is present, when no-reflow is anticipated (thrombus containing lesion, vein graft interventions, or use of the Rotablator), and when revascularizing a dominant RCA or left circumflex artery. Prophylactic insertion of a balloon pump or CPS is performed in selected patients (Chapter 6).

7. **Other Considerations.** Cardiovascular technicians and nurses must be alerted to the high-risk nature of the case. Both groins should be prepped to minimize the delay in initiating emergency IABP or CPS. We routinely apply R-2 pads to the patient prior to placing the sterile drape to expedite defibrillation.

B. INTRAPROCEDURAL CONSIDERATIONS

1. **Limiting Ischemia.** Strict attention to procedural technique is necessary to avoid inadvertent or prolonged ischemia during high-risk angioplasty.

   a. **Limiting Ischemia During Guide Catheter Engagement.** Poor guide catheter technique can induce ischemia by ostial trauma or by obstructing flow down a sidebranch (mismatch between guide and ostium or deep intubation); dampening of the arterial pressure curve and/or delayed clearance of dye from the vessel should prompt immediate repositioning of the guide or selection of an alternate catheter (e.g., short-tip, side holes, different configuration).

   b. **Limiting Ischemia During Balloon Inflations** may be achieved by using short inflations (15-30 sec.) or a perfusion balloon;[5,6] possibly by intracoronary β-blockers or calcium blockers;[7-10] or by active perfusion of autologous blood through the central lumen of the balloon (hand or power injection, roller pump).[11] If, despite these measures, ischemia precludes adequate inflation, intra-aortic balloon pumping or CPS (rarely) should be initiated before continuing the procedure. To ensure maximal perfusion of non-target vessels, the guide catheter should be disengaged from the ostium during balloon inflation. Finally, when dilating a stenosis near

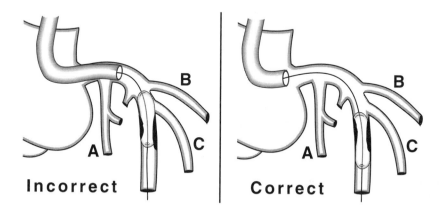

Figure 4.2   Guide Catheter and Balloon Positioning

Left panel: Incorrect technique. Deep intubation of the guide catheter obstructs flow down circumflex artery (A); mismatch between guide and proximal LAD obstructs flow down 1st diagonal (B); and poor balloon positioning obstructs flow down 2nd diagonal (C). **Right panel: Correct technique.** Guide is retracted 1-2 cm into the aorta after inflation of a properly positioned balloon. Coronary flow is maintained to branches A, B and C.

a branch-point, the balloon should be positioned to minimize obstruction of any uninvolved sidebranches (Figure 4.2). During balloon inflation, a small (3-ml) injection of contrast delivered through the guiding catheter can be used to detect impaired flow in the sidebranch; if present, prompt repositioning of the balloon is required.

2. **Assessing Results and Managing Complications.** Multiple views of the target lesion are required to accurately assess procedural outcome and exclude dissection, filling defect, residual stenosis, sidebranch occlusion, or flow impairment (Figure 1.6). Since acute closure in high-risk patients may carry in-hospital mortality rates as high as 50%, all efforts must be taken ensure an excellent angiographic result; stenting should be considered for residual diameter stenoses > 20-30%, suboptimal coronary flow, or the presence of significant dissection or thrombus. If there is haziness or dissection, repeat angiography should be performed in 15 minutes; a worsening angiographic appearance requires further intervention.

   Newer Imaging Modalities such as intravascular ultrasound (IVUS) and angioscopy may improve the operator's ability to evaluate lesion morphology, optimize procedural technique, and assess results. The advantages of IVUS include its ability to quantify lesion severity, assess lesion calcium and plaque orientation, and identify medial dissection (Chapter 31). IVUS can be used to answer the following questions: Is the lesion calcified, and if so, is the calcium superficial (amenable to Rotablator) or deep (DCA, PTCA or stent preferred)? Are further balloon inflations necessary to optimize stent expansion, apposition and symmetry? Angioscopy can identify intimal flaps and intraluminal thrombus (Chapter 32), and can be used to answer the following questions: Is thrombus present before or after intervention (i.e., are adjunctive lytics and/or prolonged heparin therapy required)? Is post-procedural haziness or filling defects due to dissection (stent indicated) or clot (stent contraindicated)? IVUS and angioscopy are valuable adjuncts during high-risk intervention, since proper device selection, optimal technique, and precise assessment of procedural results are critical to patient outcome.

3. **Adjunctive Pharmacotherapy (Chapter 34).** The most important advance surrounds the use of platelet glycoprotein receptor IIb/IIIa antagonists. Among high-risk patients (unstable angina, MI, high-risk lesion morphology) undergoing PTCA or atherectomy in the EPIC trial, use of bolus plus infusion ReoPro resulted in fewer ischemic complications at 30 days and 6 months compared to placebo. This exciting agent is detailed in Chapter 34. Other useful agents include intracoronary calcium blockers (for no-reflow and spasm) and intracoronary thrombolytics (for thrombus). New antithrombotic agents (hirudin, thromboxane receptor antagonists, serotonin inhibitors) await definition. Finally, local drug delivery systems may improve the efficacy of currently available agents (Chapter 35).

4. **Use of Regional and Systemic Support Systems.** A perfusion-balloon catheter or active hemoperfusion should be used when prolonged balloon inflations are required to treat resistant stenoses or perforations. Intra-aortic balloon pumping, which can increase coronary flow, improve ventricular functions and support the systemic circulation, is used for patients who develop

hypotension or heart failure in response to intraprocedural ischemia, and for all patients who develop acute closure and have either moderate-to-severe LV dysfunction or a large area of jeopardized myocardium. When efforts to reverse abrupt closure fail, a bailout or perfusion-balloon catheter should be placed across the lesion and IABP initiated; intermittent flushing of the bailout catheter with heparinized saline is required to prevent clotting during transport to the operating room. CPS is initiated for hypotension refractory to IABP and vasopressors, and for cardiac arrest not immediately responsive to ACLS (Chapter 6).

C. POSTPROCEDURAL CONSIDERATIONS

1. **Triage and Monitoring.** Patients should be transferred to a telemetry unit after high-risk intervention. Overnight observation in a cardiac intensive care unit is preferred if the procedure is complicated by acute closure, a suboptimal angiographic result, or the need for IABP or CPS. Complete blood counts and renal function should be monitored closely to identify bleeding and renal failure before they manifest clinically. If the procedure was uncomplicated and an excellent result was obtained, the pulmonary artery catheter and balloon pump may be removed after heparin wears off. In contrast, if the procedure was complicated by transient closure, thrombus, or slow-flow, invasive hemodynamic monitoring and support should remain in place for at least 24 hours. Due to a temporal association between heparin withdrawal and acute closure,[12] heparin should be tapered (rather than abruptly discontinued) at a time of day when emergency revascularization is feasible. Warfarin (INR 2-3) is frequently prescribed for 4-6 weeks when high-risk cases are complicated by post-procedural thrombus or suboptimal result, but there are no data to support this practice.

2. **Complications.** Recurrent chest pain associated with ECG changes or hemodynamic instability mandates immediate return to the cath lab to exclude abrupt closure. Asymptomatic hypotension may be caused by medications (sedatives, nitrates, calcium channel and β-blockers) and/or mild hypovolemia (NPO status, contrast-induced diuresis); more serious conditions such as tamponade, active retroperitoneal bleeding, and sepsis should be considered and promptly excluded.

LEFT MAIN DISEASE

Left main coronary disease is present in 7% and 15% of patients with stable and unstable angina, respectively. Among 1484 patients enrolled into the CASS Registry with > 50% obstruction of the left main, median survival was 13.3 years for the surgical group, but only 6.6 years for the medical group;[13] the survival benefit was confined mainly to patients with > 60% stenosis, particularly in the presence of LV dysfunction. In another report, 1-year survival was 95% for patients with left main disease and normal LV function, but only 61% when significant LV dysfunction was present.[14] PTCA of unprotected left main disease is technically feasible (success > 90%); however procedural & 3-year mortality for elective cases is 9% & 64%, and for acute MI is 50% & 70%![15] In contrast, Fajadet et al.[16] implanted stents in patients with unprotected (n =21) or protected (n = 13) left main disease; procedural success was 100% and stent thrombosis occurred in 3%. At 13 months, sudden death occurred in 3% and repeat PTCA for restenosis in 12%; no patient suffered an MI or required bypass surgery, and more than 90% were asymptomatic. In another report of stenting (n = 33), success was achieved in 94% and emergency CABG was required in only 3%; however, 9% of patients died within 3 months of the procedure.[17] Despite these results, unprotected left main stenosis remains a surgical disease; further studies of percutaneous intervention are required, particularly in patients who refuse surgery or who are poor surgical candidates. In contrast, when the left main is protected, catheter-based interventions can be preformed with acceptable early and late outcomes.[15]

* * * * *

REFERENCES

1. Kahn JK, Rutherford BD, McConahay DR, et al. In-hospital death following PTCA: complex patients or complex morphology. Circulation 1990;82:III-509.

2. Kimmel SE, Berlin JA, Strom BL, Laskey WK. Development and validation of a simplified predictive index for major complications in contemporary percutaneous transluminal coronary angioplasty practice. J Am Coll Cardiol 1995;26:931-938.

3. Ellis SG, Roubin GS, King SP III et al. In-hospital cardiac mortality after acute closure after coronary angioplasty: Analysis of risk factors from 8,207 procedures. J Am Coll Cardiol 1988;11:211.

4. Anto HR, Chou SY, Porush JG, et al. Infusion intravenous pyelography and renal function: Effects of hypertensic mannitol in patients with chronic renal insufficiency. Arch Intern Med 1981;141:1652.

5. Stack RS, Quigley PJ, Collins G, et al. Perfusion balloon catheter. Am J Cardiol 1988;61:77G.

6. Turi ZG, Campbell CA, Gottimukkala MV, et al. Preservation of distal coronary perfusion during prolonged balloon inflations with an autoperfusion angioplasty catheter. Circulation 1987;75:1275.

7. Zalewski A, Goldberg A, Dervan JP, et al. Myocardial protection during transient coronary artery occlusion in man: beneficial effects of regional β-adrenergic blockade. Circulation 1986;73:734.

8. Kern MJ, Pearson A, Woodruff R, et al. Hemodynamic and echocardiographic assessment of the effects of diltiazem during transient occlusion of the left anterior descending coronary artery during percutaneous transluminal coronary angioplasty. Am J Cardiol 1989;64:849.

9. Hombach V, Hopp HW, Fuchs M, et al. Beneficial effects of intracoronary nifedipine during percutaneous transluminal coronary angioplasty. Herz. 1986;11:232.

10. Hanet C, Rousseau M-F, Vincent MF, et al. Myocardial protection by intracoronary nicardipine administration during percutaneous transluminal coronary angioplasty. Am J Cardiol 1987;59;1035.

11. Banka VS, Trivedi A, Patal R, et al. Prevention of myocardial ischemia during coronary angioplasty: A simple new method for distal antegrade arterial blood perfusion. Am Heart J 1989;118:830-836.

12. Gabliani G, Deligonul U, Kern MJ, et al. Acute coronary occlusion occurring after successful percutaneous transluminal coronary angioplasty: Temporal relationship to discontinuation of anticoagulation. Am Heart J 1988;16:696.

13. Caracciolo EA, Davis KB, Sopko G, et al. Comparison of surgical and medical group survival in patients with left main coronary artery disease. Long-term CASS experience. Circulation 1995;91:2325-2334.

14. Conley MJ, Ely RI, Kisslo J, et al. The prognostic spectrum of left main stenosis. Circulation 178;57:947-952.

15. O'Keefe JH Jr., Hartzler GO, Rutherford BD, et al. Left main coronary angioplasty: early and late results of 127 acute and elective procedures. Am J Cardiol 1989;64:144-7.

16. Fajadet J, Brunel P, Jordan C, et al. Is stenting of left main coronary artery a reasonable procedure? Circulation 1995;92(8):I-355.

17. Itoh A, Colombo A, Hall P, et al. Stenting in protected and unprotected left main coronary artery: Immediate and follow-up results. J Am Coll Cardiol 1996;March Special Issue.

PTCA IN UNSTABLE ISCHEMIC SYNDROMES

Cindy L. Grines, M.D.
Gregg W. Stone, M.D.
William W. O'Neill, M.D.

ACUTE MYOCARDIAL INFARCTION

There are many deficiencies of intravenous thrombolytic therapy for acute myocardial infarction:
- Only 33% of acute MI patients receive thrombolytic therapy.
- Regardless of the dose or combination of thrombolytic agents given, most studies have demonstrated 80% patency, and only 55% of vessels achieve normal flow.
- There is a lag time to reperfusion with the median time being 45 minutes.
- No clinical markers accurately predict reperfusion.
- Patients who receive thrombolytic agents have a 15-30% incidence of recurrent ischemic events, and a 0.5-1.5% incidence of intracranial bleeding.

Because of these deficiencies, coronary angioplasty for AMI is being actively utilized. Angioplasty has been performed at different time intervals and for different reasons in acute myocardial infarction as outlined in Table 5.1.

A. **PRIMARY (DIRECT) PTCA.** Primary PTCA refers to angioplasty which is undertaken as a primary reperfusion strategy without prior thrombolytic therapy. The goal is to achieve reperfusion and salvage myocardium. There are many potential advantages and disadvantages to this approach (Table 5.2). Acute arterial patency can be achieved in 95-99% of patients. In early series, the reocclusion rate ranged between 8-15%. But with better understanding about the need for high dose heparin, aspirin, and ionic contrast media, in-hospital reocclusion has been reduced to 4-5%, and by 6 months only 9-13% of vessels have reoccluded.[1-4]

TABLE 5.1   Angioplasty in Acute MI: Various Approaches

Primary (Direct)	PTCA without prior thrombolytic therapy.
Rescue (Salvage)	PTCA after failed thrombolysis.
Immediate	PTCA immediately after successful thrombolysis.
Delayed	PTCA 1-7 days after thrombolysis.

TABLE 5.2   Primary (Direct) PTCA

Advantages Compared to Thrombolysis

- Allows reperfusion when thrombolytics contraindicated

- Early definition of coronary anatomy

- Allows risk stratification

- Superior acute vessel patency and TIMI 3 flow rates

- Reduced reocclusion

- Improved survival in high risk subjects

- Reduced reperfusion injury and myocardial rupture

- Reduced risk of intracranial hemorrhage

- Reduced rates of recurrent ischemia and reinfarction

- Shorter length of hospital stay

- Similar costs

Disadvantages Compared to Thrombolysis

- Facility constraints

- Skilled interventional cardiologist necessary

- Time delay in mobilizing lab

Low rates of recurrent ischemia and emergency CABG have been described, thus raising the question of whether on-site surgical backup is necessary. In fact, several reports are appearing describing outstanding results when primary PTCA is performed in an angiographic laboratory that does no elective PTCA. [5-8] Many studies have demonstrated serial improvement in left ventricular, and more recently, less reperfusion injury, cardiogenic shock and myocardial rupture has been described with primary PTCA compared with thrombolytics. Importantly, the prognosis of high risk patients, particularly those with cardiogenic shock, appears to be improved with primary angioplasty therapy compared to other treatment modalities.

1. **Non-Randomized Observational Series**. Twelve single centers[4,12-23] have reported their early experience in 2370 patients with primary PTCA. (Table 5.3)[23] Acute patency was restored in 93% of patients overall, with a 99% success rate in patients with single vessel disease. In these series, the mean in-hospital mortality rate after primary PTCA series averaged 7.4% which appears

TABLE 5.3. Single-center Series of Primary PTCA [23]

	n	In-Hospital Outcome %		
		Patency	Mortality	Reocclusion
Mid America [12]	1000	94	7.7	13
Brodie [13]	383	91	9	-
Beauchamp [14]	214	92	7.9	-
Nakagawa [15]	190	90	4	-
Rothbaum [16]	151	87	9	9
Miller [17]	127	92	8.6	8
Dageford [18]	65	97	1.5	9
O'Neill [4]	63	92	6.3	-
Kimura [19]	58	88	-	2
Topol [23]	47	86	6.3	13
Marco [20]	43	95	9.3	-
O'Neill [21]	29	83	6.8	8
Pooled	2370	93	7.4	10

favorable given that high risk patients including the elderly, patients with prior CABG, and those in cardiogenic shock were included. Cardiogenic shock, triple vessel disease, reduced ejection fraction, advanced age, anterior infarction, and failed PTCA have been identified as correlates of increased in-hospital mortality after primary PTCA.[24] A more recent single center experience reported a goodoutcome in 300 patients of which 62% were thrombolytic ineligible.[25] TIMI-3 flow was achieved in 95%, and mortality rates at 1 month, 1 year and 3 years was 5,9 and 13%, respectively.

The Myocardial Infarction, Triage and Intervention (MITI) investigators tracked the outcome of 3750 consecutive patients with MI at all ten hospitals in the metropolitan Seattle area having angiographic facilities over a three-year period.[26] MI was treated with thrombolytic therapy in 653 (17%) patients and primary PTCA in 441 (12%) patients. While most baseline characteristics were similar between these two groups, patients treated by PTCA were slightly more likely to be elderly, hypotensive or in shock, and not have ST-segment elevation (38 vs. 24%, p<.001). PTCA was successful in 88% of patients on a community-wide basis. In-hospital mortality was similar between patients treated with PTCA vs. thrombolysis. However, patients undergoing primary PTCA had fewer strokes (0.6 vs. 2.1%,p=.12), shorter hospital stay (7.0 vs. 8.1 days, p<.001), and

TABLE 5.4.   Primary PTCA in Thrombolytic Eligible vs Ineligible Patients [23]

	O'Keefe [12]	Brodie [13]	Pooled
Patients *n*	1000	383	1383
Thrombolytic eligible	57	74	61
Thrombolytic ineligible	43	26	39
PTCA Success*			
Thrombolytic eligible	96	92	94
Thrombolytic ineligible	92	88	90
Hospital Mortality			
Thrombolytic eligible	3	4	3
Thrombolytic ineligible	14	24	16

*Residual stenosis ≤40% (O'Keefe) or 50% (Brodie) with TIMI grade 2-3 flow

less recurrent ischemia (20 vs. 30%, p=.009). The Genentech registry has also reported their observations on primary PTCA with less favorable results. [27] Unfortunately, this registry targets hospitals with high utilization of thrombolytics, thus patients treated with primary PTCA are likely to be lytic ineligible or have other serious comorbidities. Thus, comparisons to a low-risk thrombolysis group is not warranted.

2.   **Thrombolytic Ineligible Patients**. Despite the benefits of reperfusion therapy, only a minority of patients (25-30%) are eligible to receive thrombolytic therapy. Mortality rates among patients excluded from thrombolytic trials have been far greater than those eligible for treatment. Cragg[28] analyzed 1471 patients with acute infarction admitted to our institution during the recruitment period for the TIMI-2B Study. Among the 15.6% of patients with infarction who met eligibility criteria, the in-hospital mortality rate was 3.9%. However, the mortality rate in patients who were ineligible for the study was 18.7% (p<0.001).

One of the major advantages of primary PTCA compared to thrombolytic therapy is that it may be applied to the majority of patients with MI. Angioplasty is being increasingly utilized in the management of patients ineligible for thrombolytic therapy. The results in unselected patients enrolled at two centers are outlined in Table 5.4.[12,13] Brodie reported that ineligible patients were more likely to be older, female gender, have prior MI, multivessel coronary disease, and lower ejection fraction. PTCA in lytic-ineligible patients was performed with a high success rate and resulted in improved LV function. Despite this, mortality rates remained high in lytic-ineligible patients, which appeared to be related to the underlying severity of illness.

TABLE 5.5   Outcome Based on Reperfusion Strategy Using TIMI-2B Criteria of Lytic Eligibility [32]

	Lytic Eligible			Lytic Ineligible		
	PTCA	tPA	p	PTCA	tPA	p
Number	127	117	-	68	83	-
In-hospital Events (%)						
Death	2.4	1.7	NS	2.9	13.2	.015
Reinfarction	3.1	8.5	0.7	1.5	3.6	NS
Death or reinfarction	5.5	9.4	NS	4.4	15.7	.025
Recurrent ischemia	11.8	29.0	.008	7.3	26.5	.002
Stroke	0	1.7	NS	0	6.0	.046
Intracranial bleed	0	0	NS	0	4.8	.075
Hospital stay (days)	7.3	7.9	NS	7.8	9.2	.047
6 month cumulative (%)						
Death	3.9	1.7	NS	2.9	15.7	.009
Death or reinfarction	8.7	12.8	NS	7.3	22.9	.009

In the PAMI-1 and PAMI-2 trials, lytic ineligibility was found to be predictive of a poor outcome. [2,29-31] In PAMI-1, since half the patients were randomized to tPA, the enrollment criteria required that all were lytic eligible using the expanded criteria of the 1990's, (no age limit, time extended to 12 hours, remote strokes acceptable). However, when lytic eligibility was defined according to the restrictive TIMI-2B criteria, major differences in outcome favoring PTCA were observed (Table 5.5). [25,32]

Certain subsets of lytic ineligible patients are ideally suited for primary PTCA, ie primary PTCA avoids intracranial bleeding in the elderly, provides late reperfusion with high patency rates (patency rates decline over time with thrombolytics), allows vein graft occlusions to be treated (low patency rates with IV thrombolytics due to large thrombus burden, stagnant flow preventing delivery of drug to the thrombus) and acute cath allows the diagnosis to be confirmed and treatment provided in patients without ST-elevation. (Table 5.6) [23,33] To date, randomized trials comparing PTCA to medical therapy in thrombolytic ineligible patients are limited. The 50 patient SMART trial (Study of Medicine vs Angioplasty Reperfusion Trial) found reduced ischemia and reinfarction in the PTCA arm. [34] We are in the process of completing the 200 patient MATE (Medicine versus Angiography for Thrombolytic Exclusions) trial that will address this important issue. Unfortunately, given the high success rates of PTCA, it has been difficult to convince physicians to randomize high risk patients in this study. This recruitment has been slow and enrolled patients are lower risk than anticipated.

TABLE 5.6   Primary PTCA in Saphenous Vein Graft Occlusions [23]

	n	PTCA Success (%)	In-Hospital Mortality (%)
Brodie [13]	12	75	25
O'Keefe [12]	130	90	10
Grines [33]	15	80	13
Pooled	157	87	11

3. **Cardiogenic Shock.** Given the poor outcome with thrombolysis, cardiogenic shock patients are typically taken to the catheterization laboratory for angiography, placement of intraaortic balloon pump and attempted reperfusion with PTCA or bypass surgery. Non-randomized series suggest a survival benefit with this approach. (Table 5.7).[35-52]

Based on these observations, cardiogenic shock patients treated with PTCA appear to have improved survival compared to patients treated with lytics (mortality 70%) or no therapy (mortality 90%). However, some have suggested that patients undergoing PTCA are highly selected, and patients destined to die are not taken to the lab. In the GUSTO-1 trial, using multivariate analysis to adjust for more favorable baseline characteristics in patients undergoing revascularization, an aggressive strategy of PTCA or CABG was independently associated with a reduced 30 day mortality (odds ratio 0.43, p=0.0001).[49] Unfortunately, the GUSTO trial found that early intervention was performed infrequently, and only 20% of all shock cases received balloon pumps.[53]

To date, randomized data comparing mechanical revascularization to medical therapy are not available. The ongoing SHOCK trial is a multicenter, randomized trial testing the hypothesis that emergency revascularization with PTCA or CABG will lower 30 day mortality in patients with cardiogenic shock, compared to patients who first undergo initial medical stabilization (including thrombolysis, IABP, mechanical ventilation) and later revascularization if indicated. As of December 15, 1995, 130 patients have been randomized with a target sample size of 328.

4. **Thrombolytic-Eligible Patients**
   a. **Registry Experience.** To examine the outcome of primary PTCA in lytic eligible patients, the multicenter, prospective *Primary Angioplasty Revascularization (PAR)* study performed acute catheterization in 271 and PTCA in 245 (90%) patients.[54] Patency (TIMI 2-3 flow) was achieved mechanically or spontaneously in 99%, with TIMI 3 flow in 97% of patients. Clinical outcome was favorable with recurrent ischemia in 10%, reinfarction in 3%, stroke in 1%, and death in 3.7% of patients. Follow-up catheterization at six months demonstrated persistent patency in 87%, and a striking improvement in LVEF (51.3% to 57.5%, p<.0001). [3]

TABLE 5.7 PTCA for Cardiogenic Shock

Study	n	PTCA Success (%)	Overall Survival (%)	Survival with reperfusion (%)	Survival without reperfusion (%)
Kaplan [35]	88	61	42	65	29
O'Keefe [12]	79	82	56	63	21
Lee [36]	69	71	55	69	20
Gacioch [37]	48	73	46	61	7
Bengtson [38]	46	85	54	NR	NR
Hibbard [39]	45	62	56	71	29
Moosvi [40]	38	76	53	62	22
Eltchaninoff [41]	33	76	64	76	25
Brown [42]	28	61	43	58	18
O'Neill [43]	27	88	70	75	33
Meyer [44]	25	88	53	59	0
Lee [45]	24	54	50	77	18
Brodie [13]	22	68	50	NR	NR
Seydoux [46]	21	85	57	67	0
Heuser [47]	10	60	70	100	25
Shani [48]	9	67	67	83	0
Disler [49]	7	71	43	60	0
Verna [50]	7	100	86	86	NR
Shock Registry [51]	55	69	40	NR	NR
GUSTO-1 [52]	406	NR	62	NR	39*

*reperfusion status unknown since caths not performed.

Pooling the results from the PAR registry[54] and the two centers that have reported subgroup analysis in lytic-eligible patients,[12,13] patency was achieved in 97% of the 1045 patients, with a <40-50% residual stenosis in approximately 90%, and in-hospital mortality of 3.4%. These results compare favorably to the 60-80% patency rate, 70-85% residual stenosis, 3.7-10.7% mortality and 30% late reocclusion rates reported from large thrombolytic series.[55-67]

b. **Randomized Trials.** Of course, due to selection bias, registry data may not be an accurate assessment of the efficacy of a certain treatment. Therefore, many trials were undertaken comparing primary PTCA to thrombolytics. (Tables 5.8 and 5.9)[1,29,68-73]

TABLE. 5.8   Selected Trials Comparing Primary PTCA to Thrombolytic Therapy

Trial	Design	Comments
PAMI-1 [29]	395 patients with acute MI randomized to tPA or primary PTCA. Combined endpoint: Death or recurrent MI in-hospital and at 6 months.	PTCA associated with a lower rate of stroke, recurrent ischemia, and combined MI and death; a shortened length of hospital stay was also observed. High risk patients observed the most benefit.
Zwolle trial [1]	142 patients randomized to SK or primary PTCA. Endpoint: LV ejection fraction	PTCA associated with greater patency, decreased rate of recurrent ischemia, decreased rate of recurrent MI, and increased LV ejection fraction; a shortened length of hospital stay was also observed.
Mayo Clinic trial [68]	108 patients randomized to tPA or primary PTCA. Endpoint: infarct size	PTCA associated with decreased rate of recurrent ischemia, decreased length of hospital stay, and a trend toward reduced cost. No effect on infarct size was seen.
GUSTO II-B	1100 patients randomized to accelerated tPA or PTCA with second randomization to heparin or hirudin. Endpoint: death, re-MI, stroke.	Ongoing trial to be completed in 1996.
SHOCK trial	328 Shock patients will be randomized to emergency mechanical revascularization (PTCA or CABG) vs medical stabilization (thrombolysis, IABP) with later revascularization	Ongoing trial.
AIR PAMI	430 high-risk patients who present to a hospital not equipped to do PTCA will be randomized to transfer for acute cath vs immediate thrombolytics.	To begin in 1996.

In general, these trials demonstrated that primary PTCA was superior to thrombolysis with regard to high acute patency and TIMI-3 flow rates, reduced frequency of recurrent ischemia, reocclusion, reinfarction, stroke, and death and resulted in a shorter length of hospital stay. In a metaanalysis by Michels,[73] (Table 5.9) PTCA treated patients sustained a significant reduction in death (odds ratio 0.56) and combined death and nonfatal MI (odds ratio 0.53). A poor PTCA success rate (80%) was observed in the Riberiro study, and was likely related to the fact that no aspirin was administered pre-PTCA, only 10,000 units of heparin was given, ACTs were not monitored and PTCA was performed in all patients regardless of coronary anatomy.[71] Indeed, PTCA was successful in 90% of patients "well suited", and in only 40% of patients believed not to be "well suited" for the procedure.

TABLE. 5.9 **Metaanalysis of Primary PTCA Versus Thrombolytic Therapy: Major Cardiac Events** [73]

| | Death | | | | Death or Nonfatal Reinfarction | | | |
| | 6 Weeks | | 1 Year | | 6 Weeks | | 1 Year | |
Trials	PTCA	Lytic	PTCA	Lytic	PTCA	Lytic	PTCA	Lytic
O'Neill [69]	2/29	1/27	-	-	3/29	2/27	-	-
DeWood [70]	3/46	2/44	4/46	2/44	3/46	2/44	4/46	2/44
PAMI-1 [28]	5/195	13/200	12/195	20/200	10/195	24/200	-	-
Zwolle [1]	3/152	11/149	8/152	14/149	5/152	23/149	-	-
Mayo Clinic [68]	2/47	2/56	3/47	2/56	2/47	2/56	3/47	4/56
Ribeiro [71]	3/50	1/50	3/50	2/50	5/50	2/50	4/50	3/50
Elizaga [72]	3/52	7/48	3/52	8/48	7/52	8/48	7/52	11/48
Pooled	21/571 (3.7%)	37/574 (6.4%)	33/542 (6.1%)	48/547 (8.8%)	35/571 (6.1%)	63/574 (11.0%)	18/195 (9.2%)	20/198 (10.1%)

Adapted from Michels (with permission)

O'Neill performed a pooled analysis of raw data from the PAMI-1, Mayo and Zwolle studies. [74] He found that primary PTCA was associated with a significant reduction in rates of reinfarction (2.0 vs 7.9%, p<.001), stroke (0.3 vs 2.5%, p=.007), and death (2.5 vs 6.4%, p=.008) when compared to thrombolytic treated patients. High risk patients (age > 70, anterior MI, HR > 100 or Killip class > 1) were found to have the most striking reduction in death (3.2 vs 9.8%, p=.005) and stroke (0.5 vs 3.6%, p =.04). Although low risk patients had similar low mortality rates between PTCA and lytic treated groups, a reduction in recurrent ischemia, reinfarction and shorter length of hospital stay was observed.

The mechanism of improved critical outcome with PTCA is likely to be multifactorial. It has been well established that TIMI-3 flow is an important determinant of left ventricular functional recovery and survival. [75] A metaanalysis of angiographic trials after thrombolysis [64] and the GUSTO (Global Utilization of Streptokinase and Tissue plasminogen activator for Occluded coronary arteries) angiographic substudy [75] reported acute patency rates after thrombolysis to range from 50% (with streptokinase) to 80% (after accelerated tPA) with normal antegrade flow in only 40-52% of patients. Conversely, the strategy of primary PTCA resulted in acute patency rates of 98-99%, normal flow in 93-94% of vessels and < 50% stenosis in 93-97% of patients. [1,3,4,29,68,74] Differences in rates of reocclusion may also impact on prognosis. Late angiographic follow-up has demonstrated that only 60-70% of vessels with successful thrombolysis remained patent. [76-80] In contrast, patency rates after PTCA remained high (87-91%) when measured 3-6 months after MI. (Table 5.10 and 5.11)[1,3,4]

An additional advantage is that emergency catheterization with early definition of coronary anatomy also allows the therapy to be individually tailored. In the PAMI trials, 5% of patients randomized to PTCA did not undergo the procedure due to severe multivessel or left main disease requiring bypass surgery. These patients had favorable outcomes.[29-31,5] An additional 5% had spontaneous reperfusion with no high-grade stenosis, thus avoided the complications of thrombolytics and were able to be discharged early. Moreover, use of acute catheterization to risk-stratify and triage therapy is of utmost importance. Using clinical and angiographic predictors of risk, we were able to detect an 18 fold difference in mortality between high and low risk patients enrolled in the PAMI-2 trial (p<.0001).[31]

Moreover, the PAR, PAMI-1, Mayo and Zwolle studies[1,29,68,81,82] demonstrated that the cost of primary PTCA was equal to or less than that of thrombolysis. These studies did not attempt to discharge patients early or reduce testing. The multicenter 1100 patient PAMI-2 trial performed emergency catheterization and PTCA (when indicated) and stratified patients into high and low risk groups (low-risk required age $\leq$ 70 years, 1-2 vessel disease, EF > 45%, successful PTCA of a native coronary, and no serious arrhythmias).[30] Low-risk patients were randomized to traditional care (CCU admission, 5 days hospitalization, non-invasive testing) versus accelerated care (admission to an elective PTCA unit, discharge on day 3 with no noninvasive testing).[83] Low-risk patients did very well with an in-hospital mortality rate of 0.4% (similar to elective PTCA). Early and late clinical outcomes were similar in the traditional and accelerated care groups. As expected, skipping the CCU phase of hospitalization and discharging patients early resulted in a significant $4000 cost savings. 84

TABLE 5.10   Angiographic Follow-up after Primary PTCA

	n	Time (months)	Occluded(%)	Restenosis (%)*
SAMI [4]	90	6	13	38
PAR [3]	154	6	13	45
Zwolle [1]	130	3	5	20

* Vessel patent with stenosis

TABLE 5.11   Primary PTCA: Target Vessel Revascularization after Hospital Discharge

	n	Time (months)	PTCA (n)	CABG (n)
PAR [3]	271	6	42	9
PAMI-1 [29]	175	6	24	13
MAYO [68]	47	6	2	2
ZWOLLE [1]	152	12	21	10

Since high-risk patients appear to have the greatest benefit from primary PTCA, and delayed performance of primary PTCA does not influence clinical outcomes or PTCA success rates, we have initiated the multicenter, international AIR-PAMI trial. This trial will randomize high-risk MI patients who present to a facility which cannot perform PTCA, to receive either transfer for emergency cath versus IV thrombolysis and no routine transfer. The primary endpoint is the combined occurrence of death, recurrent MI or disabling stroke, with an anticipated sample size of 430 patients.

5. **Recommendations.** Based on the available data, primary PTCA should be strongly considered in thrombolytic ineligible, high risk thrombolytic eligible patients (anterior MI, age > 70, HR > 100, BP < 100 mmHg or Killip Class > 1) and cardiogenic shock cases. Even in low risk thrombolytic eligible patients, primary PTCA should be considered since it reduces recurrent ischemia, reinfarction and length of hospital stay. No firm recommendations can be made regarding what time delay is acceptable in mobilizing the PTCA laboratory. The mean time required to perform angiography in the PAMI-1 trial was 60 minutes, and in GUSTO-2B it was reported to be 75 minutes. PTCA success and mortality rates are not dependent on time, and it appears that even a PTCA delay of ≥ 2 hours may be superior to earlier thrombolysis.

B. RESCUE (SALVAGE) PTCA FOR FAILED THROMBOLYSIS (TABLE 5.12)

1. **Observational Series**. Patients with an occluded infarct artery (TIMI 0-1 flow) or suboptimal flow (TIMI-2 flow) 90 minutes after thrombolytic therapy have worse left ventricular function, an increased incidence of mechanical defects, and increased early mortality.[75] Rescue PTCA is performed in this group to establish reperfusion, salvage myocardium, and improve healing.

In an early meta-analysis of 12 rescue PTCA studies[85-94] (Table 5.12), acute patency was restored by PTCA in 71-100% of occluded coronary arteries after failed thrombolysis (mean 80%). However, 18% of vessels reoccluded and LVEF failed to improve by hospital discharge. The in-hospital mortality in these patients averaged 10.6%.

TABLE 5.12   RESCUE CORONARY ANGIOPLASTY [85]

Study	n	In-Hospital Outcome (%)		
		Success	Reocclusion	Mortality
Topol [85]	86	73	29	10.4
Califf [86]	52	85	10	-
Belenkie [85]	16	81	-	6.7
Fung [87]	13	92	16	7.6
Topol [103]	22	86	3	0
Grines [89]	12	100	8	-
Holmes [90]	34	71	-	11
Grines [91]	10	90	12	10
O'Connor [92]	90	89	14	17
Baim [93]	37	92	26	5.4
Whitlow [94]	44	85	27	-
Ellis [85]	24	78	20	13
Belenkie [100]	28	89	-	14
Abbottsmith [95]	192	88	21	9.9
GUSTO [98]	214	90	12	-
CORAMI [101]	72	90	7	4
RESCUE [99]	78	92	8	5

Adapted with permission *from* Ellis [85]

Abbottsmith performed a post-hoc analysis of patients from the first 5 TAMI trials, and found that the in-hospital and late mortality of patients who left the cath lab with a patent infarct artery were similar in groups who had reperfusion established by successful thrombolysis (n=607) or by rescue PTCA after failed thrombolysis (n=169).[95] However, patients requiring rescue PTCA to achieve patency had a 2-fold greater rate of reocclusion, which was associated with less regional and global LV functional recovery. Moreover, in patients who failed rescue PTCA, the mortality was 39%.

In the TIMI-4 trial, rescue PTCA was attempted in 57 patients, and was successful in 88%.[96] In-hospital death, reocclusion, recurrent MI, CHF, shock and LVEF were similar in the 50 patients in whom rescue PTCA was successful and the 310 patients not undergoing immediate PTCA. Patients who failed rescue PTCA, however, had a 30% mortality rate.

In the largest observational series of rescue PTCA, 270 patients underwent rescue PTCA after failed streptokinase.[97] PTCA success was 91.5% but reocclusion and mortality rates were higher in patients with TIMI 0-2 flow compared to those with TIMI 3 flow after PTCA (reocclusion 28.8 vs 16%, p =.009, death 28.6 vs 3.9%, P =.001). As in other studies, PTCA failure occurred predominantly in patients with cardiogenic shock or multivessel coronary disease.

Although rescue PTCA studies demonstrated that PTCA success was independent of the type of lytic agent used, reocclusion was observed to be highest with tPA in early studies, (ranging between 20-30%). With greater understanding of the importance of aspirin, high dose heparin, and monitoring ACT's, reocclusion rates after rescue PTCA appear to be decreasing. In the GUSTO angiographic substudy, 214 patients underwent rescue PTCA and there was no difference in immediate patency or in-hospital reocclusion between the various thrombolytic regimens.[98] Likewise, reocclusion at 24 hours occurred in only 4% of patients in the TIMI-4 study.[96]

2. **Randomized Trials**. The results of a few randomized trials of rescue PTCA have been reported. [62,99-101] The TAMI-5 Study Group[69] randomized 575 thrombolytic patients to either immediate cath with rescue PTCA for failed thrombolysis, versus a deferred predischarge catheterization strategy. Rescue PTCA was performed in 18% of the immediate group, with an 83% success rate. As a result, 96% of the immediate cath group left the cath lab with a patent infarct artery, and greater predischarge patency (94 vs. 90%, p=.065), improved regional motion in the infarct zone, and a reduced rate of recurrent ischemia was observed. Acute catheterization appeared to be safe, with similar nadir hematocrit and transfusion rates between the 2 groups.

In the multicenter, international Randomized Evaluation of Salvage angioplasty with Combined Utilization of Endpoints (RESCUE) study, 151 anterior MI patients with angiographically documented TIMI grade 0-1 flow after lytic therapy were randomized to rescue PTCA vs. medical therapy.[99] The benefits of rescue PTCA were most likely underestimated by this study due to the exclusion of patients with prior MI by protocol, and investigator bias to dilate (and therefore not to randomize, n = 134) other high risk patients, such as those with ongoing ischemia, hemodynamic compromise or proximal LAD occlusion. Despite this, at 30 days, the patients undergoing rescue PTCA had a higher exercise LVEF (45 vs. 40%, p=.04), and a reduction in the combined endpoint of death or class III-IV CHF (6.4 vs. 16.6%, p=.05). These differences were apparent out to 1 year of follow-up.

Thus, a strategy of immediate catheterization followed by rescue PTCA for failed thrombolysis can be performed safely, has a high success rate, improves regional wall motion, exercise LV function, and may reduce the risk of CHF, shock or death in patients with a large amount of myocardium at risk. The prognosis of patients in whom rescue PTCA is successful appears to be improved, and similar to that following successful thrombolysis. Patients requiring rescue PTCA, however, remain at increased risk for reocclusion and early death, especially if unsuccessful. The high rates of death and reocclusion after rescue PTCA may partly be explained by selection of a high-risk group of patients who have already demonstrated resistance to pharmacologic reperfusion, possibly due to hypotension, large thrombus burden, or platelet rich thrombi - factors unfavorable to the performance of PTCA. To address these issues, the *Rescue PAMI* Study Group plans to investigate the role of the new glycoprotein IIb/IIIa receptor antagonist, 7E3, in a prospective, randomized, multicenter trial of PTCA in patients who have TIMI 0-2 flow after thrombolysis. Additionally, the RESCUE-2 study plans to randomize patients with TIMI-2 flow after thrombolysis to PTCA versus medical therapy.

3. **Recommendations**: Since clinical signs of reperfusion are not precise, we perform catheterization in any thrombolytic patient with ongoing chest pain, hemodynamic problems, or an asymptomatic patient who is less than 12 hours from MI onset with persistent ST elevation in anterior leads, or multiple ECG leads. PTCA is undertaken if the vessel has TIMI 0-1 flow (in an asymptomatic patient), or any significant lesion regardless of TIMI flow, in a symptomatic patient.

C. IMMEDIATE PTCA IN ASYMPTOMATIC PATIENTS FOLLOWING SUCCESSFUL THROMBOLYSIS

Following successful thrombolysis, a high-grade residual stenosis is present in the majority of patients and "immediate PTCA" is performed in hope of preventing reocclusion and augmenting recovery of ventricular function.

1. **Randomized Trials** There have been several randomized trials investigating the role of immediate PTCA after successful thrombolysis. (Table 5.13)[62,73,100,102-104] These studies demonstrated that routine performance of immediate PTCA in patients with successful thrombolysis was associated with a higher transfusion rate and need for emergency CABG, a trend toward increased mortality, and no improvement in pre-discharge ejection fraction.

2. **Limitations of studies**. Several limitations of these studies, however, should be mentioned. In only one of the studies did patients undergoing immediate PTCA routinely receive pre-procedural aspirin, the lack of which is known to increase the risk of acute vessel closure following elective PTCA. Only 10,000 units of heparin were administered and ACT's were not monitored. Immediate PTCA was performed on modest (>60%) stenoses; it is unknown whether restricting PTCA to vessels with high grade residual stenoses (≥90%) or TIMI-2 flow which are prone to reocclusion[79,105] and associated with a worse clinical outcome, would have altered the results.

3. **Recommendations**. Based on these data, it is our approach to avoid PTCA after successful thrombolysis unless the patient demonstrates ongoing ischemia, hemodynamic instability, a subtotal occlusion or TIMI-2 flow. If at the time of catheterization the patient's symptoms have resolved and TIMI grade 3 flow is present, PTCA is usually not performed (if the patient has received thrombolytics).

TABLE 5.13   Trials Comparing Immediate PTCA to Conservative Therapy after Thrombolysis [73]

Trials	Death				Death or Nonfatal Reinfarction			
	At 6 Weeks		At 1 Year		At 6 Weeks		At 1 Year	
	Inv	Cons	Inv	Cons	Inv	Cons	Inv	Cons
Immediate vs no PTCA								
Erbel [73]	12/103	17/103	18/103	22/103	25/103	34/103	32/103	40/103
ECSG [104]	12/183	5/184	17/183	10/184	20/183	17/184	29/183	31/184
TAMI-1 Pilot [103]	1/15	0/13	-	-	1/15	2/13	-	-
TAMI-5 [62]	16/287	13/288	24/287	20/288	21/287	24/288	33/287	34/288
TIMI-2A [102]	15/195	17/197	16/195	20/197	26/195	26/197	30/195	31/197
Total	56/783 (7.2%)	52/785 (6.6%)	75/765 (9.8%)	72/785 (9.2%)	93/783 (11.9%)	103/785 (13.1%)	124/768 (16.1%)	136/772 (17.6%)
Immediate vs delayed PTCA								
TAMI-1 [103]	3/99	1/98	6/99	2/98	3/99†	1/98	6/99†	2/98†
TIMI-2A [102]	15/195	11/194	16/195	15/194	26/195	17/194	30/195	25/194
Belenkie [100]	1/50	1/39	-	-	4/50	1/39	-	-
Total	19/344 (5.5%)	13/331 (3.9%)	22/294 (7.5%)	17/292 (5.8%)	33/344 (9.6%)	19/331 (5.7%)	36/294 (12.2%)	27/292 (9.2%)

Abbreviations: Inv = invasive, Cons = conservative
Adapted with permission from Michels [73]

TABLE 5.14   Delayed PTCA After Thrombolysis

Study	n	Drug	LVEF (%)		Reinfarction (%)		Mortality (%)	
			Inv	Cons	Inv	Cons	Inv	Cons
TIMI-2B [106]	3262	rPA	50	50	5.9	5.4	5.2	4.6
SWIFT [107]	800	APSAC	52	51	12.1	8.2	2.7	3.3
Barbash [108]	194	tPA	50	49	-	-	8.2	3.8
Van den Brand [109]	218	tPA	51	50	2.7	1.0	1.8	2.9
Ozbek [110]	324	SK	55	55	11.3	16.8	8.8	6.0

Abbreviations: Inv = Invasive strategy (routine predischarge angioscopy with PTCA if appropriate), Cons = Conservative strategy (angiography/PTCA only for spontaneous or inducible ischemia

D. DELAYED PTCA IN ASYMPTOMATIC PATIENTS FOLLOWING SUCCESSFUL THROMBOLYSIS. Delayed PTCA refers to angioplasty performed electively one to seven days after thrombolysis in infarct vessels that are patent but contain a stenosis. As with immediate PTCA, the goal of this approach is to reduce residual stenosis in the hopes of preventing reocclusion and augmenting recovery of ventricular function.

1. **Randomized Trials.** Two large trials[106,107] and several smaller studies[108-110] have compared the invasive and conservative approaches. (Table 5.14) There were no differences between the invasive and conservative approaches with regard to the endpoints of death, reinfarction, or LVEF. In the TIMI-2B trial, predischarge exercise testing was more frequently positive with the conservative approach (18 vs. 13%, p<.001), and at six weeks the increase in LVEF from rest to exercise was less (2.3 vs. 3.3%, p=.02).[106] Subset analysis of the TIMI-2B trial[111] revealed higher in-hospital mortality in patients with prior MI treated conservatively (12 vs. 4%, p<.001), but lower in-hospital mortality in diabetic patients without prior MI treated conservatively (4 vs. 15%, p<.001). The TIMI investigators concluded that the invasive approach offered no significant advantages over the conservative approach (except possibly in patients with prior MI), and was more complex and costly.

2. **Limitations of studies.** Several limitations in study design may have contributed to the results of the TIMI-2B study: 1) The intention to treat analysis may have masked any beneficial effect of delayed PTCA. Protocol PTCA was only performed in 54% of patients in the "invasive" arm, vs. 13% in the "conservative" arm. Given this relatively small difference, any favorable effects of the PTCA procedure would tend to be attenuated by the patients in each arm not undergoing PTCA in an intention to treat analysis. 2) 40% of the deaths occurred within 24 hours and 69% of deaths occurred in patients who never received PTCA or CABG, thus were entirely unrelated to the revascularization strategy. In fact, if one reviews the data based on the treatment received,

regardless of the randomization strategy, if mechanical revascularization was performed, the mortality rate was lower (2.6 vs 6.7%, p =.0001) (Table 5.15) 3) Patients undergoing PTCA received inadequate doses of heparin and aspirin, which may have contributed to the high PTCA complication rates. After decreasing the therapeutic intravenous heparin drip rate by 50% 2-3 hours before catheterization, only a 5000 unit heparin bolus was given during PTCA and ACTs were not monitored. In addition, patients were not given aspirin until after 24 hours and the dose was only 81mg/day. As the majority of PTCA procedures were performed between 18 and 24 hours, many patients underwent dilatation without effective anti-platelet coverage. 4) Total occlusions, which were found in 12% of infarct vessels, were not dilated by protocol, thus the groups most likely to benefit were not treated.

3. **Recommendations**. Although the available data do not support the performance of delayed PTCA in an asymptomatic patient post lysis, due to the significant limitations of the studies and the high (25-30%) late reocclusion rate after thrombolysis, revascularization may be warranted in the following situations:

   a. History of prior MI
   b. TIMI 2 flow
   c. Multivessel coronary disease
   d. Stenosis ≥ 90% supplying a moderate or large amount of myocardium
   e. Physiologic significance of lesion documented in the lab by intravascular ultrasound or doppler.

TABLE 5.15   TIMI 2-B Mortality [106]

	Invasive		Conservative		
		Mortality		**Mortality**	
	n	**(%)**	*n*	**(%)**	**P**
Intention to treat	1636	5.2	1626	4.6	NS
Received assigned therapy	1084	2.4	1319	5	.0009
Did not receive assigned therapy	552	10.7	307	3.3	.0001

Regardless of randomization strategy, if mechanical revascularization was performed, the mortality was lower (2.6 vs 6.7%, p = .0001)

E. DELAYED PTCA OF AN OCCLUDED VESSEL IN ASYMPTOMATIC PATIENTS

1. **Observational trials.** After failed thrombolysis, successful delayed PTCA of the occluded infarct related artery may result in improved exercise LVEF,[112] and improved LV volumes.[114] A patent infarct vessel has been demonstrated to improve survival independent of myocardial salvage.[115-117] This has been attributed to improved infarct healing resulting in less left ventricular dilatation, fewer aneurysms, reduced thrombus formation, and decreased arrhythmogenesis.

2. **Randomized trials.** The TAMI-6 trial randomized a small cohort (n=71) of patients with an occluded vessel at 48 hours to PTCA versus conservative care.[118] Although the rest and exercise LVEF was greater in the PTCA group at 6 weeks, this benefit was not sustained and a high reocclusion rate (40%) was noted by 6 months..

3. **Recommendations.** Due to the limited data available, firm recommendations cannot be given. We tend to perform late PTCA of an occluded vessel in an asymptomatic patient if the vessel supplies a large amount of myocardium or if there are collaterals or any LV contractility that indicates the myocardium may be viable. Given the high reocclusion rates, we are more likely to give prolonged anticoagulation, ticlopidine or utilize coronary stents.

F. PTCA FOR POST MI ISCHEMIA

1. **Randomized trials.** PTCA has been commonly used for post MI ischemia after thrombolytic therapy. To determine its clinical benefit, the DANAMI study[119] enrolled 1008 patients less than 70 years of age who had post MI angina or an abnormal exercise test after thrombolysis. Patients were randomized to receive a mechanical intervention (n=503) vs conservative therapy (n=505). Among patients randomized to an intervention, catheterization demonstrated significant disease in 92%, and 85% underwent either PTCA or CABG. These procedures were performed with low complication rates as demonstrated in Table 5.16 and resulted in improved clinical outcome out to 24 months follow-up (Table 5.17).

2. **Recommendations.** Patients with post MI angina or an abnormal stress test should undergo catheterization and mechanical revascularization with PTCA or CABG if a significant lesion is present.

TABLE 5.16   DANAMI Revascularization Strategy [119]

	PTCA (n=274)	CABG (n=176)
Randomized to procedure	18 days	38 days
Procedural MI (%)	0.7	1.2
Death [6]	0	1.2
Stroke (%)	0	0.6

TABLE 5.17 DANAMI Clinical Events [119]

	Interventional (%)	Conservative (%)	p
Anti ischemic drugs			
3 mos	56	81	.001
6 mos	49	79	.001
12 mos	43	75	.001
Hosp. for unstable angina			
3 mos	22	52	.001
6 mos	23	58	.001
12 mos	22	43	.001
Major events at 24 mos			
MI	5.6	10.5	.004
Death	3.6	4.6	.45

UNSTABLE ANGINA

Many patients with unstable angina can be successfully managed with medical therapy alone. However, in-hospital death (1%) and infarction (7-9%) rates, and 1-year mortality (8-18%) and infarction (14-22%) rates remain substantial.[120] As our understanding of the pathophysiology of unstable angina has broadened, the interventional approach to these patients has undergone evolution.

A. **PATHOPHYSIOLOGY.** Coronary thrombus plaque rupture and plaque hemorrhage are observed commonly in patients who die from unstable angina.[121] It has been demonstrated that patients with a history of antecedent angina are more likely to have critical atherosclerotic coronary disease. Conversely, patients who present with de novo unstable angina generally have ulceration and thrombus. Angiographic studies performed within the early hours of presentation have demonstrated a high incidence of intracoronary thrombus and plaque rupture, depicted as complex lesions containing irregular, ulcerated borders with overhangs or haziness. Many of these culprit lesions tend to improve with time and have variably been attributed to intrinsic fibrinolysis, treatment with aspirin and heparin, and plaque remodeling. Thrombolytic therapy may also improve the angiographic appearance if an intracoronary thrombus is documented. Unfortunately, after thrombolysis, clinical improvement has been variable, is not predicted by angiographic improvement increases the rate of infarction , thus thrombolytics are not recommended in unstable angina patients.[120]

B. SUCCESS AND COMPLICATION RATES OF PTCA IN UNSTABLE ANGINA. There have been many reports of successful coronary angioplasty in patients with unstable angina. Although the technical success rate among unstable angina patients is similar to chronic angina patients, the incidence of periprocedural complications is increased. (Table 5.18)[122-127] However, the procedural risk depends upon the type of unstable angina. Patients with repeated episodes of rest angina associated with ST segment or T wave changes have a worse prognosis with medical therapy[120] and more complications with PTCA (Table 5.19)[127-136] and new devices.[137-139]

TABLE 5.18   PTCA For Stable Versus Unstable Angina [137]

Investigators	Angina Type	n	In-Hospital Outcome (%)			
			Success	CABG	MI	Death
Faxon [137]	Stable	214	64	-	-	0.4
	Unstable	442	61	-	-	0.9
Perry [128]	Stable	175	86	3.8	5	1
	Unstable	105	87	3.8	9	1
Kamp [137]	Stable	506	83	9.2	4.3	0.6
	Unstable	334	87	10	9	0
Myler [124]	Stable	1315	88	3.8	2.3	0.2
	Unstable	807	84	5.1	3.6	0.2
Rupprecht [130]	Stable	406	85	0.5	1	0
	Unstable	202	83	2	3.5	1
Bentivoglio [129]	Stable	768	77	2.2	2	0.5
	Unstable	952	79	4.4	3.3	1.3
Stammen [125]	Stable	790	94	-	-	0.3
	Unstable	631	92	-	-	0.1

Adapted with permission from Bengtson and Wilson. [137]

TABLE 5.19 PTCA For Initially Stabilized vs Refractory Unstable Angina [122]

Study	n	Success (%)	In-Hospital Outcome (%)		
			Death	MI	CABG
Stabilized					
Steffenio [123]	89	90	0	5	5
Myler [124]	220	85	0	6.6	6.1
Stammen [125]	631	91	0.3	3.6	4.7
Medically Refractory					
Plokke [127]	469	88	1.1	4.9	3
DeFeyter [126]	114	90	0.9	7	7.9
Morrison [131]	56	84	3.6	7.2	9
Myler [124]	310	79	0.3	6.5	9.4
Rupprecht [130]	202	83	2.0	6.5	7.9
TAUSA [132]	469	95	0	2/3	3.6
EPIC [133]	489	-	1.7	5.0	4.7
Williams [134]	444	96	0.5	2.7	1.4
Bittl [135]	4098	NR	0.3	3.5	1.7
Serruys [136]	1141	92	0.2	3.3	1.6

Adapted with permission from DeFeyter and Serruys [122]

PTCA complication rates may be decreasing in recent years. In fact, the TAUSA trial found that the rate of abrupt closure was 9.3% in the early phase and 1.6% in the latter phase of the trial, p = .07. [132] Williams demonstrated PTCA success of 96% in the TIMI-3B trial and few complications occurred within 24 hours of the procedure (death 0.5%, MI 2.7%, CABG 1.4%, stroke 0.09%, any event 3.8%). [134] Retrospective reviews have suggested that the risk of PTCA may be decreased in patients who have been medically stabilized first. These studies have severe limitations in that more critical patients have a higher event rate regardless of therapy, and it is likely that medically refractory unstable angina was the reason for earlier PTCA. Furthermore, in a pre-specified subgroup analysis to assess the efficacy of heparin infusions prior to PTCA, no benefit was found in reducing abrupt closure, post PTCA ischemia or need for CABG. [135] Until the cost effectiveness of prolonged anticoagulation can be firmly established, it is difficult to endorse this approach.

C.   **COMPARISONS BETWEEN MEDICAL THERAPY, PTCA AND CABG IN UNSTABLE ANGINA PATIENTS**

1.   **Medical therapy compared to CABG.**[120] Two randomized trials compared medical and surgical therapy in unstable angina. The National Cooperative Study Group randomized 288 patients between 1972 and 1976 at nine academic centers. The Veterans Administration Cooperative Study randomized 468 patients between 1976 and 1982 at 12 VA hospitals. Both studies included patients with progressive or rest angina accompanied by ST and T wave changes. Patients over age 70 or with a recent MI were excluded.

In the National Cooperative Study, hospital mortality was similar for medicine and CABG groups (3 vs 5%). Follow-up to 30 months failed to show any differences in survival between the therapies. In the VA study, survival to 2 years was the same for medicine and CABG overall and in subgroups defined by number of diseased vessels. A post-hoc analysis of patients with depressed LV function, however, showed a significant survival advantage with CABG. All randomized trials of CABG versus medicine (including those in stable angina) have found improved symptom relief and functional capacity with CABG.

The Duke registry compared 5-year survival with medicine, PTCA, and CABG in 9,263 patients with unstable angina (defined as symptoms requiring hospital admission for control and to rule out MI) treated between 1984 and 1990. In this nonrandomized comparison, after adjustments for baseline differences, patients with three-vessel disease or two-vessel disease with a proximal severe (≥ 95%) LAD artery stenosis, surgical survival at 5 years was significantly better than medicine. A similar trend in favor of CABG was found in comparison with PTCA. In less severe two-vessel CAD, revascularization improved survival relative to medicine, and there was a trend for PTCA to provide better survival results (due to lower procedural mortality) than CABG. In one-vessel disease, all therapies were associated with high 5-year survival rates with no significant differences among groups.

2.   **Medical therapy compared to PTCA (Tables 5.20 and 5.21)**
The TIMI-3B trial enrolled 1473 patients with rest angina and ECG changes or non-Q MI.[142] Patients were randomized to receive tPA or placebo with a second randomization to early catheterization versus conservative care. The use of tPA increased the risk of MI and hemorrhagic stroke, and in the 471 patients who underwent PTCA, it increased the risk of major cardiac events (11 vs 4%, p = .06). Although there were no differences in death or MI between invasive and conservative groups, the invasive strategy allowed earlier discharge, fewer readmissions and reduced need for antianginal medicines. (Table 5.20) Furthermore, the conservative arm ultimately required cath in 57% and revascularization in 40% before hospital discharge. (Table 5.21) By one year, cath was performed in 73% and revascularization in 58% of conservative patients.[143] Thus, there is no advantage to a conservative approach and the majority of patients ultimately require an intervention.

TABLE 5.20   Outcome After Invasive Vs. Conservative Management of Unstable Angina: TIMI-3B [142]

	Invasive (n=740)	Conservative (n-733)	P
Death (%)	2.4	2.5	NS
Nonfatal MI (%)	5.1	5.7	NS
⊕ Stress at 6 wks (%)	8.6	10.0	NS
Hospital stay (days)	10.2	10.9	.01
Rehosp. In 6 wks (%)	7.8	14.1	.001
# Rehosp. days	365	930	.001
2 or more antianginal meds (%)	43.8	52.0	.02

Adapted with permission from reference 142.

TABLE 5.21 Invasive Vs. Conservative Management of Unstable Angina: Procedural Utilization in TIMI-3B [143]

	Invasive (%)	Conservative (%)	P
Catheterization			
Initial Hosp.	98	57	.001
6 weeks	98	64	.001
1 year	99	73	.001
PTCA			
Initial Hosp.	37	23	.001
6 weeks	38	26	.001
1 year	39	32	.001
CABG			
Initial Hosp.	24	18	.003
6 weeks	25	23	.17
1 year	30	30	.50
PTCA or CABG			
Initial Hosp.	60	40	.001
6 weeks	61	48	.001
1 year	64	58	.001

Adapted with permission from Anderson. [143]

3. **PTCA compared to CABG (Table 5.22).** Direct comparisons of PTCA and CABG in unstable angina patients are limited. Most randomized trials enrolled a relatively small proportion of patients with unstable angina and did not report the outcomes in this subgroup of patients.[144-148] In the 1829 patient BARI trial, 64% of the patients had unstable angina.[149] Rates of death or Q-wave MI by 5 years were similar in unstable angina patients treated with PTCA or surgery. Furthermore, the outcomes did not differ based on lesion morphology, the presence or absence of multivessel disease or LV dysfunction.

To further investigate the best means of revascularization in unstable angina patients, an ongoing 14 center VA cooperative trial is randomizing patients with medically refractory unstable angina to receive either PTCA or CABG.

DEFICIENCIES OF PTCA FOR UNSTABLE ISCHEMIC SYNDROMES

A. **REPERFUSION ARRHYTHMIAS.** Profound hypotension and bradycardia may develop after recanalization of an occluded coronary artery, especially the RCA.[150] When the vagal afferent fibers are stimulated, bradycardia and hypotension (the Bezold-Jarisch reflex) may occur. Sudden ventricular fibrillation may also occur following RCA reperfusion.

Concern has been voiced that reperfusion arrhythmias may be more common after primary PTCA compared with thrombolytic-mediated reperfusion. Bates[151] reported more arrhythmias occurred after direct PTCA than with intracoronary SK. In 83 patients, Gacioch[152] reported a high incidence of major adverse events shortly after PTCA-mediated reperfusion, and found that dilatation of the RCA compared with the LAD was associated with a greater need for CPR (16 vs 2%) and sustained hypotension requiring inotropic agents or an IABP (11 vs 3%). However, only 16% of these patients had primary PTCA; 84% underwent dilation after failed thrombolysis (rescue PTCA), thus representing a highly selected group of patients resistant to reperfusion.

In contrast, Kahn[153] reporting on 250 patients who underwent primary PTCA, found that while minor catheterization laboratory events were frequent and more common with right than left coronary PTCA, major events (death, CPR, defibrillation, cardioversion, IABP, or urgent surgery) were uncommon, occurring primarily in patients with cardiogenic shock. In addition, major adverse events were unrelated to the infarct-related artery, occurring in 8% of RCA infarcts, 10% of LAD infarcts, and 8% of left circumflex artery (LCX) infarcts. The PAR registry reported that sustained hypotension, bradyarrhythmias, or the need for CPR occurred in 16% of RCA infarcts compared to 5% of patients with other infarct arteries.[154]

TABLE 5.22   PTCA vs CABG for Unstable Angina

Study	n	Unstable Angina(%)	Results
CABRI [144]	1054	15	No difference in death or MI at 1 year overall. *
RITA [145]	1011	59	No difference in death or MI at 2 years overall. *
EAST [146]	392	60	No difference in death, MI or ischemia by thallium at 3 years. *
GABI [147]	359	14	↑Risk of MI with CABG *
ERACI [148]	127	83	No difference in death or MI at 1 year overall. *
BARI [149]	1829	64	No difference in death/QMI at 5 years overall, or in subgroup with unstable angina.
VA	700	100	Ongoing trial in 14 VA hospitals comparing PTCA to CABG in patients with medically refractory unstable angina.

* No data reported in subgroup with unstable angina.

In the PAMI-I trial,[29] ventricular fibrillation occurred in 6.7% of PTCA treated patients, and was more common in patients with inferior versus anterior MI (9.7 vs 1.4%, p = 0.03). Given animal studies showing the high potential of arrhythmias with rapid reperfusion, and clinical studies demonstrating the ability of beta blockers to reduce fatal arrhythmias in post infarct patients, slow reperfusion and IV β-blockers were adopted in the PAMI-2 study. This resulted in a significant reduction in ventricular fibrillation (3.8 vs 6.7% in PAMI-1, P = .01).[30]

Recommendations. Although data are limited in PTCA mediated reperfusion trials, based on animal studies, thrombolytic series and our experience, we recommend the following:
a. IV beta blockade prior to PTCA
b. Slow reperfusion with the wire, allowing reperfusion arrhythmias to resolve prior to balloon inflation.
c. Low osmolar, ionic contrast (ioxaglate) in patients with arrhythmias or severe LV dysfunction
d. Continuous monitoring of O_2 sats, using pulse oximeter
e. Adequate hydration prior to reperfusion of RCA
f. Correction of metabolic abnormalities

B. BLEEDING COMPLICATIONS. Although use of primary PTCA is superior to thrombolytics in reducing life-threatening bleeding ie) intracranial or gastrointestional, the need for blood transfusion is reported to be as high as 12-14%.[29,30,54,1] Many of these transfusions occurred in association with the use of thrombolytics, bypass surgery or prolonged anticoagulation with indwelling sheaths. In the PAMI-2 study, low risk patients received 48 hours of heparin with a 12 hour taper prior to discontinuation, and the transfusion rate was only 3%.[83]

Recommendations: Avoid adjunctive lytics, prolonged anticoagulation and remove sheaths as early as possible. We are testing local infusion of heparin and the use of the heparin-coated stent in MI pilot studies, where by protocol no additional heparin is administered after the PTCA procedure. This approach should dramatically reduce bleeding complictions.

C. **ISCHEMIC COMPLICATIONS.** The prognosis of patients developing recurrent ischemia is ominous. Ohman[154] found in-hospital reinfarction to be the second most common cause of death after thrombolytic therapy, with the mortality rate increasing from 4.0% to 12.8% if early reocclusion developed. Early reocclusion also resulted in an increase in heart failure, sustained hypotension, respiratory failure, and heart block. In the PAMI-1 trial,[155] patients with recurrent ischemia were significantly more likely to develop heart failure and pulmonary edema, sustained hypotension requiring IABP, respiratory failure and intubation, ventricular tachycardia, heart block, and cardiac arrest. Patients with recurrent ischemia also required a higher rate of repeat catheterization and revascularization procedures, prolonging the hospital stay by 2 days and resulting in $7800 of additional hospital charges.

Compared to treatment with thrombolytic therapy, primary PTCA is superior at reducing ischemia (10.6 vs 31.4%), and reinfarction (1.9 vs 8.1%). Pooling data from the PAR and PAMI studies, only 15.7% of patients after the index procedure require repeat catheterization and 5.6% required PTCA. [29,54] The low rate of recurrent ischemia after primary PTCA may be attributed to the routine use of aspirin prior to PTCA, aggressive heparinization, establishment of wide patency of the infarct-related artery with brisk antegrade flow, and avoidance of adjunctive thrombolysis.

Despite these advantages over thrombolysis, PTCA still has significant limitations as follows:
- Recurrent ischemia still occurs in 10-15% of patients after successful primary PTCA before hospital discharge, frequently resulting in hemodynamic and arrhythmic complications or reinfarction. Recurrent ischemia usually necessitates repeat catheterization and revascularization procedures, prolongs the hospital stay and increases costs. In the PAMI-2 database, the presence of EF < 45%, 3 vessel disease, dissection or residual stenosis ≥ 30% following primary PTCA was highly predictive of important ischemic events.[156]

- When compared to elective cases, PTCA performed in the setting of unstable angina or AMI is associated with an increased risk of abrupt closure resulting in recurrent MI or death. Silent or clinically apparent infarct artery reocclusion after primary PTCA occurs in 5% of vessels prior to hospital discharge.[2] Reocclusion of the infarct-related vessel after successful rescue PTCA is as high as 29%.[95]

- By 6 months, reocclusion (TIMI 0-1 flow) has occurred in 10-15% of patients and restenosis with a patent (TIMI 2-3 flow) vessel in 40%. This is a major cause of patient morbidity and mortality in the first 6 months after successful primary PTCA and necessitates frequent repeat revascularization procedures.[1,3,4,157] (Tables 5.10, 5.11)

DEVICES AND DRUGS TO FURTHER IMPROVE OUTCOME WITH PERCUTANEOUS REVASCULARIZATION FOR MI OR UNSTABLE ANGINA (TABLE 5.23)

A. **INTRAAORTIC BALLOON PUMP.** The concept of balloon pumping was based on early studies which demonstrated reduced reocclusion rates (2-8%) compared to 18-21% without IABP, and improved LV function.[158,159] The multicenter PAMI-2 trial performed emergency catheterization and PTCA (when indicated) and stratified patients into high and low risk groups (high-risk required age > 70 years, 3 vessel disease, EF < 45%, suboptimal PTCA vein graft culprit or no serious arrhythmias).[2] High-risk patients were randomized to receive IABP for 36-48 hours (n=211) versus no IABP (n=226). Although IABP treated patients had reductions in ischemia (11.6 vs 17.8%, p=.07) and re-PTCA (8.2 vs 14.2%, p=.05), there was no reduction in the predefined endpoints of death, recurrent MI, CHF, stroke, or in-hospital reocclusion (6.2 vs 8%, p =.46) on routine predischarge angiography. Furthermore, LV function at 1 and 6 weeks was similar between the two groups.[160] In a post-hoc analysis, we found that if 2 or more high-risk factors were present, IABP reduced the composite endpoint (primarily due to a deduction in CHF).[170] Based on these data, we are using IABP only in patients who have severe LV dysfunction or hypotension. We place stents for suboptimal PTCA results (stenosis > 30% or dissection) that may predispose patients to recurrent ischemia.

B. **DIRECTIONAL CORONARY ATHERECTOMY.**
   1. **Observational Trials.** Case series have documented successful use of directional coronary atherectomy (DCA) in thrombotic lesions. These small case series must be put into the perspective of the larger reports. In the NACI registry, the outcome of DCA in 147 lesions in 170 patients with recent MI (<30 days) was compared to 490 lesions in 438 patients without prior MI.[171] Patients with recent MI were more likely to have thrombus present (19 vs 6%) and reduced LVEF (49 vs 61%), but less likely to have lesion calcification (9 vs 18%). DCA in patients with recent MI resulted in reduced clinical success (83 vs 88%, p< .01), with greater rates of dissection (7 vs 3%, p< .05), abrupt closure (5 vs 1%, p<.05), and major procedural complications (3.4 vs 1.1%, p <.07). The clinical success rate increased from 77% for DCA attempted 1-9 days post MI, to 90% for DCA attempted 10-19 and 20-30 days post MI, respectively (p=.07) . Robertson [172]reported 62 post MI patients who underwent DCA and compared them to 393 non MI patients. The MI patients treated with DCA had a significant increase in abrupt closure, need for CABG and a trend for more distal embolization. Timing of the DCA procedure relative to the infarction did not affect complication rates. Abelmeguid also reported the results of DCA in patients with unstable angina.[173] Results of atherectomy were compared between three groups: patients with stable angina (n=77),

TABLE 5.23   Devices for Unstable Ischemic Syndromes

Device	Results
Intraaortic Balloon Pump	• Reduces clinical ischemia, but not reinfarction or reocclusion after primary PTCA • Reduces CHF in patients with two or more high-risk features.
Directional Atherectomy	• ↑ abrupt closure, MI, distal embolization compared to PTCA
TEC Atherectomy	• No comparative trials available • Extracts thrombus, but high restenosis rates
Rotablator Atherectomy	• Theoretically contraindicated, but no data available
Stents	• No comparative trials available • High success rates and few complications in observational series
Laser	• Limited data available
Local Drug Delivery	• Local heparin inhibits platelet deposition in animals, studies in MI patients ongoing

patients with progressive angina (n=110) and patients with post infarction angina or rest angina (n=100). Angiographic thrombus was only identified in 7% of lesions (2.6% stable, 10% progressive, 7% rest). DCA in rest pain or post infarction patients was associated with reduced success (93 vs 99%, p=0.04) and higher risk of major complication (9.7 vs 1.1%, p=0.04).

2. **Randomized trials.** In the CAVEAT trial, 65% of the patients randomized to DCA had unstable angina (46% with angina at rest, 18% post infarction). DCA was associated with higher frequency of non Q-wave MI (5.9 vs 2.5%, p=0.006) and higher frequency of MI at six month follow-up (8.2 vs 3.8%, p=0.0031).[174]

3. **Recommendations.** The mechanism of the higher complication rate is unknown, but likely to be due to the rigid bulky device which may create hemostasis during the procedure, embolize thrombus, and perform deep cuts leading to more intense platelet deposition. Based on these data, we do not recommend DCA in the acute or post MI patient, unless an occlusive lesion cannot be treated with a balloon or other device.

C. TEC ATHERECTOMY

1. **Non-randomized series**. The transluminal extraction catheter (TEC) with its suction-extraction cutting apparatus may be useful in patients with MI and large thrombus burden or totally occluded vein grafts.[175,176] Larkin et al reported that TEC atherectomy was feasible in 17 of 19 patients with MI who had either contraindications to or had failed thrombolysis.[177] Procedural success was obtained in 16 patients (94%), with 1 in-hospital reocclusion.

   We prospectively evaluated extraction atherectomy in 100 high-risk patients with acute myocardial infarction including patients with shock, thrombolytic failure, thrombolytic ineligibility, and previous bypass surgery.[178,179] The use of the TEC device was associated with high success rates (94%) and a low incidence of procedural complications Ninety-five percent of patients left the hospital with a patent infarct vessel and patency was maintained in 90% at six month angiographic follow-up. Despite the low in-hospital mortality of 5% (2% in patients without cardiogenic shock), clinical and angiographic restenosis rates in the six month follow-up period were high, 38 and 59% respectively.

2. **Randomized Studies**. A multicenter randomized trial comparing TEC and PTCA in unstable angina or MI patients with native coronary lesions has been initiated, (TOPIT-TEC Or PTCA In Thrombus). As of January 1996, 150 patients have been enrolled.

3. **Recommendations**. Given the increased equipment costs, larger sheath sizes and technical expertise required for the TEC device, as well as concern over coronary dissection, we reserve TEC atherectomy for unstable patients who present with a degenerated vein graft or a native coronary which contains a large thrombus in a relatively straight proximal or mid segment of large caliber ($\geq$ 2.8 mm diameter)

D. ROTABLATOR ATHERECTOMY.

No data are available in MI or unstable angina patients. Due to concern over distal embolization of thrombus in these clinical situations, rotablator is not recommended unless the lesion is rigid and cannot be dilated with high pressure balloons or excimer laser.

E. STENTS (Table 5.24).

In the past, the presence of intracoronary thrombus has been considered a contraindication for stenting. However, despite initial concerns about using stents in the setting of thrombus, the initial experience appears to be favorable. These results are likely due to the ability of stents to achieve a large lumen and reduce dissection planes, both of which would reduce shear forces and platelet thrombus deposition. Importantly, within the PAMI-2 database the presence of dissection post PTCA or residual stenosis > 30% was highly predictive of recurrent ischemic events.[156] Therefore, coronary stenting may be of great benefit in improving clinical outcome and the need for repeat revascularization in unstable angina and MI patients.

1. **Observational Series**. Malosky et al reviewed the results of Palmaz-Schatz stenting in 105 patients with unstable angina versus stable angina.[180] The overall success rate was 90% (stable angina 88%

versus unstable angina 90%) and rate of subacute thrombosis was 4% (stable angina 2% versus unstable angina 6%, p = NS). The restenosis rate was 28% in stable angina patients and 26% in unstable angina patients.

Bouvagnot[181] compared 234 patients who received stents for unstable angina to 124 patients stented with stable angina. Stents were placed for dissection in 49 vs 38% of patients, respectively, p =.0001. Although in-hospital complications were slightly higher in the unstable angina group, these did not achieve statistical significance (stent thrombosis 3.8 vs 0.8%, death 1.7 vs 0%, emergency CABG 1.3 vs 0%, vascular surgery 1.3 vs 0%). Stenting has been performed in MI patients with increasing enthusiasm, with surprisingly good results, as outlined in Table 5.24.[181-186] However, due to concern about stent thrombosis, prolonged anticoagulants have been administered to most patients.

To further reduce the risk of stent thrombosis, a heparin-coated stent has been developed. In an in-vitro model of pulsatile blood flow, platelet deposition was reduced by 95% with the heparin coated J&J stent compared to the non-coated stent (p< .005)[187]. In non-atherosclerotic pigs which were pretreated with aspirin and IV heparin, by 4-12 weeks the heparin coated stent resulted in 0% thrombosis compared to 37% in stents that were not heparin coated (p<.01) The Benestent II pilot study treated 200 patients with the heparin coated stent.[188] No patient experienced subacute thrombosis and the angiographic restenosis rate at 6 months was reported to be only 13%. Therefore, the heparin coated stent is less thrombogenic and may be ideally suited for use in unstable lesions. This stent will be tested in a multicenter, international PAMI trial involving patients with MI < 12 hours in symptom onset, to begin in 1996.

2. **Randomized Trials.** To date, no randomized data are available in MI or unstable angina patients. After a 100 patient pilot study using the heparin coated stent for "primary stenting" in MI, we plan to perform a randomized trial comparing the heparin coated stent with primary PTCA. Six month follow-up angiography will allow determination of reocclusion and restenosis rates.

3. **Recommendations**. Due to the increased equipment costs, and potential risk of stent thrombosis, many physicians have questioned the appropriateness of stenting in low-risk patients with a good PTCA result. We currently recommend consideration of stenting in patients who have a high ischemic risk after PTCA for AMI, ie residual stenosis > 30%, dissection, 3 vessel disease, LV dysfunction as long as the vessel caliber is ≥ 3 mm and the lesion can be covered with ≤ 2 stents, in the absence of huge thrombi or no reflow.

F. **LASER .** Although the excimer laser has been utilized in patients with thrombus , higher embolization rates observed, and data regarding its use in MI patients are limited. Conversely, the mid-infrared wavelength of the holmium: YAG laser closely corresponds to the high water content of fresh thrombus, and has been used in some MI patients.[189-191] De Marchena performed holmium laser in 3 patients with contraindications to thrombolysis, successfully restoring TIMI grade 3 flow in all.[190] No

TABLE 5.24 **Stents for AMI**

Series	n	Population	Results
Neumann [182]	74	Dissection and < TIMI 3 flow after PTCA for AMI ASA, ticlid +/- coumadin	TIMI 3 flow achieved in 100% 9.6% reocclusion
Monassier [183]	311	Heterogeneous group, 35% stent < 24 hrs from MI ASA, ticlid, IV heparin x 72 hrsthen LMWH 7-14 days	Success 97% Stent thrombosis 1.5% Death 3%
Castiglioni *	51	Stent for suboptimal result ASA, ticlid	Success 93% Stent thrombosis 7.1%
Bouvagnot *	33	Stent for suboptimal result after primary PTCA Ticlid & LMWH	Stent thrombosis 3% Death 9% Predictors of cardiac complications: EF, prior MI, artery size, TIMI flow grade
Grinfeld *	16	Stent for suboptimal result ≤ 12 hrs from MI	Predischarge cath: TIMI 3 flow in 100%
Benzuly [185]	31	Heterogeneous group Stent for suboptimal result	Stent thrombosis 2.8%
Medina *	31	Stent ≤ 6 hrs from MI	TIMI 3 flow in 100% 6 month angiographic restenosis rate 19%
Repetto *	51	Primary stenting Rescue stenting after failed lytics	Success 96% Stent thrombosis 6% No deaths
Benzuly *	24	Primary stenting ASA, ticlid, coumadin	Success 100% 1 death 1 stent thrombosis
Stone *	91	J&J primary stenting in MI 0-12 hrs	Ongoing multicenter pilot study No reinfarctions or death, 1 patient with stent thrombosis
Grines	100	Primary stenting 0-12 hrs using heparin coated stent ASA, ticlid No heparin or coumadin	Multicenter international pilot study. Followed by randomized trial comparing heparin coated J&J stent to PTCA. To begin in 1996

*Personal communication

patient developed in-hospital reocclusion. Topaz performed holmium laser in 25 patients with MI who either had contraindications to or had failed thrombolysis with a procedural success rate of 95%.).[191] Unlike chronic atherosclerosis, the size of the channel created after lasing in the presence of thrombus was noted to frequently be larger than the catheter diameter, consistent with "laser thrombolysis". However, adjunctive PTCA was required in all patients.

Recommendations. While the solid state nature of the holmium laser system facilitates rapid set-up and deployment, some delay is inevitable, the cost is increased, and "blind" lasing across a total occlusion without visualization of the distal vessel is potentially hazardous. Further studies will be required to establish a role for holmium laser thrombolysis as an adjunct to PTCA in MI.

G. **THERMAL BALLOON ANGIOPLASTY.** Controlled photothermal warming of a complex plaque during or after PTCA may "weld" or seal dissections, diminish elastic recoil, and reduce the thrombogenicity at the PTCA site by desiccating thrombus and thermally denaturing or cross-linking thrombogenic proteins.[193] Thermal balloon angioplasty using a continuous wave ND:YAG laser as the energy source has been extensively studied, and was found to be effective in treating abrupt closure after PTCA.[194-196] Unfortunately, the laser-balloon angioplasty project was terminated after reports of high restenosis rates. Heat may also be applied during balloon angioplasty through radiofrequency, ultrasonic or chemical means. Whether newer radiofrequency "pyroplasty" systems can obtain the same effects with less restenosis by operating on a lower thermal curve is currently under study, although restenosis rates remain high in preliminary reports.[197-198]

H. **LOCAL DRUG DELIVERY.** Heparin infused locally into the vessel wall adheres to and permeates the intima of arteries resulting in a high concentration locally that persists for several hours to days. When heparin is infused locally after balloon injury in an animal model, platelet deposition is reduced by 60% at 30 minutes, with a 39% reduction persisting for at least 12 hours.[199] A variety of different delivery devices Channelled Balloon, Hydrogel, Dispatch, and an inotophoretic catheter used to infuse local heparin have consistently demonstrated reduced platelet deposition, thus the findings appear to be believable and reproducible.[200-203] Potential benefits to local heparin infusion may include a reduction in recurrent ischemia, reocclusion or late restenosis. In fact, local heparin infusions in animals have been demonstrated to reduce intimal hyperplasia.[201,204] Moreover, in a series of 38 patients who received local heparin during PTCA, angiographic restenosis occurred in only 7%.[205] An additional benefit of local heparin delivery is the potential to reduce the dose and duration of systemic heparin, thus potentially reducing bleeding complications. We are currently investigating the safety and efficacy of local heparin infusion (4000 units) in MI patients in a multicenter pilot study.

Local infusion of urokinase is also undergoing evaluation. Steg[206] randomized patients to local urokinase (n=14) versus saline (n=14) during PTCA for MI. Although the local urokinase appeared to reduce angiographic evidence of thrombus, there were no differences in PTCA success or clinical outcome. Furthermore, reocclusion was nonsignificantly increased in the urokinase group (14 vs 0%).

I. **OTHER NEW DEVICES.** Therapeutic ultrasound energy may be particularly efficient in ablating fresh thrombus while at the same time producing coronary vasodilation.[207-208] In a series of 11 MI patients, Hann[209] demonstrated resolution of angiographically visible clots, however TIMI-3 flow was restored in only 3 patients. All patients required PTCA with success achieved in 11 of 12 cases.

J. **SYSTEMIC DRUGS**

1. **Antiplatelet Agents**

    a. **Aspirin.** Aspirin is targeted only toward one of many different pathways leading to platelet activation. Significantly, all agonists can independently expose the GP IIb/IIIa receptor, and platelet aggregation can occur even if the arachidonic acid pathway is completely blocked with aspirin).[210] A high dose of aspirin[211] and a chewable or intravenous route of administration[212] appear to reduce platelet aggregation and thrombus formation more quickly and effectively. However, despite aspirin therapy, patients with unstable angina or MI have heightened platelet activity and enhanced propensity for platelet thrombus formation on an injured artery.[213] We have all our patients chew at least 325 mg aspirin in the emergency room.

    b. **Ticlopidine** is a more potent antiplatelet agent than aspirin. Ticlid inhibits binding of fibrinogen to the platelet GP IIb/IIIa receptor, and is 85% effective at inhibiting platelet aggregation). Although ticlopidine exerts its maximal antiplatelet effect at 3-5 days, antiplatelet effects can be detected within hours of ingestion. Moreover, loading with 500 mg BID for the first 2-3 days allows greater platelet inhibition than the conventional 250 mg dose, with differences detectable within the first day of administration.[215] In randomized trials compared to aspirin, ticlopidine reduced the stroke rate in patients with transient ischemic attacks, and reduced the rate of MI and rest angina in patients with unstable angina.[216] There are now studies suggesting that aspirin and ticlid act synergistically. Aspirin and ticlopidine were found to have a synergistic effect in reducing coronary platelet deposition[217] and in humans has been shown to attenuate the post-PTCA thrombin generation.[218] Additional advantages include its wide utilization in tens of thousands of patients and low cost. We are currently employing both aspirin and ticlopidine pre-and for 1 month post intervention in our PAMI trials of PTCA or stenting for MI.

    c. **Glycoprotein IIb/IIIa Receptor Antagonists**. The newest antiplatelet agents block the GPIIb/IIIa receptor, leading to a dose dependent inhibition of platelet aggregation.

        1. **7E3 (ReoPro).** The EPIC (Evaluation of 7E3 in the Prevention of Ischemic Complications) trial evaluated 2099 high risk PTCA patients (unstable angina, MI or high risk coronary morphology).[219,220] Among the 64 patients enrolled for primary PTCA (n=42) or rescue PTCA (n=22), the acute and 6 month ischemic endpoints were reduced in the 7E3 group.[221] Among the 489 patients with unstable or post MI angina, the rate of MI was 1.8% vs 9% in 7E3 and placebo groups, respectively.[222] Although the early rate of death or revascularization was no different, by 6 months, a significant difference in mortality rate favoring 7E3 was observed (1.8% vs 6.6%, p =.038). However, the beneficial effects of 7E3 were achieved at the risk of increased major bleeding (14% vs 7%) and high

pharmaceutical costs ($1300/dose).

Since 7E3 was found to increase the ACTs by 40 seconds, it was thought that a lower heparin dose may have reduced bleeding.[223] The follow-up EPILOG study utilized medium and low dose heparin with 7E3 compared to placebo. This demonstrated a therapeutic benefit (reduction in asymptomatic CK elevation) with no increased risk of bleeding.[224] Although data have not been published, reportedly, there was no difference in the rate of recurrent ischemia, clinical MI, need for emergency bypass or death.

Preliminary results from the CAPTURE, in which patients with medically-refractory unstable angina were randomized to 7E3 vs. placebo, reportedly indicate a beneficial effect for 7E3 for the combined endpoint of in-hospital ischemic complications.

Despite these benefits, most physicians are not utilizing 7E3 prophylactically for all high-risk patients due to high cost. Michelstein reported 16 patients who received 7E3 only after a thrombus was observed post PTCA, with resolution of thrombus and improvement in TIMI flow.[225] They concluded that prophylactic administration of 7E3 may not be necessary, and confining its use to patients with post PTCA thrombosis may be the most cost effective approach. ReoPro is discussed in detail in Chapter 34.

2. **Integrelin.** The investigational peptide Integrelin (COR Therapeutics) was tested in a 4000 patient PTCA trial.[226] No significant differences in death, MI, urgent revascularization or need for stenting was observed between placebo and Integrelin groups. Although it was proposed that too low of a dose was utilized, the clinical endpoints were actually slightly higher in the "high" dose Integrelin arm. To date, trials utilizing this drug during PTCA for AMI or high risk unstable angina patients have not been performed.

3. **MK-383.** MK-383 (Merck) is an investigational nonpeptide inhibitor of fibrinogen binding to the platelet GP IIb/IIIa receptor. Based on pilot data in high risk PTCA patients,[227] a multicenter trial comparing MK-383 to placebo in 2000 unstable angina or MI patients undergoing PTCA was undertaken. Enrollment into the study is now complete, and results will be available shortly.

2. **Heparin** Several randomized trials have clearly shown the benefit of IV heparin (with or without aspirin) on the acute outcome of unstable angina. Although the benefit in MI patients is less well established, it is customary to administer heparin in these patients as well. However, the dose, duration of treatment and method of discontinuation merit review.

   a. **Pre-PTCA.** Retrospective studies have suggested that prolonged heparinization (3-7 days) in patients with unstable angina improve the safety of PTCA.[124,228-232] These studies have severe limitations since more critical patients have a higher event rate regardless of therapy, and it is likely that medically refractory unstable angina was the reason for the earlier PTCA. In a pre-specified subgroup analysis accessing the efficacy of heparin infusions prior to PTCA, no benefit was found in reducing abrupt closure, post PTCA ischemia or need for CABG.[233] Delaying PTCA for several days is simply not practical in this era of cost containment. In unstable angina patients, we generally perform the PTCA at a time that is convenient for the operator without consideration of the duration of anticoagulation.

In acute MI patients we administer heparin in the emergency room, prior to mobilizing the cath lab. In the PAMI-1 and PAMI-2 trials, a bolus of 10,000 units was recommended. Even with a 60 minute delay in performing angiography, only 20% of infarct arteries were patent.[29,234] Thus, 10,000 units of heparin did not appear to improve the rate of reperfusion over what would be expected spontaneously. Verheugt utilized the dose commonly used for bypass surgery (300 units/Kg - which resulted in doses between 10,000 and 40,000 units).[235] This megadose of heparin resulted in patency in 56% of patients within 90 minutes. Thus, high dose heparin appears quite promising. We are using the 300 units/Kg dose prior to transfer for emergency PTCA in our AIR PAMI trial.

b. **During PTCA.** Maintaining an ACT of 300 seconds for the entire duration of the procedure (not just initially) appears to be adequate to reduce the risk of abrupt closure in elective cases.[236] However, we have noted 40-60 sec variations in ACT measurements, making us uncomfortable with a single ACT measurement of 300 sec. Furthermore, it is well known that unstable patients are hypercoagulable, and there is increasing evidence that the ACT should be maintained much higher than 300 sec.

Independent investigators have found that an ACT of 300 did not predict suppression of intravascular thrombin activity in humans, and this resistance was predictive of acute ischemic events following PTCA.[237,238] In the CAVEAT trial, heparin resistance (as assessed by ACT, adjusted for heparin dose and body size) was a strong predictor of major cardiac events.[239] In another study, low dose heparin enhanced and high dose heparin inhibited platelet activation and aggregation in humans.[240] In a 4000 patients trial of PTCA for unstable angina, higher levels of anticoagulation reduced ischemic events.[241] In fact, for each 10 second increase in ACT, abrupt closure was decreased by 1.3% (p = .04), even up to ACTs of 400 sec.

In a study of 1290 PTCA patients, Narins[242] found that patients with abrupt closure had a significantly lower ACT (346 vs 376 sec, p = .009) compared to patients without abrupt closure. There was an inverse linear relationship between abrupt closure and ACTs, p = .018). Hillegass found that higher ACTs increased bleeding, but they were also associated with reduced ischemic events.[243] A risk/benefit analysis suggested that the optimal ACT range was between 425-525 sec.

The EPIC trial showed improved outcome in the 7E3 group, but this group also had a mean ACT 40 seconds higher than the placebo group.[223] It is possible that some of the improved outcome may have been due to potentiation of heparin activity.

Recommendations. We recommend high dose heparin to achieve an ACT between 350-400 seconds. This approach has been used in the PAMI trials, with subsequent low ischemic events. ACTs must be checked every 20 minutes and additional heparin given to maintain this ACT for the entire duration of the procedure. Care must be given not to underdose patients who are brought to the lab with IV heparin infusing. Studies have shown that despite higher initial ACTs, the procedural heparin requirements were no different than patients not on a continuous infusion (12,000 units to achieve ACT of only 300)[244]

c.   **Post PTCA.** Few data exist regarding the optimal dose and duration of heparin infusion after PTCA for AMI or unstable angina. Although commonly used, it is not known whether a prolonged infusion is necessary. In the PAMI-1 trial, patients were treated for 3-5 days and experienced a transfusion rate of 14%.[29] A small study evaluated short (24 hrs) versus prolonged heparin (72 hrs) after successful reperfusion in acute myocardial infarction.[246] It showed that low risk patients with successful PTCA mediated reperfusion were not protected against rethrombosis with prolonged heparin and experienced more bleeding complications. They concluded that heparin therapy > 24 hours may not be beneficial. In the PAMI-2 trial, low risk patients were treated with 48 hours of full-dose and 12 hours of half dose heparin. These patients did exceedingly well (mortality 0.4%, reinfarction or acute reocclusion 3%), and could be discharged by the third hospital day.[83]

IV heparin should not be abruptly stopped. It was documented in numerous studies that a rebound hypercoagulable state occurred with the abrupt discontinuation of IV heparin, resulting in an increased risk of reinfarction.[246-250] Based on these observations, in the PAMI trials we have tapered heparin to half-dose for 12 hours prior to discontinuation.

3.   **Direct thrombin inhibitors** are not dependent on anti-thrombin III for their anticoagulant action, thus they are better inhibitors of fibrin-bound thrombin and are not inactivated by platelet factor 4 or heparinase. Furthermore, there is less variability in anticoagulant response to a given dose. Since thrombin is the most potent platelet activator, better thrombin inhibition should theoretically improve PTCA outcome.

a.   **Hirudin** is a peptide derived from the medicinal leech. Hirudin reduced platelet deposition and restenosis in animal models. In a randomized trial comparing it to heparin in 1141 unstable angina patients undergoing PTCA, the results were equivocal.[136] Although ischemic events within the first 96 hours were higher in the heparin group compared to the 2 hirudin groups (11.0 vs 7.9 vs 5.6%, p = .03), this benefit was not sustained. At 7 months, the frequency of angina, major cardiac events, and minimal luminal diameter on follow-up angiography were similar between the groups. The GUSTO 2-B substudy of primary PTCA has also randomized patients to receive either heparin or hirudin. Results are anticipated shortly.

b.   **Hirulog** is a synthetic peptide. It was compared to heparin in a trial of 4098 patients undergoing PTCA for unstable or post MI angina).[135] For the overall study, hirulog did not reduce ischemic events (11.4 vs 12.2%), but did lower the incidence of bleeding (3.8 vs 9.8%, p < .001). In a subgroup analysis of patients with post MI angina, hirulog was associated with reduced early ischemic events, however, this benefit was not sustained at 6 months.

4.   **Thrombolytics (Table 5.25).**   To investigate the role of thrombolytic therapy for unstable angina, a number of investigators have performed angiograms before and after administration of a thrombolytic agent. In these small series, it appeared that thrombolytic drugs may improve resolution of intracoronary thrombus, but some lesions may become more severely stenosed or totally occluded. Considering all thrombolytic trials in unstable angina patients reported to date, it appears that clinical improvement is not predicted accurately by improvements in angiographic luminal diameter.   In fact, a metaanalysis of large randomized, placebo controlled trials demonstrated that thrombolytics increase the risk of myocardial infarction by 1.7% when applied to unstable angina patients.[120]   Likewise, every randomized trial involving PTCA patients demonstrated a worse outcome with empiric infusion of thrombolytics. (Table 5.25)[4,156,251-255]

Spielberg et al[251] compared four different PTCA regimens in 660 consecutive patients, many of whom had chronic stable angina.   One treatment strategy administering small doses of intracoronary urokinase (1670 to 6670 units) during the PTCA procedure, resulted in an increased incidence of abrupt closure. In the larger, multicenter TAUSA trial, 469 patients with unstable angina, non-Q MI or post MI angina were randomized to receive IC urokinase 250,000-500,000 units vs placebo during PTCA[254]. UK was associated with a worse outcome in the overall population. Furthermore, patients with angiographic features most likely to benefit from lytics (complex lesions, filling defects), were also found to have a higher risk of abrupt closure with urokinase.[255]   Similarly, worse clinical and angiographic outcomes were observed with thrombolytics in the TIMI-2B, SAMI and PAMI-2 trials.[4,156,253]

The mechanism by which thrombolytics may induce abrupt closure is not well defined. In vitro studies have demonstrated enhanced platelet aggregation during thrombolytic infusion.[256-258] Intimal splitting occurs in most vessels following successful PTCA. It may be associated with excessive bleeding in the plaque and media of the vessel.[259-262] In the absence of fibrinolytic agents, the intima may adhere to the vessel by prolonged balloon inflations and activation of the coagulation system.   This repair mechanism may be altered by intracoronary or systemic fibrinolysis. In autopsy series of patients who died after PTCA combined with thrombolysis, extensive intramural hemorrhage was found in the dilated segment.[260-262] In these autopsy series, no patient had intraplaque bleeding following PTCA in the absence of thrombolytics.

TABLE 5.25 Effect of Lytics On PTCA Outcome in Unstable Angina or MI Patients

Author	n	Lytic	Dose (units)	Results
Spielberg [251]	660	UK	1670-6670 IC	Increased abrupt closure with UK
TAUSA Pilot [252]	66	UK	150,000 IC	No difference in abrupt closure
TAUSA [254,255]	469	UK	250-500,000 IC	Overall: Increased acute closure with UK (10.2 vs 4.3%, p=0.02) and major cardiac events (12.9 vs 6.3%, p=0.02) Complex Lesions: Increased acute closure with UK (15 vs 5.9%, p=0.03) Filling Defects: Nonsignificant increase in acute closure with UK (18.8 vs 8.3%)
TIMI-2B [253]	471	tPA	80mg IV	In pts pretreated with tPA 1-2 days before PTCA, increased risk of abrupt closure/MI/CABG/death (11.0 vs 4.0, p=0.06)
O'Neill [4]	122	SK	1.5 MU IV	SK associated with increased risk of emergency CABG (10.3 vs 1.6, p=0.03), transfusion (39 vs 8%, p=.0001), ↑ hospital stay and cost.
PAMI-2 [156]	172	UK	Variable doses	Post PTCA thrombus not predictive of in-hospital ischemia. When thrombus was treated with IC lytics, trend for a higher rate of ischemia (18.4 vs 10.6% p=0.10) despite controlling for other predictors of ischemia in a multivariate analysis.

5. **Contrast Agents.** Ionic contrast agents are preferred for PTCA in unstable ischemic syndromes. Ionic contrast has been shown to prolong PTT, clotting times, inhibit platelet aggregation and degranulation and shorten the time to thrombolysis. Numerous obervational studies as well as randomized trials have demonstrated a reduced rate of abrupt closure, no reflow, recurrent ischemia and MI with ionic compared to non ionic contrast.[263-265]

We use ionic contrast for all unstable ischemic interventions. High osmolar ionic agents are used for most cases, and the low osmolar ionic agent, Hexabrix is used for patients with hemodynamic instability or arrhythmias.

K. **EMERGENCY CABG**. Potential indications for emergency CABG in the setting of acute MI are described in Table 5.26.

TABLE 5.26 INDICATIONS FOR EMERGENCY SURGERY FOR ACUTE MI

- Left main stenosis > 50% with LAD or circumflex infarct vessel.

- Left main stenosis > 75% with right coronary infarct vessel.

- Severe proximal multivessel disease not suitable for PTCA, particularly if the infarct vessel is patent.

- Severe multivessel disease with cardiogenic shock.

- Failed thrombolytic and/or mechanical reperfusion with infarct duration <6 hours, a large amount of jeopardized myocardium, and ongoing pain.

CLINICAL APPROACH TO THE ACUTE MI OR UNSTABLE PATIENT

All MI patients presenting within 12 hours of symptom onset with ongoing ischemia benefit from reperfusion therapy; if a skilled interventionalist and cath lab team are available, the optimal reperfusion strategy in MI is emergent PTCA. If the cath lab is not available and the patient is eligible for thrombolysis, intravenous thrombolytic therapy should be administered. In the event of a large infarction, continued or recurrent ischemia, hemodynamic instability, or shock, catheterization should be performed even if interhospital transfer is required. Our recommendations include:

- Chewable aspirin 325mg, ticlopidine 500 mg PO, IV heparin (ACT 350-400), and IV β - blockers
- Ionic contrast (low osmolar ionic agent ioxaglate for hemodynamic instability)
- Defer PTCA in high-risk lesions with TIMI-3 flow unless absolutely necessary
- PTCA of culprit vessel only (goal < 30% stenosis with TIMI grade 3 flow)
- Stent for severe dissection (vessel ≥ 3mm)
- Large intracoronary thrombus: Avoid lytics; Prolonged inflations, slightly oversized balloon, low pressure; consider TEC, Reopro, local infusion of heparin
- Treat no-reflow with IC NTG, Verapamil; Adenosine may be useful
- IABP for continued ischemia, hypotension, pulmonary edema, LV dysfunction and multivessel disease
- Consider bypass surgery for high risk anatomy not amenable to PTCA

REFERENCES

1.   Zijlstra F, Jan de Boaer M, Moorntje JCA, Reiffer S, Reiber JHC, Suryapranata H. A comparison of immediate coronary angioplasty with intravenous streptokinase in acute myocardial infarction. N Engl J Med 1993;328:680-684.

2.   Griffin J, Grines CL, Marsales D, et al. A prospective, randomized trial evaluating the prophylactic use of balloon pumping in high risk myocardial infarction patients: PAMI-2. J Am Coll Cardiol 1995;25:86A.

3.   Brodie BR, Grines CL, Ivanhoe R, Knopf W, Taylor G, O'Keefe J, Weintraub RA, Berdan LG, Tcheng JE, Woodlief LH, Califf RM, O'Neill WW. Six-month clinical and angiographic follow-up after direct angioplasty for acute myocardial infarction. Circulation 1994;25:156-162.

4.   O'Neill WW, Weintraub R, Grines CL, Meany TB, Brodie BR, Friedman HZ, Ramos RG, Gangadharan V, Levin RN, Choksi N, Westveer DC, Strzelecki RN, Timmis GC. A prospective placebo-controlled randomized trial of intravenous streptokinase and angioplasty therapy of acute myocardial infarction. Circulation 1992;86:1710-1717.

5.   Weaver WD, Parsons L, Every N. Primary coronary angiopalsty in hospitals with and without surgery backup. J Invas Cardiol 1995;7:34F-39F

6.   Ayres M. Coronary angioplasty for acute myocardial infarction in hospitals without cardiac surgery. J Invas Cardiol 1995;7:40F-46F.

7.   Weaver W, Parsons L, Martin JS, Every N. Direct PTCA for treatment of acute myocardial infarction: A community experience in hospitals with and without surgical back-up. Circulation 1995;92:I-138.

8.   Wharton TP, Schmitz JM, Fedele FA, McNamara NS, Gladstone AR, Jacobs MI. Primary angioplasty in cute myocardial infarction at community hospitals without cardiac surgery: Experience in 195 cases. Circulation 1995;92:I-138.

9.   Ohnishi Y, Saffitz J, Sobel B, Coor P, Goldstein J. Primary angioplasty minimizes reperfusion injury and enhances recovery of myocardial function compared with thrombolysis. J Am Coll Cardiol 1995:219A.

10.   Kinn J, Benzuly K, Sachs D, O'Neill W. Primary angioplaty results in less myocardial rupture than thrombolytics in patients recently treated for acute myocardial infarction. Circ 1995;92:I-139.

11.   Krikorian R, Vacek J, Rosamont T, Beauchamp G. Timing, mode and predictors of death after direct angioplasty for acute myocardial infarction. J Am Coll Cardiol 1995:296A.

12.   O'Keefe JO, Bailey WL, Rutherford BD, Hartzler GO. Primary angioplasty for acute myocardial infarction in 1000 consecutive patients. Am J. Cardiol 1993;k72:107-G-115G.

13.   Brodie BR, Weintraub RA, Stuckey TD, et al. Outcomes of direct coronary angioplasty for acute myocardial infarction in candidates and non-candidates for thrombolytic therapy. Am J Cardiol 1991;67:7-12.

14.   Beauchamp GD, Vacek JL, Robuck W. Management comparison for acute myocardial infarction: direct angioplasty versus sequential thrombolysis-angioplasty. Am Heart J 1990;120:237-242.

15.   Nakagawa Y, Iwasaki Y, Takeshi, Nobuyoshi M. Serial angiographic follow-up after successful direct angioplasty for acute myocardial infarction; single center experience. Circulation 1993;88(Suppl I):I-106 (abstr).

16.   Rothbaum DA, Linnemeier TJ, Landin RJ, et al. Emergency percutaneous transluminal coronary angioplasty in acute myocardial infarction: a 3 year experience. J Am Coll Cardiol 1987;10:264-272.

17.   Miller PF, Brodie BR, Weintraub RA, et al. Emergency coronary angioplasty for acute myocardial infrction. Arch Intern Med 1987;147:1565-1570.

18.   Dageford DA, Genovely HC, Goodin RR, Allen RD. Emergency percutaneous transluminal coronary angiopalsty in acute myocardial ifnarction. J Kentucky Med Assn 1987;85:368-372.

19.   Kimura T, Nosaka H, Ueno K, Nobuyoshi M. Role of coronary angioplasty in acute myocardial infarction. Circulation 1986;74(Suppl II):II-22(abstr).

20.   Marco J, Caster L, Szatmary LJ, Fajadet J. Emergency percutaneous transluminal coronary angioplasty without thrombolysis as initial therapy in acute myocardial infarction. Int J Cardiol 1987;15:55-63.

21.   O'Neill W, Timmis GC, Bourdillon PD, et al. A prospective randomized clinical trial of intracoronary streptokinase versus coronary angioplasty for acute myocardial infarction. N Engl J Med 1986;314:812-818.

22.   Stone GW, Rutherford BD, McConahay DR, et al. Direct coronary angioplasty in acute myocardial infarction: outcome in patients with single vessel disease. J Am Coll Cardiol 1990;15:534-43.

23.   Stone GW, Grines CL, Topol EJ. Update on percutaneous transluminal coronary angioplasty for acute myocardial infarction. Book chapter. Current Review of Interventional Cardiology. Ed. E. Topol, M.D., P. Serruys, M.D., Current Medicine, Philadelphia, PA, 1995.

24.   Stone CW, Grines CL, Browne KF, Marco J, Rothbaum D, O'Keefe J, Hartzler GO, Overlie P, Donohue B, Chelliah N, Timmis GC,

Vlietstra R, Strzelecki M, Puchrowicz-Ochocki S, O'Neill WW. Predictors of in-hospital and 6 month outcome after acute myocrdial infarction in the reperfusion era: The Primary Angioplasty in Myocardial Infarction (PAMI) trial. J Am Coll Cardiol 1995;25:370-377.

25. Waldecker B, Waas W, Haberbosch W, Voss R, Kistler P, Tillmanns H. Long-term follow-up (2.5 years) of 300 consecutive patients with primary angioplasty for acute myocardial infarction. Circulation 1995;92:I-461.

26. Maynard C, Weaver D, Litwin PE, et al. Hospital mortality in acute myocardial infarction in the era of reperfusion therapy (the Myocardial Infarction Triage and Intervention Project). Am J Cardiol 1993;72:877-82.

27. Rogers WJ, Chandra NC, Gore JM for the NMRI Investigators. National registry of myocardial infarction (NMRI): What have we leaned from the first 100,000 patients? J Am Coll Cardiol 1993;21:349A.

28. Cragg DR, Friedman HZ, Bonema JD, et al. Outcome of patients with acute myocardial infarction who are ineligible for thrombolytic therapy. Ann Int Med 1991;115:173-177.

29. Grines CL, Browne KF, Marco J, Rothbaum D, Stone GW, O'Keefe J, Overlie P, Donohue B, Chelliah N, Timmis GC, Vlietstra RE, Strzelecki M, Puchrowicz-Ochocki S, O'Neill W. A comparison of immediate angioplasty with thrombolytic therapy for acute myocardial infarction. N Engl J Med 1993;328:673-679.

30. Grines CL, Griffin JJ, Brodie BR, Stone GW, Donohue BC, Balestrini CE, Wharton TP, Spain MG, Shimshak T, Jones D, Mason D, Sachs D, O'Neill WW. The second Primary Angioplasty for Myocardial Infarction study (PAMI-II): Preliminary Report. Circulation 1994;90:I-433.

31. Grines C, Marsalese D, Brodie B, Griffin J, Donohue B, Sampaolesi A, Costantini C, Stone G, Spain M, Jones D, Sachs D, Mason D, O'Neill W. Acute cath provides the best method of risk stratifying MI patients. Circulation, 1995;92:I-531.

32. Stone GW, Grines CL, Browne KF, Marco J, Rothbaum D, O'Keefe J, Overlie P, Donohue B, Puchrowicz S, O'Neill WW. Outcome of different reperfusion strategies in thrombolytic "eligible" versus "ineligible" patients with acute myocardial infarction. J Am Coll Cardiol February 1995;401A.

33. Grines CL, Booth D, Nissen S, Gurley J, Bennett K, O'Connor WN, DeMaria A. Mechanism of acute myocardial infarction in patients with prior coronary artery bypass grafting and therapeutic implications. Am J Cardiol 1990;65:1292-96.

34. McKendall GR, Drew TM, Kelsey SF, et al. What is the optimal treatment for thrombolytic ineligible AMI Preliminary results of the Study of Medicine vs. Angioplasty Reperfusion Trial (SMART). J Am Coll Cardiol 1994;1A-484A:225A.

35. Kaplan AJ, Bengtson JR, Aronson LG, et al. Reperfusion improves survival in patients with cardiogenic shock after acute myocardial infarction. J Am Coll Cardiol 1990;15:155 (abstr).

36. Lee L, Erbel R, Brown TM, et al. Multicenter registry of angioplasty therapy of cardiogenic shock: initial and long-term survival. J Am Coll Cardiol 1991;17:599-603.

37. Gacioch GM, Ellis SG, Lee L, et al. Cardiogenic shock complicating acute myocardial infarction: the use of coronary angioplaty and the integration of the new support devices into patient management. J Am Coll Cardiol 1992;19:647-653.

38. Bengtson JR, Kaplan AJ, Pieper KS, et al. Prognosis in cardiogenic shock aftr acute myocardial infarction in the interventioanl era. J Am Coll Caridol 1992;20:1482-1489.

39. Hibbard MD, Holmes DR, Gersh BJ, Reeder GS. Coronary angioplasty for acute myocardial infarction complicated by cardiogenic shock. Circulation 1990;82:III-511.

40. Moosvi AR, Villaneuva L, Gheorghiade M, et al. Early revascularization improves survival in cardiogenic shock. Circulation 1990;82:III-308.

41. Eltchaninoff H, Simpendorfer C, Whitlow PL. Coronary angioplasty improves both early and 1 year survival in acute myocardial infarction complicated by cardiogenic shock. J Am Coll Cardiol 1991;17:167.

42. Brown TM, Lannone LA, Gordon DF, et al. Percutaneous myocardial reperfusion reduces mortality in acute myocardial infarction complicated by cardiogenic shock. Circulation 1995;72:III-309.

43. O'Neill WW, Erbel R, Laufer N, et al. Coronary angioplasty therapy of cardiogenic shock complicating acute myocardial infarction. Circulation 1995;72:III-309.

44. Meyer P, Blanc P, Badouy M, Morand P. Treatment de choc cardiogenique primaire par angioplastie transluminale coronarienne a la phase aigue de l'Infarctus. Arch Mal Coeur 1990;83:329-334.

45. Lee L, Bates ER, Pitt B, Walton JA, et al. Percutaneous transluminal coronary angioplasty improves survival in acute myocardial infarction complicated by cardiogenic shock. Circulation 1988;78:145-151.

46. Seydoux C, Goy J-J, Beuret P, et al. Effectiveness of percutaneous transluminal coronary angioplasty in cardiogenic shock during acute myocardial infarction. Am J Cardiol 1992;68:968-969.

47. Heuser RR, Maddoux GL, Goss JE, et al. Coronary angioplasty in the treatment of cardiogenic shock: the therapy of choice. J Am Coll cardiol 1986;7:219.

48. Shani J, Rivera M, Geengart A, et al. Percutaneous transluminal coronary angioplasty in cardiogenic shock. J Am Coll Cardiol 1986;7:149.

49. Disler L, Haitas B, Benjamin J, et al. Cardiogenic shock in evolving myocardial infarction: treatment by angioplaty and streptokinase. Heart Lung 1987;16:649.

50. Verna E, Repetto S, Boscarina M, et al. Emergency coronary angioplasty in patients with severe left ventricular dysfunction of cardiogenic shock after acute myocardial infarction. Eur Heart J 1989;10:958-966.

51. Hochman JS, Boland J, Sleeper LA, Porway M, Brinker J, Col J, Jacobs A, slater J, Miller D, Wasserman H, Menegus MA, Talley D, McKinlay S, Sanborn T, LeJemtel T, and the SHOCK Registry Investigators. Current spectrum of cardiogenic shock and effect of early revascularization on mortality. Circulation 1995;91:372-881.

52. Holmes DR, Bates ER, Kleiman NS, Sadowski Z, Horgan JHS, Morris DC, Califf RM, Berger PB, Topol EJ. Contemporary reperfusion therapy for cardiogenic shock: The GUSTO-I trial experience. J Am Coll Cardiol 1995;26:668-674.

53. Anderson RD, Stebbins AL, Bates E, Stomel R, Granger CB, Ohman EM. Underutilization of aortic counterpulsation in patients with cardiogenic shock: Observations from the GUSTO-1 study. Circulation 1995;92:I-139.

54. O'Neill WW, Brodie BR, Ivanhoe R, Knopf W, Taylor G, O'Keefe J, Grines CL, Weintraub R, Sickinger B, Berdan LG, Tcheng JE, Woodlief LG, Strzelecki M, Hartzler G, Califf RM. Primary Coronary Angioplasty for Acute Myocardial Infarction (The Primary Angioplasty Registry). Am J Cardiol 1994;73:627-634.

55. Gruppo Italiano per lo Studio della Streptochinasi nell'Infarto Miocardico (GISSI): Effectiveness of intravenous thrombolytic treatment in acute myocardial infarction. Lancet 1986;1:397-402.

56. ISIS-2 (Second International Study Group of Infarct Survival) collaborative group: Randomized trial of intravenous streptokinase, oral aspirin, both, or neither among 17,187 cases of suspected acute myocardial infarction. Lancet 1988;2:349-360.

57. Wilcox RG, Olsson CG, Skene AM, Von Der Lippe G, Jensen G, Hampton JR. Trial of tissue plasminogen activator for mortality reduction in acute myocardial infarction. Anglo Scandinavian Study of Early Thrombolysis (ASSET). Lancet 1988;2:525-530.

58. AIMS Trial Study Group: Effect of intravenous APSAC on mortality after acute myocardial infarction: Preliminary report of a placebo-controlled clinical trial. Lancet 1988;1:515-549.

59. Chesebro JH, Knatterud G, Roberts R, et al. Thrombolysis in Myocardial Infarction (TIMI) Trial, phase I: a comparison between intravenous tissue plasminogen activator and intravenous streptokinase. Circulation 1987;76:142-154.

60. Topol EJ, Califf RM, George BS, Kereiakes DJ, Lee KL. Insights derived from the Thrombolysis and Angioplasty in Myocardial Infarction (TAMI) trials. J Am Coll Cardiol 1988;12:24A-31A.

61. Grines CL, Nissen SE, Booth DC, et al. A prospective, randomized trial comparing half-dose tissue-type plasminogen activator with streptokinase to full-dose tissue-type plasminogen activator. Circulation 1991;84:540-549.

62. Califf RM, Topol EJ, Stack RS, et al. Evaluation of combination thrombolytic therapy and timing of cardiac catheterization in acute myocardial infarction: results of Thrombolysis and Angioplasty in Myocardial Infarction-Phase 5 randomized trial. Circulation 1991;83:1543-1556.

63. Carney RJ, Murphy GA, Brandt TR, et al. Randomized angiographic trial of recombinant tissue-type plasminogen activator (alteplase) in myocardial infarction. J Am Coll Cardiol 1992;20:17-23.

64. Granger CB, Ohman EM, Bates E. Pooled analysis of angiographic patency rates from thrombolytic therapy trials. Circulation 1992;86(suppl I):I-269(abstr).

65. Kennedy JW, Martin GV, Davis KB, et al. The Western Washington Intravenous Streptokinase in Acute Myocardial Infarction randomized trial. Circulation 1988;77:345-352.

66. Schroder R, Neuhaus K-L, Leizorovicz A, Linderer T, Tebbe U. A prospective placebo-controlled double-blind multicenter trial of intravenous streptokinase in acute myocardial infarction (ISAM): long-term mortality and morbidity. J Am Coll Cardiol 1987;9:197-203.

67. Meinertz T, Kasper W, Schumacher M, Just H. The German multicenter trial of anisoylated plasminogen streptokinase activator complex versus heparin for acute myocardial infarction. Am J Cardiol 1988;62:347-351.

68. Gibbons RJ, Holmes DR, Reeder GS, Bailey KR, Hopenspirger MR, Gersh BJ. Immediate angioplasty compared with the administration of a thrombolytic agent followed by conservative treatment for myocardial infarction. N Engl J Med 1993;328:685-691.

69. O'Neill W, Timmis GC, Bourdillon PD, Lai P, Ganghadarhan V, Walton J, Ramos R, Laufer N, Gordon S, Schork MA, Pitt B. A prospective randomized clinical trial of intracoronary streptokinase versus coronary angioplasty for acute myocardial infarction. N Engl J Med 1986;31:812-818.

70. DeWood MA, Fisher MJ, for the Spokane Heart Research Group. Direct PTCA versus intravenous rtPA in acute myocardial infarction: Preliminary results from a prospective randomized trial. Circulation 1989;80:II-418.

71. Ribeiro EE, Silva LA, Carneiro R, D'Oliveria LG, Gasquez A, Jose GA, Tavares JR, Petrizzo A, Torossian S, Duprat R, Buffolo E, Ellis SG. Randomized trial of direct coronary angioplasty versus intravenous streptokinase in acute myocardial infarction. J Am Coll Cardiol 1993;88:I-411.

72. Elizaga J, Garcia EJ, Delcan JL, Garcia-Robles JA, Bueno H, Soriano J, Abeytua M, Lopez-Bescos L. Primary coronary angioplasty versus systemic thrombolysis in acute anterior myocardial infarction: in-hospital results from a prospective randomized trial. Circulation 1993;88:I-411.

73. Michels KB, Yusif S. Does PTCA in acute myocardial infarction affect mortality and reinfarction rates? A quantitative overview (meta-analysis) of the randomized clinical trials. Circulation 1995;91:476-485.

74. O'Neill WW, de Boaer MJ, Gibbons RJ, Holmes DR, Timmis GC, Sachs D, Griens CL, Zijlstra F. Data from three prospective randomized clinical trials of thrombolytic versus angioplasty therapy of acute myocardial infarction. Preliminary results from a pooled analysis. Book chapter in <u>Primary Coronary Angioplasty in Acute Myocardial Infarction</u>. Ed. Menko Jan de Boer, Proefschrift Rotterdam: Erasmus University, 1994, pp. 165-171.

75. The GUSTO Angiographic Investigators. The effects of tissue plasminogen activator, streptokinase, or both on coronary-artery patency, ventricular function, and survival after acute myocardial infarction. N Engl J Med 1993;329:1615-1622.

76. Topol EJ, Califf RM, Vandormael M, et al, the the Thrombolysis and Angioplasty in Myocardial Infarction (TAMI-6) Study Group. A randomized trial of late reperfusion therapy for acute myocardial infarction. Circulation 1992;85:2090-2099.

77. Meijer A, Verheugt FWA, Werter CJPJ, Lie KI, vander Pol JMJ, van Eenige MJ. Aspirin versus coumadin in the prevention of reocclusion and recurrent ischemia after successful thrombolysis: A prospective placebo-controlled angiographic study. Results of the APRICOT study. Circulation 1993;87:1524-1530.

78. Meijer A, Verheugt F, Eenigem M, Werter C. Left ventricular function at 3 months after successful thrombolysis. Impact of reocclusion without reinfarction on ejection fraction, regional function and remodeling. Circulation 1994;90:1706-1714.

79. Veen G, Meyer A, Verheugt F, et al. Culprit lesion morphology and stenosis severity in the prediction of reocclusion after coronary thrombolysis: Angiographic results of the APRICOT study. J Am Coll Cardiol 1993;22:1755-62.

80. White H, French J, Hamer A, et al. Frequent reocclusion of patent infarct-related arteries between 4 weeks and 1 year: Effects of antiplatelet therapy. J Am Coll Cardiol 1995;25:218-23.

81. Mark DB, O'Neill WW, Brodie B, Ivanhoe R, Knopf W, Taylor G, O'Keefe JH, Grines CL, Davidson-Ray L, Knight JD, Califf RM. Baseline and six-month costs of primary angiopalty therapy for acute myocardial infarction: Results from the primary angioplasty registry. J Am Coll Cardiol 1995;26:688-695.

82. Eckleberg T, Vlietstra R, Brenner A, Grines C, O'Neill W, Browne K. Cost comparison of primary angioplasty versus thrombolytic therapy for acute myocardial infarction. J Am Coll Cardiol 1993;21:347A.

83. Brodie B, Grines CL, Spain M, et al. A prospective, randomized trial evaluating early discharge (day 3) without non-invasive risk stratification in low risk patients with acute myocardial infarction: PAMI-2. J Am Coll Cardiol 1995;25:5A.

84. Donohue BC, O'Neill WW, Jackson EJ, Brodie B, Griffin J, Balestrini C, Stone G, Wharton T, Jones DE, Grines CL. Cost analysis of different management strategies for myocardial infarction. American College of Cardiology. 1996, abstract, in pess.

85. Ellis SG, Vande Weft F, DaSilva ER, et al. Present status of rescue coronary angioplasty: Current polarization of opinion and randomized trials. J Am Coll Cardiol 1992;19:681-686.

86. Califf RM, Topol EJ, George BS, et al. Characteristics and outcomes of patients in whom reperfusion with tissue-type plasminogen activator fails: results of the Thrombolysis and Angioplasty in Myocardial Infarction TAMI) trial. Circulation 1988;77:1090-1099.

87. Fung AY, Lai P, Topol EJ, et al. Value of percutaneous transluminal coronary angioplasty after unsuccessful intravenous streptokinase therapy in acute myocardial infarction. Am J Cardiol 1986;58:686-691.

88. Topol EJ, Califf RM, George BS, et al and the TAMI Study Group. Coronary arterial thrombolysis with combined infusion of recombinant tissue-type plasminogen activator and urokinase in patients with acute myocardial infarction. Circulation 1988;77:1100-1107.

89. Grines CL, Nissen SE, Booth DC, et al and the KAMIT study group. A new thrombolytic regimen for acute myocardial infarction using combination half dose tissue-type plasminogen activator with full dose streptokinase: a pilot study. J Am Coll Cardiol 1989;14:573-580.

90. Holmes DR, Gersh BJ, Baily KR, et al. "Rescue" percutaneous transluminal coronary angioplasty after failed thrombolytic therapy: 4-year follow-up. J Am Coll Cardiol 1989;13:193 (abstr).

91. Grines CL, Nissen SE, Booth DC, et al and the Kentucky Acute Myocardial Infarction Trial (KAMIT) Group. A prospective, randomized trial comparing combination half-dose tissue-type plasminogen activator and streptokinase with full-dose tissue-type plasminogen activator. Circulation 1991;84:540-549.

92. O'Connor CM, Mark DB, Hinohara T, et al. Rescue coronary angioplasty after failure of intravenous streptokinase in acute myocardial infarction: in-hospital and long-term outcomes. J Invasive Cardiol 1989;1:85-95.

93. Baim DS, Diver DJ, Knatterud GL and the TIMI II-A Investigators. PTCA "salvage" for thrombolytic failures: implications from TIMI II-A. Circulation 1988;78(Suppl II):II-112(abstr).

94. Whitlow PL. Catheterization/rescue angioplasty following thrombolysis (CRAFT) study: results of rescue angioplasty. Circulation 1990;82(Suppl III):III-308(abstr).

95. Abbottsmith CW, Topol EJ, George BS, et al. Fate of patients with acute myocardial infarction with patency of the infarct-related vessel achieved with successful thrombolysis versus rescue angioplasty. J Am Coll Cardiol 1990;16:770-778.

96. Gibson CM, Cannon CP, Piana RN, et al. Rescue PTCA in the TIMI 4 trial. J Am Coll Cardiol 1994;1A-484A:225A.

97.   Wnqk A, Krupa H, Gasior M, Kalarus Z, Borkowski B, Wqs T, Lekston A, Wester A, Chodor P, Pasyk S. Results of rescue-angioplasty after unsuccessful intracoronary streptokinase therapy in patients with acute myocardial infarction. European Congress of Cardiology, abstract, 1995.

98.   Ross AM, Reiner JS, Thompson MA, et al. Immediate and follow-up procedural outcome of 214 patients undergoing rescue PTCA in the GUSTO trial: no effect of the lytic agent. Circulation 1993;88(Suppl I):I-410(abstr).

99.   Ellis SG, Riberiero da Silva E, Heyndrickx G, Talley D, Cernigliaro C, Steg G, Spaulding C, Nobuyoshi M, Erbel R, Vassanelli C, Topol EJ. Randomized comparison of rescue angioplasty with conservative management of patients with early failure of thrombolysis for acute anterior myocardial infarction.

100. Belenkie I, Traboulsi M, Hall CA, Hansen JL, Roth DL, Manyari D, Filipchuck NG, Schnurr LR, Rosenal TW, Smith ER, Knudtson M. Rescue angioplasty during myocardial infarction has a beneficial effect on mortality: A tenable hypothesis. Can J Cardiol 1992;8:357-362.

101. The CORAMI Study Group. Outcome of attempted rescue coronary angiopalsty after failed thrombolysis for acute myocardial infarction. Am J of Cardiol 1994;74:172174.

102. Rogers WJ, Baim DS, Gore JM, et al for the TIMI-IIA Investigators. Comparison of immediate invasive, delayed invasive, and conservative strategies after tissue-type plasminogen activator. Circulation 1990;81:1457-1476.

103. Topol EJ, Califf RM, George BS, et al and the Thrombolysis and Angioplasty in Myocardial Infarction Study Group. A randomized trial of immediate versus delayed elective angioplasty after intravenous tissue plasminogen activator in acute myocardial infrction. N Engl J Med 1987;317:581-588.

104. Simoons ML, Arnold AET, Bertriu A, et al. Thrombolysis with tissue plasminogen activator in acute myocardial infarction: No additional benefit from immediate percutaneous coronary angioplasty. Lancet 1988;1:197-202.

105. Gibson C, Cannon C, Piana R. Angiographic predictors of reocclusion after thrombolysis: Results from the thrombolysis in myocardial infarction (TIMI-4) trial. J Am Coll Cardiol 1995;25:589-9.

106. The TIMI Study Group. Comparison of invasive and conservative strategies after treatment with intravenous tissue plasminogen activator in acute myocardial infarction. Results of the Thrombolysis in Myocardial Infarction (TIMI) Phase II Trial. N Engl J Med 1989;320:

107. SWIFT (Should We Intervene Following Thrombolysis?) Trial Study Group. SWIFT trial of delayed elective intervention vs. Conservative treatment after thrombolysis with anistreplase in acute myocardial infarction. Br Med J 1991;302:5550560.

108. Barbash GI, Roth A, Hod H, et al. Randomized controlled trial of late in-hospital angiography and angioplasty versus conservative management after treatment with recombinant tissue-type plasminogen activator in acute myocardial infarction. Am J Cardiol 1990;66:538-545.

109. Van den Brand MJ, Betrui A, Bescos LL, et al. Randomized trial of deferred angioplasty after thrombolysis for acute myocardial infarction. Coronary Artery Disease 1992;3:393-401.

110. Ozbek C, Dyckmans J, Sen S, et al. Comparison of invasive and conservative strategies after treatment with streptokinase in acute myocardial infrction: results of a randomized trial (SIAM). J Am Coll Cardiol 1990;15:63A (abstr).

111. Mueller HS, Cohen LS, Braunwald E, et al, for the TIMI Investigators. Predictors of early morbidity and mortality after thrombolytic therapy of acute myocardial infarction. Analyses of patient subgroups in the Thrombolysis in Myocardial Infarction (TIMI) Trial, Phase II. Circulation 1992;85:1254-1264.

112. Guerci AD, Gerstenblith G, Brinker JA, et al. A randomized trial of intravenous tissue plasminogen activator for acute myocardial infarction with subsequent randomization to elective coronary angioplasty. N Engl J Med 1987;317:1613-1618.

113. Danchin N, Angioi M, Cardar R, et al. Late percutaneous recanalization of chronic total coronary occlusion after myocrdial infarction improves global and regional left ventricular function and avoids remodeling in the absence of subsequent reocclusion. Circulation 1995;92:I-74.

114. Meneveau N, Bassard J, Lablanche J, et al. Late reopening with angioplasty of totally occluded infarct related arteries prevents LV remodelling after myocardial infarction. Presented at the European Congress of Cardiology, 1995

115. Van de Werf F. Discrepancies between the effects of coronary reperfusion on survival and left ventricular function. Lancet 1989;I:1367-1369.

116. Galvani M, Ottani F, Ferrini D, Sorbello F, Rusticali F. Patency of the infarct-related artery and left ventricular function as the major determinants of survival after Q-wave acute myocardial infarction. Am J Cardiol 1993;71:I-7.

117. Anderson JL. Overview of patency as an endpoint of thrombolytic therapy. Am J Cardiol 1991;67:11-16E.

118. Topol EJ, Califf RM, Vandormael M, Grines CL, George BS, Sanz ML, Wall T, O'Brien M, Schwaiger M, Aguirre FV, Young S. Popma JJ, Lee KL, Ellis SG and the Thrombolysis and Angioplasty in Myocardial Infarction-6 Study Group. A randomized trial of late reperfusion therapy for acute myocardial infarction. Circulation 1992,85:2090-2099.

119. DANAMI Study. Results presented at the American Heart Association, 1995 Plenary Session.

120. Braunwald E, Mark DB, Jones RH, Cheitlin MD, Fuster V, McCauley K, Edwards C, Green LA, Mushlin AL, Swain JA, Smith EE, Cowan M, Rose GC, Concannon CA, Grines CL, Brown L, Lytle BW, Goldman LA, Topol EJ, Willerson JT, Brown J, Archibald

N. Unstable Angina: Diagnosis and Management - Clinical Practice Guidelines. U.S. Department of Health and Human Services. AHCPR Publication No. 94-0682, March 15, 1994.

121. Roberts W, Kragel A, Gertz S, Roberts S. Coronary arteries in unstable angina, acute myocardial infarction and sudden coronary death. Am J Cardiol 1994;127:1588-1593.

122. DeFeyter P, Serruys P. Percutaneous transluminal coronary angioplasty for unstable angina. Chapter in <u>Textbook of Interventional Cardiology</u>. Ed. EJ Topol, M.D. W.B. Saunders Co., 1994, p. 274.

123. Steffenino G, Meier B, Finci L, et al. Follow-up results of treatment of unstable angina by coronary angioplasty. Br Heart J, 1987; 57:416.

124. Myler RK, Shaw RE, Stertzer SH, et al. Unstable angina and coronary angioplasty. Curculation 1990;82:II-88-95.

125. Stammen F, De Scheerder I, Glazier JJ, et al. Immediate and follow-up results of the conservative coronary angioplasty strategy of unstable angina pectoris. Am J Cardiol 1992;69:1533.

126. de Feyter PJ, Suryapranata H, Serruys PW, et al. Coronary angioplasty for unstable angina: Immediate and late results in 200 consecutive patients with identification of risk factors for unfavorable early and late outcome. J Am Coll Cardiol 1988;12:324.

127. Plokker HWT, Ernst SMPG, Bal ET, et al. Percutaneous transluminal coronary angioplasty in patients with unstable angina pectoris refractory to medical therapy. Cathet Cardiovasc Diagn 1988;14:15.

128. Perry RA, Seth A, Hunt A, et al. Coronary angioplasty in unstable angina and stable angina: A comparison of success and complications. Br Heart J 1988;60:367.

129. Bentivoglio LG, Holubkov R, Kelsey SF et al. Short and long term outcome of percutaneous transluminal coronary angioplasty in unstable versus stable angina pectoris: A report of the 1985-1986 NHLBI PTCA Registry. Cathet Cardiovasc Diagn 1991;23:227.

130. Rupprecht HJ, Brennecke R, Kottmeyer M, Bernhard G, Erbel R, Pop T, Meyer R. Short and long-term outcome after PTCA in patients with stable and unstable angina. Eur Heart J 1990;11:964.

131. Morrison DA. Coronary angioplasty for medically refractory unstable angina within 30 days of acute myocardial infarction. Am Heart J 1990;120:256.

132. Ambrose J, Almeida O, Sharma S, et al. Adjunctive thrombolytic therapy during angioplasty for ischemic rest angina. Results of the TAUSA trial. Circulation 1994;90:69-77.

133. Lincoff A, Califf R, Anderson K, et al. Striking clinical benefit with platelet GPIIb/IIIa inhibition by C7E3 among patients with unstable angina: Outcome of the EPIC trial. Circulation 1994;90:I-21.

134. Williams D, Sharaf B, Braunwald E, et al. Percutaneous transluminal coronary angioplasty (PTCA) for acute myocardial ischemia: The TIMI-3 experience. Circulation 1994;90:I-433.

135. Bittl J, Strong J, Brinker J, et al. Treatment with Bivalirudin (Hirulog) as compared with heparin during coronary angioplasty for unstable or post ibnfarciton angina. N Engl J Med 1995;333:764-9.

136. Serruys P, Herrman J, Simon R, et al. A comparison of Hirudin with heparin in the prevention of restenosis after coronary angioplasty. N Engl J Med 1995;333:757-63.

137. Bengtson J, Wilson J. Interventions in unstable angina. Chapter in <u>Interventional Cardiovascular Medicine - Prinicples and Practice</u>. Eds. Roubin, Califf, O'Neill, Phillips, Stack. Churchill Livingstone, Inc. New York, New York, 1996.

138. Chuang Y, Popma J, Satler et al. Increasing angina predicts an unfavorable outcome after new device angioplasty. J Am Coll Cardiol 1994:289A.

139. Hong M, Popma J, Wong S, et al. Incidence of and factors associated with abrupt closure in patients undergoing elective, new device angioplasty in native coronary arteries. J Am Coll Cardiol 1995;122A.

140. Harrington R, Holmes D, Berdan L, et al. Clinical characteristics and outcomes of patients with unstable angina undergoing percutaneous intervention in CAVEAT. J Am Coll Cardiol 1994;288A.

141. Ambrose J, Almeida D, Ratner D, et al. Heparin administered prior to angioplasty does not decrease angioplasty complications. Circulation 1994;90:I-374.

142. TIMI-3B Investigators. Effects of tissue plasminogen activator and a comparison of early invasive and conservative strategies in unstable angina and non Q-wave myocardial infarction. Circulation 1994;89:1545-1556.

143. Anderson H, Cannon C, Stone P, et al. One year results of the thrombolysis in myocardial infarction (TIMI)3B clinical trial. J Am Coll Cardiol 1995;26:1643-1650.

144. CABRI Trial Partipants. First-year results of CABRI (Coronary Angiolsty vs Bypass Revascularisation Investigation). Lancet 1995;346:1179-84.

145. RITA Trial Participants. Coronary angioplasty versus coronary artery bypass surgery: The Randomised Intervention Treatment of Angina (RITA) trial. Lancet 1993;343:573-80.

146. King SB, Lembo NJ, Kosinski AS, et al. A randomised trial comparing coronary angioplasty with coronary bypass surgery. N Engl J Med 1994;331:1044-50.

147. Hamm CW, Riemers J, Ischinger T, et al. A randomised study of coronary angioplasty compared with bypass surgery in patients

with symptomatic multi-vessel coronary disease. N Engl J Med 1994;331:1037-1043.

148. Rodriguez A, Boullon F, Prez-Balino N, et al. Argentine randomised trial of percutaneous transluminal coronary angioplasty versus coronary artery bypass surgery in multi-vessel disease (ERACI): in-hospital results and 1-yer follow-up. J Am Coll Cardiol 1993;22:1060-67.

149. Bypass Angioplasty Revascularization Investigation (BARI). N Engl J Med 1996, in press.

150. Kaplan B, Safian R, Grines C, et al. Differences in outcome after angioplasty for AMI: The left anterior descending artery vs the right coronary. J Am Coll Cardio 1996, abstract, in press.

151. Bates ER. Reperfusion therapy in inferior myocardial infarction. J Am Coll Cardiol 1988;12:44A-51A.

152. Gacioch GM, Topol EJ. Sudden paradoxic clinical deterioration during angioplasty of the occluded right coronary artery in acute myocardial infarction. J Am Coll Cardiol 1989;14:1202-9.

153. Kahn JK, Rutherford BD, McConahay DR, et al. Catheterization laboratory events and hospital outcome with direct angioplsty for acute myocardial infarction. Circulation 1990;82:1910-1915.

154. Ohman EM, Califf RM, Topol EJ, et al. Consequences of reocclusion after successful reperfusion therapy in acute myocardial infarction. Circulation 1990;82:781-91.

155. Stone GW, Griens CL, Browne KF, Marco J, Rothbaum D, O'Keefe J, Hartzler GO, Overlie P, Donohue B, Chelliah N, Vlietstra R, Puchrowicz-Ochocki S, O'Neill WW. Implications of recurrent ischemia after reperfusion therapy in acute myocardial infarction: A comparison of thrombytic therapy and primary angioplsty. J Am Coll Cardiol 1995;26:66-72.

156. Grines C, Brodie B, Griffin J, Donohue B, Sampaoiesi A, Costantini C, Sachs D, Wharton T, Esente P, Spain M, Stone G. Which primary PTCA patients may benefit from new technologies? Circulation, 1995;92:I-146.

157. Nunn C, O'Neill W, Rothbaum D, O'Keefe J, Overlie P, Donohue B, Mason D, Catlin T, Grines C. Primary angioplasty for myocardial infarction improves long-term survival : PAMI-1 follow-up. J Am Coll Cardiol 1996;abstract, in press.

158. Ohman GM, George B, White C, et al. Use of aortic counterppulsation to improve sustained coronary patency during acute MI. Results of a randomized trial. Circulation 1994;90:792-799.

159. Ishihara M, Sato H, Tateishi H, et al. Intraaortic balloon pumping as the postangioplasty strategy in acute myocardial infarction. Am Heart J 1991;122:385-389.

160. Grines CL, Brodie BR, Griffin JJ, Donohue BC, Costantini C, Balestrini C, Stone G, Jones DE, Sachs D, O'Neill WW. Prophylactic intraaortic balloon pumping for acute myocardial infarction does not improve left ventricular function. J Am Coll Cardiol 1996, abstract, in press.

170. Stone GW, Marsalese D, Brodie B, Griffin J, Donohue B, Costantini C, Balestrini C, Wharton

171. Ghazzal ZMB, Hinohara T, Scott NA, et al. Directional coronary atherectomy in patients with recent myocardial infarction: a NACI Registry report. J Am Coll Cardiol 1993;21:32A.

172. Robertson G, hinohara T, Vetters J, et al. Directional coronary atherectomy for patients with recent myocardial infarction. J Am Coll Cardiol 1994:219A.

173. Abdelmeguid A. Sapp S, Lynch D, et al. Immediate and follow-up results of directional coronary atherectomy for the treatment of unstable angina. Circulation 1993;88:I-496.

174. Topol EJ, Leya F, Pinkerton CA, et al. A comparison of directional atherectomy with coronary angioplasty in patients with coronary artery disease. N Engl J Med 1993;329:221-7.

175. Smucker ML, Sarnat WS, Kil D, Scherb DE, Howard PF. Salvage from cardiogenic shock by atherectomy after failed emergency coronary artery angioplasty. Cath Cardiovasc Diagn 1990;21:23-5.

176. Lasorda DM, Incorvati DL, Randall RR. Extraction atherectomy during myocardial infarction in a patient with prior coronary artery bypass surgery. Cath Cardiovasc Diag 1992;26:117-121.

177. Larkin TJ, Niemyski PR, Parker MA, Kramer BL. Primary and rescue extraction atherectomy in patients with acute myocrdial infarction. Circulation 1991;84:II-537.

178. Larkin TJ, O'Neill WW, Safian RD, Schreiber TL, May MA, Kazziha S, Niemyski PR, Parker MA, Kramer BL, Grines CL. A prospective study of transluminal extraction atherectomy in high risk patients with acute myocardial infarction. J Am Coll Cardiol 1994;226A.

179. Kaplan BM, O'Neill WW, Safian RD, Schreiber TL, Larkin TJ, Dooris M, May M, Grines CL. Clinical and angiographic follow-up to a prospective study of transluminal extraction atherectomy in high risk patients with acute myocardial infarction. J Am Coll Cardiol, 1995:331A.

180. Malosky S, Hirschfeld J, Herman H. Comparison of results of intracoronary stenting in patients with unstable vs stable angina. Cath and CV Diagn 1994;31:95-101.

181. Levy G, deBoisgelin, Volpiliere R, Bouvagnet P. Intracoronary stenting in direct infarct angioplasty: Is it dangerous? Circulation 1995;92:I-139.

182. Neumann F, Walter H, Schmitt C, Alt E, Schomig. Coronary stenting as an adjunct to direct balloon angioplasty in acute myocardial

infarction. Circulation 1995;92:I-609.

183. Monassier J, Elias J, Raynaud P, Joly P. Results of early (<24hrs) and late (>24hrs) implantation of coronary stents in acute myocardial infarction. Circulation 1995;92:I-609.

184. Guameri E, Schatz R, Sklar M, et al. Acute coronary syndromes: Is it safe to stent? Circulation 1995;92:I-616.

185. Benzuly K, Goldstein J, Almany S, et al. Feasibility of stenting in acute myocardial infarction. Circulation 1995;92:I-616

186. Stone G, Personal communication, January, 1996.

187. Van der Giessen WJ, Hardhammar P, Van Beusekom MM, et al. Reduction of thrombotic events using heparin-coated Palmaz-Schatz stents. Circulation 1993;88:I-661.

188. Serruys PW, Emanuelsson H, van der Giessen W, Lunn AC, Kiemeney F, Macaya C, Rutsch W, Heyndrickx G, Suryapranata H, Legrand V, Goy JJ, Materne P, Bonnier H, Morice M-C, Fajadet J, Belardi J, Colombo An, Garcia E, Ruygrok P, de Jaegere P, Morel M-A. Heparin-coated Palmaz-Schatz stents in human coronary arteries. Circulation 1996;93:412-422.

189. Topaz O. Holmium laser coronary thromboysis - a new treatment modality for revascularization in acute myocardial infarction: Review. J Clin Laser Med & Surg 1992;10:427-31.

190. De Marchena E, Mallon S, Posada JD, et al. Direct holmium laser-assisted balloon angioplasty in acute myocardial infarction. Am J Cardiol 1993;71:1223-5.

191. Topaz O, Rozenbaum EA, Battista S, Peterson C, Wysham DG. Laser facilitated angioplasty and thrombolysis in acute myocardial infarction complicated by prolonged or recurrent chest pain. Cath Cardiovasc Diag 1993;28:7-16.

192. Topaz O, Minisi A, Luxenberg M, et al. Laser angioplasty for lesions unsuitable for PTCA in acute myocardial infarction: Quantitative coronary angiography and clinical results. Circulation 1994;90:I-434.

193. Spears JR, Kundu SK, McMath LP. Laser balloon angioplasty: Potential for the reduction of the thrombogenicity of the injured arterial wall and for local application of bioprotective materials. J Am Coll Cardiol 1991;17:179B-188B.

194. Spears JR, Dsgisn TF, Douglas JS, et al. Multicenter acute and chronic results of laser balloon angioplasty for refractory abrupt closure after PTCA. Circulation 1991;84:II-517.

195. Reis GJ, Pomerantz RM, Jenkins RD, et al. Laser balloon angioplasty: clinical, angiographic and histologic results. J Am Coll Cardiol 1991;18:193-202.

196. Schwartz L, Andrus S, Sinclair IN, et al. Restenosis following laser balloon angioplasty - a randomized pilot multicenter trial. Circulation 1991;84:II-361.

197. Makowski S, O'Neill B, Sarkis A, et al. Physiological low stress angioplasty at 60° C. Initial results and 6 month follow-up. J Am Coll Cardiol 1993;21:440A.

198. Saito S, Arai H, Kim K, et al. Initial experience of unipolar radio-frequency hot balloon angiopalsty for bail-out from abrupt coronary closure after conventional balloon angioplasty. J Am Coll Cardiol 1993;21:338A.

199. Moura A, Lam JYT, Hebert D, Letchacovski G, Robitaille D, Grant G, Kaplan A. Local heparin delivery decreases the thrombogenicity of the balloon-injured artery. Circulation 1994;90:I-449.

200. Thomas CN, Barry JJ, King SB, Scott NA. Local delivery with heparin with a PTCA infusion balloon inhibits platelet-dependent thrombosis. J Am Coll Cardiol 1994;23:4A.

201. Azrin MA, Mitchel JF, Fram DB, Pedersen CA, Cartun RW, Barry JJ, Bow LM, Waters D, McKay RG. Decreased platelet deposition and smooth muscle cell proliferation following intramural heparin delivery with hydrogel-coated balloons. Circulation 1994;90:433-441.

202. Fram DB, Mitchel JF, Azrin MA, Schwedick MW, Waters DD, McKay RG. Local heparin delivery in porcine coronary arteries with the Dispatch catheter delivery, washout and effect on platelet deposition following balloon angioplasty. Circulation 1994;90:I-493.

203. Mitchel JF, Azrin MA, Schwedick MW, Bow LM, Waters DD, McKay RG. Local delivery of heparin with a novel iontophoretic catheter - quantitative heparin delivery and effect on platelet depositon following balloon angioplasty. Circulation 1994;90:I-492.

204. Lopez-Sendon J, Sobrino N, Gamallo C, Lorenzo A, Jimenez J, Calvo L, Sobrino JA, Rico J, de Miguel E. Locally delivered heparin reduces intimal hyperplasian and lumen stenosis following arterial balloon injury in swine. European Heart J 1993;14:191.

205. Camenzind E, van der giesen W, Ligthart J, Ruygrok P, de Jaegere P, de Feyter P, Serruys PW. Local, low pressure heparin delivery following angioplasty in man: the solution to restenosis? J Am Col Cardiol 1995:376A.

206. Steg P, Spaulding C, Makowski S, et al. A double blind randomized trial of hydrogel balloon delivery of urokinase during primary angioplasty for acute myocardial infarction. Circulation 1995;92:

207. Hartnell GG, Saxton JM, Friedl SE, et al. Ultasonic thrombus ablation: in vitro assessment of a novel device for intracoronary use. J Interven Cardiol 1993;6:69-76.

208. Steffen W, Luo H, Nita H, et al. Catheter delivered therapeutic ultrasound recanalizes thrombotically occluded canine coronary arteries. J Am Coll Cardiol 1993;k21:338A.

209. Hamm C, Steffen W, Reimers J, et al. Ultrasound induced thrombolysis in patients with acute myocardial infarctions. Circulation 1995;92:I-416.

210. Coller BS. Platelets and thrombolytic therapy. N Engl J Med 1990;322:33-42.

211. Lacoste L, Lam JYT, Letchacovski G. Comparative antithrombotic efficacy of aspirin: 80mg vs 325mg daily. Circulation 1994;90:I-552.

212. Dabaghi SF, Damat S, Hendricks O, Payne J, Kleiman NS. Low dose aspirin inhibits in vitro platelet aggregation within minutes after ingestion. Circulation 1992;86:I-261.

213. Lacoste L, Lam JYT. Enhanced platelet thrombus formation in unstable angina. Circulation 1994;90:1374.

214. Hardisty RM, Powling MJ, Nokes TJC. The action of ticlopidine on human platelets; studies on aggregation, secretion, calcium mobilization, and membrane glycoproteins. Thromb Haemost. 1990;64:105-115.

215. Khurana S, Westley S, Mattson J, Safian R. Is it possible to expedite the antiplatelet effect of ticlopidine? Presented at the TCT, February, 1996.

216. Sadowski Z, Kuczak D, Dyduszynski. Comparison of ticlopidine and aspirin in unstable angina, presented at European Congress of Cardiology, 1995.

217. Jeong M, Owen W, Staabon, et al. Does ticlopidine effect platelet deposition and acute stent thrombosis? Circulation 1995;92:I-489.

218. Gregorini L, Marco J, Fajadet J, et al. Ticlopidine alternates post-angioplasty thrombin generation . Circulation 1995;92:I-608.

219. EPIC Investigators. Use of a monoclonal antibody directed against the platelet glycoprotein IIb/IIIa receptor in high-risk coronary angioplasty. N Engl J Med 1994;330:956-961.

220. Topol EJ, Califf RM, Weisman HF, Ellis SG, Tcheng JE, Worley S, Ivanhoe R, George BS, Fintel D, Weston M, Sigmon K, Anderson KM, Lee KL, Willerson JT; on behalf of the EPIC investigators. Randomised trial of coronary intervention with antibody against platelet IIb/IIIa integrin for reduction of clinical restenosis: Results at six months. Lancet 1994;343:881-886.

221. Lefkovits J, Ivanhoe R, Anderson K, et al. Platelet IIb/IIIa receptor inhibition during PTCA for acute myocaridal infarction: Insights from the EPIC trial. Circulation 1994;90:I-564.

222. Linoff AM, Califf R, Anderson , et al. Striking clinical benefit with platelet Iib/IIIa inhibition by C7E3 among patients with unstable angina: Outcome in the EPIC trial. Circulation 1994;90:I-21.

223. Moliterno D, Califf R, Anderson K, et al. Activated clotting time is increased during coronary interventions with platelet IIb/IIIa antagonism: Results from the EPIC trial. J Am Coll Cardiol 1994:106A.

224. EPILOGUE study results. Press release, December, 1995.

225. Muhlestein J, Gomez M, Karagounish L. Rescue ReoPro: Acute utilization of Abciximab for the dissolution of coronary thrombus developing as a complication of coronary angioplasty. Circualtion 1995;92:I-607.

226. Tcheng J, Lincoff AM, Sigmon K. Platelet glyprotein IIb/IIIa inhibition with integrelin during PTCA: The Impact II trial. Circulation 1995;92:I-543.

227. Kereiakes D, Kleiman N, Ambrose J. A dosing study in high risk PTCA of MK-383, a platelet IIb/IIIa antagonist. Circulation 1994;90:I-21.

228. Hettleman BD, Aplin RA, Sullivan PR, et al: Three days of heparin pretreatment reduces major complications of coronary angioplasty in patients with unstable angina . J Am Coll Cardiol 1990;15:154.

229. Lasky MAL, Deutsch E, Barnathan E, et al. Influence of heparin therapy on percutaneous transluminal coronary angioplasty outcome in unstable angina pectoris. Am J Cardiol 1990;65:1425.

230. Pow TK, Varricchione TR, Jacobs AK, et al. Does pretreatment with heparin prevent abrupt closure following PTCA? J Am Coll Cardiol 1988;11:238A.

231. Lukas MA, Deutsch E, Hirschfeld JW, et al. Influence of heparin on percutaneous transluminal coronary angioplasty outcome in patients with coronary arterial thrombus. Am J Cardiol 1990;65:179.

232. Myler RK, Shaw RE, Stertzer SH, et al. Unstable angina and coronary angioplasty. Circulation 1990;82:II-95.

233. Ambrose J, Almeida D, Ratner D, et al. Heparin administered prior to angioplasty does not decrease angioplasty complications. TAUSA trial results. Circulation 1994;90:I-374.

234. Wharton TP, Marsalese D, Brodie BR, Griffin JJ, Donohue BC, Costantini CRF, Balestrini CE, Stone GW, Esente P, Moses J, McNamara NS, Jones D, Sachs D, Grines CL. How often do infarct-related arteries show early perfusion without prior thrombolytic therapy, and should these vessels be dilated acutely? Results from PAMI-2. Circulation 1995:92:I-530.

235. Verheugt F, Marsh R, Veen G. Megadose bolus heparin as reperfusion therapy for acute myocardial infarction: Results of the HEAP pilot study. Circulation 1995;92:I-41.

236. Ferguson J, Dougherty K, Gaos C, et al. Relation between procedural activated coagulation time and outcome after percutaneous transluminal coronary angioplasty. J Am Coll Caridol 1994;23:1061-1065.

237. Snitzer R, Hiremath Y, Lee J, et al. Suppression of intracoronary thrombin activity by weight-adjusted heparin administration during coronary interventions. Circulation 1995;92:I-609.

238. Winters K, Oltrona L, Hiremath Y, et al. Heparin-resistant thrombin activity is associated with acute ischemic events during high risk coronary interventions. Circulation 1995;92:I-608.

239. Harrington Ra, Leimberer JD, Berdan L, Topol EJ, Califf RM for the CAVEAT Investigators. The ACT index: A method for stratifying likelihood of success and risk of acute complications in coronary intervention. Circulation 1993;88:I-208.

240. Naqvi T, Ivy P, Linn P, et al. Low dose heparin enhances and high dose heparin suppresses platelet P-selection expression and platelet aggregation. Circulation 1995;92:I-673.

241. Ahmed W, Meckel C, Grines C, et al. Relation between ischemic complications and activated clotting times during coronary angioplasty: Different profiles for heparin and Hirulog. Circulation 1995;92:I-608.

242. Nairns CR, Hillegass WG, Nelson CL, et al. Activated clotting time predicts abrupt closure risk during angioplasty. J Am Coll Cardiol 1994;23:470A.

243. Hillegass W, Narins C, Brott B, et al. Activated clotting time predicts bleeding complications from angioplasty. J Am Coll Cardiol 1994;184A.

244. Blumenthal R, Wolff M, Resar J, et al. Preprocedural anticoagulation does not reduce angioplasty heparin requirments. Am Heart J 1993;125:1221.

245. Kander NH, Holland KJ, Pitt B, Topol EJ. A randomized pilot trial of brief versus prolonged heparin after succerssful reperfusion in acute myocardial infarction. Am J Cardiol 1990;65:139-142.

246. Granger C, Armstrong P. For the GUSTO IIa investigators. Reinfarction following discontinuation of intravenous heparin or hirudin for unstable angina and acute myocardial infarction. Circulation 1995;92:I-460.

247. Granger C, Miller J, Bovill E, et al. Rebound increase in thrombin generation and activity after cessation of intravenous heparin in patients with acute coronary syndromes. Circulation 1995;91:1929-35.

248. Flather M, Weitz J, Campeau J, et al. Evidence for rebound activation of the coagulation system after cessation of intravenous anticoagulant therapy for acute MI. Circulation 1995;92:I-485.

249. Strony J, Ahmed W, Meckel C, et al. Clinical evidence for thrombin rebound after stopping heparin but not hirulog. Circulation 1995;92:I-609.

250. Khan M, Sepulveda J, Jeroudi M, et al. Rebound increase in thrombin activity with associated decrease in antithrombin III levels after PTCA. Circulation 1995;92:I-785

251. Spielberg C, Schnitzer L, Linderer T, et al. Influence of catheter technology and adjuvant medication on acute complications in percutaneous coronary angioplasty. Cathet Cardiovasc Diagn, 1990;21:72.

252. Ambrose JA, Torre SR, Sharma SK, et al. Adjuvant urokinase for PTCA in unstable angina: final angiographic results of TAUSA pilot study. Circulation, 1991;84:II-590.

253. Buller CE, Fung AY, Thompson CR, Ricci DR, Thompson B, Schrachtman M, Williams DO. Does pre-treatment with tPA improve safety of coronary angioplasty in acute coronary syndrome? Results from TIMI II-B. Circulation 1994;90:I-22.

254. Ambrose JA, Almeida OD, Sharma SK, Torre SR, Marmur JD, Israel DH, Ratner DE, Weiss MB, Hjemdahl-Monsen CE, Myler TK, Moses J, Unterecker WJ, Grunwald AM, Garrett JS, Cowley MJ, Anwar A, Sobolski J for the TAUSA Investigators. Adjunctive thrombolytic therapy during angioplasty for ischemic rest angina. Results of the TAUSA Trial. Circulation 1994;90:69-77.

255. Mehran R, Ambrose JA, Bongu RM, Almeida OD, Israel DH, Torre S, Sharma SK, Ratner ED for the TAUSA study group. Angioplasty of complex lesions in ischemic rest angina: Results of the Thrombolysis and Angioplasty in UnStable Angina (TAUSA) trial. J am coll cardiol 1995;26:961-966.

256. Kerins DM, Roy L, FitzGerald GA, Pitzgerald DJ. Platelet and vascular function during coronary thrombolysis with tissue-type plasminogen activator. Circulation, 1989;80:1718.

257. Bennett WR, Yawn DH, Migliore PJ, et al. Activation of the complement system by recombinant tissue plasminogen activator. J Am Coll cardiol, 1987;10:627.

258. Fitzgerald DJ, Roy L, Wright F, Fitzgerald GA. Functional significance of platelet activation following coronary thrombolysis. Circulation, 1987;76:IV-153.

259. Castaneda-Zuniga WR, Sibley R, Amplatz K. The pathologic basis of angioplasty. Angiology, 1984;35:195.

260. Kohchi K, Taebayashi S, Block PC. Arterial changes after percutaneous transluminal coronary angioplasty: results at autopsy. J Am Coll cardiol, 1987;10:592.

261. Waller BF, Rothbaum DA, Pinkerton CA, et al. Status of the myocardium and infarct-related coronary artery in 19 necropsy patients with acute recanalization using pharmacologic (streptokinase, r-tissue plasminogen activator), mechanical (percutaneous transluminal coronary angioplasty) or combined types of reperfusion therapy. J Am Coll Cardiol, 1987;9:785.

262. Colavita PG, Ideker RE, Reimer KA, et al. The spectrum of pathology associated with percutaneous transluminal coronary angioplasty during acute myocardial infarction. J Am Coll Cardiol, 1986;8:855.

263. Grines C, Schreiber T, Savas V, et al. A randomized trial of low osmolar ionic versus nonionic contrast media in patients with acute myocardial infarction or unstable angina undergoing PTCA. J Am Coll Cardiol 1996, in press.

264. Piessens JH, Stammen F, Brolix MC, et al. Effects of an ionic versus a nonionic low osmolar contrast agent on the thrombotic complications of coronary angioplasty. Catheterization and Cardiovascular Diagnosis 1993;28:99-105.

265. Aguirre F, Topol EJ, Donohue T. Impact of ionic and non inoic contrast media on post PTCA ischemic complications: Results from the EPIC trial. J Am Coll Cardiol 1995;25:8A.

INTERVENTIONAL STRATEGIES IN PATIENTS WITH LEFT VENTRICULAR DYSFUNCTION

Steven L. Almany, M.D.

When angioplasty was originally introduced in the late 1970's, it was estimated that only 5% of patients with coronary artery disease would be acceptable candidates.[1] Absolute contraindications to angioplasty included the presence of multivessel disease and severe left ventricular (LV) dysfunction. Since then, the development of circulatory support systems, advances in catheter technology, and increased operator experience have extended the application of percutaneous techniques. It is estimated that more than 500,000 percutaneous interventions will occur in 1996 in the United States alone.

A. **HISTORICAL RESULTS.** There are limited published data regarding PTCA in patients with LV dysfunction (LV ejection fraction <40%) (Table 6.1). In general these patients are older; more commonly have a history of previous myocardial infarction, coronary artery bypass grafting, multivessel disease; and are more symptomatic than patients with normal LV function. Patients with coronary artery disease and LV dysfunction treated medically have 4-year survival rates of 35 to 60%.[9] The nonrandomized Coronary Artery Surgery Study Registry (CASS) reported a 4-year survival of 72% after CABG compared to 61% after medical therapy in patients with LV ejection fraction < 35%.[10] Patients

Table 6.1. PTCA in Patients with Left Ventricular Dysfunction.

Series	EF (%)	N	Success (%)	Complications (%) D / MI / CABG	Follow-up
Eltchaninoff[5] (1994)	< 40	343	95	2.6 / 2.6 / 3.2	36 mos: Death (18%), repeat PTCA (13%), CABG (9.4%)
Holmes[7] (1993)	< 45	1802	-	0.8 / 4.9 / 4.5	Survival (87%), EFS (77%)
Terrien[8] (1993)	< 31	72	-	11 / - / -	29 mos: Survival (70%)
Serota[3] (1991)	< 40	73	85	5 / - / -	Survival: 1 yr (79%); 5 yr: (57%)
Stevens[2] (1991)	< 40	845	93	4 / - / 2	33 mos: CABG (15%), repeat PTCA (27%); Survival: 1 yr (87%), 4 yr (69%)
O'Keefe[6] (1991)	< 40	100	-	3 / - / -	Survival: 1 yr (84%) 5 yr (66%); EFS: 1 yr (75%), 5 yr (40%)
Kohli[4] (1990)	< 35	61	90	3.2 / 5 / 5	21 mos: Death (23%), EFS (51%)

Abbreviations: EF = LV ejection fraction; MI = myocardial infarction; CABG = coronary artery bypass grafting; EFS = event-free survival; - = not reported

Table 6.2. CABG in Patients with Left Ventricular Dysfunction

Series	EF (%)	N	Complications (%) D / MI	Follow-up
BARI[16] (1995)	< 50	-	- / -	5-year survival: no difference between CABG and PTCA
Veterans[14] (1995)	< 50	150	- / -	Survival: 7 yr (74%); 11 yr (53%)
Elefteriades[15] (1993)	< 30	83	8.4 / -	Survival: 1 yr (87%); 3 yr (80%)
O'Keefe[6] (1991)	< 40	100	5 / -	Survival: 1 yr (91%); 5 yr (77%)
CASS[9] (1983)	< 36	231	6.9 / 10.8	5 yr survival (63%)
Hochberg[11] (1983)	< 40	466	- / -	3 yr survival: EF <20% (15%); EF 20-39% (60%)
Rahimtoola[13] (1983)	-	520	2 / -	Survival: 1 yr (91%); 5 yr (79%)

Abbreviations: EF = LV ejection fraction; - = not reported; MI = myocardial infarction; CABG = coronary artery bypass grafting; EFS = event-free survival; - = not reported; CASS = Coronary Artery Surgery Study; BARI = Bypass Angioplasty Revascularization Intervention.

with LV dysfunction and 1- or 2- vessel disease had better total survival after PTCA or CABG compared to medical therapy, but there was no difference in event-free survival.[11] Although comparisons between nonrandomized studies are difficult, PTCA (Table 6.1) appears comparable to CABG (Table 6.2) in patients with LV dysfunction.

B. DETERMINATION OF NEED FOR SUPPORTED ANGIOPLASTY. Before considering percutaneous interventions in patients with LV dysfunction, the hemodynamic significance of target lesions and the viability of the myocardial perfusion bed must be assessed. One method of assessing the hemodynamic importance of "culprit" lesions is the jeopardy score, which is correlated with the risk of death after abrupt closure.   In this scoring system (Figure 6.1) the coronary tree is divided into 6 segments of equal myocardial perfusion.[17] A score of 0.5 is given for each segment of hypokinetic myocardium and a score of 1.0 is given to each area that is akinetic or dyskinetic. "Closure score" is the sum of the 6 areas if the target vessel became occluded during PTCA (assuming the myocardium perfused by that vessel would become akinetic).[18] On the basis of clinical and angiographic descriptors outlined in Table 6.3, we select patients for supported angioplasty. As demonstrated in Table 6.4, systemic and regional mechanical support systems are available, as well as pharmacologic methods for attenuating myocardial ischemia.

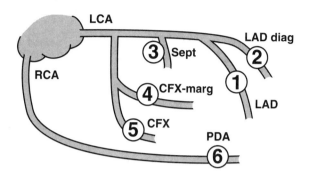

Figure 6.1 Jeopardy Score

Six arterial segments are used to calculate the jeopardy score, which considers the total region of jeopardized myocardium (supplied by the target vessel and providing collaterals to other regions) and the degree of baseline LV dysfunction. Scoring system:

- 1 point: for each myocardial region supplied by the target lesion.
- 1 point: for each myocardial region supplied by a vessel with diameter stenosis $\geq$ 70%.
- 0.5 point: for each myocardial region that is hypokinetic at baseline and not supplied by a vessel with significant stenosis.

Table 6.3. Potential Candidates for Supported Angioplasty

- Target vessel supplies the majority of viable myocardium.
- Ejection fraction < 20-30%.
- Jeopardy score > 3.
- Cardiogenic shock and multivessel disease.

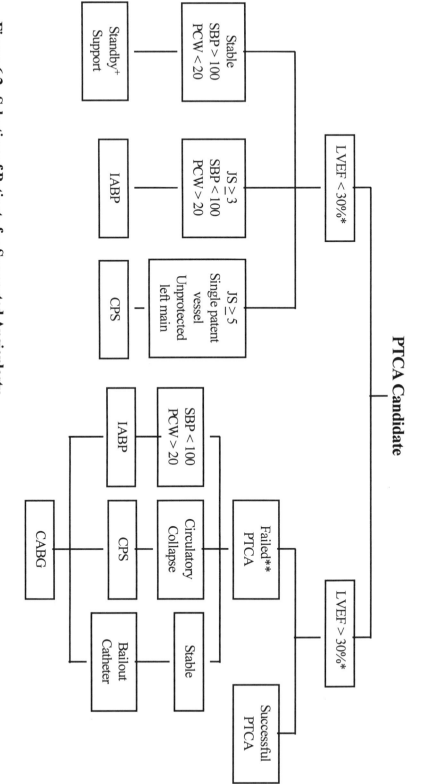

Figure 6.2. Selection of Patients for Supported Angioplasty

Abbreviations: LVEF = left ventricular ejection fraction; SBP = systolic blood pressure; PCW = pulmonary capillary wedge pressure; JS = jeopardy score; IABP = intra-aortic balloon pump; CPS = percutaneous cardiopulmonary bypass support; CABG = emergency coronary artery bypass grafting

* Autoperfusion balloons may be useful.

** Bailout catheters are recommended if emergency CABG is needed.

\+ Standby implies contralateral femoral vascular access; IABP or CPS ready if needed.

Table 6.4. Overview of Supported Angioplasty

I. Systemic Support

Intra-Aortic Balloon Pump (IABP)	**Advantages**: Extensive clinical experience. Provides afterload reduction. May result in improved outcome for selected high-risk PTCA patients and for those unable to be weaned from CPS. **Disadvantages**: Requires stable cardiac rhythm for optimal function. Probable slight increase in vascular complications.
Percutaneous Cardiopulmonary Bypass Support (CPS)	**Advantages**: Provides systemic support independent of ventricular function or cardiac rhythm. **Disadvantages**: Does not prevent myocardial ischemia during balloon inflation (or during acute closure). Not intended for long term support. Does not unload ventricle.
Ventricular Assist Devices	**Advantages**: Systemic support independent of ventricular function or cardiac rhythm. Long-term support possible. **Disadvantages**: Surgical placement required. Limited clinical experience.
Left Atrial-Femoral Bypass	**Advantages**: Systemic support independent of ventricular function or cardiac rhythm. Able to provide support for longer periods than CPS. **Disadvantages**: Requires transseptal puncture. Limited clinical experience. Limited flow rates.

II. Regional Myocardial Support

Autoperfusion Catheters	**Advantages**: Allows better tolerance of prolonged balloon inflations. Better outcome for patients with abrupt closure. **Disadvantages**: Large profile limits access to distal lesions or tortuous vessels. Requires mean arterial pressure >65mmHg for effective passive perfusion.
Active Hemoperfusion	**Advantages**: Less ischemia during balloon inflations. **Disadvantages**: Limit clinical experience. Potential for hemolysis at high flow rates.
Coronary Sinus Retroperfusion	**Advantages**: Improves myocardial oxygenation during inflations. Retrograde delivery of drugs possible. Does not require crossing lesion. **Disadvantages**: Requires separate venipuncture (usually internal jugular). Not consistently effective for right coronary and circumflex arteries. Coronary sinus rupture may occur. Placement may be difficult. Not widely available.
Perfluorochemicals	**Advantages**: High oxygen carrying capacity. Low viscosity. Hemolysis absent at high flow rates. **Disadvantages**: Removed from commercial market in 1995, Expensive. Time required for thawing. Increased incidence of pulmonary edema.
Adjunctive Pharmacotherapy	**Advantages**: Ease of administration. **Disadvantages**: Least effective of all local approaches.

SYSTEMIC SUPPORT

A. INTRA-AORTIC BALLOON COUNTERPULSATION

1. **Description.** Intra-aortic balloon counterpulsation (IABP) is the most commonly used method of cardiac support, and consists of an inflatable 40cc balloon attached to an external control console; 32 cc balloons are recommended in patients less than 62-inches tall. Positioned just distal to the origin of the left subclavian artery, the balloon is triggered to inflate with helium immediately after aortic valve closure, causing an increase in aortic diastolic pressure. This results in an increase in aortic diastolic pressure and coronary blood flow. The balloon is deflated as the aortic valve opens in early systole, markedly decreasing resistance to ventricular ejection (afterload) and improving stroke work.

    a. **Preparation of the IABP.** A one-way valve is connected to the helium port of the IABP. All air is aspirated from the balloon by applying negative pressure to the one-way valve. A 0.030-inch J-tipped IABP wire is next inserted through the central lumen after removing the stylet and flushing the catheter.

    b. **Access Site Evaluation.** In a non-emergent setting, the aorto-iliac system should be assessed for severe tortuosity or high-grade obstruction by contrast injection.

    c. **Arterial Access.** The femoral artery is predilated with an 8F sheath to facilitate atraumatic insertion of the larger 9.5-10.5 IABP sheath. Although the pre-packaged IABP wire can be used to introduce the IABP sheath into the femoral artery, we prefer a 0.035- or 0.038-inch wire for extra support.

    d. **Balloon Pump Insertion.** After removing the internal dilator, the IABP is inserted into the sheath. Prior to advancing the balloon, the IABP guidewire is extended beyond the distal end of the balloon and the system is advanced into position. If resistance is met during balloon advancement, the wire is removed and the location of the balloon is checked by a hand injection of contrast through the distal lumen. In patients with small or diseased iliofemoral systems, an 8.5F IABP without a central lumen may be used with a "peel away" femoral sheath.

    e. **Balloon Pump Positioning.** The guidewire is advanced into the ascending aortic arch as the balloon is positioned approximately 2cm below the left subclavian artery. Proper position is confirmed by the presence of an adequate arterial wave form, augmentation of diastolic pressure, and afterload reduction. Adequate balloon positioning and full inflation should be confirmed under fluoroscopy. If incomplete filling is detected, refilling of the balloon should be performed by depressing the "autofill" button. If the balloon remains unwrapped, a brief hand injection and aspiration of 30cc of helium may be attempted.

3. **Advantages.** IABPs decrease myocardial oxygen demand, increase coronary perfusion pressure (by augmenting diastolic blood pressure and decreasing left ventricular filling pressure), and increase cardiac output by 20-39%.[19] It is easily placed in 90% of patients, and prolonged treatment is possible.

4. **Disadvantages.** IABPs were previously associated with a high incidence of vascular complications (9-43%), including AV fistulae, pseudoaneurysms, iliofemoral thrombosis and local bleeding. In contrast, the PAMI-2 study found no increase in vascular complications in patients randomized to IABP after PTCA for acute MI. Complications are more common in patients with pre-existing vascular disease, diabetics, and females (4 times more common than men); however, complication rates are not affected by age, adequacy of anticoagulation, or body surface area.[20] Effective diastolic augmentation requires a stable cardiac rhythm.[21] Moderate hemolysis and thrombocytopenia are common, although platelet counts below 50,000 are quite unusual.

5. **Outcome.** Several small studies suggest that prophylactic placement of an IABP may allow successful revascularization in over 95% of high-risk patients.[22,23] In the setting of abrupt closure, IABPs were associated with hemodynamic stabilization and resolution of ST segment changes.[24] Although some studies suggest that an IABP during infarct angioplasty results in fewer reocclusions and improved ventricular function,[25-27] the PAMI-2 Trial shows no difference in reocclusion, reinfarction , death or LV function at 1 and 6 months in high risk patients with or without IABP. Less well established roles for IABP include mitigation of myocardial necrosis during acute myocardial infarction[28] and the treatment of intractable ventricular arrhythmias due to ischemia.[29]

6. **Applications.** Prophylactic IABP should be considered in selected high risk patients,[22] refractory angina,[30] cardiogenic shock,[31] and failure to wean from percutaneous cardiopulmonary support (Figure 6.2).[32]

B. PERCUTANEOUS CARDIOPULMONARY SUPPORT (CPS)

1. **Description.** Femoral vein-femoral artery bypass has been employed by surgeons for over thirty years. Advances in technology and design have led to the development of a portable system, allowing extended application to patients undergoing high risk percutaneous revascularization procedures.[33] The cardiopulmonary support system (CPS) collects venous blood from a cannula within the right atrium, pumping it through a semipermeable membrane oxygenator and heat exchanger and then returning it to the arterial system via a cannula in the femoral artery (Figure 6.3).

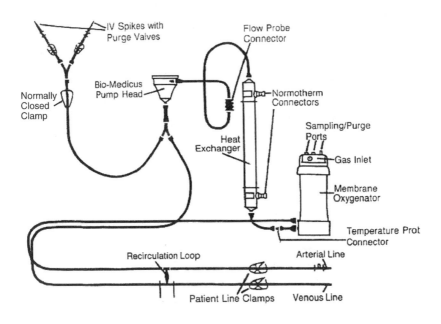

Figure 6.3   CPS Circuitry

2. **Technique of Cardiopulmonary Support**

    a. **Obtain Vascular Access** in the right femoral artery and vein.

    b. **Optimize Volume Status.** A pulmonary artery catheter is inserted to optimize filling pressures and cardiac output prior to beginning CPS. Systemic and pulmonary artery pressures are recorded continuously during the procedure.

    c. **Evaluate Suitability of Peripheral Vasculature.** Because of the large caliber of the CPS sheaths, patency, size and tortuosity in the aorto-iliac system must be determined by angiography before placement of cannulae. It is essential that the arterial cannula not be inserted into the superficial femoral or profunda femoral artery due to the increased risk of vascular complications.

    d. **Venous Cannula Insertion.** An 0.038-inch Amplatz or other stiff wire is inserted through the venous sheath and positioned under fluoroscopy at the junction between the right atrium and inferior vena cava. The femoral vein is progressively dilated with 8F, 12F and 14F dilators.

The CPS venous cannula (18F or 20F depending on body size and desired flow) is inserted under fluoroscopy and positioned in the right atrium. The guidewire and internal dilator are removed as the patient performs the Valsalva maneuver ensuring that external air is not introduced into the system. The thumb-clamp is applied, and the cannula is sutured to the skin to prevent migration.

e. **Arterial Cannula Insertion.** As with venous cannula placement, 8F, 12F and 14F dilators are inserted into the common femoral artery over a stiff guidewire. The arterial cannula is advanced under fluoroscopy to a position between the renal arteries and aortic bifurcation. The guidewire and internal dilator are removed and the thumb clamp applied. This must be performed quickly to minimize blood loss. The cannula is sutured to the skin.

f. **Anticoagulation.** Intravenous heparin, 300 U/kg (average 20,000-25,000 units) is given as a bolus. ACT should be >400 seconds while on CPS. Pre-PTCA transfusions should be considered in patients undergoing CPS if hemoglobin <10gm/dl.

g. **Connect Cannulae to the CPS Console.** Hold the polyvinyl chloride (PVC) venous cannula tubing vertically in the left hand and the PVC tubing from the venous port of the CPS console vertically in the right hand, side by side. An assistant fills both ends of the tubing with saline and the two ends are quickly connected, minimizing air trapping. The thumb clamp is released and the perfusionist vents any air trapped in the venous line through the console. The same steps are followed for the arterial cannula; it is absolutely critical that no air is trapped in the arterial line before releasing the thumb clamp.

h. **Initiate CPS Flow and Perform PTCA.** Monitored continuously by a perfusionist, CPS flow is rapidly increased to an average rate of 3-5L/min. Maximum flow rates are dependent on the size of the CPS cannulae (18F=3-5L/min, 22F= 4-7L/min) and volume status. Pulmonary capillary wedge pressure should be maintained above 5mmHg and mean arterial pressure between 60-80mmHg.

I. **After CPS Has Been Discontinued,** the thumb clamps are reapplied to both arterial and venous cannulae, the PVC tubing is cut just proximal to the clamps, and the plunger from a 5cc syringe is inserted into the cut end of the PVC tubing connected to the cannulae. The cannulae are sutured in place, and the patient is transferred to the cardiac care unit for observation.

3. **Special Considerations**

a. **Hypotension.** Hypotension is very common within the first few minutes of CPS and usually responds to a bolus of normal saline (100-300 cc) rather than increasing the flow rate. Hypotension occurs secondary to a decrease in systemic vascular resistance from CPS-induced volume shifts or vasodilation. On occasion, decreasing CPS flow may improve systemic vascular resistance and restore blood pressure. When vasopressors are required, Neosynephrine (1 mg) can be given directly thorough the CPS unit. Vibration in the venous line is frequently caused by either volume depletion or excessive flow.

b. **Weaning.** Following conclusion of the case, CPS is gradually weaned by decreasing flow rates. On occasion, placement of an IABP is required for hemodynamic support during the CPS weaning process. The IABP can usually be discontinued 4-12 hrs later, following recovery from PTCA-induced myocardial stunning or CPS-induced production of myocardial depressant factors.

c. **Cannulae Removal.** Arterial and venous cannulae are removed 4-6 hours after the last heparin dose; protamine is not used. Initially, manual pressure is applied for 5-20 minutes, followed by placement of a compression device. Surgical removal is recommended when manual compression is not possible (e.g. poor patient cooperation) or continued anticoagulation is required (e.g. suboptimal post-PTCA angiographic result). Pressure should be sufficient to maintain hemostasis without loss of pedal Doppler signals; pressure is gradually released over several hours once the ACT falls below 150 seconds. Total compression time up to 18 hours is frequently required. If adequate hemostasis is achieved, the heparin may be restarted and continued until therapeutic prothrombin times are achieved. Coumadin therapy is recommended for 1-6 months following CPS to reduce the risk of iliofemoral venous thrombosis.

4. **Advantages.** CPS provides excellent systemic perfusion independent of ventricular function or intrinsic cardiac rhythm. Patient perception of chest pain is less common in CPS-supported patients, allowing for prolonged balloon inflations.[34]

5. **Disadvantages.** The most significant deficiency of CPS-supported angioplasty is that myocardial ischemia still occurs distal to the inflated balloon; regional wall motion abnormalities and anaerobic metabolism occur during balloon inflation despite CPS.[35] CPS cannot be continued > 6 hrs because of the onset of disseminated intravascular coagulation and hemolysis, third-spacing of fluids, and the development of hypokalemia and hypomagnesemia. Other disadvantages include vascular injury, large heparin requirements, the need for a perfusionist, and the need for surgical removal of lines or prolonged compression. Other effects include an immediate fall in hemoglobin ≥ 3g/dl due to the dilutional effect of pump priming; suppression of respiratory drive; inadequate CNS perfusion; and varying degrees of aortic insufficiency. Peripheral vascular complications include bleeding, pseudoaneurysm, AV fistula, and arterial occlusion. Transfusion rates in the 1989 CPS registry varied from 25% after percutaneous CPS to 76% after cutdown techniques.[36]

Table 6.5. High-Risk PTCA: Indications for CPS

Probably indicated

· Cath lab hemodynamic collapse

Possible indications

· Poor LV function (EF <20-30%)

· Large area of myocardium at risk

· PTCA of unprotected left main

Contraindication

· Peripheral vascular disease

· Moderate to severe aortic insufficiency

6. **Outcome**. The National Registry of Supported Angioplasty has collected data on patients undergoing elective supported angioplasty. Patients with poor LV function (EF <20%), single patient coronary vessel, and inoperable patients underwent CPS-supported angioplasty with an in-hospital mortality rate of 6%. Over >90% of these patients improved by at least one anginal class.[37] Thus, CPS-supported angioplasty can be performed with a high degree of success and low mortality in selected patients. Patients who experienced cardiac arrest or cardiogenic shock and were immediately placed on CPS (within 15 minutes) and then revascularized (PTCA or CABG) had a survival rate of 48%. CPS in these cases was superior to other hemodynamic support systems.[38]

7. **Indications (Table 6.5).** Because of the many drawbacks associated with prophylactic CPS, standby CPS has emerged as an accepted support strategy (Figure 6.2). When this approach is employed, 5-6F sheaths are usually placed in the left femoral artery and vein after angiographic views demonstrate their suitability for CPS cannulae placement. Experienced operators can usually prime the support system and insert cannulas in less than 5 minutes.[39] Data from the registry indicate that only 5-10% of patients with standby CPS will actually require initiation of circulatory support. Mortality rates in patients who undergo standby CPS (6%) are similar to those in whom prophylactic placement was performed. Several reports suggest that patient outcome improves when CPS is initiated within 10 minutes of cardiac arrest unresponsive to conventional ACLS measures.

C. VENTRICULAR ASSIST DEVICES

1. **Description.** There are limited data on the use of adjunctive assist devices during high-risk angioplasty.[40] The Hemopump (Nimbus® left ventricular assist device) utilizes the Archimedes screw principle to create antegrade aortic flow while decompressing the left ventricle. The screw is encased in a flexible tube that is inserted and removed surgically through the femoral artery. The Hemopump lies across the aortic valve and generates flow up to 3.5L/minute. The system is highly

dependent upon adequate pulmonary venous return.

2.   **Advantages.** The system is light (less than 25 lbs), does not require a membrane oxygenator, may be run on rechargeable batteries, and results in marked left ventricular unloading. It appears to lack the fluid and coagulation abnormalities of prolonged CPS. Systemic support is achieved independent of ventricular function or cardiac rhythm. The cable drive shaft is 11F and has been well tolerated during periods of prolonged support without limb ischemia. Long term support is possible and the system requires only low-dose heparin.

3.   **Disadvantages.** Surgical placement is required. Complications include cannulae migration, coagulopathy, emboli, arrhythmias and sepsis. Contraindications to the Hemopump include the presence of aortic dissection, significant peripheral vascular disease, moderate-severe aortic insufficiency, significant aortic stenosis, or the presence of a left ventricular thrombus.

4.   **Outcome.** Animal studies suggest that the Hemopump can be used for several weeks without significant clinical or biochemical sequelae.[41]   When compared to intra-aortic balloon counterpulsation in dogs, the Hemopump was better able to maintain aortic pressure, unload the left ventricle, and reduce dyskinesis of the ischemic region during balloon inflation.[42] Hemodynamic measurements obtained during Hemopump supported angioplasty demonstrated a 23% improvement in cardiac index and a 17% reduction in pulmonary capillary wedge pressure. Hematological complications were limited to mild hemolysis and moderate thrombocytopenia. A 14F device was been associated with severe hemolysis.

5.   **Applications.** Current indications for this investigational device include inability to wean from CPS, intractable cardiogenic shock, and as a bridge to cardiac transplantation.

D. LEFT ATRIAL-FEMORAL ARTERY BYPASS

1.   **Description.** Involves placement of a 21F catheter into the left atrium (by transseptal technique), which returns blood to a femoral artery catheter.[43] The system is highly dependent upon adequate pulmonary venous return.

2.   **Advantages.** It allows unloading of the left ventricle, but does not require use of a membrane oxygenator; longer support is possible compared to CPS.

3.   **Disadvantages.** This device requires transseptal puncture; left-to-right heart shunting has been recognized. It is less effective when the clinical picture is complicated by pulmonary edema or severe right heart failure and has limited flow rates (4.5L/min) secondary to use of roller pumps.

REGIONAL MYOCARDIAL SUPPORT

A. AUTOPERFUSION CATHETERS. Many patients are unable to tolerate balloon inflations due to severe angina, arrhythmias, and/or hemodynamic instability. Autoperfusion catheters allow safe and effective management of these patients.

1. Description. There are several types of perfusion balloon catheters (see Chapter 1, Chapter 35). All except the Scimed Dispatch have sideholes permitting passive blood flow during balloon inflation. The Dispatch catheter consists of an over-the-wire catheter with a spiral inflation coil wrapped around a non-porous polyurethane sheath. When the spiral inflation coil is inflated, it forms an internal lumen that allows antegrade blood flow (60-100 cc/min); it can also be used for local drug delivery (see Chapter 39).

2. Technique. These catheters are inserted over 0.014-0.018-inch guidewires; because of their large profile and limited trackability, they may be difficult to place in tortuous vessels or distal coronary segments. Once properly positioned, the balloon is inflated to 6 atmospheres; higher inflation pressures may impair blood flow. The guidewire is withdrawn proximal to the sideholes and the central lumen intermittently flushed with heparinized saline to prevent thrombosis. The guiding catheter is retracted to allow blood to enter the proximal side holes. Distal flow is directly related to the perfusion pressure; rates as high as 40-60 ml/min have been reported.[44] Hypotension must be corrected as flow rates are dependent on arterial pressure; fluids, IABP or vasopressors may be necessary. "Bail-out" catheters have a similar design to autoperfusion catheters except they lack a balloon at their distal end. Use of this catheter is confined to failed angioplasty while preparing for emergency surgical revascularization. Flow rates are similar to those achieved with autoperfusion balloon catheters.

3. Advantages. Subjective and objective evidence of ischemia, ST segment shifts, and segmental wall motion abnormalities improve with autoperfusion catheters.[45] In a nonrandomized series of 31 patients in whom abrupt closure developed after coronary angioplasty, the bail-out catheter was successfully placed before surgery in 61%. Among those in whom a bailout catheter could be properly positioned, there was a lower incidence of Q wave infarction (9% vs. 75%), less ST segment elevation, and greater subsequent use of internal mammary grafts.[46]

4. Disadvantages. The large profile often limits catheter placement to proximal and mid-coronary vessel segments, and relatively inflexible shaft contributes to the difficulty navigating tortuous vessels.

5. Applications. Perfusion balloons are indicated when PTCA results in severe symptoms or hemodynamic instability, or when prolonged balloon inflations are required (e.g. in treating suboptimal angiographic outcomes, including coronary dissections and acute closure).

B. ACTIVE CORONARY HEMOPERFUSION. In addition to passive perfusion with autoperfusion balloon catheters, other techniques actively deliver autologous blood into the distal coronary bed. These systems actively deliver oxygenated blood obtained from the side arm of an arterial sheath via hand injection, roller pump or power injector. Use of active hemoperfusion during balloon inflation has resulted in fewer subjective and objective manifestations of ischemia.

C. PERFLUOROCHEMICALS. Fluosol® was taken off the commercial market in 1995. Randomized trials demonstrated that fluorocarbons have the potential to relieve or prevent regional ischemia.[42-48] However, other studies have shown that autologous blood infusion may be just as effective.[49]

D. CORONARY SINUS RETROPERFUSION. The concept of coronary vein perfusion was advanced in the early 1940's when Beck and colleagues surgically interposed a vein graft between the aorta and coronary sinus. This technique allowed blood to travel through the coronary sinus retrograde into ischemic myocardium resulting in improved patient symptomatology. However, myocardial edema and hemorrhage led to a marked decline in enthusiasm. Percutaneous coronary sinus retroperfusion was later developed as a method for delivering oxygenated blood to the myocardial bed during balloon inflation.

1. **Description.** The retroperfusion catheter consists of a triple lumen 8.5F radio-opaque catheter with a balloon 10 mm from the distal end. Arterial blood is pumped from the femoral artery to the coronary sinus. The 7 or 8F arterial cannula is connected to the console, which can deliver flow rates up to 250 ml/minute.[50] The coronary sinus balloon is synchronized with the R wave of the electrocardiogram, preventing regurgitation of arterial blood into the right atrium during systole.

2. **Technique.** Cannulation of the coronary sinus is usually performed via the right internal jugular or subclavian vein under fluoroscopic guidance. For optimal retroperfusion of the LAD territory, the catheter should be advanced into the distal segment of great cardiac vein.

3. **Advantages.** It allows for retrograde delivery of pharmacologic agents and does not require crossing diseased coronary arterial segments.[51] When used in the setting of high risk angioplasty, it has been shown to reduce wall motion abnormalities, ST segment changes, and allow longer inflations; there was no difference in hemodynamic performance or angina.[52-53]

4. **Disadvantages.** Inability to cannulate the coronary sinus precludes its use in 10-15% of patients.[54] It does not provide systemic support and is not consistently effective for the circumflex and right coronary arteries. Infrequent complications include transient atrial fibrillation, hematoma, and coronary sinus staining.[55]

5. **Outcome.** In 28 patients who underwent LAD angioplasty, retroperfusion was successfully performed in 87%.[49] The incidence of balloon-induced angina was reduced by 50%.[55]

6. **Applications.** Coronary sinus retroperfusion allows regional support and subselective administration of pharmacologic agents during complex PTCA of the LAD.

E. PHARMACOTHERAPY. Although definitive data are lacking, nitroglycerin, beta blockers and calcium channel antagonists reduce myocardial oxygen consumption; none augment collateral flow.

1. **Beta Blockers.** These agents delay the onset of ischemia and may allow for longer balloon inflations.[56] In patients demonstrating evidence of high adrenergic tone (i.e., hypertension, tachycardia) supplemental use of intravenous beta blockers (e.g., Metoprolol 5mg q 5 min. x 3, Propranolol 1-2 mg or Esmolol 0.15mg/kg) may allow for longer inflation times; however PTCA-induced bradycardia may be accentuated.

2. **Calcium Channel Antagonists and Nitrates.** Pre- and intra-procedural calcium channel antagonists and nitrates are routinely administered during angioplasty. These agents have been shown to delay the onset of angina, electrocardiographic evidence of ischemia and blunt the increase in left ventricular-end-diastolic pressure during balloon inflation.[57]

* * * * *

REFERENCES

1. Gruentzig AR, Senning A, Siegenthaler WE. Nonoperative dilation of coronary artery stenosis: percutaneous transluminal coronary angioplasty. N Engl J Med 1979;301:61-68.

2. Stevens T, Kahn JK, McCallister BD, et al. Safety and efficacy of percutaneous transluminal coronary angioplasty in patients with left ventricular dysfunction. Am J Cardio 1991;68:313-319.

3. Serota H, Deligonul U, Lee WH, et al. Predictors of cardiac survival after percutaneous transluminal coronary angioplasty in patients with severe left ventricular dysfunction. Am J Cardiol 1991;67:367-372.

4. Kohli RS, DiSciascio G, Cowley MJ, et al. Coronary angioplasty in patients with severe left ventricular dysfunction. J Am Coll Cardiol 1990;16:807-811.

5. Eltchaninoff H, Franco I, Whitlow PK, et al. Late results of coronary angioplasty in patients with left ventricular ejection fractions < or =40%. Am J Cardiol 1994;73:1047-52.

6. O'Keefe JH, Allan JJ, McCallister, et al. Angioplasty versus bypass surgery for multivessel coronary artery disease with left ventricular ejection fraction < 40%. Am J Cardiol 1993;71:897-901.

7. Holmes DR, Detre KM, Williams DO, et al. Long term outcome of patients with depressed left ventricular function undergoing percutaneous transluminal coronary angioplasty. The NHLBI PTCA Registry. Circulation 1993;87:21-9.

8. Terrien EF, Siegel N, O'Neill WW, et al. Angioplasty in patients with severe left ventricular dysfunction an analysis of immediate and long term survival. J Am Coll Cardio. Feb 1993 21:2:272A.

9. Pigott JD, Kouchoukos NT, Oberman A, et al. Late results of surgical and medical therapy for patients with coronary artery disease and depressed left ventricular function. J Am Coll Cardiol 1985;5:1036-1045.

10. Alderman EL, Fisher LD, Litwin P, et al. Results of coronary artery surgery in patients with poor left ventricular function (CASS). Circulation 1983;68:785-795.

11. Miller TD, Christian TF, Taliercio CP, et al. Impaired left ventricular function, one- or two-vessel coronary artery disease, and severe ischemia: outcome with medical therapy versus revascularization. Mayo Clin Proc 1994;69:626-31.

12. Hochberg MS, Parsonnet V, et al. Coronary artery bypass grafting in patients with ejection fractions below forty percent. J Thorac Cardiovasc Surg 1983;86:519-527.

13. Rahimtoola SH, Nunley D, Grunkemeier G, et al. Ten year survival after coronary artery bypass surgery for unstable angina. N Engl J Med 1983;308:676-681.

14. The Veterans Administration Coronary Artery Bypass Surgery Cooperative Group. Eleven year survival in the Veterans Administration trial of coronary bypass surgery for stable angina. N Engl J Med 1995;311:1333-1339.

15. Elefteriades JA, Tolis G, Levi E, et al. Coronary artery bypass grafting in severe left ventricular dysfunction: excellent survival with improved ejection fraction and functional state. J Am Coll Cardiol 1993;22:1411-7.

16. BARI Investigators. The bypass angioplasty revascularization investigation (BARI): five year mortality and morbidity in a randomized study comparing CABG and PTCA in patients with multivessel coronary artery disease. N Engl J Med (in-press).

17. Califf R, Phillips H, Hindman M, et al. Prognostic value of a coronary artery jeopardy score. J Am Coll Cardiol 1985;5:1055-63.

18. Ellis SG, Roubin GS, King SB III, et al. In-hospital cardiac mortality after acute closure after coronary angioplasty: analysis of risk factors from 8207 procedures. J Am Coll Cardiol 1988;11:211-216.

19. Kaltenbach M, Gruentzig A, Rentrop P, et al. In: Transluminal Coronary Angioplasty and Intracoronary Thrombolysis, 1982;145-150.

20. Alderman JD, Gabliani GI, McCabe CH, et al. Incidence and management of limb ischemia with percutaneous wire-guided intraaortic balloon catheters. J Am Coll Cardiol 1987;9:524-530.

21. Fuchs RM, Brin KP, Brinker JA, et al. Augmentation of regional coronary blood flow by intra-aortic balloon counterpulsation in patients with unstable angina. Circulation 1983;68:117-123.

22. Kahn JK, Rutherford BD, McConahay DR, et al. Supported "high risk" coronary angioplasty using intraaortic balloon pump counterpulsation. J Am Coll Cardiol 1990;15:1151-1155.

23. Meany TB, Pavlides G, Cragg D, et al. Prophylactic percutaneous cardio- pulmonary bypass versus intraaortic balloon pump support for high risk angioplasty. J Am Coll Cardiol 1992;19:349A.

24. Murphy DA, Craver JM, Jones EL, et al. Surgical management of acute myocardial ischemia following percutaneous transluminal coronary angioplasty. J Thorac Cardiovasc Surg 1984;87:332-339.

25. Ishihara M, Sato H, Tateishi H, et al. Intraaortic balloon pumping as the postangioplasty strategy in acute myocardial infarction. Am Heart J 1991;122:385-388.

26. Ohman EM, George BS, White CJ, et al. Use of aortic counterpulsation to improve sustained coronary artery patency during acute myocardial infarction. Results of a randomized trial. Circulation 1994;90:792-9.

27. Ohman EM, Califf RM, George BS, et al. The use of intraaortic balloon pumping as an adjunct to reperfusion therapy in acute myocardial infarction. Am Heart J 1991; :895-901.

28. Leinbach RC, et al. Early intraaortic balloon pumping for anterior myocardial infarction without shock. Circulation 1978;58:204.

29. Hanson EC, et al. Control of post infarction ventricular irritability with intraaortic balloon pump. Circulation 1978;62:30.

30. Aroesty J, Weintraub R, Paulin S, et al. Medically refractory unstable angina pectoris. Ii. Hemodynamic and angiographic effects of intraaortic balloon counterpulsation. Am J Cardiol 1979;43:887.

31. DeWood MA, Notske RN, Hensley GR, et al. Intraaortic balloon counterpulsation with and without reperfusion for myocardial infarction shock. Circulation 1980;61:1105-1112.

32. Tomasso CL. Use of percutaneously inserted cardiopulmonary bypass in the cardiac catheterization laboratory. Cathet Cardiovasc Diagn 1990;20:32-38.

33. Sturm JT, McGee MG, Fuhrman TM, et al. Treatment of postoperative low output syndrome with intraaortic balloon pumping: experience with 419 patients. Am J Cardiol 1980;45:1033-1036.

34. Vogel RA, Shawl F, Tommaso C, et al. Initial report of the national registry of elective cardiopulmonary bypass supported coronary angioplasty. J Am Coll Cardiol 1990;15:23-29.

35. Stack RK, Pavlides GS, Miller R, et al. Hemodynamic and metabolic effects of venoarterial cardiopulmonary support in coronary artery disease. Am J Cardiol 1991;67:1344-1348.

36. Vogel RA et al. Textbook of Interventional Cardiology 1994.

37. Shawl FA, et al. Cardiopulmonary bypass supported PTCA: long term follow-up of 85 consecutive patients. Circulation 1990;82:III-653A.

38. Overlie PA, Walter PD, Hurd HP, et al. Emergency cardiopulmonary support with circulatory support devices. Cardiology 1994;84(3):231-7.

39. Overlie PA. Emergency use of portable cardiopulmonary bypass. Cathet Cardiovasc Diagn 1990;20:27-31.

40. Loisance D, Dubois-Rande JL, et al. Prophylactic use of Hemopump in high risk coronary angiography. J Am Coll Cardiol 1990;15:249A.

41. Wampler RK, Moise JC, Frazier OH, et al. In vivo evaluation of a peripheral vascular access axial flow blood pump. Trns Am Soc Artif Intern Organs Trans 1988;34:450-454.

42. Smalling RW, Cassidy DB, Merhige M, et al. Improved hemodynamic and left ventricular unloading during acute ischemia using the Hemopump left ventricular assist device compared to intra aortic balloon counterpulsation. J Am Coll Cardiol 1989;13:160A.

43. Babic UU, Grujicic S, Djurisic Z, et al. Percutaneous left atrial aortic bypass with a roller pump. Circulation 1989;80:II-272.

44. Stack RS, Quigley PJ, Collins G, et al. Perfusion balloon catheter. Am J Cardiol 1988;61:77G-80G.

45. Turi ZG, Campbell CA, Gottimukkala MV, et al. Preservation of distal coronary perfusion during prolonged balloon inflation with an autoperfusion angioplasty catheter. Circulation 1987;75:1273-1280.

46. Banka VS, Trivedi A, Patel R, et al. Prevention of myocardial ischemia during coronary angioplasty: a simple new method for distal antegrade arterial blood perfusion. Am Heart J 1989;118:830-836.

47. Bell MR, Nishimura RA, Holmes DR, et al. Does intracoronary infusion of Fluosol-Da.. 20% prevent left ventricular diastolic dysfunction during coronary balloon angioplasty? J Am Coll Cardiol 1990;16;4:959-966.

48. Robalino BD, Marwick T, Lafont A, et al. Protection against ischemia during prolonged balloon inflation by distal coronary perfusion with use of an autoperfusion catheter or Fluosol. J Am Coll Cardiol 1992;20:1378-84.

49. Christensen CW, Reeves WC, Lassar TA, et al. Inadequate subendocardial oxygen delivery during perfluorocarbon perfusion in a canine model of ischemia. Am Heart J 1988;115:30-37.

50. Hajduczki I, Kar S, Areeda J, et al. Reversal of chronic regional myocardial dysfunction (hibernating myocardium) by synchronized diastolic coronary venous retroperfusion during coronary angioplasty. J Am Coll Cardiol 1990;15:238-242.

51. Drury JK, Yamazaki S, Fishbein MC, et al. Synchronized diastolic coronary venous retroperfusion: results of a preclinical safety and efficacy study. J Am Coll Cardiol 1985;6:328-335.

52. Incorvati RL, Tauberg SG, Pecora MJ, et al. Clinical applications of coronary sinus retroperfusion during high risk percutaneous transluminal coronary angioplasty. J Am Coll Cardiol 1993;22:127-34.

53. Nanto S, Nishida K, Hirayama A, et al. Supported angioplasty with synchronized retroperfusion in high risk patients with left main trunk or near left main trunk obstruction. Am Heart J 1993;125:301-9.

54. Carday E, Kar S, Drury JK, et al. Coronary venous retroperfusion for support of ischemic myocardium. Cardiovascular Rev Rep 1988:9:50-53.

55. Kar S, et al. Reduction of PTCA induced ischemia by Synchronized Coronary Venous Retroperfusion: Results of a Multicenter Clinical Trial. J Am Coll Cardiol 1990;15:250A.

56. Zalewski A, Goldberg S, Dervan JP, et al. Myocardial protection during coronary occlusion in man: beneficial effects of regional b blockade. J Am Coll Cardiol 1985;5:445.

57. Zalewski A, Savage M, Goldberg S. Protection of the ischemic myocardium during percutaneous transluminal coronary angioplasty. Am J Cardiol 1988;61:54-60G.

REVASCULARIZATION BASED ON PATIENT CHARACTERISTICS

Joel K. Kahn, M.D.
Mark Freed, M.D.

YOUNG PATIENTS (AGE < 40 YEARS)

A. **BACKGROUND.** Although coronary artery disease typically occurs with advancing age, 3-6% of patients are less than 40 years old. Compared to older patients, young patients typically have more cardiac risk factors and less extensive disease. Coronary artery bypass grafting (CABG) can be performed with high success and excellent results (acute mortality 0-2%); however, since young patients may develop saphenous vein graft failure and require reoperation, CABG is a less-than-ideal method of revascularization. Catheter-based intervention may offer a more attractive alternative to CABG in younger patients.

B. **BALLOON ANGIOPLASTY.** Patients as young as 15 years old have been treated by PTCA;[1] larger series indicate that PTCA can be performed with success rates of 86-96% and major complication rates of 0-12% (Table 7.1).

Table 7.1. PTCA in Young Patients: Acute Outcome

Series	Age	N	Success (%)	Complications (%) D / Q-MI / CABG	Other
Mehan[2] (1994)	≤ 40	89	90	0 / 0 / 0	5-yr survival (100%). Follow-up at 30 mos: CABG (5%); re-PTCA (34%)
	> 40	1916	86	5 / 1 / 1	
Buffett[3] (1994)	< 40	140	86	5.7 / 6.4 / 0	10-yr survival (96%); return to work (93%); restenosis (28%)
Kofflard[4] (1993)	<35	57	92	3.4 / 1.7 / 1.7	5-yr survival (87%). Follow-up at 4 yrs: MI (14%); CABG (11%); re-PTCA (32%)
Stone[5] (1989)	≤ 35	71	96	0 / 1 / 0	3-yr survival (98%)

Abbreviations: D = in-hospital death; MI = in-hospital Q-wave myocardial infarction; CABG = emergency coronary artery bypass grafting

C. **FOLLOW-UP.** Among successfully treated patients followed over 3-5 years, repeat PTCA was required in approximately 30%, survival was 87-100%, and more than 80% were asymptomatic[3,5] and working.[5]

D. **CONCLUSIONS.** Balloon angioplasty has a high success rate, acceptable complication rates (although mortality rates up to 5.7% have been reported[5]), excellent longterm survival, and may be preferred over surgical revascularization for young patients with coronary disease. The need for repeat PTCA (for restenosis or new disease) is similar to other PTCA patients.

ELDERLY PATIENTS (AGE 65-75 YEARS)

A. **BACKGROUND.** In 1990, the United States Census estimated that 25% of 31 million people over the age of 65 years had symptomatic coronary artery disease. Within the next 30 years, this number is expected to increase by 65%. From 1987 to 1990, the rates of PTCA and CABG among the elderly have increased by 55% and 18%, respectively.

B. **PROCEDURAL RESULTS.** Compared to younger patients, elderly patients undergoing coronary revascularization are more often female, and more likely to have diffuse disease, calcified lesions, unstable angina, prior MI, comorbid conditions, and low ejection fractions. Nevertheless, elective use of CABG (Table 7. 2), PTCA (Tables 7.2, 7.3) and new devices (Table 7.4) can be performed with success rates > 90% and major complication rates of 3-13%. However, the elderly are at increased risk of death after acute closure; there is also a 2-3 fold risk of peripheral vascular complications (pseudoaneurysm, AV fistula, large hematoma) and blood transfusions.

C. **FOLLOW-UP.** More than 75% of successfully revascularized elderly patients are less symptomatic. One and 3-year survival rates are 95% and 90% respectively, with late MI in ~ 5%, late CABG in 15%, and late PTCA in 20% — similar to other PTCA patients.

D. **APPROACH.** Patients between the ages of 65-75 with symptomatic coronary artery disease should be offered percutaneous or surgical revascularization. CABG and PTCA achieve similar longterm survival rates. However, PTCA is associated with less in-hospital morbidity and mortality, but more repeat procedures are needed to treat recurrent angina. Many patients with 1- or 2-vessel disease can be treated equally well by either technique, but patients with anatomical features unsuitable for PTCA or severe 3-vessel disease (especially with LV dysfunction) should be referred for CABG. When percutaneous intervention is performed, it is important to pay special attention to volume status, contrast load, renal function, bleeding and peripheral vascular complications to minimize morbidity and mortality (Table 7.5).

Table 7.2. Effect of Age on Coronary Revascularization

Series	Modality	Age	N	Complications (%) D / Q-MI / CABG	Other
Hannan[6] (1994)	CABG[†]	40-49	2448	1.1 / - / -	Older cohorts include more
		50-59	6118	1.7 / - / -	females, emergency surgery,
		60-64	5352	2.2 / - / -	unstable angina, previous
		65-69	6268	2.8 / - / -	CABG, CHF, renal failure, EF
		70-74	5563	3.4 / - / -	< 20%, previous stroke,
		75-79	3561	5.3 / - / -	peripheral vascular disease
		≥ 80	1372	8.3 / - / -	
					5-yr survival (%):
O'Keefe[7] (1994)	CABG	> 70	195	9 / 6 / 5	65
	PTCA	> 70	195	2 / 1 / 0	63

				Mortality (%)	
				30-day	4-year
Peterson[8] (1994)	PTCA*	65-69	93,077	2.1	5.2
		70-74	71,389	3.0	7.3
		75-79	42,246	4.6	10.9
		≥ 80	19,203	7.8	17.3
		Overall	225,915	3.3	8.0
	CABG*	65-69	142,080	4.3	8.0
		70-74	121,323	5.7	10.9
		75-79	70,861	7.4	14.2
		≥ 80	23,620	10.6	19.5
		Overall	357,885	5.8	11.0

Series	Modality	Age	N	Complications (%) D / Q-MI / CABG	3-yr survival (%):
Mick[9] (1991)	CABG	≥ 80	142	6 / 4 / 4	87
	PTCA	≥ 80	53	2 / 6 / 0	81

Abbreviations: D = in-hospital death; MI = in-hospital Q-wave myocardial infarction; CABG = emergency coronary artery bypass grafting; - = not reported
† From the New York State Cardiac Surgery Reporting Center (CSRC) file
* From the Medicare Provider Analysis and Review (MEDPAR) file

Table 7.3. PTCA For Patients Over Age 65: Acute Outcome

Series	Age	N	Success (%)	Complications (%) D / Q-MI / CABG	Comments
					Vascular repair (%):
Lindsay[10]*	55-64	914	93	0.5 / 0.3 / 3.7	1
(1994)	65-74	996	92	1.1 / 0.5 / 2.2	1.9
	≥ 75	474	94	2.1 / 1.3 / 3.6	3.6
Burstein[11]	< 50	172	-	0.7 / - / 4.7	
(1994)	50-69	938	-	1.3 / - / 3.5	
	≥ 70	622	-	3.6 / - / 2.1	
					Mortality (%)
					<u>1-yr</u> <u>3-yr</u>
Jollis[12]†	65-69	-	-	1.8 / - / -	5.2 10.4
(1995)	>80	20,006	-	7 / - / -	17 29.6
	Age 82††	-	-	- / - / -	7.7 23.6
Thompson[13]					In-hosp. + 6 mo. death/MI
(1994)					(%)
1980-89	> 65	982	88	3.3 / 3.9 / -	10.3
1990-92	> 65	768	94	1.4 / 2.2 / -	9.9
Little[14]	< 80	500	88	0.2 / 1.4 / 2.6	Octogenarians: 1- and 3-yr
(1993)	> 80	118	89	2.1 / 0.8 / 0.8	survival (76%, 61%)
					3-yr survival (%):
Foreman[15]	60-69	570	88	2 / 6 / 5	96
(1992)	70-79	270	88	2 / 5 / 4	80
	≥ 80	67	84	6 / 5 / 2	72
ten Berg[16]	> 75	212	91	1.9 / 3.3 / 0.9	7-yr event-free survival
(1992)					(52%); recurrent angina (75%)
Thompson[17]					EFS (%)
(1991)					1-yr / 3-yr / 5-yr
	65-69	326	82	1.2 / 2.7 / 10.7	74 / 60 / 51
	70-74	233	82	2.2 / 4.3 / 9	72 / 55 / 48
	≥ 75	193	93	6.2 / 6.7 / 3	58 / 36 / 24

Abbreviations: D = in-hospital death; MI = in-hospital Q-wave myocardial infarction; CABG = emergency coronary artery bypass grafting; EFS = event-free survival (no death, MI, CABG, PTCA, angina); - = not reported

*   New devices in 35%

†   From the Medicare Provider Analysis and Review (MEDPAR) file

††   US population

Table 7.4. New Interventional Devices in the Elderly

Series	Modality	Age	N	Success[†] (%)	Complications (%)[*] D / Q-MI / CABG	Other
Lefevre[32] (1996)	Stent	≥75	245	-	-	1-mo. follow-up: D (3%), MI (1.6%), subacute closure (1.6%), vascular complications (2.1).
Yokoi[18] (1995)	PSS	65-69	131	96	0.8 / 0.8 / 0	6-12 mo. EFS (%) :81
		70-74	126	94	1.6 / 1.6 / 2.4	84
		≥ 75	74	86	4.1 / 1.4 / 1.4	75
Fishman[19] (1995)	DCA + Stent	< 70	388	96	0.8	
		≥ 70	116	91	3.5	
Movsowitz[20] (1994)	DCA	< 65	222	96	5.7	Transfusion required in 17% of patients ≥ 75 yrs. Trend toward more groin complications in elderly.
		66-75	101	88	10.9	
		≥ 75	50	95	9.5	
Elliott[21] (1994)	PTCA	>70	443	92	4.3	Vascular complications (%): 13
	DCA	>70	56	98	1.8	9
	ROTA	>70	91	97	2.2	14
	Stent	>70	29	86	13.8	45
Henson[22] (1993)	ROTA	< 70	298	95	3	1-yr EFS for age ≥ 70 (84%).
		73-79	136	96	1.7	
		≥ 80	29	88	8.3	

Abbreviations: D = in-hospital death; MI = in-hospital Q-wave myocardial infarction; CABG = emergency coronary artery bypass grafting; ROTA = Rotablator Atherectomy; DCA = Directional Coronary Atherectomy; PSS = Palmaz Schatz Stent; EFS = event-free survival (without death, MI, CABG, re-PTCA); not reported
†   Device + adjunctive PTCA as needed
*   Single number denotes overall complication rate

ELDERLY PATIENTS (AGE > 80 YEARS)

A. **BYPASS SURGERY.** In-hospital mortality is 5-10% in octogenarians undergoing CABG, and another 5% develop perioperative MI or stroke (Table 7.2). In addition to advanced age, risk factors for operative mortality include female gender, unstable angina, diabetes mellitus, smoking, poor ejection fraction, and severe angina. Five-year survival ranges from 60-85%; 30% of late deaths are due to noncardiac causes. At 1-year follow-up, up to 90% of patients are in functional Class 1 or 2.

Table 7.5. Important Considerations for Patients Undergoing Coronary intervention

Patient Group	Measure
All patients	• Ensure euvolmia • Check hemoglobin, platelets, electrolytes, neurologic and peripheral vascular status • Obtain venous access • Consider substituting antihistamines for sedatives in the elderly • Have a pacemaker on standby • Remove sheaths as soon as possible after the case • Promote early ambulation • Remove bladder catheter early • Prescribe support stockings if prolonged bedrest • Simplify medical regimen and educate patient prior to discharge
EF < 40% or culprit supplies large myocardial territory	• Perform angiography to evaluate peripheral vessels for IABP or CPS • Obtain contralateral arterial access using a 5F sheath for rapid insertion of IABP or CPS • Use perfusion balloon when feasible • Perform culprit vessel angioplasty; stage remaining stenoses
Suboptimal result or large contrast load	• Stage the procedure
Unstable ischemic syndrome	• Perform culprit vessel angioplasty; stage remaining stenoses

Abbreviations: IABP = intraaortic balloon pump, CPS = percutaneous cardiopulmonary bypass, EF = ejection fraction

B. **BALLOON ANGIOPLASTY.** Procedural success can be achieved in 85% of patients > 80 years old (Table 7.6). Compared to younger patients, octogenarians have more acute complications and late cardiac death. Among 17 patients > 90 years old treated with PTCA, 41% died during 1-year follow-up.[32] Nevertheless, 87% of patients in one study were subjectively improved after PTCA, 33% were more physically active, and 55% required less medication.[28] Three-year survival rates of 80-91% have been reported,[27,28] and > 90% of longterm survivors indicated a high level of satisfaction with their quality of life and health status.[14]

C. **CONCLUSIONS.** When medical therapy fails to control anginal symptoms in octogenarians, PTCA can be performed with high success rates, but acute ischemic complications occur more often than in younger patients. Short-term follow-up reveals relief of angina but frequent late cardiac events. Preliminary reports using new devices suggest lower success and a higher incidence of ischemic, vascular and bleeding complications compared to PTCA. When percutaneous intervention is performed, it is important to pay special attention to volume status, contrast load, renal function, bleeding and peripheral vascular complications to minimize morbidity and mortality (Table 7.5).

Table 7.6. PTCA For Patients Over Age 80: Acute Outcome

Series	N	Success (%)	Complications (%) D / Q-MI / CABG
Jollis[12] (1995)	20,006*	-	7 / - / -
Weyrens[23] (1994)	26	65	23 / 4 / -
Little[14] (1993)	118	89	2 / 1 / 1
Forman[15] (1992)	67	84	6 / 5 / 2
Santana[24] (1992)	53+	83	15 / 4 / -
Bedotto[25] (1991)	111	91	6 / 3 / 0
Jackman[26] (1991)	31	90	6 / 6 / 10
Myler[27] (1991)	74	80	1 / 0 / 4
Jeroudi[28] (1990)	54	91	4 / 4 / 0
Patron[29] (1990)	53	83	2 / 5 / 7
Rich[30] (1990)	22	86	0 / 14 / 0
Kern[31] (1988)	21	67	19 / 0 / 14

Abbreviations: D = in-hospital death, MI = in-hospital Q-wave myocardial infarction, CABG = emergency coronary artery bypass grafting; - = not reported
* From the Medicare Provider Analysis and Review (MEDPAR) file
+ All patients had unstable angina

FEMALE PATIENTS

A. **BACKGROUND.** Many studies suggest differences in the prevalence, manifestations, diagnosis, and prognosis of coronary artery disease between men and women.[33-35] Reports on the safety and efficacy of CABG during the 1980's indicated a higher procedural mortality in women. Many centers have recently reported acute and longterm outcomes for females undergoing percutaneous therapy.

B. **BALLOON ANGIOPLASTY.** Several studies suggest that females have a higher in-hospital mortality than males (Table 7.7). However, females are older, and have a higher prevalence of diabetes

Table 7.7. Effect of Gender on PTCA Outcome

Series	Gender	N	Success (%)	Complications (%) D / Q-MI / CABG
Stone[36] (1995)	Male Female	145[++] 50[++]	90 80	2.1 / 2.8[@] / - 4.0 / 2.0[@] / -
Malenka[37] (1995)	Male Female	11,493 5472	94 95	0.7 / MI or CABG: 4.5 1.6 / MI or CABG: 5.0
Weintraub[38] (1994)	Male Female	7940 2845	90 91	0.1 / 0.8 / 2 0.7 / 1 / 2
Arnold[39] (1994)	Male Female	3726 1274	93 94	0.3 / 0.4 / 4.5 1.1 / 0.4 / 5
Cavero[40] (1994)	Male Female	340[†] 340[†]	- -	Females had higher in-hospital mortality but similar total and event-free survival
				Mortality (%) 30-day / 1-year
Peterson[8][*] (1994)	Male Female	129,675 96,240	- -	3.0 / 7.8 3.8 / 8.2
Bell[42] (1993)	Male Female	1508 593	90 87	3.1 / 0.6 / 2.1 5.4 / 0.7 / 2.9
Kahn[43] (1992)	Male Female	7142 2033	95 95	0.8 / 1.4 / 1.6 1.4 / 1.7 / 1.6

Abbreviations: D = in-hospital death; MI = in-hospital Q-wave myocardial infarction; CABG = emergency coronary artery bypass grafting; - = not reported
† Multivessel PTCA or CABG; * From the Medicare Provider Analysis and Review (MEDPAR) file
++ Primary PTCA for acute MI   @ In-hospital reinfarction

mellitus, hypertension, unstable angina, and prior MI. After accounting for these differences, female gender little or no independent effect on outcome.

C. **FOLLOW-UP.** Compared to males, females had similar survival and <u>better</u> event-free survival (freedom from death, MI, repeat PTCA, or CABG).[38,39] Mayo Clinic investigators found no differences between sexes with regard to 5-year infarct-free survival, although females had less late CABG.[44]

D. **NEW DEVICES (Table 7.8).** Acute success and longterm survival rates similar for females and males. However, females appear to be at increased risk for major ischemic complications, possibly due to greater comorbidity and lower body surface area.

E. **CONCLUSIONS.** In-hospital mortality is higher for women undergoing PTCA, but is largely related to older age, advanced angina class, small body habitus, and comorbid conditions. Longterm results are similar to men.

AFRICAN-AMERICANS

A. **BACKGROUND.** African-Americans have a higher prevalence of coronary risk factors and greater cardiac mortality than the general population.[55] CABG is equally effective among black and white patients in reducing symptoms and improving survival.[56]

B. **CORONARY INTERVENTION (Table 7.9).** Despite greater comorbidity and coronary risk factors among blacks, results from the 1985-1986 NHLBI PTCA Registry indicate that PTCA outcome is independent of race.[57] In a report using new devices, procedure-related death was higher among blacks, which may have been due to a higher prevalence of comorbid conditions.[58]

C. **FOLLOW-UP.** One and 5-year survival and event-free survival rates were similar between black and white patients subjected to new device angioplasty[58] or PTCA[57] (Table 7.9). More than 80% of patients have improved anginal status; repeat PTCA is required in 20-25%, which is similar to the general population.

D. **CONCLUSIONS.** Despite the presence of greater comorbidity, African-Americans demonstrate excellent acute and longterm results after percutaneous therapy.

Table 7.8. Effect of Gender on New Device Outcome

Series	Modality	Gender	N	Results
Hermiller[86] (1996)	Bailout Stent	Male Female	606 270	Females with similar ischemic complications but more vascular complications (13% vs. 5%).
Fenton[45] (1995)	PSS (STRESS trial)	Male Female	170 35	Females with similar 8-month event-free survival (83% vs. 80%), restenosis (36% vs. 30%), target lesion revascularization (14%), but females were older, had smaller vessels, and developed more peripheral vascular complications (14% vs. 5%).
Fishman[19] (1995)	Stent or DCA	Male Female	413 91	Females with lower procedural success (89% vs. 96%), similar major complications (~1%), and greater peripheral vascular complications (25% vs. 9%).
Baumbach[46] (1994)	ELCA	Male Female	1156 365	Females with 2.5-fold increase in severe dissection and 2.4-fold increase in perforation.
Combs[47] (1994)	PTCA + DCA	Male Female	982 406	Females with more acute closure (5.2% vs 2.7%). Emergency CABG and procedural success rates equivalent.
Dean[48] (1994)	GRS	Male Female	947 400	Females with similar procedural success, and 30-day and 6-month event-free survival. Females with a 2-fold increase in bleeding complications.
Ellis[49] (1994)	ROTA	Male Female	243 82	Females with 2.4-fold increase in procedural failure and 3.0-fold increase in ischemic complications.
Bowling[50] (1993)	New Devices	Male Female	446 150	Females with more perforation (3.6% vs. 1.2%), transfusion (10.7% vs. 4.3%), Q-MI (6.7% vs. 2.7%), and death (4.7% vs 1.3%) despite fewer comorbidities.
Casale[51] (1993)	ROTA	Male Female	1951 785	Females with lower success (93% vs. 95%) and more ischemic complication (12.5% vs 7.4%), but were older, and had more diabetes, unstable angina, and calcified lesions.
Scott[57] (1993)	PTCA	Male Female	337 160	Females with higher success (91% vs. 88%), similar major complications, similar total and event-free survival at 8-years.
Henson[52] (1993)	New Devices	Male Female	752 262	Similar success (~94%) and 1-year event-free survival (~72%).
Movsowitz[54] (1993)	DCA	Male Female	281 137	Females with lower procedural success (68% vs. 80%), primarily due to the inability to engage the ostium with the guiding catheter and the inability to cross the lesion with the device due to smaller vessel size.

Abbreviations: See Table 7.4

Table 7.9. Coronary Intervention in African-Americans

Series	Modality	Group	N	Success (%)	Complications (%) D / Q-MI / CABG			Other
Scott[57] (1994)	PTCA	Black White	76 1939	76* 79	0 / 7 / 4 1 / 5 / 4			5-yr outcome (black/white; %): death (11/10), MI (13/14), CABG (20/19), re-PTCA (25/28), asymptomatic (66/81).
Chuang[58] (1994)	New Devices	Black White	169 1955	92 91	4.1 / 1.2 / 2.4 0.6 / 0.9 / 3.4			1-year outcome (black/white;%): Death (1.5/1.6), MI (0.8/1.4), CABG (9/8), re-PTCA (21/18).
Scott[59] (1993)	PTCA	Black ♂ Black ♀	337 160	88 91	0.6 / 2.1 / 4.8 1.9 / 0.4 / 4.4			No difference in 8-yr survival (~ 79%) and event-free survival (~ 35%) between men and women.

Abbreviations: D = in-hospital death; MI = in-hospital Q-wave myocardial infarction; CABG = emergency coronary artery bypass grafting

* Clinical success: Residual diameter stenosis < 50% without death, MI, or emergency CABG.

DIABETICS

A. BACKGROUND. Compared to nondiabetics, patients with diabetes mellitus have a 2-3 fold higher rate of coronary disease, and are at increased risk of myocardial infarction, congestive heart failure and cardiac mortality.

B. BYPASS SURGERY. Compared to nondiabetics, patients with diabetes have more in-hospital deaths and strokes, lower longterm survival, and more late MI, CABG, and PTCA (Table 7.10).[60,61] Approximately 20-25% of diabetics die within 5 years of CABG. Even after correction for differences in baseline characteristics (unstable angina, lower EF, multivessel disease, other comorbidity), diabetes mellitus is still an independent predictor of adverse outcome.

C. BALLOON ANGIOPLASTY

1. **Procedural Results (Table 7.10).** Approximately 10-20% patients submitted for coronary intervention have diabetes mellitus. Most PTCA series indicate similar success rates (~ 90%) among diabetics and nondiabetics,[62-64] despite more unstable angina, prior MI, prior CABG, peripheral vascular disease, coronary calcification, and lower ejection fractions in diabetics.[65]

2. **Follow-up.** As shown in Table 7.10, diabetes have reduced longterm survival, more ischemic cardiac events, and require more target lesion revascularization after PTCA.[60,62,63,65] Potential factors include the presence of more diffuse disease; greater propensity for plaque rupture and hypercoagulablity (increased blood viscosity, platelet aggregability and production of procoagulant factors; decreased synthesis of prostacyclin; impaired fibrinolysis). The impact of diabetes mellitus on restenosis remains unresolved; some reports indicate higher restenosis rates,[66-68] while others do not.[69-71] In the Bypass Angioplasty Revascularization Intervention (BARI) trial, PTCA patients with diabetes had higher 5-year mortality compared to CABG patients with diabetes (35% vs. 19%, $p = 0.0024$).[60]

D. CONCLUSIONS.
Compared to nondiabetics, diabetics undergoing PTCA have similar angiographic success but a trend toward higher in-hospital complications; longterm survival after percutaneous or surgical revascularization is reduced. CABG may be preferable to PTCA for diabetic patients who meet the other entry criteria for the BARI trial. Adequate hydration and attention to limited contrast loads are especially important for diabetics patients, who may be at increased risk of contrast-induced acute renal failure. Given the high mortality rates following revascularization, aggressive risk factor modification is recommended to retard progressive disease at non-PTCA sites.

CHRONIC DIALYSIS PATIENTS

A. BACKGROUND.
Coronary artery disease is responsible for > 40% of deaths among patients with end-stage renal disease. CABG is feasible for patients on dialysis, but operative mortality is increased.[72,73]

B. BALLOON ANGIOPLASTY.
As shown in Table 7.11, lesion success (< 50% residual stenosis) can be achieved in ~ 90% of cases, but major ischemic complications and entry-site (groin) hematomas may be increased, especially in those > 65 years of age.[74]

C. FOLLOW-UP.
Compared to the general PTCA population, dialysis patients have a higher incidence of recurrent cardiac events (50-80%) and restenosis (>50%) over 6-24 month follow-up.

D. CONCLUSIONS. PTCA of chronic dialysis patients is associated with high rates of ischemic and vascular complications, and frequent clinical recurrence. In the largest report to date, patients on hemodialysis undergoing PTCA or CABG had 2-3 fold higher mortality at 1 and 12 months compared to the general PTCA population.[74] Until further data are available (e.g., use of stents), both percutaneous and surgical revascularization of hemodialysis patients must be approached with caution.

Table 7.10. Revascularization of Patients with Diabetes Mellitus

Series	Group	N	Success (%)	Complications (%) D / Q-MI / CABG	Other
BARI trial[60] (1995)	PTCA Diabetic CABG Diabetic	174 183	- -	0.6 / - / - 1.2 / - / -	5-year outcomes (PTCA vs. CABG) (%): death (35/19), repeat revascularization (62/8).
Weintraub[61] (1995)	CABG Diabetic CABG Nondiabetic	2372 10,291	- -	4.2 / - / - 1.8 / - / -	Diabetics with ↑ stroke (3.1% vs. 1.5%), 5-yr mortality (26% vs. 13%), and 10-yr mortality (50% vs. 28%). Diabetics with ↑ late MI, CABG/PTCA
Stein[62] (1995)	PTCA Diabetic PTCA Nondiabetic	1133 9300	87 89	0.4 / 0.6 / 2.3 0.3 / 0.9 / 2.1	5-yr outcomes (diabetics/nondiabetics) (%): death (17/7), MI (19/11), CABG (23/14), PTCA (43/32), EFS (36/53).
Faxon[63] (1995)	PTCA Diabetic PTCA Nondiabetic	280 1833	85 87	3.2 / - / - 0.5 / - / -	8-yr outcome (diabetic/nondiabetic) (%): death (31/15), MI (30/18), CABG (34/26). Diabetics with 75% ↑ risk of death after controlling for baseline differences.
Tan[64] (1995)	PTCA Diabetic PTCA Nondiabetic	57 674	93 90	- -	
Bailey[65] (1993)	PTCA Diabetic PTCA Nondiabetic	2043 10,178	- -	1.9 / 1.6 / 1.8 0.8 / 1.2 / 1.4	Longterm survival, EFS, and target lesion revascularization all worse in diabetics.

Abbreviations: D = in-hospital death; MI = in-hospital Q-wave myocardial infarction; CABG = emergency coronary artery bypass grafting; EFS = event-free survival (without death, MI, CABG, or re-PTCA); - = not reported
+   Multivessel PTCA
*   Receiving oral hypoglycemics or insulin

Table 7.11. PTCA for Chronic Dialysis Patients

Series	Mode	Group	N	Success (%)	Complications (%) D / Q-MI / CABG
					Mortality 30-d / 1-yr (%)
Ahmed[74+]	CABG	Dialysis	168	-	8.9 / 32.1
(1995)	PTCA	Dialysis	202	-	5.4 / 31.7
	PTCA	No dialysis	58,837	-	2.8 / 7.6
Reusser[73]	PTCA	Dialysis	13	92	0 / 8 / 8
(1994)	PTCA	No dialysis*	13	100	0 / 0 / 0
Kahn[72]	PTCA	Dialysis	17	88	12 / 12 / 0
(1990)					

Abbreviations: D = in-hospital death; MI = in-hospital Q-wave myocardial infarction; CABG = emergency coronary artery bypass grafting; - = not reported
* Matched control
+ From the 1988-1991 Medicare Provider Analysis and Review (MEPAR)

CARDIAC TRANSPLANT PATIENTS

A. BACKGROUND. Coronary artery disease is the leading cause of death among patients who survive more than one year after cardiac transplantation, and affects 20 - 40% of allografts 1 - 5 years after transplantation. Angiographic abnormalities range from focal stenoses to diffuse involvement of the entire epicardial and coronary circulation. Because allograft hearts are denervated, angina pectoris is distinctly uncommon — clinical presentations typically include myocardial infarction, heart failure, or sudden death. Unfortunately, medical therapy and surgical revascularization are relatively ineffective: Medical therapy is empiric and consists of risk factor modification, immunosuppressive and antiplatelet agents, diet, and exercise. Diltiazem (30-90 mg orally 3 times/day)[75] and lipid lowering agents may retard the progression of coronary disease and are uniformly recommended. Surgical options include: 1) bypass surgery, which is limited in the short-term by poor wound healing and infection, and in the longterm by disease progression; and 2) re-transplantation, which is associated with significant postoperative mortality and a 50% recurrence rate. A growing number of patients with allograft vasculopathy are now being managed percutaneously.

B. PROCEDURAL RESULTS (Table 7.12). PTCA (and atherectomy) have been applied to small numbers of patients. Combined data show PTCA success in 91% with in-hospital mortality in 5%.

Table 7.12. Coronary Intervention For Cardiac Transplant Patients

Series	Modality	N	Success (%)	Complications (%) D / Q-MI / CABG	Other
Halle[76] (1995)	PTCA	66	94	8 / - / -	Allograft survival[†] 61% at 19 mos.
	DCA	11	82	18 / - / -	82% at 8 mos.
	CABG	12	-	33 / - / -	58% at 9 mos.
Swan[77] (1993)	PTCA	13	92	0 / 0 / 0	
Sandhu[78] (1992)	PTCA	13	85	0 / 0 / 0	
Mullins[79] (1992)	PTCA	10	75	0 / 0 / 0	

Abbreviations: D = in-hospital death; MI = in-hospital Q-wave myocardial infarction; CABG = emergency coronary artery bypass grafting; - = not reported
† Allograft survival = freedom from death or retransplantation

C. **FOLLOW-UP.** In the multicenter report,[76] 39% of PTCA patients died or required retransplantation at 19 months, and actuarial survival at 5-years was only 30%. Restenosis rates have ranged from 33-55%.

D. **CONCLUSIONS.** PTCA can be performed with acceptable success and complication rates for cardiac transplant patients with focal or tubular stenoses, although repeat intervention is often required to treat restenotic and new lesions. Data on restenosis are incomplete. New device angioplasty, while feasible, awaits further study.

SILENT ISCHEMIA

A. **BACKGROUND.** The presence of silent ischemia increases the risk of adverse cardiac events.[45] Findings from the Asymptomatic Cardiac Ischemia Pilot (ACIP) trial suggest that compared to medical therapy alone, revascularization may improve the extent and frequency of exercise-induced ischemia,[80] anginal status and 1-year survival.[81,82]

B. **PROCEDURAL RESULTS.** The results of PTCA in patients with silent ischemia are shown in Table 7.13.

Table 7.13. PTCA for Patients with Silent Ischemia

Series	N	Success (%)	Complications (%) D / Q-MI / CABG
Knatterud[83] (1994)	103	81	0 / 1 / 2
Stone[84] (1989)	50	95	0 / 0 / 2

Abbreviations: D = in-hospital death; MI = in-hospital Q-wave myocardial infarction; CABG = emergency coronary artery bypass grafting

C. **FOLLOW-UP.** Following successful PTCA, objective evidence of ischemia was alleviated in 53-93% of patients at 3-6 months;[83,84] 3-year total and infarct-free survival was 98% and 96%, respectively.[83]

D. **CONCLUSIONS.** Elective PTCA on patients with silent ischemia is safe and effective. The ACIP and other ongoing randomized trials will determine whether suppression of silent ischemia by PTCA or bypass surgery improves longterm outcome.

* * * * *

REFERENCES

1. Kahn JW, Hartzler GO. Saphenous vein graft angioplasty in a teenager. Am J Cardiol 1990;65:25-260.

2. Mehan V, Urban P, et al. Coronary angioplasty in the young: Procedural results and late outcome. J Invas Cardiol 1994;6:202-208.

3. Buffet P, Colasante B, et al. Long-term follow-up after coronary angioplasty in patients younger than 40 years of age. Am Heart J 1994;127:509-513.

4. Kofflard M, van Dombur R, van den Brand M, de Jaegere P. 5-year follow-up of coronary angioplasty in patients aged 35 years or younger. Circulation 1994;88(Part II):I-218.

5. Stone GW, Ligon RW, Rutherford BD, et al. Short-term outcome and long-term follow-up following coronary angioplasty in the young patient: An 8-year experience. Am Heart J 1989;118:873-877.

6. Hannan E, and Burke J. Effect of age on mortality in coronary artery bypass surgery in New York, 1991-1992. Am Heart J 1994;128:1184-91.

7. O'Keefe J, Sutton M, et al. Coronary angioplasty versus bypass surgery in patients >70 years old matched for ventricular function. J Am Coll Cardiol 1994;24:425-430.

8. Peterson ED, Gollis JG, Bebchuk JD, DeLong ER, et al. Chances in mortality after myocardial revascularization in the elderly. The National Medicare experience. Ann Intern Med. 1994;121:919-927.

9. Mick MJ, Simpfendorfer C, et al. Early and late results of coronary angioplasty and bypass in octogenarians. Am J Cardiol 1991;68:1316-1320.

10. Lindsay J, Reddy V, et al. Morbidity and mortality rates in elderly patients undergoing percutaneous coronary transluminal angioplasty. Am Heart J 1994;128:697-702.

11. Burnstein S, Sun GW, Hammer JS, Mann JD, et al. Adjusted influence of age and gender on PTCA outcomes and hospital resource consumption. J Am Coll Cardiol 1994;March Special Issue:223A.

12. Jollis JG, Peterson ED, Bebchuk JD, DeLong ER, et al. Coronary angioplasty in 20,006 patients over age 80 in the United States. J Am Coll Cardiol 1995; March Special Issue:47A.

13. Thompson RC, Holmes DR, Grill DR, Bailey KR. Changing outcome of angioplasty in elderly. J Am Coll Cardiol 1996;27:8-14.

14. Little T, Milner M, Lee K, Contantine J, Pichard AD, Lindsay JJ. Late outcome and quality of life following percutaneous transluminal coronary angioplasty in octogenarians. Cathet Cardiovasc Diagn 1993;29:261-266.

15. Forman DE, Berman AD, McCabe CH, et al. PTCA in the elderly: The "young-old" versus the "old-old". J Am Geriatr Soc 1992;40:19-22.

16. ten Berg J, Bal E, et al. Initial and long-term results of percutaneous transluminal coronary angioplasty in patients 75 years of age and older. Cathet Cardiovasc Diagn 1992;26:165-170.

17. Thompson RC, Holmes DR, Gersh B, Mock MB. Percutaneous transluminal coronary angioplasty in the elderly: Early and long-term results. J Am Coll Cardiol 1991;17(6):1245-1250.

18. Yokoi H, Kimur T, Sawada Y, Nosaka H, et al. Efficacy and safety of Palmaz-Schatz stent in elderly ($\geq$ 75 years old) patients: Early and follow-up results. J Am Coll Cardiol 1995; March Special Issue:47A.

19. Fishman RF, Kuntz RE, Carrozza JP, et al. Acute and long-term results of coronary atherectomy in women and the elderly. Circulation (in-press).

20. Movsowitz H, Manginas A, et al. Directional coronary atherectomy can be successfully performed in the elderly. Am J Cardiol 1994;31:261-263.

21. Elliot JM, MacIsaac AI, Lefkovits J, Horrigan MCG, Franco I, Whitlow PL. New coronary devices in the elderly: Comparison with angioplasty. Circulation 1994;90:4 (Part II):I-333.

22. Henson, K. D., J. J. Popma, et al. Comparison of results of rotational coronary atherectomy in three age groups (<70,70 to 79 and >80 years). Am J Cardiol 1993;71:862-864.

23. Weyrens F, Goldberg I, et al. Percutaneous transluminal coronary angioplasty in patients aged >90 years. Am J Cardiol 1994;74:397-398.

24.   Santana J, Haft J, LaMarche N, Goldstein J. Coronary angioplasty in patients eighty years of age or older. Am Heart J 1992;124:13-18.

25.   Bedotto JB, Rutherford BD, McConahay DR, et al. Results of multivessel percutaneous transluminal coronary angioplasty in persons aged 65 years and older. Am J Cardiol 1991;67:1051-1055.

26.   Jackman JD, Navetta FI, Smith JE, et al. Percutaneous transluminal coronary angioplasty in octogenarians as an effective therapy for angina pectoris. Am J Cardiol 1991;116-119.

27.   Myler RK, Webb JG, Nguyen KPV, et al. Coronary angioplasty in octogenarians: Comparison to coronary bypass surgery. Cath Cardiovasc Diagn 1991;23:3-9.

28.   Jeroudi OM, Kleiman NS, Minor ST, et al. Percutaneous transluminal coronary angioplasty in octogenarians. Ann Intern Med 1990;113:423-428.

29.   Rizo-Patron C, Hamad N, Paulus R, et al. Percutaneous transluminal coronary angioplasty in octogenarians with unstable coronary syndromes. Am J Cardiol 1990;66:857-858

30.   Rich JJ, Crispino CM, Saporito JJ, et al. Percutaneous transluminal coronary angioplasty in octogenarians. Am J Cardiol 1988;61:457-458.

31.   Kern MJ, Deligonoul U, Galan K, et al. Percutaneous transluminal coronary angioplasty in octogenarians. Am J Cardiol 1988;61:457-458.

32.   Weyrens EJ, Goldenberg I, Fishman MJ, et al. Percutaneous transluminal coronary angioplasty in patients aged > 90 years. Am J Cardiol 1994;74:397-398.

33.   Lerner DJ, Kannel WB. Patterns of coronary heart disease morbidity and mortality in the sexes: A 26-year follow-up of the Framingham population. Am Heart J 1986;111:383-390.

34.   Harper R, Kennedy G, DeSanctis R, et al. The incidence and pattern of angina prior to acute myocardial infarction: A study of 577 cases. Am Heart J 1979;97:178-183.

35.   Weiner DA, Ryan TJ, McCabe CH, et al. Exercise stress testing: Correlations among history of angina, ST-segment response and prevalence of coronary-artery disease in the Coronary Artery Surgery Study (CASS). N Engl J Med 1979;301:230-235.

36.   Stone G, Grines C, Browne K, et al. Comparison of in-hospital outcome in men versus women treated by either thrombolytic therapy or primary coronary angioplasty for acute myocardial infarction. Am J Cardiol 1995;75:987-992.

37.   Malenka DJ, O'Connor GAT, Robb J, Kellett M Jr., et al. Is female gender a risk factor for adverse outcomes following PTCA? Circulation 1995;92:I-437.

38.   Weintraub WS, Wenger NK, Kosinski AS, et al. Percutaneous transluminal coronary angioplasty in women compared with men. J Am Coll Cardiol 1994;24:81-90.

39.   Arnold A, Mick M, et al. Gender differences for coronary angioplasty. Am J Cardiol 1994;74:18-21.

40.   Cavero PG, O'Keefe JH, McCallister B, Cochran V, et al. Effect of gender on early and longterm outcome after multiple vessel revascularization with coronary bypass surgery or balloon angioplasty. J Am Coll Cardiol 1994;March Special Issue:351A.

41.   Kelsey S, James M, Holubkov AL, Holubkov R. Results of percutaneous transluminal coronary angioplasty in women. 1985-1986 National Heart, Lung, and Blood Institute's Coronary Angioplasty Registry. Circulation 1993;87:720-727.

42.   Bell MR, Holmes DR, Berger PB, et al. The changing in-hospital mortality in women undergoing percutaneous transluminal coronary angioplasty. JAMA 1993;269:2091-2095.

43.   Kahn JK, Rutherford BD, McConahay DR, et al. Comparison of procedural results and risks of coronary in men and women for conditions other than acute myocardial infarction. Am J Cardiol 1992;69:1241-1242.

44.   Bell M, Grill D, Garratt K, Berger P, Gersh B, Holmes D. Long-term outcome of women compared with men after successful coronary angioplasty. Circulation 1995;91:2876-2881.

45.   Erne P, Evequoz D, Zuber M, Yoon S, Burckhardt D. Swiss interventional study on silent ischemia II (SWISSI II): Study design and preliminary results. Circulation 1995;92:I-80.

46.   Baumbach A, Bittl J, Fleck E, et al. Acute complications of excimer laser coronary angioplasty: A detailed analysis of multicenter results. J Am Coll Cardiol 1994;23:1305-1313.

47.   Combs WG, Rothenberg MD, Burke JA, et al. Gender does not influence the morbidty and mortality associated with diagnostic and interventional cardiac catheterization procedures. J Am Coll Cardiol 1994;March Special Issue:401A.

48.   Dean LS, Voorhees WD, Sutor C, Roubin GS. Female gender: A risk factor for complications following intracoronary stenting? A Cook multicenter Registry Report. Circulation 1994;90:4 (Part II):I-620.

49.   Ellis, S., J. Popma, et al. Relation of clinical presentation, stenosis morphology, and operator technique to the procedural results of rotational atherectomy-facilitated angioplasty. Circulation 1994;89:882-892.

50.   Bowling BA, May M, Lichtenberg A, et al. Clinical and angiographic outcome of new interventional devices in men and women. Circulation 1994;88 (4) (Part II):I-448.

51.   Casale PN, Marco J, Warth D, Buchbinder M. Women have a lower success rate and higher complication rate with percutaneous rotational atherectomy. Circulation 1994;88 (4) (Part II):I-448.

52.   Henson KD, Popma JJ, Satler LF, Kent KM, et al. Late clinical outcome after new device angioplasty in women. J Am Coll Cardiol 1993;21:2:233A.

53.   Mehta S, Margolis JR, Bejarano J, et al. Acute and long-term results with new devices do not demonstrate significant gender differences: Results from the NACI Registry. Circulation 1994;88(44):I-448.

54.   Movsowitz H, Emmi R, Manginas A, et al. Does female gender affect the success rate and outcome of directional coronary atherectomy? Circulation 1994;88(4):I-448.

55.   Sempos C, Cooper R, Kovear MD, McMullen M. Divergence of the recent trends in coronary mortality for the four major race-sex groups in the United States. Am J Public Health 1988;78:1422-1427.

56.   Maynard C, Fisher LD, Passamani ER. Survival of black persons compared with white persons in the Coronary Artery Surgery Study (CASS). Am J Cardiol 1987;60:513-518.

57.   Scott, N, Kelsey S, et al. Percutaneous transluminal coronary angioplasty in African-American patients (The National Heart, Lung, and Blood Institute 1985-1986 percutaneous transluminal coronary angioplasty registry). Am J Cardiol 1994;73:1141-1146.

58.   Chuang YC, Merritt AJ, Popma JJ, Bucher TA, et al. Do racial differences affect outcome after new device angioplasty? J Am Coll Cardiol 1994;Special Issue:301A.

59.   Scott NA, Capers Q, Weintraub WS, Liberman HA, et al. In hospital and long term outcome of PTCA in African-American women and men. Circulation 1994;88 (4) (Part II):I-448.

60.   The BARI Investigators. The Bypass Angioplasty Revascularization Investigation (BARI): five year mortality and morbidity in a randomized study comparing CABG and PTCA in patients with multivessel coronary disease. N Engl J Med 1996 (Submitted).

61.   Uthoff K, Schuerholz T, Mügge A, Schaefers JH, et al. Coronary revascularization in renal risk patients —coronary angioplasty (PTCA) or coronary artery bypass grafting (CABG)? Circulation 1995;92:I-643.

62.   Stein B, Weintraub W, et al. Influence of diabetes mellitus on early and late outcome after percutaneous transluminal coronary angioplasty. Circulation 1995;91:979-989.

63.   Faxon DP, Kip KE, Currier JW, Yeh W, et al. Diabetics have a significantly poorer eight year outcome after angioplasty. Circulation 1995;92:I-76.

64.   Tan K, Sulke N, et al. Clinical and lesion morphologic determinants of coronary angioplasty success and complications: Current experience. J Am Coll Cardiol 1995;25:855-65.

65.   Bailey WL, Westerhausen DR, Rutherford BD, McConahay DR, et al. Characteristics and long term outcomes of diabetic patients presenting for coronary angioplasty. J Am Coll Cardiol 1993;21:2:273A.

66.   Carrozza J, Kuntz R, et al. Angiographic and clinical outcome of intracoronary stenting: Immediate and long-term results from a large single-center experience. J Am Coll Cardiol 1992;20:328-337.

67.   Rensing BJ, Hermans WR, Strauss BH, Serruys PW. Regional differences in elastic recoil after percutaneous transluminal coronary angioplasty: A quantitative angiographic study. J Am Coll Cardiol 1991;17:34B-8B.

68.   Weintraub WS, Kosinski AS, Brown CL, King SB III. Can restenosis after coronary angioplasty be predicted from clinical variables? J Am Coll Cardiol 1993;21:6-14.

69.   Levin GN, Leya F, Keeler G, Berdan LG, Jacobs AK. The impact of diabetes mellitus on restenosis following directional coronary atherectomy and PTCA: A report from CAVEAT-1. Circulation 1994;90:4 (Part II):I-652.

70.   Faxon DP. Effect of high dose angiotensin-converting enzyme inhibition on restenosis: Final results of the MARCATOR

study, a multicenter, double-blind, placebo-controlled trial of cilazapril. J Am Coll Cardiol 1995;2:362-9.

71.   Bourassa MG, Lesperance J, Eastwood C, et al. Clinical, physiologic, anatomic and procedural factors predictive of restenosis after percutaneous transluminal coronary angioplasty. J Am Coll Cardiol 1991;18:368-76.

72.   Kahn JK, Rutherford BD, McConahay DR, et al. Short and longterm outcome of percutaneous transluminal coronary angioplasty in chronic dialysis patients. Am Heart J 1990;119:484-489.

73.   Reusser LM, Osborn LA, White HJ, et al. Increased morbidity after coronary angioplasty in patients on chronic hemodialysis. Am J Cardiol 1994;73:965-6.

74.   Ahmed WH, Pashos CL, Ayanian JZ, Bittle JA. 30-day and one-year mortality in hemodialysis patients undergoing coronary revascularization: Results from a national cohort. Circulation 1995;92:I-75.

75.   Schroeder J, Gao SZ, et al. A preliminary study of diltiazem in the prevention of coronary artery disease in heart-transplant recipients. N Engl J Med 1993;328:164-170.

76.   Halle A, DiSciascio G, et al. Coronary angioplasty, atherectomy and bypass surgery in cardiac transplant recipients. J Am Coll Cardiol 1995;26:120-8.

77.   Swan JW, Norell M, Yacoub M, et al. Coronary angioplasty in cardiac transplant recipients. Eur Heart J 1993;14:65-70.

78.   Sandhu JS, Uretsky BF, Reddy S, et al. Potential limitations of percutaneous transluminal coronary angioplasty in heart transplant recipients. Am J Cardiol 1992;69:1234-1237.

79.   Mullins PA, Shapiro LM, Aravot DA, et al. Experience of percutaneous transluminal coronary angioplasty in orthotopic transplant recipients. Eur Heart J 1991;12:1205-1207.

80.   Chaitman B, Stone P, Knatterud G, et al. Asymptomatic cardiac ischemia pilot (ACIP) study: Impact of anti-ischemia therapy on 12-week rest electrocardiogram and exercise test outcomes. J Am Coll Cardiol 1995;26(3):585-593.

81.   Rogers W, Bourassa M, Andrews T, et al. Asymptomatic cardiac ischemia pilot (ACIP) study: Outcome at 1-year for patients with asymptomatic cardiac ischemia randomized to medical therapy or revascularization. J Am Coll Cardiol 1995;26(3):594-605.

82.   Bourassa M, Pepine C, Forman S, et al. Asymptomatic cardiac ischemia pilot (ACIP) study: Effects of coronary angioplasty and coronary artery bypass graft surgery on recurrent angina and ischemia. J Am Coll Cardiol 1995;26(3):606-614.

83.   Knatterud GL, Bourassa MG, Pepine CJ, et al. Effects of treatment strategies to suppress ischemia in patients with coronary artery disease: 12-week results of the Asymptomatic Cardiac Ischemia Pilot (ACIP) study. J Am Coll Cardiol 1994;24:11-20.

84.   Stone GW, Spaude D, Ligon RW, et al. Usefulness of percutaneous transluminal coronary angioplasty in alleviating silent myocardial ischemia in patients with absent or minimal painful myocardial ischemia. Am J Cardiol 1989;64:560-564.

85.   Lefevre T, Morice MC, Labrunie B, et al. Coronary stenting in elderly patients. Results from the stent without coumadin French Registry. J Am Coll Cardiol 1996; March Special Issue:975-71.

86.   Hermiller J, Fry E, Berkompas D, et al. Effect of gender on acute outcome following intracoronary bailout stenting. J Invas Cardiol 1996;8.

OVERVIEW OF INTERVENTIONAL DEVICES

Robert D. Safian, M.D.
Mark Freed, M.D.

Several interventional devices are now widely used for percutaneous coronary revascularization, including balloon angioplasty, atherectomy, lasers, and stents (Tables 8.1-8.4). Although non-balloon devices have been developed to address the known limitations of PTCA, with few exceptions, no clear advantage over PTCA has been demonstrated. Nevertheless, certain commercially-available devices or device combinations may have value for treating selected lesion morphologies and angiographic complications.

A. LIMITATIONS OF INTERVENTIONAL DEVICES (Table 8.5)

1. **Failure to Cross a Chronic Total Occlusion with a Guidewire** is quite common and precludes PTCA, atherectomy, lasers, and stenting. Potential strategies for addressing this problem include prolonged infusions of thrombolytic drugs (Chapter 9), and investigational devices such as rotational angioplasty (ROTACS), vibrational angioplasty, and the excimer laser guidewire (Chapter 16). In contrast, failure to cross a subtotal occlusion is extremely rare, is usually due to severe target vessel tortuosity, and can usually be managed by the use of special guidewire and guiding catheter techniques (Chapter 16).

2. **Failure to Cross a Lesion with a Device.** Once the target lesion has been crossed with a guidewire, percutaneous intervention may be unsuccessful due to the inability to access the lesion with the intended device. These failures may be due to proximal vessel tortuosity (Chapter 11) or severe lesion calcification (Chapter 12), precluding passage of inflexible devices such as DCA or stents; these cases can often be managed by PTCA. At times, severe lesion rigidity or calcification precludes passage of even low-profile balloons. Such failures can often be treated by Rotablator atherectomy (Chapter 27) or the excimer laser (Chapter 30), followed by definitive lumen enlargement with DCA, stents, or PTCA.

3. **Failure to Dilate or Deploy a Device.** Once a target lesion has been crossed with a guidewire and the intended device has been properly positioned, failure of intervention may be due to the inability to fully dilate or deploy the device. In some PTCA cases, extreme lesion rigidity precludes full balloon expansion despite high pressure balloons; such failures can often be treated by the use of a parallel guidewire external to the balloon ("force-focused angioplasty," Chapter 12), Rotablator (Chapter 27), excimer laser (Chapter 30), or DCA (Chapter 28). In other cases, full balloon expansion is readily achieved, but significant elastic recoil limits adequate lumen enlargement (Chapter 13); this problem can often be managed by the Rotablator (Chapter 27), DCA (Chapter 28), or stents (Chapter 26). In unusual cases, severe degrees of elastic recoil may complicate DCA or stent procedures, necessitating the use of multiple overlapping stents.

4. **Dissection & Abrupt Closure.** Severe dissection and abrupt closure complicate 2-10% of PTCA procedures, increasing the risk of death, MI, and emergency bypass surgery (Chapter 20). Neither

Table 8.1. Interventional Devices

Percutaneous transluminal coronary angioplasty (PTCA) *

Atherectomy devices
    Directional coronary atherectomy (DCA)*
    Transluminal extraction catheter (TEC)*
    High-speed mechanical rotational atherectomy (MRA; Rotablator)*
    Pullback atherectomy catheter (PAC)
    Rotary atherectomy system

Lasers
    Excimer laser coronary angioplasty (ELCA)*
    Infrared laser coronary angioplasty (ILCA)
    Excimer laser guidewire

Stents
    Gianturco-Roubin stent (Flexstent)*
    Palmaz-Schatz stent *
    Microstent
    Multilink stent
    Cordis stent
    Nir stent
    Wallstent
    Strecker stent **

Thermal Devices
    Laser balloon angioplasty **
    Physiologic low-stress angioplasty (PLOSA)
    Radiofreqeuncy balloon

Other Devices
    Hydrolyzer
    Angiojet
    Therapeutic ultrasound
    Vibrational angioplasty
    Cutting balloon angioplasty
    Low-speed rotational angioplasty catheter system (ROTACS)

---

*   FDA approved
**   Removed from market

laser nor atherectomy has been shown to lower the incidence of abrupt closure or associated clinical complications. In contrast, the coronary stent has proven to be highly effective in reversing abrupt closure and improving clinical outcome (Chapter 26); stent thrombosis, however, negates

Table 8.2. Coronary Atherectomy Devices: Technical Features

	Atherectomy Method		
	Directional	**Rotational**	**Extractional**
Names:	Directional coronary atherectomy (DCA) AtheroCath	Rotablator; Mechanical rotational atherectomy (MRA); Percutaneous transluminal coronary rotational ablation (PTCRA)	Transluminal Extraction Catheter (TEC)
Description:	Nonflexible housing with window on one side and balloon on other side. Cup-shaped cutter inside housing is connected to a drive cable. Hollow nosecone is tapered, acts as a specimen collection chamber.	Spindle-shaped, diamond coated brass burr connected to a flexible drive housed in 4F Teflon sheath. Compressed air turbine controls speed of rotation.	Two stainless steel conical cutting blades attached to a hollow torque tube. Vacuum bottle creates constant suction during cutting.
Method of Action	Atheroma situated in cutting window is excised and stored in nosecone collection chamber for retrieval; "Dotter" and angioplasty effects also operative	Preferential pulverization of hard atheromatous tissue and relative sparing of plaque-free wall. Particles pass through coronary microcirculation.	Simultaneous excision and aspiration of particulate slurry (atheroma, clot, saline).
Rotational speed	1500-2000 rpm. Controlled by hand-held, battery-powered, motor drive unit; speed not adjustable	150,000-200,000 rpm. Controlled by compressed air turbine, speed adjustable by foot pedal.	750 rpm. Controlled by trigger on hand-held, battery-powered motor drive unit; speed not adjustable
Saline irrigation during device activation	No.	Yes. Lubricates and cools rotation system.	Yes. Creates particulate effluent for aspiration.
Cutter movement	Rotating cutter moves forward in stationary housing; Excision during cutter advancement.	Rotating burr tracks through lesion over guidewire; Pulverization during burr advancement.	Rotating cutter tracks through lesion over guidewire; Cutting during advancement.
Adjunctive PTCA	70 - 90%	> 90%	> 90%
FDA Status	Approved	Approved	Approved

some of this beneficial effect. In highly selected focal dissections, DCA may be used to excise obstructing intimal flaps and reverse abrupt closure (Chapter 28).

5. **Recurrent Ischemia and Restenosis.** Restenosis is the most important longterm limitation of percutaneous intervention. Compared to PTCA, laser and atherectomy have not been shown to favorably impact restenosis.[1-3] While stents demonstrated a modest reduction in restenosis compared to PTCA, these results were achieved at higher cost, increased length of stay, and more bleeding and vascular complications (Chapter 26).[4,5] Studies of "optimal" atherectomy and stenting are in progress (Chapters 26, 28).

B. EVALUATION OF INTERVENTIONAL DEVICES (Table 8.6)

1. **Procedural Success.** The "preferred" definition of procedural success is final diameter stenosis < 50% in the absence of a major complication (death, Q-wave MI, or emergency CABG). Nevertheless, other definitions are frequently used, including angiographic success (final diameter stenosis < 50%), device success (decrease in diameter stenosis > 20%), and clinical success (procedure success without an early clinical event). It is important to verify that similar definitions are used when comparing different studies. When two devices are used in succession to treat a lesion (e.g., Rotablator followed by adjunctive PTCA for calcified stenoses), "procedural success" frequently refers to final outcome. In reality, four outcomes are possible (Figure 8.1): (1) device success and PTCA success; (2) device success and PTCA failure; (3) device failure and PTCA

Table 8.3. Coronary Laser Systems: Technical Features

	Excimer Laser	Holmium/TM
Description	Multi-element fiber passes over 0.018" guidewire. Short (2 to 3 sec) laser bursts; Adjunctive PTCA required in most cases; tissue contact not required.	Multi-element fiber passess over 0.18" guidewire. Tissue contact not required.
Mechanism	Vaporization; acoustic shock or pressure waves. Minimal thermal effects.	Vaporization; acoustic shock or pressure waves. Minimal thermal effects.
Laser Characteristics: Media Wavelength Mode	Xenon Chloride Ultraviolet Pulsed	Holmium/TM:YAG Infrared Pulsed
FDA Status	Approved	Investigational

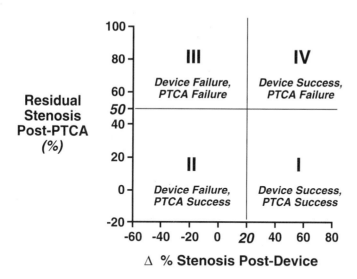

Figure 8.1 Angiographic Outcomes after Interventions with Devices and Adjunctive PTCA

success; and (4) device failure and PTCA failure. There is ongoing debate as to whether angiographic and clinical outcomes should be reported after each device, or only from the final result. The problem in reporting results only at the end of the procedure is that it overestimates the value of a bad device that is salvaged by a good device, and underestimates the value of a good device that is followed by a bad device. Furthermore, prognostic information may be lost when results are not recorded after each device; even when salvaged by PTCA, abrupt closure after TEC, ELCA, or Rotablator strongly predicted subsequent ischemic complications.[7]

2. **Assessment of Lumen Enlargement.** Conventional measures of lumen enlargement include absolute lumen dimensions (minimal lumen diameter, reference diameter) and percent diameter stenosis. However, use of these measures is confounded by several factors, including differences in device size, vessel size, and device "efficiency" (i.e., ratio of final lumen diameter-to-device diameter. Available studies suggest that the efficiency of lumen enlargement for some lasers, atherectomy devices, and stents is superior to PTCA; however, the magnitude of lumen enlargement (assessed by absolute dimensions and diameter stenosis) is limited by the small sizes of devices (particularly for ELCA, TEC, and Rotablator).[9]

3. **Relationship Between Immediate Lumen Enlargement and Late Outcome.** Several studies suggest an inverse relationship between post-procedural lumen diameter and angiographic

Table 8.4. Intracoronary Stents: Technical Features

	Wallstent* (Schneider)	Palmaz-Schatz ** (Johnson & Johnson)	Gianturco-Roubin (Cook)	MultiLink (ACS)
Design	Self expanding	Balloon expandable	Balloon expandable	Balloon expandable
Configuration	Woven wire mesh	Slotted tube	Flexible wire	Slotted tube with loops and bridges
Material	Stainless steel	Stainless steel	Stainless steel	Stainless steel
Strut diameter (mm/inch)	0.08/0.003	0.08/0.003	0.15/0.006	0.05/0.002
Delivery sheath	Yes	Yes	No	Yes
Length (mm)	15-43	15	12,20	15
Metal surface area (%)	10-15	12	10	10-15
Maximum guidewire (in)	0.018	0.014	0.018	0.014
Minimum guide ID (in)	0.077	0.084	0.086	0.075
Expanded diameter (mm)	3.5-6.0	3.0-5.0	2.0-4.5	3.0-3.85
Radio-opacity (Fluoroscopy)	Poor	Poor	Poor	Fair
Deployment pressure (ATM)	---	6-8	4-7	9

*   Less-shortening Wallstent-=second generation prototype; Less metal surface, shortens by 25%.
**   Biliary stents and peripheral stents have been used in large coronary arteries and saphenous vein grafts
***   Monorail design will accept a 0.014-inch guidewire
****   The Strecker stent (Boston Scientific) was withdrawn from the market.

restenosis (i.e., "bigger is better").[10,11] While these studies found that device type itself had little if any impact on restenosis, other studies suggest the contrary: In the ERBAC trial, a trend toward *more* restenosis was observed in the Rotablator and excimer laser groups (vs. PTCA) despite *larger* post-procedural lumen diameters.[3] Very high (> 70%) restenosis rates were also reported after laser balloon angioplasty despite excellent initial lumen enlargement. A recent study of matched lesions also suggested that DCA may result in more intimal hyperplasia than PTCA.[12] In CAVEAT-I, despite greater acute gain and a larger final lumen, DCA patients had a higher incidence of *late* myocardial infarction compared to PTCA patients. Collectively, these data suggest that the final lumen diameter and possibly the device type (i.e., type of vessel injury) impact on late lumen dimensions and restenosis. Furthermore, attainment of a larger post-procedural lumen diameter does not ensure a lower incidence of cardiac events or restenosis.

Table 8.4. Intracoronary Stents: Technical Features (con't)

Self-Expanding Stent (SciMed)	MicroStent-II (AVE)	Wiktor (Medtronic)	Nir**** (SciMed)	Cordis
Self expanding	Balloon expandable	Balloon expandable	Balloon expandable	Balloon expandable
Slotted tube	Coil wire	Flexible wire	Wire mesh	Coil wire
Stainless steel	Stainless steel	Tantalum	Stainless steel	Tantalum
0.13/0.005	0.20/0.008	0.13/0.005	0.08/0.003	0.13/0.005
Yes	No	No	No	No
14, 20, 30	6-36	16	9, 16, 32	18
20	8.5	7-9	14-19	15
NA	0.014	0.018***	0.014	0.018
0.072	0.072	0.082	0.065	0.072
2.75-4.25	2.5-4.5	2.5-4.0	2.0-5.0	3.0-4.0
NA	Good	Good	Fair	Good
---	9-12	6	8	8

*	Less-shortening Wallstent-=second generation prototype; Less metal surface, shortens by 25%.
**	Biliary stents and peripheral stents have been used in large coronary arteries and saphenous vein grafts
***	Monorail design will accept a 0.014-inch guidewire
****	The Strecker stent (Boston Scientific) was withdrawn from the market.

4. **Cost.** Compared to PTCA, atherectomy, lasers, and stents are associated with higher procedural and total hospital costs, and longer lengths of stay.[17-22] Detailed studies of cost-effectiveness of interventional devices are anxiously awaited.

Table 8.5. Limitations of Interventional Devices

- ▸ Failure to cross lesion with a guidewire
- ▸ Failure to cross lesion with a device
- ▸ Failure to dilate or deploy a device
- ▸ Dissection/abrupt closure
- ▸ Recurrent ischemia and restenosis

Table 8.6. Efficacy and Safety of Interventional Devices

	PTCA	DCA	TEC	ROTA	ELCA	Stent
Success	≥ 90%	-	-	-	-	-
Acute Closure	4-5%	-	-	-	-	↓
Dissection	30%	↓↓	↑	↓	↑	↓↓
Spasm	1-2%	-	↑	↑	↑	↓
MI: Q-wave	1%	-	-	-	-	-
non Q-wave	1-2%	↑	-	↑	-	-
CABG	2%	-	-	-	-	-
Death	<1%	-	-	-	-	-
Perforation	0.3%	↑	↑	↑	↑	-
Restenosis	30-50%	-	-	-	-	↓
Adjunctive PTCA	NA	70-80*	90	90	90	100

Abbreviations: DCA = Directional Coronary Atherectomy; TEC = Transluminal Extraction Catheter Atherectomy; ROTA = Rotablator; ELCA = Excimer-Laser Coronary Angioplasty; LBA = Thermal-Laser balloon angioplasty; NA = not applicable
- equivalent rate/risk
↑ increased risk
↓ decreased risk
* optimal atherectomy technique

5. **Complications.** Multicenter prospective randomized studies show no difference in major in-hospital complications (death, Q-wave MI, emergency CABG) between new devices and PTCA.[1-5] In contrast, the incidence of non-Q-wave MI was higher after DCA compared to PTCA in both CAVEAT-I and CAVEAT-II.

C. **IMPORTANT CONSIDERATIONS IN USING INTERVENTIONAL DEVICES.** Over the last 5 years, enormous experience has been achieved with newer atherectomy, laser, and stent devices. Despite this experience, definitive guidelines and recommendations remain elusive, and further studies are in progress to help define their roles. In the meantime, currently available data suggest that use of a lesion-specific, multi-device approach may optimize results and decrease complications.
   1. **Facilitated Lumen Enlargement.** There is a growing impression among interventionalists that sequential use of two different devices may improve procedural outcome compared to using one device. When atherectomy or laser angioplasty is followed by PTCA, this approach has been

called *facilitated angioplasty*;[31] the use of two different nonballoon devices (e.g., Rotablator, TEC, or ELCA followed by DCA or stent) has been called *transcatheter device synergy*.[32] These concepts, in which the first device renders the lesion more responsive to the actions of the second, although interesting mechanistically, have not been shown to be superior to PTCA alone. In a study of Rotablator or DCA followed by PTCA, intravascular ultrasound failed to demonstrate facilitated PTCA.[33] However, in another study, facilitated lumen enlargement was identified for adjunctive PTCA after Rotablator, TEC, and ELCA, but only for certain lesion morphologies.[31] Facilitated lumen enlargement is only one aspect of the broader concept of "facilitated intervention," which considers the impact of two or more devices used in succession on procedural complications, late outcome, and cost.

2. **Lesion-Specific Approach to Coronary Intervention (Table 8.7).** Current studies have failed to demonstrate major differences in overall outcome between patients treated with PTCA vs. other laser and atherectomy devices. Nevertheless, it is possible that certain lesion subsets might be more amenable to some devices than others. There have been numerous cases of successful ELCA and MRA after failed PTCA for rigid or nondilatable lesions,[34-39] as well as successful DCA and stenting after failed PTCA for elastic recoil,[40-45] but these failures are relatively uncommon and quite unpredictable.[46] ELCA was initially proposed for long lesions, but recent studies revealed that ELCA increased the risk of adverse clinical events[47] and restenosis[48] compared to PTCA. Recent studies suggest that the greatest degree of facilitated lumen enlargement is achieved with ELCA, TEC, or Rotablator (followed by adjunctive PTCA) for ostial lesions; the incremental gain in lumen diameter was 21-41% compared to PTCA alone. Although laser and atherectomy devices appear to have fairly narrow "niche" applications (see Chapters 27-29), coronary stents appear to have superior results compared to PTCA for a broad range of lesion morphologies in vessels $\geq$ 3 mm in diameter (Chapter 26). Stents may ultimately account for at least 50% of all percutaneous interventions.

3. **Adjunctive Imaging Techniques.** Intravascular ultrasound, coronary angioscopy, and the intracoronary Doppler flowire may have important uses as adjuncts to percutaneous intervention. Intravascular ultrasound (Chapter 31) is useful for assessing vessel dimensions prior to and following intervention, identifying the extent and distribution of calcification, and possibly optimizing stenting, Rotablator, and DCA. Coronary angioscopy (Chapter 32) is superior to angiography in evaluating intraluminal thrombus and dissection, and may optimize interventions in vein grafts. Finally, Doppler flow measurements (Chapter 33) may be valuable for assessing the physiologic response to catheter-based intervention and predicting complications. All of these techniques may be used to evaluate "borderline lesions" prior to intervention and suboptimal or hazy results after intervention, and to assist in decision-making (e.g., device selection, need for further intervention).

Table 8.7. Interventional Devices: Lesion-Specific Indications

Lesion Morphology	PTCA	Stent	DCA	ROTA	TEC	ELCA
Elective Use:						
Eccentric	+	+	+	+	-	-
Ulcerated	+	+	+	+	-	-
Ostial	-	+	+	+	+	+
Total occlusion	+	+	+/-	+/-	+/-	+/-
Bifurcation	+	+/-	+	+/-	-	-
Diffuse Disease	+	-	-	+/-	-	+/-
Thrombus	+	-	+/-	-	+	+/-
Severe angle	+	-	-	-	-	-
Suboptimal PTCA:						
Focal dissection	+	+	+	-	-	-
Long dissection	+	+/-	-	-	-	-
Elastic	-	+	+	-	-	-
Rigid	-	-	+	+	-	+/-

Abbreviations: PTCA = percutaneous transluminal coronary angioplasty; DCA = directional coronary atherectomy; ROTA = Rotablator; ELCA = excimer laster coronary angioplasty; TEC = transluminal extraction catheter
+ Favorable
- Unfavorable

4. **Adjunctive Pharmacotherapy.** While aspirin and heparin remain the mainstays of interventional pharmacotherapy, recent data suggest an emerging role for ticlopidine (aspirin-allergy, stent implantation), platelet IIb/IIIa receptor antagonists (high-risk intervention) (Chapter 34), superselective infusions of thrombolytics (chronic total occlusion) (Chapter 16), and intracoronary calcium blockers (no-reflow) (Chapter 21). Local drug delivery systems may further improve the efficacy of adjunctive medical therapy (Chapter 35). New antithrombins (e.g., hirudin) are under intense investigation, while the role of serotonin antagonists, thromboxane inhibitors, and protein C blockers await determination.[49-54]

D. **NEW INVESTIGATIONAL DEVICES**. There continues to be enormous interest in the development of new interventional devices, which will hopefully solve some of the residual problems associated with existing techniques. These devices are in varying stages of preclinical and clinical evaluation; at the present time, there are insufficient data to make recommendations about their use. Nevertheless, here is a brief description of some of the more promising devices:

1. **Hydrolyzer.** The Cordis Hydrolyzer is a hydrodynamic thrombectomy catheter that relies on the Venturi principle for aspiration and removal of intraluminal thrombus and debris. Experimental and preliminary clinical studies in Europe suggest a possible role for this device in degenerated vein grafts and thrombus-containing lesions.[55,56]

2. **AngioJet (Figure 8.2).** The POSSIS AngioJet is another hydrodynamic thrombectomy catheter; it removes thrombus through a Venturi effect created by high-pressure saline jets from the tip of this 5F over-the-wire catheter. Preliminary data from the VeGAS-I Pilot study revealed successful reduction in thrombotic obstructions in 14/15 (93%) cases; diameter stenosis decreased from 91% to 44% after the AngioJet.[7] This device may have an important role in the treatment of thrombus-containing lesions prior to PTCA, DCA, or stents.

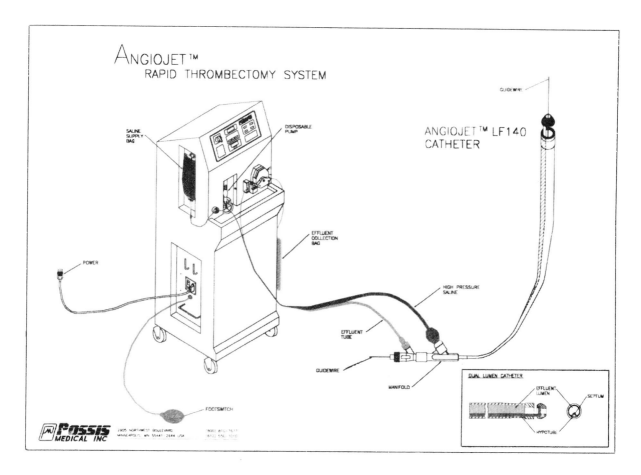

Figure 8.2 POSSIS AngioJet: System Setup

3. **Therapeutic Ultrasound (Figure 8.3).** Potential applications for cardiovascular ultrasound include valvuloplasty, angioplasty, cardiopulmonary bypass, pacing, defibrillation, and controlled drug release.[57] In the peripheral and coronary circulations, ultrasound has been used to recanalize atherosclerotic vessels (Chapter 16)[58-60] and to ablate thrombus.[61,62] The ability of ultrasound to treat coronary obstruction is currently under evaluation in the prospective multicenter CRUSADE study;[63] preliminary data suggest the need for adjunctive PTCA in virtually all lesions.[64]

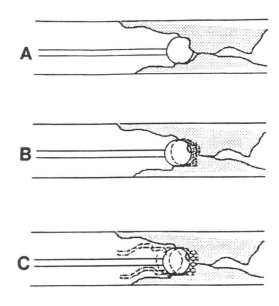

Figure 8.3   Ultrasound Angioplasty

Oscillations of the ultrasound catheter produce microcavitations, resulting in fragmentation of plaque.

4. **Radiofrequency & Thermal Angioplasty Devices (Figure 8.4).** The prototype thermal angioplasty device was laser balloon angioplasty (LBA), which relied on Nd: YAG laser to heat the arterial wall through an inflated angioplasty balloon. Although LBA was useful for decreasing elastic recoil and sealing dissections,[65,66] restenosis rates were unacceptable (> 70%) and the device was withdrawn from the market. Other thermal angioplasty devices have been developed which rely on radiofrequency (100 kHz-300 MHZ)[67-70] or microwave (2450 MHZ)[71] energy to heat the vascular wall to 50-100° C. Experimental and clinical studies suggest that these thermal devices may be useful for decreasing elastic recoil,[67,68] sealing dissections,[67,68,72] and desiccating thrombus. Restenosis, however, occurs in at least 50% of lesions and remains a significant problem.[67,68] Physiologic low stress angioplasty (PLOSA) relies on the application of radiofrequency-induced

heat (60°C) and low inflation pressures (2-5 atm) to remodel the arterial wall;[73] immediate angiographic results and restenosis are similar to those of LBA.[74] Finally, thermal angioplasty may have a role in the delivery and application of materials or drugs to the arterial wall for the prevention of intimal proliferation and thrombosis.[75]

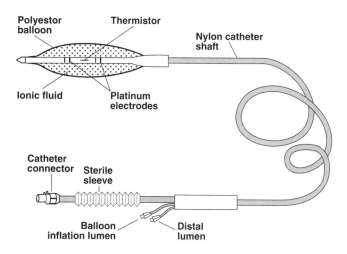

Figure 8.4   Radiofrequency Angioplasty: Catheter Design

5. **Vibrational Angioplasty.** The vibrational angioplasty system consists of a steerable angioplasty guidewire connected to a motor and gearing system; once activated, the guidewire oscillates at 100-500 Hz as it is slowly advanced through the lesion. Preliminary studies in humans suggest that this device may be useful for chronic occlusions that cannot be crossed with a conventional guidewire;[76,77] in one such report, vibrational angioplasty successfully recanalized 67% of resistant lesions.[78]

6. **Cutting Balloon Angioplasty (Figure 8.5).** The cutting balloon is a conventional angioplasty balloon with 3-4 longitudinal microtomes, which focally incise plaque during balloon inflation. A prospective randomized trial is currently underway to determine whether controlled "scores" in the atheroma facilitate balloon-mediated lumen enlargement.[79-81] The principles of cutting balloon angioplasty are similar to those of force-focused angioplasty using a parallel guidewire technique.[82]

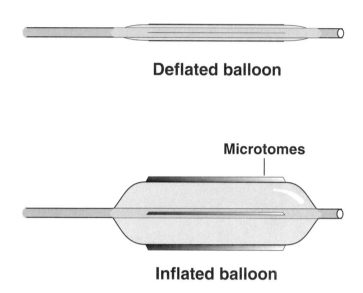

Deflated balloon

Microtomes

Inflated balloon

Figure 8.5   Cutting Balloon Angioplasty

The razor-sharp microtomes are not exposed when the balloon is deflated.

7. **Pullback Atherectomy Catheter (PAC) (Figure 8.6).** The Pullback atherectomy catheter is an over-the-wire cutting and collecting device that consists of an inner movable catheter with a tapered, hollow collecting chamber; a flexible outer closing catheter; and a stainless steel cutting blade. The inner catheter (i.e., cutting blade) is powered by a hand-held motor drive unit and rotates at 2000 rpm. After the device crosses the target lesion (in the closed position), the outer catheter is retracted proximally, the cutting blades are activated, and the inner movable collecting chamber is pulled back through the lesion. This device may permit atherectomy without the problems of distal embolization (seen with the Rotablator) or blood loss (seen with TEC); however, the device is rigid and has a large profile, which may limit its use. Further studies are in progress in the United States and Europe.[83]

8. **Rotary Atherectomy System (RAS) (Figure 8.7).** The rotary atherectomy system consists of a spiral guidewire with a floppy tip (which is advanced over a conventional angioplasty guidewire), a rotating cutting catheter (which is advanced over the spiral wire), and a hand-held motor unit. The system functions as an auger: Atherosclerotic plaque is captured on the spiral guidewire and removed as the cutting catheter is advanced over the spiral wire while rotating at 1500 rpm. Preliminary experimental and peripheral vascular studies indicate the feasibility of tissue removal, but further investigation is needed.[84,85]

Figure 8.6   Pullback Atherectomy Catheter (PAC)

A. Baseline angiogram.
B. Advance PAC past lesion (0.014-inch guidewire).
C. The "closing catheter" is retracted proximal to the lesion.
D. The "cut-collect" chamber is rotated at 2,000 RPM and slowly pulled-back across the lesion; excised tissue is stored in the "cut-collect" chamber.
E. Final angiogram.

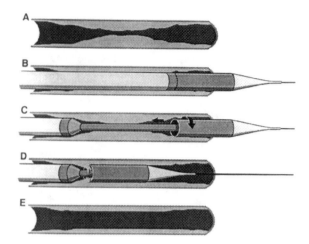

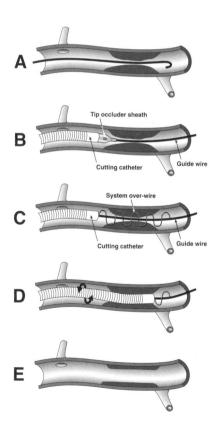

Figure 8.7   Rotary Atherectomy System (RAS)

A. Baseline angiogram.
B. The cutting catheter and tip occluder sheath are advanced up to the lesion.
C. Remove the tip occluder and advance the system-wire (auger).
D. The cutting catheter rotates over the system-wire, excising and collecting tissue.
E. Final angiogram.

9. **Low-speed Rotational Angioplasty Catheter System (ROTACS) (Figure 8.8).** ROTACS was designed as a method for recanalizing chronic total occlusions resistant to conventional PTCA guidewires. ROTACS consists a rotating catheter made up of several stainless steel coils in a helical configuration, an olive-shaped tip, and a polyethylene shielding tube that protects the proximal vessel from the rotating catheter.[86] A battery-powered motor drive rotates the ROTACS at 200 rpm as it is advanced across the lesion. This device has been successfully applied to chronic total occlusions in the peripheral and coronary circulations, and is described in greater detail in Chapter 16.[87,88]

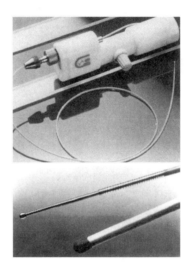

Figure 8.8   Rotational Angioplasty Catheter System (ROTACS)

10. **Excimer Laser Guidewire (Figure 8.9).** The excimer laser guidewire appears to be of value for the revascularization of chronic total occlusions. In a study of 173 chronic total occlusions, laserwire crossing was successful in 59%; final procedural success was 53%, but extravascular wire passage occurred in 24%.[89] This promising device is discussed in greater detail in Chapter 16. In contrast to the excimer laser guidewire, results using the argon laser (LASTAC) system were disappointing, prompting the manufacturer to withdraw the device.

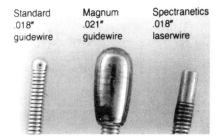

Standard
.018″
guidewire

Magnum
.021″
guidewire

Spectranetics
.018″
laserwire

Figure 8.9   Excimer Laser Guidewire

* * * * *

REFERENCES

1. Adelman A, Eric C, Kimball B, et al. A comparison of directional atherectomy with balloon angioplasty for lesions of the left anterior descending coronary artery. N Engl J Med 1993;329:228-233.
2. Topol E, Leya F, Pinkerton C, et al. A comparison of directional atherectomy with coronary angioplasty in patients with coronary artery disease. N Engl J Med 1993;329:221-227.
3. Vandormael M, Reifart N, Preusler W, et al. Six months following excimer laser angioplasty, rotational atherectomy and balloon angioplasty for complex lesions: ERBAC study. Circulation 1994;90:I-213.
4. Serruys P, deJegere P, Kiemeneij F, et al. A comparison of balloon expandable stent implantation with balloon angioplasty in patients with coronary artery disease. N Engl J Med 1994;331:489-495.
5. Fischman D, Leon M, Baim D, et al. A randomized comparison of coronary stent placement and balloon angioplasty in the treatment of coronary artery disease. N Engl J Med 1994:496-501.
6. Safian R, Freed M, Lichtenberg A, et al. Usefulness of percutaneous transluminal coronary angioplasty after new device coronary interventions. Am J Cardiol 1994;73:642-646.
7. Safian R, May M, Lichtenberg A, Schreiber T, Pavlides G. Detailed clinical and angiographic analysis of transluminal extraction coronary atherectomy for complex lesions in native coronary arteries. J Am Coll Cardiol 1995;25:848-854.
8. McCullough PA, O'Neill WW, May M, et al. Predictors of acute complications after percutaneous coronary revascularization with new devices. J Am Coll Cardiol 1995;25:122A.
9. Safian R, Freed M, Lichtenberg A, et al. Are residual stenoses after excimer laser angioplasty and coronary atherectomy due to inefficient or small devices? Comparison with balloon angioplasty. J Am Coll Cardiol 1993;22:1628-1634.
10. Kuntz RE, Safian RD, Carrozza JP, Fishman RF, Mansour M, Baim D. The importance of acute luminal diameter in determining restenosis after coronary atherectomy or stenting. Circulation 1992;86:1827-1835.
11. Kuntz R, Gibson C, Nobuyoshi M, Baim D. Generalized model of restenosis after conventional balloon angioplasty and new devices. J Am Coll Cardiol 1993;21:15-25.
12. Umans V, Melkert R, de Jaegere P, de Feyter P, Serruys P. A matched comparison of the long-term outcome of directional coronary atherectomy versus coronary stenting. J Am Coll Cardiol 1995;25:393A.
13. Foley DP, Appleman YE, Piek JJ. Comparison of angiographic restenosis propensity of excimer laser coronary angioplasty (ELCA) and balloon angioplasty (BA) in the Amsterdam Rotterdam (AMRO) trial. Circulation 1995;92:I-477.
14. Duerr RL, Topol EJ. Dissociation between minimal luminal diameter and clinical outcome at 6 month follow-up in randomized trials of percutaneous revascularization. J Am Coll Cardiol 1995;25:36A.
15. Miyazaki S, Nakao K, Itoh A, Daikoku S, et al. Correlation of residual stenosis immediately after coronary angioplasty with long-term prognosis. J Am Coll Cardiol 1995;25:269A.
16. Cohen EA, Foley B, Kimball BP, et al. Evidence for a device specific effect on late changes in lumen dimensions after directional atherectomy or intracoronary stenting. Circulation 1994;90:I-58.
17. Nino C, Freed M, Blankenship L. Procedural cost of new interventional cardiology devices. Am J Cardiol 1994;74:1165-1166.
18. Dick RJ, Popma JJ, Muller DWM, Burek KA. In-hospital costs associated with new percutaneous coronary devices. Am J Cardiol 1991;68:879-885.
19. Guzman L, Simpfendorfer C, Fix J, Franco I, Whitlow P. Comparison of costs of new atherectomy devices and balloon angioplasty for coronary artery disease. Am J Cardiol 1994;74:22-25.
20. Vandormael M, Reifart N, Preusler W, et al. In-hospital costs comparison of excimer laser angioplasty, Rotational atherectomy (Rotablator) and balloon angioplasty for complex coronary lesions: A randomized trial (ERBAC). J Am Coll Cardiol 1994;23:223A.
21. Weintraub WS, Waksman R, Bernard J, Hicks F, et al. The influence of new devices on the costs of interventional procedures. Circulation 1994;90:I-44.
22. Appleman YE, Birnie E, Piek JJ, de Feyter PJ, Koolen JJ, et al. Excimer laser angioplasty versus balloon angioplasty in longer coronary lesions: A cost-effectiveness analysis. Circulation 1995;92:I-512.
23. Adbelmeguid AE, Sapp SK, Topol EJ. Long-term outcome of transient uncomplicated in-lab coronary closure. Circulation 1994;90:I-43.
24. Waksman R, Ziyad MBG, Steenkiste AR, Detre K. Predictors and significance of myocardial infarction as a

complication of new interventional devices: Report from the NACI Registry. Circulation 1994;90:I-43.

25. Tauke JT, Kong TQ, Meyers SN, Srinivasan G, et al. Prognostic value of creatinine kinase elevation following elective coronary artery interventions. J Am Coll Cardiol 1995;25:269A.

26. Kong TQ, Tauke JT, Meyers SN, Parker MA, Davidson, CJ. Late outcomes after elective coronary angioplasty: Impact of patient characteristics, lesion morphology and creatine kinase elevation. Circulation 1995;92:I-88.

27. Tardiff BE, Granger CB, Woodlief L, Mahaffey KW, et al. Prognostic significance of post-intervention isozyme elevations. Circulation 1995;92:I-544.

28. Redwood SR, Popma JJ, Kent KM, Pichard AD, et al. "Minor" CPK-MB elevations are associated with increased late mortality following ablative new-device angioplasty in native coronary arteries. Circulation 1995;92:I-544.

29. Hong MK, Popma JJ, Wong SC, Kent KM, et al. Incidence of and factors associated with abrupt closure in patients undergoing elective, new device angioplasty in native coronary arteries. J Am Coll Cardiol 1995;25:122A.

30. McCullough PA, O'Neill WW, Hoffman M, Glazier S, et al. The "protective effect" of restenosis lesions on angiographic complications with new devices. Circulation 1995;92:I-346.

31. Safian RD, Freed M, Reddy V, Kuntz RE, Baim DS, Grines CL, O'Neill WW. Do excimer laser and rotational atherectomy facilitate balloon angioplasty? Implications for lesion-specific coronary intervention. J Am Coll Cardiol (in-press).

32. Henson KD, Flood R, Javier SP, Popma JJ, et al. Transcatheter device synergy: Use of adjunct directional atherectomy after rotational atherectomy vs. excimer laser angioplasty. J Am Coll Cardiol 1994;23:220A.

33. De Franco AC, Tuzcu EM, Moliterno DJ, Guyer S, et al. Do new interventional devices "facilitate" balloon angioplasty? Ultrasound evidence of no reduction in vessel recoil. Circulation 1994;90:I58.

34. Israel D, Marmur J, Sanborn T. Excimer laser-facilitated balloon angioplasty of a nondilatable lesion. J Am Coll Cardiol 1991;18:1118-1119.

35. Berger PB, Bresnaha J. Use of excimer laser in the treatment of chronic total occlusion of a coronary artery that cannot be crossed with a balloon catheter. Cathet Cardiovasc Diagn. 1993;28:44-46.

36. Wolfe C, Landin R, Linnemeier T, et al. Successful excimer laser angioplasty following unsuccessful primary balloon angioplasty. Cathet Cardiovasc Diagn 1993;28:273-278.

37. Rosenblum J, O'Donnell MJ, Stertzer SH, Schechtmann NS. Rotational ablation of a severely angulated stenosis previously not amenable to balloon angioplasty. Am Heart J 1991;122:1766-1768.

38. Brown RIG, Penn IM. Coronary rotational ablation for unsuccessful angioplasty due to failure to cross the stenosis with a dilatation catheter. Cathet Cardiovasc Diagn. 1992;26:110-112.

39. Rosenblum J, Stertzer S, Shaw R, et al. Rotational ablation of balloon angioplasty failures. J Inv Cardiol 1992;4:312-318.

40. Brogan W, Popma J, Pichard A, et al. Rotational coronary atherectomy after unsuccessful coronary balloon angioplasty. Am J Cardiol 1993;71:794-798.

41. McCluskey E, Cowley M, Whitlow P. Multicenter clinical experience with rescue atherectomy for failed angioplasty. Am J Cardiol 1993;72:42E-46E.

42. Hofling B, Gonschior P, Simpson L, Bauriedel G. Efficacy of directional coronary atherectomy in cases unsuitable for percutaneous transluminal coronary angioplasty (PTCA) and after unsuccessful PTCA. Am Heart J 1992;124:341-348.

43. Bergelson B, Fishman R, Tomaso C, et al. Acute and long-term outcome of failed percutaneous transluminal coronary angioplasty treated by directional coronary atherectomy. Am J Cardiol 1994;73:1224-1226.

44. Harris W, Berger P, Holmes D, Garratt K. "Rescue" directional coronary atherectomy after unsuccessful percutaneous transluminal coronary angioplasty. Mayo Clin Proc 1994;69:717-722.

45. Macaya C, Alfonso F, Iniguez A, Goicolea J. Stenting for elastic recoil during coronary angioplasty of the left main coronary artery. Am J Cardiol 1992;70:105-107.

46. Kahn JK, Hartzler GO. Frequency and causes of failure with contemporary balloon coronary angioplasty and implications for new technologies. Am J Cardiol 1990;66:858-860.

47. Appleman YE, Piek JJ, Redekop WK, deFeyter PJ, et al. Excimer laser angioplasty versus balloon angioplasty in longer coronary lesions: A multivariate analysis. Circulation 1995;92:I-74.

48. Strikwerda S, van Swijndregt EM, Foley DP, Boersma E, et al. Immediate and late outcome of excimer laser and balloon coronary angioplasty: A quantitative angiographic comparison based on matched lesions. J Am Coll Cardiol 1995;26:939-946.

49. EPIC Investigators, Topol EJ. Use of a monoclonal antibody directed against the platelet glycoprotein IIb/IIIa receptor

in high-risk coronary angioplasty. N Engl J Med 1994;330:956-61.

50. Bittl J, Strony J, Brinker J, et al. Treatment with Bivalirudin (hirulog) as compared with heparin during coronary angioplasty for unstable or postinfarction angina. N Engl J Med 1995;333:764-9.

51. Serruys P, Herrman J-P, Simon R, et al. A comparison of Hirudin with heparin in the prevention of restenosis after coronary angioplasty. N Engl J Med 1995;333:757-63.

52. Tcheng J, Harrington R, Kottke-Marchant J, Kleiman N. Multicenter, randomized, double-blind, placebo-controlled trial of the platelet integrin glycoprotein IIb/IIIa blocker integrelin in elective coronary intervention. Circulation 1995;91:2151-2157.

53. Lincoff AM, Topol EJ, Califf RM, Weisman HF, et al. Influence of platelet GP IIb/IIIa receptor inhibition with c7E3 on the sequelae of dissection during percutaneous coronary revascularization. J Am Coll Cardiol 1995;25:390A.

54. Challapalli RM, Eisenberg MJ, Sigmon K, Lemberger J. Platelet glycoprotein IIb/IIIa monoclonal antibody (c7E3) reduces distal embolization during percutaneous intervention of saphenous vein grafts. Circulation 1995;92:I-607.

55. Van Ommen V, Veen E, Daemen M, Habets J, et al. In vivo evaluation of the safety to the vessel wall of the hydrolyser (a hydrodynamic thrombectomy catheter). J Am Coll Cardiol 1994;23:406A.

56. Fajadet J, Bar O, Jordan C, Robert G, et al. Human percutaneous thrombectomy using the new hydrolyser catheter: Preliminary results in saphenous vein grafts. J Am Coll Cardiol 1994;23:220A.

57. Meltzer RS, Schwarz KQ, Mottley JG, Everbach EC. Therapeutic cardiac ultrasound. Am J Cardiol 1991;67:422-424.

58. Eccelston DS, Cumpston GN, Hodge AJ, Pearne-Rowe D, Don Michael TA. Ultrasonic coronary angioplasty during bypass grafting: A new method of atherectomy: Initial results. Circulation 1993;88:I-640.

59. Steffen W, Siegel RJ. Ultrasound angioplasty-a review. J Interven Cardiol 1993;6:77-88.

60. Ernst A, Schenk EA, Woodlock TJ. Feasibility of recanalization of human coronary arteries using high-intensity ultrasound. Am J Cardiol 1994;73:126-132.

61. Hartnell GG, Saxton JM, Friedl SE, Abela GS. Ultrasonic thrombus ablation: In vitro assessment of a novel device for intracoronary use. J Interven Cardiol 1993;6(1):69-76.

62. Hamm CW, Steffen W, Reimers J, Terres W. Ultrasound induced thrombolysis in patients with acute myocardial infarction. Circulation 1995;92:I-416.

63. Hamm CW, Bertrand ME, de Scheerder I, Gunn J, et al. Initial multicenter experience with therapeutic ultrasonic coronary angioplasty in patients. J Am Coll Cardiol 1995;25:268A.

64. Steffan W, Bertrand ME, Hamm CW, de Scheerder I, et al. Multicenter experience with therapeutic ultrasound coronary angioplasty in symptomatic patients. Circulation 1995;92:I-330.

65. Spears JR, Reyes VP, Wynne J et al. Percutaneous coronary laser balloon angioplasty: Initial results of a multicenter experience. J Am Coll Cardiol 1990;16:293.

66. Reis GJ, Pomerantz RM, Jenkins RD, et al. Laser balloon angioplasty: Clinical, angiographic and histologic results. J Am Coll Cardiol 1991;18:193.

67. Yamashita K, Satake S, Omira H, Ohtomo K. Radiofrequency thermal balloon coronary angioplasty: A new device for successful percutaneous transluminal coronary angioplasty. J Am Coll Cardiol 1994;23:336-340.

68. Saito S, Arai H, Kim K, Aoki N. Initial clinical experiences with rescue unipolar radiofreqency thermal balloon angioplasty after abrupt or threatened vessel closure complicating elective conventional balloon coronary angioplasty. J Am Coll Cardiol 1994;24:1220-8.

69. Becker GJ, Lee BI, Waller BF, Barry KJ. Radiofrequency balloon angioplasty-rationale and proof of principle. Invest. Radiology 1988;23:810-17.

70. Lee BI, Becker GJ, Waller BF, Barry KJ. Thermal compression and molding of atherosclerotic vascular tissue with use of radiofrequency energy: Implications for radiofrequency balloon angioplasty. J Am Coll Cardiol 1989;13:1167-75.

71. Walinsky P, Rose A, Martinez-Hernandez A, Smith DL. Microwave balloon angioplasty. J Inv Cardiol 1991;3:152-156.

72. Resar JR, Wolff ME, Hruban R, Brinker JA. Endoluminal sealing of vascular wall disruptions with radiofrequency-heated balloon angioplasty. Cath Cardiovasc Diagn. 1993;29:161-167.

73. Fram DB, McKay RG. "Hot" balloon angioplasty: Radiofrequency, neodymium: YAG, and microwave. In Topol EJ (ed): Textbook of Interventional Cardiology, 2nd Edition. Philadelphia, WB Sauders Company, 1994, pp 819-839.

74. Makowski S, O'Neill B, Sarkis A, et al. Physiological low stress angioplasty at 60°C. Initial results and 6 month follow-up. J Am Coll Cardiol 1993;21:440A.

75. McMath LP, Kundu SK, Spears JR: Experimental application of bioprotective materials to injured arterial surfaces with laser balloon angioplasty, abstracted. Circulation 1990;82:III-72.

76. Rees ME, Michalis LK. Vibrational coronary angioplasty for chronic total occlusions. A novel approach. J Am Coll Cardiol 1994;23:58A.

77. Rees ME, Michalis LK. Vibrational coronary angioplasty; Challenging chronic total occlusions. Preliminary clinical data. J Am Coll Cardiol 1995;25:268A.

78. Rees ME, Michalis LK. Activated-guidewire technique for treating chronic coronary artery occlusion. Lancet 1995;346:943-944.

79. Barath P, Fishbein MC, Vari S, Forrester JS. Cutting balloon: A novel approach to percutaneous angioplasty. Am J Cardiol 1991;68:1249-1252.

80. Unterberg C, Buchwald AB, Barath P, Schmidt T, et al. Cutting balloon coronary angioplasty--initial clinical experience. Clin Cardiol 1993;16:660-664.

81. Popma JJ, Knopf WD, Davidson C, Feldman RC, Eisenhauer AC, et al. Angiographic outcome after "cutting" balloon angioplasty. J Am Coll Cardiol 1995;25:268A.

82. Solar RJ, Meaney DF, Miller RT, Rahdert DA, et al. Enhanced lumen enlargement with new focused force angioplasty device. Circulation 1995;92:I-147.

83. Drexler H, Fischell TA. Initial clinical experience using a novel pullback atherectomy catheter (PAC) in the treatment of obstructive coronary artery disease. Circulation 1995;92:I-147.

84. Agmon M, Scheinowitz M, Beitner S, et al. The Bard Rotary Atherectomy System (BRAS): Initial experience in patients with peripheral vascular disease. J Interven Cardiol 1993;6:51-59.

85. Wilson BH, Tuntelder J, Thompson M, Dezern K, et al. A coring device: Intracoronary rotational excision. J Am Coll Cardiol 1994;23:406A.

86. Kaltenbach M, Vallbracht C. Reopening of chronic coronary artery occlusions by low speed rotational atherectomy. J Interven Cardiol 1989;2:137-145.

87. Kaltenbach M, Vallbracht C, Hartmann A. Recanalization of chronic coronary occlusions by low speed rotational angioplasty (ROTACS). J Interven Cardiol 1991;4:155-165.

88. Vallbracht C, Liermann D, Prignitz I, et al. Results of low speed rotational angioplasty for chronic peripheral occlusions. Am J Cardiol 1988;62:935-940.

89. Serruys PW, Hamburger J, Fleck E, Koolen JJ, Teunissen Y. Laser guidewire: A powerful tool in recanalization of chronic total coronary occlusion. Circulation 1995;92:I-76.

90. Ramee SR, Kuntz RE, Schatz RA, et al. Preliminary experience with the POSSIS coronary AngioJet rheolytic thrombectomy catheter in the VEGAS-I Pilot study. J Am Coll Cardiol;March Special Issue.

9 INTRACORONARY THROMBUS

Mark Dooris, M.B.B.S.
Cindy Grines, M.D.

Among those undergoing PTCA for medically-refractory unstable ischemic syndromes, angiographic thrombus has been observed in up to 40% of cases and in up to 90% by angioscopy.[1-4] Unfortunately, balloon dilation of thrombus-containing lesions is associated with an increased risk of acute thrombotic occlusion, emergency bypass surgery, myocardial infarction and death when compared to PTCA of non-thrombotic lesions.[5-19,123-128] Various pharmacologic and mechanical approaches have been employed, with the hope of providing safe revascularization for these patients. To date, the optimal therapy for patients with intracoronary thrombus awaits definition. Unsettled management issues include the timing of coronary intervention; the dose, route and optimal combination of antiplatelet, antithrombin and thrombolytic therapies; and the most effective mechanical revascularization strategy.

A. **DEFINITION AND DETECTION.** Since there is no uniform angiographic definition of intracoronary thrombus, the rates of intracoronary thrombus vary widely between studies. The strictest angiographic criteria require definite intraluminal globular filling defects seen in multiple angiographic views, or if the vessel is totally occluded, a convex margin that stains with contrast and persists for several cardiac cycles.[1-3] Numerous studies have demonstrated the poor sensitivity of angiography for detecting intracoronary thrombus (as low as 19%), although specificity approaches 100% when the strictest definitions are used.[12-24,123] In our experience, there is marked interobserver variability in the diagnosis of thrombus. The use of coronary angioscopy (Chapter 32) and intravascular ultrasound (Chapter 31) have extended our ability to assess normal and pathological coronary arterial segments.[10-21] Intravascular ultrasound is less useful since thrombus and "soft" plaque have similar echogenicity.[22]

Direct visualization by angioscopy provides the best method for detecting intraluminal thrombus. Red, globular, mobile thrombus was commonly found in acute MI, whereas non-occlusive, mural, irregular, white thrombus was more common in unstable angina.[13] Another study suggested that angiographic filling defects corresponded to red thrombus, whereas hazy lesions could be white thrombus, intimal disruptions or smooth plaque.[17] Preliminary studies in patients with unstable angina have confirmed that angioscopic evidence of thrombus is associated with increased risk of adverse outcome following PTCA.[16,123] However, prospective data suggest that the vast majority of patients with unstable angina and acute MI are safely treated with PTCA (Chapter 5). Furthermore, angiography remains the most widely used method for detecting thrombus.

B. **PATHOPHYSIOLOGY.** Rupture of lipid rich atheromatous plaque is the initiating event for intracoronary thrombus formation,[23-31] usually at the junction between the fibrous cap and adjacent normal vessel. Plaque rupture exposes the lipid core which appears to be most thrombogenic.[32] A complex series of events involving the vessel wall, platelets, coagulation cascade and fibrinolytic systems result in variable amounts of thrombus formation. This is particularly active in patients with unstable angina and acute myocardial infarction.[33-35] PTCA, by causing intimal and medial dissection, is itself a powerful thrombogenic stimulus and resembles the deep vascular injury of spontaneous plaque rupture.

C. **PTCA AND THROMBOTIC LESIONS (Table 9.1).** PTCA of thrombotic lesions is associated with an increased incidence acute occlusion, distal embolization and no-reflow. In one report, no-reflow occurred in 7% of patients with unstable angina and thrombus-containing lesions.[39] To date, no randomized data demonstrate benefit of any adjunctive medical therapy before, during, or after PTCA of a thrombotic lesion. Although thrombolytics were widely advocated in the past, randomized data from several trials now confirm a higher incidence of cardiac events with thrombolytics (Chapter 5).[119] 7E3 (ReoPro) has not been tested in patients with thrombotic lesions.

D. **NEW DEVICES AND THROMBOTIC LESIONS (Table 9.2).** Data from the NACI Registry demonstrated that patients with intracoronary thrombus had lower EF, more left main and 3 vessel disease, prior CABG, prior MI and unstable angina than patients without thrombus.[43] Furthermore, intracoronary thrombus was associated with a 2.8-fold higher risk of major complications. These high risk lesions dramatically influenced device selection: Thrombus was present in 2% of Rotablator, 5-11% of ELCA, 10% of DCA, and 41% of TEC cases. Outcome after new device interventions in vein grafts was related to thrombus and lesion length rather than device selection per se.[44]

1. **Directional Atherectomy (DCA).** Early studies reported greater procedural success and fewer major complications 30 patients with thrombus compared to 348 patients without thrombus.[129] Other studies have not confirmed these results: In another report, procedural success was similar in patients with and without thrombus (75% vs. 80%). but thrombus was associated with more major complications (16% vs. 8%, p=.06) and emergency CABG (10% vs. 4%, p=.03.[93] Likewise, when DCA was applied to patients with unstable angina or recent MI, an increased complication rate was observed (Chapter 5). We generally avoid DCA in lesions with significant thrombus.

2. **Rotablator.** Intracoronary thrombus is considered a contraindication to Rotablator atherectomy.

3. **Extraction Atherectomy (TEC).** TEC atherectomy is commonly used for thrombus extraction. Angioscopic studies confirm its ability to extract thrombus.[130,131] However, dissections are common, and no reflow or distal embolization occurs in 8-12% of vein grafts.[122] TEC has no beneficial impact on restenosis, but may be a useful adjunct to stenting in thrombotic vein graft lesions.[145] Al-Shaibi[132] demonstrated that in degenerated vein grafts, TEC was associated with less CK elevation compared to PTCA.

4. **Excimer Laser Angioplasty (ELCA) (Chapter 30).** Although lasers have not been shown to be thrombogenic[133] in animal models,[134] relatively few patients with angiographic thrombus have been treated.[113,114,135,136,137] In a report from the Excimer Laser Coronary Angioplasty Registry,[36] the procedural success rate was 81% in thrombotic lesions and 90% in simple lesions; ECLA resulted in distal embolization in 5.7%. Others also reported lower clinical success in thrombotic lesions

Table 9.1. Impact of Pre-Procedural Thrombus On PTCA Outcome

Series	N (Patients)	Description	Results
White[123] (1996)	74	Angioscopic thrombus: 61%. No lytics given.	Thrombus ↑ risk of in-hospital ischemia (16 vs 10%; p=.03) and major cardiac events (14 vs 2%, p=.03)
Tausa[119] (1995)	245	Randomized trial of IC UK vs. No UK	UK ↑ rate of abrupt closure (15% vs. 5.9%; p=.03) and major cardiac events (17.3% vs. 6.8%; p=.02)
Hillegass[124] (1995)	238	Unstable angina with thrombus	Unstable angina and thrombus associated with ↓ success (80%); ↑ abrupt closure (11%); ↑ CABG (9%).
	1476	Unstable angina without thrombus	PTCA outcome in unstable angina patients without thrombus similar to stable angina
	450	Stable angina	
Tan[125] (1995)	46	Thrombus: 3.6% of 1248 lesions	Thrombus ↑ risk of abrupt closure (8.7% vs 3.1%; p=.04)
Violaris[126] (1994)	159	Thrombus: 4.5% of 3529 lesions dilated.	Thrombus ↑ risk of late reocclusion (13.8 vs 5.3%, p<.001).
Tenaglia[127]	93	Thrombus: 12% of 779 lesions.	Thrombus ↑ risk of abrupt closure (6.1 fold.)
Myler[128] (1992)	82	Thrombus: 10.5% of 779 lesions.	Thrombus ↑ risk of major cardiac event (7.3% vs 1%, p>.003). All events occurred in patients utilizing urokinase.
Pavlides[56] (1991)	30	I.C. urokinase: 250,000-500,000 over 20 min. I.V. urokinase: 250,000-3MU (mean 1.4 MU) over 30-60 min in > 50% of patients.	Urokinase did not improve PTCA success, but improved cardiac event rate (19% vs 3%) with thrombus.
	27	No urokinase	
Chapekis[55] (1991)	21	Continuous urokinase via intracoronary infusion wire (120,000 U bolus, 120,000 U/hr Infusion x 24 hrs). Heparin IV: 1000 U/hr.	Distal embolization (5%). No acute closures.
Kiesz[118] (1991)	29	I.C. urokinase (250,000 U boluses over 5 min up to 1.5 M units or until thrombi resolves)	Complete resolutions of I.C. thrombus in 83%; overall PTCA success in 93%.

Table 9.1. Impact of Pre-Procedural Thrombus On PTCA Outcome

Series	N (Patients)	Description	Results
Mooney[8] (1990)	112	Aspirin, dipyridamole, nifedipine, pretreatment. Intraprocedural heparin (IV: 10,000 and IC: 3000U). Balloon: artery ration 1.2 to 1.	Acute in-lab closure in 7%. Nonobstructive residual thrombus in 24%. Emergency or elective CABG in 7%.
Lasky[45] (1990)	35	Aspirin, pre-PTCA heparin	PTCA success 94%, Acute occlusion 6%.
	18	Aspirin, No pre-PTCA heparin	PTCA success 61%, Acute occlusion 33%.
Deligonul[7] (1988)	45	Aspirin pre-procedure in 84%, heparin in 65%. IV heparin: 5-10,000 U bolus.	Distal embolization and/or thrombotic occlusion in 31%.
Segrue[6] (1986)	34	Aspirin, dipyridamole, IV heparin: 5-10,000 U bolusl, infusion x 24 hrs.	Acute occlusion in 24%.
Mabin[5] (1985)	15	Aspirin, variable IV heparin: 5200-10,000 U bolus, protamine after PTCA.	Acute occlusion in 73%.

(58% vs. 95%, p=.0001).[113] By multivariate analysis, the presence of thrombus was identified as the most important determinant of procedural failure.

5. **Stents (Chapter 26).** The presence of intraluminal thrombus has been considered a contraindication to stent insertion. However, in the Cook registry of stenting for abrupt or threatened closure, thrombus was present prior to stent deployment in 14% of patients.[76] Despite thrombus, angiographic success was achieved in 84%, and only 27% of patients had significant residual thrombus following stent placement. However, insertion of stents in small vessel (< 2.5mm) with acute closure and thrombus was associated with a mortality rate of 16% compared to 4% in patients with larger vessels. The Palmaz-Schatz and Gianturco-Roubin stents have been used in the acute MI setting with favorable angiographic and clinical results (Chapter 5).

E. INVESTIGATIONAL TECHNIQUES

1. **Catheter Aspiration** of thrombus has been described.[96]

2. **Hydrolyser Catheter.** Fajadet described vein graft thrombectomy in 7 patients utilizing the Hydrolyser catheter,[97] which is a 7F double lumen catheter which aspirates thrombus via the Venturi effect. Further investigation is planned in the United States.

Table 9.2. Impact of Thrombus On New Devices

Series	N	Device	Outcome
Grinstead[76] (1996)	109	GRS	84% angiographic success in the setting of pre-stent thrombus. Only 27% had angio evidence of post stent thrombus.
Meany[121] (1995)	183	TEC (SVG)	Angiographic success not affected by thrombus.
Dooris[96] (1995)	59	TEC (SVG)	Thrombus lowered rate of clinical success (69% vs. 88%) and ↑ angiographic and clinical complications including no reflow and Q-wave MI.
Al-Shaibi[132] (1995)	124	TEC (SVG)	TEC associated with ↓ rate of embolization and CK leak compared to PTCA.
Moses[122] (1995)	59	TEC	Thrombus was a predictor of distal embolization after TEC.
Baumbach[114] (1994)		ELCA	Thrombus associated with 6.4-fold ↓ in procedural success, (p = .007).
Estella[113] (1993)	12	ELCA	Thrombus associated with ↓ clinical success (58% vs. 95%, p < .0001).
Agrawal[138] (1994)	77	GRS	Pre-stent filling defect not predictive of stent thrombosis.
O'Neill[43] (1993)	345	All devices	Thrombus ↓ angiographic success (85% vs. 93%, p < .001), ↑ embolization (6% vs. 0.6%, p < .001) and ↑ cardiac events (9% vs. 3%, p < .001).
Emmi[93] (1993)	58	DCA	Thrombus ↑ ischemic complications (15.5% vs. 7.9%, p = .06) and emergency CABG (10.3% vs. 3.9%, p = .03)

3. **POSSIS AngioJet (Figure 8.2).** The AngioJet is a percutaneous rheolytic thrombectomy catheter that removes thrombus via the Venturi effect. The 5F double-lumen catheter is highly flexible, utilizes a 0.014 - or 0.018 inch guidewire, and requires an 8F guiding catheter (internal diameter ≥ 0.080 inches). The Angiojet has been successfully applied to thrombotic vein grafts; clinical trials are now in progress in Europe and the United States (see Chapter 8).[146]

4. **Ultrasound (Figure 8.3).** Therapeutic ultrasound energy may ablate fresh thrombus and produce coronary vasodilation.[99-101]

5. **Radiofrequency-Balloon Angioplasty (Figure 8.4).** Infrared laser or radiofrequency energy can

modify thrombus-containing lesions.[104,105] Further clinical investigations are pending.

F. PHARMACOLOGIC THERAPY OF PRE-EXISTING THROMBUS

1. **Heparin and Aspirin.** PTCA of thrombus containing lesions has been associated with acute coronary closure in up to 20% of patients.[5-7] The risk can be reduced by a 2-14 day treatment with heparin and aspirin prior to PTCA.[26,45-59] Recent data suggest that high dose intravenous heparin (ACT > 350-400 seconds) is associated with lower rates of abrupt closure. In a single report of 112 patients undergoing PTCA of thrombotic lesions, the combination of intracoronary/intravenous heparin and frequent dilatations using a slightly oversized balloon (balloon: artery ratio = 1.2:1) was associated with a low incidence of acute closure.[8] High-dose intracoronary heparin, because of its polyvalent anionic nature, may be associated with arrhythmic complications and should be diluted and infused slowly. Local delivery of 4,000 units of heparin into the vessel wall has been shown to achieve high heparin levels that persist for several days, achieving a 60% reduction in platelet deposition. The duration of heparin post procedure is unknown, but 24 to 48 hours of post procedure heparin has been used; tapering to half dose heparin for the last several hours may avoid rebound acute thrombosis.

2. **Thrombolytic Therapy.** The efficacy of thrombolysis as adjunctive therapy for thrombotic lesions is controversial. Non-randomized data suggest a role for intracoronary thrombolytic therapy when thrombus is present prior to (Table 9.1) or after PTCA (Table 9.2).[9,55-59,118] However, systemic thrombolytic therapy has consistently failed to confer a clinical benefit for unstable angina[52] and non-Q-wave myocardial infarction, despite modest angiographic improvement.[53] Thrombolytic therapy in unstable angina has produced a similar degree of angiographic resolution of thrombus as aspirin and heparin therapy.[51] The TAUSA study showed that patients with ischemic rest pain syndromes had similar outcomes with or without intracoronary urokinase.[53] In fact, the urokinase treatment group had a higher incidence of acute vessel occlusion, even in lesions that were complex or contained filling defects suggestive of thrombus.[119] Similar findings were observed in the PAMI-2 study and other clinical trials of acute MI and unstable angina (Chapter 5). Possible explanations for the disappointing results of thrombolysis include thrombolytic-induced platelet aggregation, and medial hemorrhage resulting in a more severe stenosis or bleeding complications. Based on the available data we generally avoid the use of thrombolytics before, during, and after interventional procedures unless angiographic thrombus is confirmed by angioscopy.

For chronic total occlusions, we occasionally administer prolonged (8-24 hrs), low-dose, continuous intracoronary thrombolysis (Chapter 16). This technique requires placement of a specialized infusion wire (Chapter 1) just proximal to the thrombus. Non-randomized studies suggest significant angiographic improvement and a low incidence of adverse clinical events.[9,55-61] Vein graft occlusions are often targeted for local thrombolytic infusions, but myocardial infarction (17%), reocclusion (35%), and late reocclusion (52%).[61] Bleeding complications may occur.[62,63]

The specific protocol used as our institution for prolonged selective intracoronary thrombolytic infusion is as follows (Figure 9.1):[60]

1. Aspirin 325mg po qd, started at least 2 days pre-procedure.
2. Heparin is administered (10,000 U I.V. bolus just prior to the procedure; additional heparin as necessary to achieve ACT > 300).
3. A 7F guide is advanced into the aortic root.
4. A Tuohy-Borst adapter is connected to the guide catheter and manifold.
5. The guide is securely positioned into the orifice of the occluded vessel and angiography is performed in at least two projections.
6. A .018" angioplasty guidewire is placed into an end-hole infusion wire (SOS or Cragg wire) (see Chapter 1).
7. The infusion wire is advanced into the occluded vessel.
8. The guidewire is positioned as far as possible into the occluded vessel; the infusion catheter is then advanced over the wire until it reaches the occlusion.
9. The guidewire is then removed and a stopcock is attached to the end of the infusion catheter to permit urokinase infusion.
10. Bubbles are slowly aspirated and contrast is injected to assure intraluminal position. Heparin is then flushed through the infusion wire and guide.
11. Depending on the dose and duration of infusion, 0.5-2 million units of urokinase are reconstituted in 100-200cc of saline. We infuse urokinase (50,000-100,000 u/hr) through the guide and infusion wire for 8 hrs.
12. IV heparin (bolus and continuous infusion) is administered to achieve (ACT 200-300) throughout the period of intracoronary thrombolysis.
13. An intravenous broad spectrum antibiotic is continued while catheters are in place.
14. The patient is monitored in a coronary care unit during infusion.
15. The patient is returned to the lab after the infusion is complete. Repeat angiograms are obtained, and PTCA is then performed using standard techniques. Re-bolus with heparin to achieve ACT > 350 sec.
16. If PTCA is successful, heparin is continued for 6-24 hrs prior to removing sheaths. Coumadin is initiated and IV or subcutaneous heparin is continued until PT is 18-20 sec.

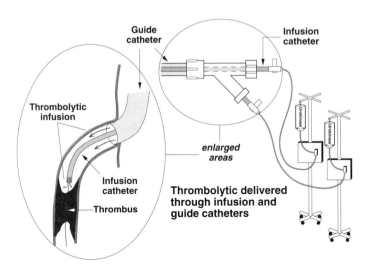

Figure 9.1 Setup for Intracoronary Thrombolytic Infusion

3. **Novel Antiplatelet and Antithrombotic Drugs.** Several highly potent antiplatelet and antithrombin agents are currently under (Chapters 5 and 34). No data are yet available with regard to their efficacy in thrombotic lesions. However, "off-label" use of intravenous or intracoronary ReoPro (7E3) has been described for PTCA complicated by thrombosis, with successful resolution of thrombus.[139]

4. **Local Drug Delivery.** To avoid cost and side effects of systemic therapy, local delivery of heparin or thrombolytics is under investigation (Chapters 5 and 35).

G. **POST-PTCA THROMBUS.** The detection of post-procedural thrombus is difficult; most often "haziness" is due to intimal dissection. Thrombolytic therapy has been used in several small series with equivocal results (Table 9.3). Utilization of stents for suboptimal results, intracoronary or local infusions of heparin, and "rescue" ReoPro[139] should be considered (Chapter 20).

H. **STENT THROMBOSIS (Chapter 26).** Stent thrombosis is usually a manifestation of suboptimal stent deployment, due to incomplete expansion, inadequate apposition, or unstented residual disease or dissection. If stent thrombosis occurs, remedial causes should be sought and corrected. Potential treatment approaches are discussed in Chapter 26.

Table 9.3   PTCA Outcome: Impact of Post-Procedural Thrombus

Series	N (Pts.)	Adjunctive Therapy	Results
Muhlestein[135] (1995)	16	Post PTCA IV ReoPro	Decrease in thrombus score and increase in TIMI flow; procedural success in 100%.
Grines[120] (1995)	172	IC lytics in 34 (20%)	Primary PTCA for AMI:, post-PTCA thrombus not predictive of ischemic events; trend for ↑ ischemia if lytics given (18.4 vs 10.6%; p = .10).
Chapekis[55] (1991)	12	Continuous urokinase via intracoronary infusion wire (120,000 U bolus, 120,000 U/hr Infusion x 24 hrs). Heparin IV: 1000 U/hr.	Acute closure in 8%.
Herrmann[56] (1990)	55	rt-PA (I.C. 20 mg bolus followed by 50 mg/60-120 min IV)	Emergency CABG lower in rt-PA group (1.8%) compared to PTCA group (6.8%, n=59)
Schieman[9] (1990)	48	I.C. urokinase 100,000-250,000 units (mean 141,000) over 20-65 minutes (mean 34 min.). Continuous post-procedural heparin infusion and aspirin x 5 days.	No recurrent ischemic events requiring PTCA. No procedure-related MI or deaths prior to discharge.
Pavlides[141] (1991)	256	Urokinase	Trend for ↑ major cardiac event rate (21% vs 9%, p=.1) when used for post-PTCA abrupt closure.
Lincoff[140] (1992)	43	I.C. urokinase. tPA used in 43 of 109 cases of abrupt closure.	PTCA success in 44%, not related to use of lytics. Predictors of success were prolonged inflations and stents.
deFeyter[142] (1991)	34	I.C. urokinase	Success in 65%
Haft[143] (1990)	36	I.C. urokinase or tPA	Success in 72%
Gulba[144] (1990)	27	I.C. and IV tPA	Initial success in 82% but 55%; reoccluded within 36 hrs.

* * * * *

REFERENCES

1. Ambrose JA, Winters SL, Stern A, et al. Angiographic Morphology and the Pathogenesis of Unstable Angina Pectoris. J Am Coll Cardiol 1985;5:609-616.
2. Fuster V, Badimon L, Badimon J, et al. The Pathogenesis of Coronary Artery Disease and the Acute Coronary Syndromes. N Eng J Med 1992;326:242-250.
3. Cowley MJ, DiSciascio G, Vetrovec GW. Coronary Thrombus in Unstable Angina: Angiographic Observations and Clinical Relevance. In Hugenholtz PG and Goldman BG (eds): Unstable Angina: Current Concepatients and Management. Schattauer Press, Stuttgart, 1985;95-102.
4. Gotoh K, Minamino T, Katoh O, et al. The Role of Intracoronary Thrombus in Unstable Angina: Angiographic Assessment and Thrombolytic Therapy During Ongoing Anginal Attacks. Circulation 1988;77:526-534.
5. Mabin TA, Holmes DR, Smith HC. Intracoronary Thrombus Role in Coronary Occlusion Complicating PTCA. J Am Coll Cardiol 1985;5:198-202.
6. Sugrue DR, Holmes DR, Smith HC. Coronary Artery Thrombus as a Risk Factor for Acute Vessel Occlusion During PTCA: Improved Results. Br Heart J 1986;53:62-66.
7. Deligonul V, Gabliani GI, Caroles DG, et al. PTCA in Patients with Intracoronary Thrombus. Am J Cardiol 1988;62:474-476.
8. Mooney MR, Fishman-Mooney J, Goldenberg I, et al. Percutaneous Transluminal Coronary Angioplasty in the Setting of Large Intracoronary Thrombus. Am J Cardiol 1990;65:427-431.
9. Schieman G, Cohen BM, Kozina J, et al. Intracoronary Urokinase for Intracoronary Thrombus Accumulation Complicating Percutaneous Transluminal Coronary Angioplasty in Acute Ischemic Syndromes. Circulation 1990;82:2052-2060.
10. Yanagida S, Mizuno K, Miyamolo A: Comparison of Findings Between Coronary Angiography and Angioscopy. Circulation 1989;80 (Supp II):376.
11. Ramee SR, White CJ, Collins TJ, et al. Percutaneous Angioscopy During Coronary Angioplasty Using a Steerable Microangioscope. J Am Coll Cardiol 1991;17:100-105.
12. Mizuno K, Satumora K, Miyamoto A, et al. Angioscopic Evaluation of Coronary-Artery Thrombi in Acute Coronary Syndromes. New Engl J Med 1992;326:287-291.
13. Mizuno K, Miyamoto A, Satomura K, et al. Angioscopic coronary macromorphology in patients with acute coronary disorders. Lancet 1991,337:809-812.
14. Mizuno K, Hikita H, Miyamoto A, Satomura K, et al. The pathogenesis of an impending infarction and its treatment - an angioscopic analysis. Jpn Circ J 1992, 56:1160-5.
15. Hombach V, Hoher M, Kochs M, Eggeling T, et al. Pathophysiology of unstable angina pectoris-correlations with coronary angioscopic imaging. Eur Heart J 1988,;9:40-5.
16. Waxsman S, Sassower M, Zarich S, et al. Angioscopy can Identify lesion specific predictors of early adverse outcome following PTCA in patients with unstable angina. Circulation 1994;90:I-490.
17. Manzo K, Netso R, Sassower M, Leeman D, et al. Coronary lesion morphology by angioscopy vs angiography: the ability to detect thrombi. J Am Coll Cardiol 1994: 955-4023.
18. Annex BH, Ajluni SC, Larkin TJ, O'Neill WW, Safian RD. Angioscopic guided interventions in a saphenous vein bypass graft. Cathet Cardiovasc Diagn 1994;31:330-3.
19. den Heijer P, Foley D, Escaned J, Hillege HL, Serruys PW, Lie KI. Angioscopic versus angiographic detection of intimal dissection and intracoronary thrombus. J Am Coll Cardiol 1994;955-100.
20. Sherman CT, Litvack F, Grundfest W, Lee M, et al. Coronary angioscopy in patients with unstable angina pectoris. N Engl J Med 1986, 315:913-9.
21. den Heijer P, van Dijk RB, Hillege HL, et al. Serial angioscopic and angiographic observations during the first hour after successful coronary angioplasty: A preamble to a multicenter trial addressing angioscopic markers for restenosis. Am Heart J 1994;128:656-63.
22. Siegel RJ, Fischbein MC, Chae JS, Helfant RH, Hickey A, Forrester JS. Comparative studies of angioscopy and ultrasound for the evaluation of arterial disease. Echocardiography 1990;7:495-502.
23. Chesebro J, Zoldhelyi P, Fuster V: Pathogenesis of Thrombosis in Unstable Angina. Am J Cardiol 1991;68:2B-10B.
24. Fuster V, Lewis A. Conner Memorial Lecture. Mechanisms leading to myocardial infarction: insights from studies of vascular biology. Circulation 1994;90:2126-2146.

25. Kawai C. Pathogenesis of acute myocardial infarction: novel regulatory system of bioactive substances in the vessel wall. Circulation 1994; 90:1033-1043.

26. Jang Y, Lincoff AM, Plow EF, Topol EJ. Cellular adhesion molecules in coronary artery disease. J Am Coll Cardiol 1994;24:1591-601.

27. Lefkovits J, Topol EJ. Direct thrombin inhibitors in cardiovascular medicine. Circulation 1994; 90:1522-1536.

28. Davies MJ, Thomas, AC. Plaque Fissuring--The Cause of Acute Myocardial Infarction, Sudden Ischemic Death, and Crescendo Angina. Br Heart J 1985;53:363-373.

29. Falk E. Plaque Rupture with Severe Pre-Existing Stenosis Precipitating Coronary Thrombosis. Characteristics of Coronary Atherosclerotic Plaques Underlying Fatal Occlusive Thrombi. Br Heart 1983;50:127-134.

30. Davies MJ, Bland JM, Hangartner JRW, et al. Factors influencing the Presence of Absence of Acute Coronary Artery Thrombi in Sudden Ischemic Death. Eur Heart J 1989;10:203-208.

31. Badimon L, Badimon JJ, Gahez A, et al. Influence of Arterial Damage and Wall Shear Forces on Platelet Deposition. Ex Vivo Study U.A. Swine Model. Arteriosclerosis 1986;6:312-330.

32. Fernandez-Ortiz A, Badimon JJ, Falk E, et al. Characterization of the relative thrombogenicity of atherosclerotic plaque components: implications for consequences of plaque rupture. J Am Coll Cardiol 1994;23:1562-9.

33. Merlini PA, Bauer KA, Oltrona L, Ardissino D, Cattaneo M, Belli C, Manucci PM, Resenberg RD. Persistent activation of coagulation mechanisms in unstable angina and myocardial infarction. Circulation 1994;90:61-68.

34. Theroux PR, Latour JG, Leger-Gautier C, De Lara J. Fibrinopeptide A plasma levels and platelet factor 4 in unstable angina pectoris. Circulation 1987;75:156-162.

35. Kruskal JB, Commerford PJ, Franks JJ, Kirsch RE. Fibrin and fibrin-related antigens in patients with stable and unstable angina. N Engl J Med 1987;317:1361-1365.

36. Gold GH, Gimple LW, Yasuda T, et al. Pharmacodynamic study of F (ab')2 fragments of murine monoclonal antibody 7E3 directed against human platelet glycoprotein IIb/IIIa in patients with unstable angina pectoris. J Clin Invest 1990;86:651-9.

37. Kleiman NS, Ohman EM, Ellis SG, et al. Profound inhibition of platelet aggregation with monoclonal antibody 7E3 Fab following thrombolytic therapy: results of the TAMI 8 Pilot study. Circulation 1993;86:I-260.

38. The EPIC Investigators. Use of a monoclonal antibody directed against the platelet glycoprotein IIb/IIIa receptor in high-risk coronary angioplasty. N Engl J Med 1994;330:956-61.

39. Wilson RF, Lesser JR, Laxson DD, et al. Intense Microvascular Constriction After Angioplasty of Acute Thrombotic Coronary Arterial Lesions. Lancet 1989:801-811.

40. Abbo KM, Kazziha S, Byrd D, Dooris M, et al. Clinical and Angiographic Features of the No-reflow Phenomenon. J Am Coll Cardiol 1994:296A.

41. Piana RN, Palk GY, Mosucci M, Cohen DJ, et al. Incidence and treatment of "no-reflow" after percutaneous coronary intervention. Circulation 1994;89:2514-2518.

42. Weyrens FJ, Mooney J, Mooney MR. Intracoronary diltiazem improves distal microvascular spasm following coronary interventions. Cathet Cardiovasc 1994,32:84.

43. O'Neill WW, Sketch MH Jr, Steenkiste A, Detre K. New Device Intervention in the treatment of intracoronary thrombus: report of the NACI registry. Circulation 1993;88: I-595.

44. Sketch MH Jr, Davidson CJ, Popma J, et al. Morphologic and quantitative predictors of acute outcome with new devices in saphenous vein grafts. J Am Coll Cardiol 1994; 90:219A.

45. Laskey MAL, Deutsch E, Barnathan E, et al. Influence of Heparin Therapy on Percutaneous Transluminal Coronary Angioplasty Outcome in Unstable Angina Pectoris. Am J Cardiol 1990;65:1425-1429.

46. Myler RK, Shaw NE, Stertzer SH, et al. Unstable Angina and Coronary Angioplasty. Circulation 1990;82:88-95.

47. Hettleman BD, Aplin RA, Sullivan PR, et al. Three Days of Heparin Pretreatment Reduces Major Complications of Coronary Angioplasty in Patients with Unstable Angina. J Am Coll Cardiol 1990;15:154A.

48. Pow TK, Varricchione TR, Jacobs AK, et al. Does Pretreatment with Heparin Prevent Abrupt Closure Following PTCA? J Am Coll Cardiol 1988;11:238A.

49. Lukas MA, Deutsch E, Hirshfeld JW Jr, et al. Influence of Heparin Therapy on Percutaneous Transluminal Coronary Angioplasty Outcome in Patients with Coronary Arterial Thrombus. Am J Cardiol 1990;65:179-182.

50. Friedman HZ, Cragg DR, Glazier SM, Gangadharan V, et al. Randomized prospective evaluation of prolonged versus abbreviated intravenous heparin therapy after coronary angioplasty. J Am Coll Cardiol 1994;24:1214-1219.

51. The TIMI IIIA Investigators. Early effects of tissue-type plasminogen activator added to conventional therapy on the culprit coronary lesion in patients presenting with ischemic cardiac pain at rest. Results of the Thrombolysis in

Myocardial Ischemia (TIMI IIIA) Trial. Circulation 1993;87:38-52.

52.   The TIMI IIIB Investigators. Effects of tissue plasminogen activator and a comparison of early invasive and conservative strategies in unstable angina and non Q wave myocardial infarction: results of the TIMI IIIB trial. Circulation 1994;89:1545-1556.

53.   Ambrose JA, Almeida OD, Sharma SK, et al. Adjunctive thrombolytic therapy during angioplasty for ischemic rest angina. Results of the TAUSA trial. Circulation 1994;90:69-77.

54.   Vaitkus PT, Laskey WK. Efficacy of adjunctive thrombolytic therapy in percutaneous transluminal coronary angioplasty. J Am Coll Cardiol 1994;24:1415-23.

55.   Chapekis AT, George BS, Candela RJ. Rapid thrombus dissolution by continuous infusion of urokinase through an intracoronary perfusion wire prior to and following PTCA: results in native coronaries and patent saphenous vein grafts. Cathet Cardiovasc Diagn 1991;23:89-92.

56.   Pavlides GS, Schreiber TL, Gangadharan V, et al. Safety and Efficacy of Urokinase During Elective Coronary Angioplasty. Am Heart J 1991;121:731-736.

57.   Suryapranata H, DeFeyter PJ, Serruys PW. Coronary Angioplasty in Patients with Unstable Angina Pectoris: Is There a Role for Thrombolysis? J Am Coll Cardiol 1988;12:69A-77A.

58.   Goudreau E, DiSciascio G, Vetrovec GW, et al. Intracoronary Urokinase as an Adjunct to Percutaneous Transluminal Coronary Angioplasty in Patients with Complex Coronary Narrowings or Angioplasty - Induced Complications. Am J Cardiol 1992;69:57-62.

59.   Ambrose J, Torre S, Sharma S, et al. Adjunctive Urokinase for PTCA in Unstable Angina. Circulation 1991;84:590.

60.   Grines, C, Ajluni S, Savas V, Samyn J, Pavlides G, et al. William Beaumont Hospital, Royal Oak, Michigan. Prolonged Urokinase Infusion for Chronic Total Native Coronary Occlusions. J Am Coll Cardiol 1996;March Speciall Issue.

61.   Hartmann JR, Mc Keever LS, Stamato NJ, et al. Recanalization of chronically occluded aortocoronary saphenous vein bypass grafts by extended infusion of urokinase: initial results and short term clinical follow-up. J Am Coll Cardiol 1991;18:1517-1523.

62.   Taylor MA, Santoran EC, Aji J, Eldredge WJ, et al. Intracerebral hemorrhage complicating urokinase infusion into an occluded aortocoronary bypass graft. Cathet Cardiovasc Diagn 1994;31:206-210.

63.   Brown DL, Topol EJ. Stroke complicating percutaneous coronary revascularization. Am J Cardiol 1993;72:1207-1209.

64.   Topol EJ, Fuster V, Harrington RA, Califf RM, et al. Recombinant hirudin for unstable angina pectoris: a multicenter randomized trial. Circulation 1994;89:1557-1566.

65.   Topol EJ, Bonan R, Jewitt D, Sigwart U, et al. Use of direct antithrombin, hirulog, in place of heparin during angioplasty. Circulation 1993;87:1622-1629.

66.   van den Bos AA, Deckers JW, Heyndricks GR, et al. Safety and efficacy of recombinant hirudin (CGP 393) versus heparin in patients with stable angina pectoris undergoing coronary angioplasty. Circulation 1993;88:2058-2066.

67.   Antmann EM, for TIMI 9A Investigators. Hirudin in Acute Myocardial Infarction. A safety report from the Thrombolysis in Myocardial Ischemia (TIMI) 9A Trial. Circulation 1994;90:1624-30.

68.   Neuhaus KL, Essen RV, Tebbe U, Jessel A, et al. Safety observations from the pilot phase of the randomized r-hirudin for improvement of thrombolysis (HIT-III) study. A study of the Arbeitsgemeinschaft Leitender Kardiologischer Krankenhausarzte (ALKK). Circulation 1994;90:1638-42.

69.   The Global Use of Strategies to Open Occluded Coronary Arteries (GUSTO) II Investigators. Randomized trial of intravenous heparin versus recombinant hirudin for acute coronary syndromes. Circulation 1994;90:1631-7.

70.   Lincoff AM, Topol EJ, Ellis SG. Local drug delivery systems for the prevention of restenosis. Circulation 1994;90:2070-2084.

71.   Nunes GL, Hanson SR, King SB 3rd, et al. Local delivery of a synthetic antithrombin with a hydrogel-coated angioplasty balloon catheter inhibits platelet-dependent thrombosis. J Am Coll Cardiol 1994;23:1578-83.

72.   McKay R, Fram DB, Hirst JA, Klernan FJ, et al. Treatment of intracoronary thrombus with local urokinase using a new, site-specific drug delivery system: the Dispatch catheter. Cathet Cardiovasc Diagn 1994;33:181-88.

73.   Fram DB, Aretz T, Azrin MA, Mitchel JF,et al. Localized intramural drug delivery during balloon angioplasty using hydrogel-coated balloons and pressure augmented diffusion. J Am Coll Cardiol 1994;23:1570-7.

74.   Plante S, Dupuis G, Mongeau CJ, Durand P. Porous balloon catheters for local delivery: assessment of vascular damage in a rabbit iliac angioplasty model. J Am Coll Cardiol 1994;24:820-4.

75.   Hong MK, Wong SC, Popma JJ, Kent KM, et al. A dual-purpose angioplasty-drug infusion catheter for treatment

of intragraft thrombus. Cathet Cardiovasc Diagn 1994;32:193-5.

76. Grinstead WC, Kleiman NS, Marks GF, et al. Stenting of coronary arteries containing thrombus: Angiographic and clinical outcomes of 109 patients from the Gianturco-Roubin Flex-Stent™ Registry. J Am Coll Cardiol 1996 (in-press).

77. Gershony G, Glass PR. Coronary thrombosis: a novel catheter based approach to treatment. Cathet Cardiovasc Diagn 1994;31:147-149.

78. O'Neill WW, Kramer BL, Sketch MH et al. Mechanical extraction atherectomy. Report of the US Transluminal Extraction Catheter Investigation. Circulation 1992;86:I-79.

79. Annex BH, Larkin TJ, Safian RD. Evaluation of intracoronary thrombus by percutaneous coronary angioscopy before and after transluminal extraction atherectomy. Am J Cardiol 1994;74:606-609.

80. Dooris M, May M, Grines CL, Pavlides GS, et al. Comparative results of transluminal extraction atherectomy in saphenous vein graft lesions with and without thrombus. J Am Coll Cardiol 1995;25:1700-1705.

81. Safian RD, Grines CL, May MA, Lichtenberg A, et al. Clinical and angiographic results of transluminal extraction coronary atherectomy in saphenous vein bypass grafts. Circulation 1994;89:302-312.

82. Popma JJ, Leon MB, Mintz GS, Kent KH, et al. Results of coronary angioplasty using the Transluminal Extraction Catheter. Am J Cardiol 1992;70:1526-32.

83. Hong MK, Popma JJ, Pichard AD, Kent et al. Clinical significance of distal embolization after Transluminal Extraction Atherectomy in diffusely diseased saphenous vein grafts. Am Heart J 1994;127:1496-503.

84. Moses JW, Tierstein PS, Sketch MH, et al. Angiographic determinants of risk and outcome of coronary embolus and myocardial infarction (MI) with the Transluminal Extraction Catheter (TEC): A report from the New Approaches for Coronary Intervention (NACI) Registry. (abstr) J Am Coll Cardiol 1994;March Special Issue:219A.

85. Larkin TJ, O'Neill WW, Safian RD, et al. A prospective study of transluminal extraction atherectomy in high risk patients with acute myocardial infarction. (abstract) J Am Coll Cardiol 1994;March Special Issue:226A.

86. Cowley MJ, Whitlow PL, Baim DS, et al. Directional coronary atherectomy of saphenous vein graft narrowings: multicenter investigational experience. Am J Cardiol 1993;72:30E-34E17.

87. Cowley MJ. DiSciascio G. Experience with directional atherectomy since pre-market approval. Am J Cardiol 1993;72:12E-20E.

88. Sabri MN, Johnson D, Warner M, Cowley MJ. Intracoronary thrombolysis followed by directional atherectomy. A combined approach for thrombotic vein graft lesions considered unsuitable for angioplasty. Cathet Cardiovasc Diagn 1992;26:15-18.

89. Saito S, Arai H, Kim K, Aoki N, et al. Primary directional atherectomy for acute myocardial infarction. Cathet Cardiovasc Diagn 1994;32:44-48.

90. Topol EJ, Leya F, Pinkerton CA, et al. A comparison of directional atherectomy with coronary angioplasty in patients with coronary artery disease. N Engl J Med 1993;329:221-7.

91. Adelman AG, Cohen EA, Kimball BP, et al. A comparison of directional atherectomy with balloon angioplasty for lesions of the left anterior descending coronary artery. N Engl J Med 1993;329:228-33.

92. Abdelmeguid AE, Ellis SG, Sapp SK, et al. Directional coronary atherectomy in unstable angina pectoris. J Am Coll Cardiol 1994;24:46-54.

93. Emmi R, Movsowitz H, Manginas A, Wells E, et al. Directional coronary atherectomy in lesions with co-existing thrombus. Circulation 1993;88:I-596.

94. Serruys PW, de Jaegere P, Kiemeneij F, et al. A comparison of balloon-expandable stent implantation with balloon angioplasty in patients with coronary artery disease. N Engl J Med 1994;331:489-95.

95. Fischman DL, Leon MB, Baim DS et al. A randomized comparison of coronary stent placement and balloon angioplasty in the treatment of coronary artery disease. N Engl J Med 1994;331:496-501.

96. Dooris M, Grines CL. Successful reversal of cardiogenic shock precipitated by saphenous vein graft distal embolization using aspiration thrombectomy. Cathet Cardiovasc Diagns 1994;33:267-71.

97. Fajadet J, Bar O, Jordan C, Robert G, et al. Human percutaneous thrombectomy using the new Hydrolyser catheter: preliminary results in saphenous vein grafts. J Am Coll Cardiol 1994;March Special Issue:220A.

98. Tomaru T, Geschwind HJ, Boussignac G, et al. Comparison of Ablation Efficacy of Excimer, Pulsed Dye and Holmium YAG Laser Relevant to Shock Waves. Circulation 1991;84:423.

99. Hartnell GG, Saxton JM, Friedl SE, Abela GS, Rosenchein U. Ultrasound thrombus ablation: in vitro assessment of a novel device for intracoronary use. J Interven Cardiol 1993;6:69-76.

100. Siegel RJ, Gunn J, Ahsan A, Fiscbein MC, et al. Use of therapeutic ultrasound in percutaneous coronary angioplasty.

Experimental in vitro and initial clinical experience. Circulation 1994;89:1587-92.

101. Gal D, Monteverde C, Hogan J, et al. In Vivo Assessment of Ultrasound Angioplasty of Fibrotic Total Occlusions. Circulation 1991;84:II-422.

102. Spears JR, Safian RD, Douglas, et al. and LBA Study Group. Multicenter Acute and Chronic Results of Laser Balloon Angioplasty for Refractory Abrupt Closure After PTCA. Circulation 1991;84:II-517.

103. Schwartz L, Andrus S, Sinclair IN, et al. Restenosis Following Laser Balloon Coronary Angioplasty: Results of a Randomized Pilot Multicenter Trial. Circulation 1991;84:II-361.

104. Nardone D, Bravette B, Shi Y, et al. Effect of Microwave Thermal Angioplasty on Intracoronary Thrombus. Circualtion 1991;84:II-300.

105. Yamashita K, Satake S, Ohira H, Ohtomo K. Radiofrequency thermal balloon coronary angioplasty: a new device for successful percutaneous transluminal coronary angioplasty. J Am Coll Cardiol 1994;23:336-40.

106. Leon MB, Wong SC, Pichard A. Balloon expandable stent implantation in saphenous vein grafts. In hermann HC, Hirshfeld JW (eds). Clinical use of the Palmaz Schatz Intracoronary Stent. Futura Publishing /Company Inc. 1993;111-121.

107. Hermann HC, Buchbinder M, Cleman MW, et al. Emergent use of balloon expandable coronary artery stenting for failed PTCA. Circulation 1992;86:812-819.

108. Piana RN, Moscucci M, Cohen DJ, Kugelmass AD, et al. Palmas-Schatz stenting for treatment of focal vein graft stenosis: immediate results and long-term outcome. J Am Coll Cardiol 1994;23:1296-304.

109. Ho D, Roubin G. Gianturco Roubin coronary flexible coil stent: present state of the art. J Interven Cardiol 1994;7:303-316.

110. Wong PHC, Wong CM. Intracoronary stenting in acute myocardial infarction. Cathet Cardiovasc Diagn 1994;33:39-45.

111. Cannon AD, Roubin GS, Macander PJ, Agrawal SK. Intracoronary stenting as an adjunct to acute myocardial infarction. J Invas Cardiol 1991;3:255-258.

112. Malosky SA, Hirshfeld JW, Hermann HC. Comparison of results of intracoronary stenting in patients with unstable angina vs stable angina. Cathet Cardiovasc Diagn 1994;31:95-101.

113. Estella P, Ryan TJ Jr, Landzberg JC, Bittl JA. Excimer laser assisted coronary angioplasty for lesions containing thrombus. J Am Coll Cardiol 1993;21:1550-6.

114. Baumbach A, Oswald H, Kvasnika J, Fleck E, et al. Clinical results of coronary excimer laser angioplasty: report from the European Coronary Excimer Laser Angioplasty Registry. Eur Heart J 1994;15:89-95.

115. Fischman DL, Savage MP, Goldberg S. Coronary stent thrombosis. In Hermann HC, Hirschfeld JW (Eds). Clinical use of the Palmaz Schatz Intracoronary Stent. Futura Publishing Company Inc. 1993;125-135.

116. Hall P, Colombo A, Almagor Y, Maiello L, et al. Preliminary experience with intravascular ultrasound guided Palmaz-Schatz coronary stenting. The acute and short-term results in a consecutive series of patients. J Interven Cardiol 1994;7:141-159.

117. Schomig A, Kastrai A, Mudra H, Blasim R, et al. Four-year experience with Palmaz-Schatz stenting in coronary angioplasty complicated by dissection with threatened or persistent vessel closure. Circulation 1994;90:2716-2724.

118. Kiesz R, Hennecken J, Bailey S. Bolus administration of intracoronary urokinase during PTCA in the presence of intracoronary thrombus. Circulation 1991;84:II-346.

119. Mehran R, Ambrose JA, Bongu M, et al. Angioplasty of complex lesions in ischemic rest angina: Results of the thrombolysis and angioplasty in unstable angina (TAUSA) trial. J Am Coll Cardiol 1995;26:961-966.

120. Grines C, Brodi B, Griffin J, Donohue B, et al. Which primary PTCA patients may benefit from new technologies? Circulation 1995;92:I-146.

121. Meany T, Leon M, Kramer B, Margolis J, et al. Transluminal extraction catheter for the treatment of diseased saphenous vein grafts: A multicenter experience. Cathet Cardiovasc Diagn 1995;34:112-120.

122. Moses J, Yeh W, Popma J, Sketch M, NACI Investigators. Predictors of distal embolization with the TEC catheter: a NACI registry report. J Am Coll Cardiol 1995;92:I-329.

123. White CJ, Ramee SR, Collins TJ, et al. Coronary thrombi increase PTCA risk: Angioscopy as a clinical tool. Circulation 1996;93:253-258.

124. Hillegass WB, Ohman EM, O'Hanesian MA, et al. The effect of preprocedural intracoronary thrombus on patient outcome after percutaneous coronary intervention. J Am Coll Cardiol 1995;March Special Issue:94A.

125. Tan K, Sulke N, Taub N, Sowton E. Clinical and lesion morphologic determinants of coronary angioplasty success and complications: Current experience. J Am Coll Cardiol 1995;25:855-65.

126. Violaris AG, Herrman JP, Melkert R, et al. Does local thrombus formation increase long term luminal renarrowing following PTCA? A quantitative angiographic analysis. J Am Coll Cardiol 1994;March Special Issue:139A.

127. Tenaglia A, Fortin D, Califf R, Frid D, et al. Predicting the risk of abrupt vessel closure after angioplasty in an individual patient. J Am Coll Cardiol 1994;24:1004-11.

128. Myler R, Shaw R, Stertzer S, Hecht H, et al. Lesion morphology and coronary angioplasty: Current experience and analysis. J Am Coll Cardiol 1992;19:1641-52

129. Holmes DR, Ellis SG, Garratt KN. Directional coronary atherectomy for thrombus containing lesions: Improved outcome. Circulation 1991;84:II-26.

130. Annex BH, Larkin TJ, O'Neill WW, Safian RD. Evaluation of thrombus removal by transluminal extraction atherectomy by percutaneous coronary angioscopy. Am J Cardiol 74:606-609.

131. Kaplan B, Safian RD, Goldstein JA, Grines CL, O'Neill WW. Efficacy of angioscopy in determining the effectiveness of intracoronary urokinase and TEC atherectomy thrombus removal from an occluded saphenous vein graft prior to stent implantation. Cathet Cardiovasc Diagn 1995;36:335-337.

132. Al-Shaibi KF, Goods C, Jain S, Negus B, et al. Does transluminal extraction atherectomy reduce distal embolization in saphenous vein grafts? Circulation 1995;92:I-329.

133. Tomaru T, Nakamura F, Yanagisawa-Miwa A, et al. Reduced vasoreactivity and thrombogenicity with pulsed laser angioplasty: Comparison with balloon angioplasty. J Intervn Cardiol 1995;8:6:643-651.

134. Shefer A, Forrester JS, Litvack F. Recanalization of acute thrombus: Comparison of acute success and short-term patency after excimer laser coronary angioplasty, balloon angioplasty and intracoronary thrombolysis in pigs. J Am Coll Cardiol 1991;17:205A.

135. Cook Sl, Eigler NL, Shefer A, et al. Percutaneous excimer laser coronary angioplasty in lesions not ideal for balloon angioplasty. Circulation 1991;84:632-43.

136. Klein LW, Litvack F, Holmes D, et al. Prospective multicenter anlaysis of excimer laser coronary angioplasty (ELCA) in stenoses with complex morphology. J Am Coll Cardiol 1991:448A.

137. Chasteney EA, Ravichandran PS, Furnany AP, et al. Laser thrombolysis for bypass graft thrombosis. J Am Coll Cardiol 1994;March Special Issue:374A.

138. Agrawal SK, Ho DSW, Liu M, Iyer S, et al. Predictors of thrombotic complications after placement of the flexible coil stent. Am J Cardiology Vol. 73; 1216-1219.

139. Muhlestein JB, Gomez MA, Karagounis L, Anderson G. "Rescue ReoPro": Acute utilization of Abciximab for the dissolution of coronary thrombus developing as a complication of coronary angioplasty. Circulation 1995;92:I-607.

140. Lincoff AM, Popma JJ, Ellis SG, et al. Abrupt vessel closure complicating coronary angioplasty: Clinical, angiographic and therapeutic profile. J Am Coll Cardiol 19:926, 1992.

141. Pavlides G, Schreiber TL, Gangadharan V, et al. Safety and efficacy of urokinase during elective coronary angioplasty. Am Heart J 121:731, 1991.

142. de Feyter PJ, van den Brand M, Jaarman G, et al. Acute coronary artery occlusion during and after percutaneous transluminal coronary angioplasty. Circulation 83:927, 1991.

143. Haft JI, Goldstein JE, Homoud MK, et al. PTCA following myocardial infarction: Use of bailout fibrinolysis to improve results. Am Heart J 120:243, 1990.

144. Gulba DC, Daniel WG, Simon R, et al. Role of thrombolysis and thrombin in patients with acute coronary occlusion during percutaneous transluminal coronary angioplasty. J Am Coll Cardiol 16:563, 1990.

145. Hong M, Wong S, Popma J, et al. Favorable results of debulking followed by immediate adjunct stent therapy for high risk saphenous vein graft lesions. J Am Coll Cardiol March Special Issue, 1996.

146. Ramee S, Kuntz R, Schatz R, et al. Preliminary experience with the POSSIS coronary AngioJet Rheolytic Thrombectomy Catheter in the VeGAS I Pilot Study. J Am Coll Cardiol March Special Issue, 1996.

10 BIFURCATION STENOSIS

Patrick Koller, M.D.
Robert D. Safian, M.D.

A. **DESCRIPTION.** A true bifurcation lesion is defined as the presence of a stenosis >50% involving both a parent vessel and the ostium of its sidebranch. Vessel bifurcations may be predisposed to atherosclerosis as turbulent flow and increased shear stress favor abnormal interactions between the endothelium, lipoproteins, and cellular elements.[1] Although true bifurcation lesions account for only 4-16% of PTCA procedures, the vast majority (74-87%) involve the LAD-diagonal bifurcation; ~ 20% of parent vessel lesions undergoing angioplasty have mildly diseased sidebranches (< 50% obstruction).[2-5] Although bifurcation lesions were originally considered a contraindication to PTCA due to the risk of sidebranch occlusion, PTCA is commonly applied to a wide variety of vessel bifurcations (Figure 10.1) with high success and acceptable complication rates. In addition, new device techniques (e.g., bifurcation DCA, kissing stents) have been developed in the hope of improving acute and longterm outcome.

B. **APPROACH TO BIFURCATION LESIONS**

1. **Need for Sidebranch Protection.** The likelihood of significant sidebranch narrowing or closure depends on whether the branch originates from the primary lesion and the degree to which its ostium is narrowed (Tables 10.1, 10.2). Branch vessels that do not originate from the parent vessel (but may be transiently occluded during balloon inflation) are at low risk for sidebranch occlusion.[6] However, if the sidebranch originates from the parent lesion, the risk of occlusion increases progressively if the sidebranch contains an ostial stenosis < 50%; the sidebranch contains a nonostial stenosis > 50%; and the sidebranch has an ostial stenosis > 50%. In one study, branch-ostial stenoses ≤ 50% had a 12% risk of narrowing compared to 41% with ostial stenoses > 50%.[7]

Table 10.1. Parent Vessel-Side Branch Relationships[2,4,6,8,9]

Anatomy	Risk of side branch occlusion	Technical difficulty in passing a wire into branch	Protection required
Branch uninvolved by parent vessel lesion but in jeopardy due to transient occlusion during balloon inflation (Type 2B, 3B)	Low (< 1%)	Low	No
Branch originates from diseased parent vessel segment; branch is normal (Type 1B)	Moderate (1-10%)	Low-Moderate	Probably yes; depends on vessel size, distribution
Ostium of branch vessel > 50% stenosis (Type 1A, 2A, 3A)	High (14-35%)	High	Yes

When the primary atheroma obstructs both parent vessel and sidebranch ostium by > 50%, there is a high incidence of branch occlusion (14-34%) [4,6,8] or narrowing (27-41%) [7-9] unless protected by a guidewire (Figure 10.2). Predictors of sidebranch occlusion include significant branch-ostial stenosis, parent vessel dissection, and unstable angina; factors not predictive of sidebranch occlusion include branch vessel caliber, parent vessel PTCA success, and anatomic location of the branch. [3,4,9,10] Table 10.2 summarizes the need for sidebranch protection.

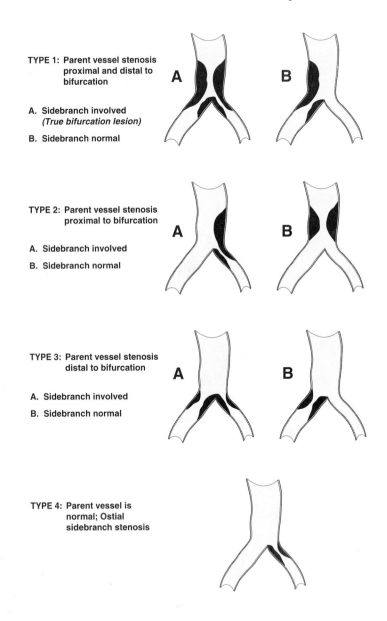

TYPE 1: Parent vessel stenosis proximal and distal to bifurcation

A. Sidebranch involved *(True bifurcation lesion)*

B. Sidebranch normal

TYPE 2: Parent vessel stenosis proximal to bifurcation

A. Sidebranch involved

B. Sidebranch normal

TYPE 3: Parent vessel stenosis distal to bifurcation

A. Sidebranch involved

B. Sidebranch normal

TYPE 4: Parent vessel is normal; Ostial sidebranch stenosis

Figure 10.1 Classification of Bifurcation Lesions

Table 10.2. Need for Sidebranch Protection

Sidebranch Protection Recommended		
	1.	Any sidebranch > 2.0 mm in diameter that has an ostial stenosis ≥ 50% and originates from the parent vessel lesion (Figure 10.1; Types 1A, 2A, 3A). "True" bifurcation lesions (Figure 10.1; Type 1A) are associated with a high incidence of sidebranch occlusion and a low salvage rate when left unprotected.
	2.	Any sidebranch > 2 mm in diameter (without ostial stenosis) originates from the parent vessel lesion (Figure 10.1; Type 1B). Although it is usually possible to retrieve these occluded sidebranches, their large caliber justifies protection. In such lesions, a double guidewire approach is reasonable; if sidebranch occlusion occurs, sequential PTCA or a kissing balloon technique may be employed.
Protection Probably Not Necessary*		
	1.	The sidebranch is normal and does not originate from the parent vessel lesion (Figure 10.1; Type 2B, 3B). Even though the sidebranch may be transiently covered by the inflated balloon in the parent vessel, the risk of occlusion is low.
	2.	The sidebranch is < 1.5 mm in diameter and would not receive a bypass graft during CABG.
	3.	The sidebranch supplies a small amount of viable myocardium.
	4.	Isolated stenoses of the origin of the sidebranch usually do not require protection of the parent vessel (Figure 10.1; Type 4).

* In these lesions, it may be reasonable to leave the sidebranch unprotected; if sidebranch occlusion does occur, it can be retrieved by conventional PTCA, depending on the clinical situation, or not retrieved at all.

2. PTCA TECHNIQUES (Table 10.3)

a. **Double Guiding Catheter Technique.** This outdated approach was initially recommended before the availability of low-profile balloons and large-lumen 7F and 8F guiding catheters. It involves placement of two guiding catheters (via two arterial punctures) in the aortic root, and requires separate engagement and retraction of each guide to permit sequential advancement of each guidewire and balloon system.

b. **Single Guiding Catheter Technique.** Virtually all 8F giant-lumen (internal diameter ≥ 0.084-inch) guiding catheters can most accommodate balloons and guidewires needed for bifurcation angioplasty, even when two 0.014-inch over-the-wire systems are used. Regardless of the approach (sequential or kissing balloons), use of a 3-way Touhy-Borst adapter is recommended. To minimize the risk of guidewire entanglement, parent vessel

Table 10.3. Technical Approaches to Bifurcation Angioplasty

Approach	Advantages	Disadvantages
Guiding Catheter Technique		
Two-guide approach	• Large variety of dilatation catheters to choose from • Excellent visualization	• Two arterial punctures • More procedural complexity • Potential ostial injury
One-guide approach	• One access site • Fewer catheter engagements; less risk of ostial injury • Less time consuming	• More limited choice of balloons, wires • Visualization may be impaired
Protection Technique		
Double-guidewire	• Maintain continuous access to both vessels • Less obstruction to coronary flow from a guidewire than a balloon • Better contrast opacification • Less expensive if the same balloon can be used for both branches	• Increases chance of wire entanglement
Double balloon-on-the-wire	• Allows immediate PTCA of branch if needed • Balloon serves as a "stent" during sequential dilatations	• Increases chance of wire entanglement • Cannot upsize or exchange without giving up wire position and must recross lesion with wire • May impair contrast opacification
Double balloon over-the-wire	• Maintains guidewire access in the parent vessel • Allows immediate PTCA of sidebranch for abrupt closure	• Increases chance of wire entanglement • May impair contrast opacification
Inflation Technique		
Sequential balloon inflation	• Requires less intracoronary hardware • Can use same balloon for both vessels	• Increases chance of wire entanglement • Does not eliminate "snow-plow" or shifting plaque • Single balloon may not match diameter of parent vessel proximal and distal to branch
Kissing balloon inflations	• Minimizes "snow-plow" and shifting plaque • Allows PTCA of large caliber proximal vessel without overdilating smaller vessel distal to bifurcation	• More complex procedure • Increases chance of wire entanglement • May overdilate parent vessel proximal to bifurcation

and sidebranch guidewires should be advanced simultaneously to the tip of the guide catheter, the more difficult lesion wired first, and guidewire rotation limited to < 180°. If both vessels are angulated or tortuous, the larger vessel should be wired first. Balloon diameters should be selected to match the caliber of the disease-free segment of each vessel just beyond the bifurcation; deliberate undersizing increases the risk of procedural failure, while oversizing increases the risk of complications. In general, bifurcation lesions may be approached with double guidewires and sequential PTCA, or double guidewires and kissing balloons.

1. **Double Guidewire, Sequential PTCA.** This approach, which involves placing guidewires in both parent vessel and sidebranch before balloon inflation, maintains continuous access to limbs of the bifurcation (in the event acute closure occurs or balloon/device exchange is needed), but does not prevent shifting-plaque or sidebranch narrowing. Monorail balloons, over-the-wire balloons, fixed wire-balloons, or any combination of the above may be used. Initial use of bare guidewires allows excellent visualization during contrast injections and is a popular approach. Once both guidewires are in place, the parent vessel and sidebranch are dilated in sequential fashion; the same balloon may be used if the bifurcation limbs are the same diameter. While a balloon on-the-wire system can be used, the sidebranch cannot be protected if balloon upsizing is necessary; when used to dilate the parent or branch, it is best to advance the balloon beyond the lesion (to assess the angiographic result) before removing it. Use of a tapered balloon (Chapter 15) may provide a more uniform balloon-to-artery ratio proximal and distal to the bifurcation (Types 1B, 2A; Figure 10.1).[42]

2. **Kissing Balloon Technique.** Simultaneous "kissing-balloon" inflations are preferable to prevent "shifting plaque" and "snow-plow" injury (Figure 10.2). By performing simultaneous inflations, adequate dilatation of the proximal vessel can be achieved without oversizing the balloon relative to the smaller distal vessels (Figure 10.3). Low-pressure inflations (1-4 atmospheres) are performed initially; higher pressures may be used if the angiographic result is suboptimal.

3. **DCA TECHNIQUE.** Bifurcation DCA can be performed using "kissing" or sequential guidewires (Figure 10.4).[13,16,17,18,20] Sequential intervention is recommended, using either DCA of the parent vessel and PTCA of the sidebranch, or DCA of both vessels (Chapter 28). Nitinol wires are resistant to damage during DCA and should be used for the kissing wire technique;[15] when this technique is used, the AtheroCath should be rotated < 180° to prevent wire entanglement. Predilation of sidebranches with ostial disease is sometimes recommended to reduce the risk of sidebranch occlusion during DCA of the parent vessel; when sidebranch predilation is performed, balloon inflation pressures < 2 atm should be used to reduce the risk of shifting plaque.

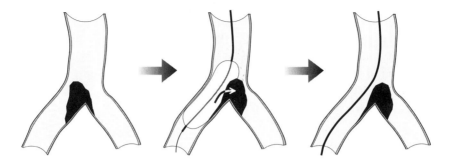

Figure 10.2 "Snow-Plow" Effect

During PTCA of the parent vessel, shifting plaque causes sidebranch narrowing. Simultaneous dilatation of both limbs of the bifurcation ("kissing-balloon" technique) is often required when the snow-plow effect complicates PTCA.

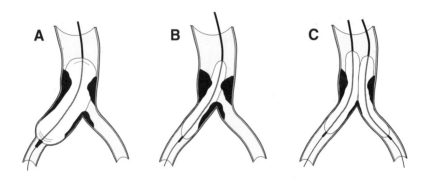

Figure 10.3 Bifurcation Stenosis Requiring Simultaneous Balloon Inflations

When the target lesion extends from a large proximal vessel segment to a smaller distal (post-bifurcation) vessel, "kissing" balloon inflations are usually necessary.
A.   Sizing the balloon to the proximal vessel results in overdilating the distal vessel.
B.   Sizing the balloon to the distal vessel results in underdilating the proximal vessel.
C.   Kissing balloon inflations allow adequate dilatation of both proximal and distal vessel segments.

4.   **STENT TECHNIQUE.** Experimental data have shown that flow into nondiseased sidebranches is well-preserved after stent placement,[33] and several angiographic studies suggest a low incidence of sidebranch occlusion. Nevertheless, stents should be used cautiously in patients with stenoses involving significant sidebranches.[35] Even though sidebranches may still be accessible to PTCA after implantation of a Gianturco-Roubin or other coil stents,[45] added technical expertise is required for successful salvage. In addition, attempts to cross the struts of slotted tubular (e.g., Palmaz-Schatz) stents may increase the risk of balloon entrapment. When a parent lesion requires intervention but has a sidebranch, the decision to perform stenting is predicated on the need for

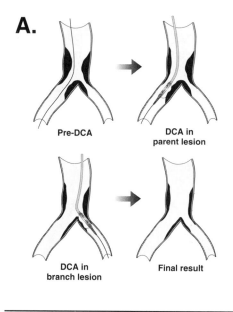

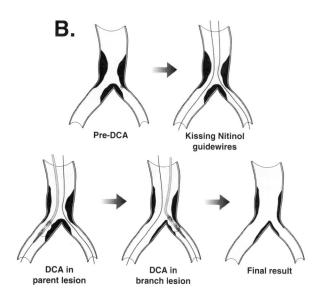

Figure 10.4 Bifurcation Lesions: DCA Techniques

A. Sequential guidewires and sequential DCA.
B. Kissing nitinol guidewires and sequential DCA.

immediate revascularization of the sidebranch, the likelihood of future revascularization, the size of the sidebranch, and the size of the myocardium served by that branch. In general, jeopardy of acute marginal branches of the RCA, small diagonal branches of the LAD, and small obtuse marginal branches of the left circumflex artery may not represent significant contraindications to stent placement. In some anatomically suitable vessels (i.e., parent and branch vessels ≥ 3 mm with focal stenoses), there are now several reports of "kissing" stents; these techniques are technically demanding and should be reserved for operators with extensive stent experience (Figure 10.5)[31,32] — half disarticulated stents may be employed, but must be mounted on low-profile balloons without the delivery sheath.[31, 32]

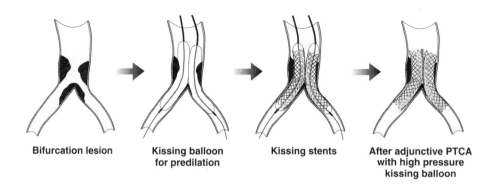

Bifurcation lesion   **Kissing balloon**   **Kissing stents**   **After adjunctive PTCA**
                 for predilation   **with high pressure**
                                                                  kissing balloon

Figure 10.5 Bifurcation Lesions: Stent Technique

C. PROCEDURAL RESULTS

1. **PTCA (Table 10.4).** Although successful dilation can be achieved in 87-100% of parent vessel lesions, successful sidebranch revascularization occurs less often (76-89%).[2-5,8-10] In addition to the usual risks of PTCA, bifurcation angioplasty is associated with the additional risk of sidebranch occlusion, incomplete dilation due to the "snow-plow" effect (Figure 10.2), and retrograde propagation of dissection from sidebranch to parent vessel. Branch occlusion may be silent or associated with chest pain, hemodynamic instability and/or malignant arrhythmias depending upon the vessel caliber, presence and adequacy of collaterals, other coronary disease, and left ventricular function. Causes of sidebranch occlusion include snow-plow injury, dissection, spasm, and/or thrombosis.

2. **Directional Atherectomy (DCA) (Table 10.5).** Observational studies report that sidebranch occlusion occurs in 0.7-7.7% of unselected lesions,[14,21-29] and up to 37% of bifurcation lesions treated by DCA.[18] Fortunately, most sidebranch closures can be salvaged by PTCA. Much like PTCA, baseline narrowing of the sidebranch origin increases the risk of sidebranch occlusion during DCA.[20] In highly selected bifurcation lesions, high procedural success (91-100%) and low

Table 10.4. Results of PTCA for Bifurcation Lesions

Series	Sidebranch Protected	N	Success (%)	Complications (%)	Restenosis (%)
Tan[42] (1995)	Bifurcation - Yes	135	95	2.2*	-
	Bifurcation - No	52	85	3.8*	-
	Non-bifurcation	970	93	3.4*	-
Lewis[19][†] (1993)	Bifurcation	-	74	3.7	Angiographic (61%)
	Non-bifurcation	-	86	6.1	(52%)
Myler[5] (1992)	Bifurcation - Yes	17	94	0	-
	Bifurcation - No	106	89	3.8	-
	Non-bifurcation	656	95	1.4	-
Ciampricotti[4] (1992)	Bifurcation - No	22	95	0	-
Weinstein[8] (1991)	Bifurcation - Yes	35	97	0	Clinical (42%)
	Bifurcation - No	21	76	0	Clinical (16%)
Renkin[2] (1991)	Bifurcation - Yes	34	97	2.9	Angiographic (37%)**
	Bifurcation - No	8	88	12.5	
Thomas[11] (1988)	Bifurcation - Yes	54	87	6.0	Clinical (30%)
George[3] (1986)	Bifurcation - Yes	52	98	3.8	Angiographic (53%) Clinical (32%)

Abbreviations: - = not reported
* complications reflect the incidence of abrupt closure
** overall restenosis rate for all lesions
† Coronary Angioplasty versus Excisional Atherectomy Trial (CAVEAT)

major complication rates (0-3%) have been reported.[14,17,18] In one study, transient sidebranch occlusion occurred in 37%; after salvage PTCA or DCA, final diameter stenosis was 6-12% in the parent vessel and 0-17% in the sidebranch.[18] In CAVEAT-I, compared to bifurcation lesions treated by PTCA, DCA led to higher success (88% vs. 74%, p < 0.001) and less restenosis (50% vs. 61%, p < 0.001), but more ischemic complications (9.5% vs. 3.7%, p < 0.001).

3. **Stents.** Although stents should be used cautiously in lesions with large sidebranches (Chapter 26), high success and acceptable complication rates have been reported. In one study, Gianturco-Roubin stenting resulted in reappearance of sidebranches which were initially occluded after PTCA — the incidence of sidebranch occlusion was 6-18% after initial PTCA but rare after stenting.[34]

Table 10.5. Results of DCA in Bifurcation Lesions

Series	N	Success (%)	MC (%)	SBO (%)
Miguel[new-3] (1994)	122	-	0.8	17
Lewis[19][†] (1993)	-	88	9.5	50
Mansour[17] (1992)	8	100	0	0
Hinohara[14] (1991)	22	91	4.5	-

Abbreviations: MC = major in-hospital complications (death, Q-wave myocardial infarction, emergency coronary artery bypass grafting); SBO = sidebranch occlusion; - = not reported

†   Coronary Angioplasty versus Excisional Atherectomy Trial (CAVEAT); success (90%), MC (8.2%), SBO (50%) for non-bifurcation lesions

Another study of the Palmaz-Schatz stent revealed sidebranch occlusion in 10%; two-thirds were associated with initial PTCA and one-third was associated with subsequent stenting.[38] The management of sidebranch occlusion is less complicated after the Gianturco-Roubin stent, since wires and balloons may be passed through the stent coils and into the affected branch. PTCA salvage through slotted stents is feasible, but low-profile balloons are necessary to reduce the risk of balloon entrapment.[35] In a report of 43 cases of sidebranch narrowing treated by PTCA through Palmaz-Schatz and Gianturco-Roubin stent struts or articulation sites, success was achieved in 84% and there were no cases of balloon entrapment.[45] Late (8-month) follow-up after stenting across sidebranches revealed progression and regression of sidebranch narrowing in 19% and 26%, respectively.[39] In another study, all occluded sidebranches after stenting were patent at 6 months.[38] Limited data are available concerning the use of kissing stents; Colombo et al.[43] treated 18 major bifurcation lesions with kissing stents; procedural success was 89%, but ischemic complications and stent thrombosis occurred in 11% and 6%, respectively.[43]

4. **Other Devices.** The application of ELCA, Rotablator, or TEC to true bifurcation lesions is generally not recommended because of the inability to protect the diseased sidebranch and an increased risk of procedural complications and reduced clinical success.[36,40,41]

5. **Retrieval of Occluded Sidebranches.** Salvage rates depend on whether the affected sidebranch contains a high-grade ostial stenosis, and whether the branch was initially protected by a second wire. Acutely occluded sidebranches without ostial stenoses can be reopened in 75-100% of cases, although salvage rates < 50% have been reported when the ostium of the sidebranch contains a significant stenosis.[4,8,11] In another report, sidebranch retrieval was successful in 10/11 (91%) protected sidebranch occlusions compared to 11/34 (32%) unprotected branches.[8] When attempting

to salvage an occluded sidebranch, excessive or forceful sidebranch probing increases the risk of traumatizing the parent vessel lesion and should be avoided. In addition, it is imperative to protect the parent vessel with a guidewire in the event of parent vessel closure. In a report of 15 patients with sidebranch occlusion, 67% demonstrated spontaneous recanalization at 6-month follow-up angiography; if this phenomenon occurs early, it may explain the low incidence of myocardial infarction after refractory sidebranch occlusion.[13]

6.   **Parent Vessel Closure.** Sustained patency of the parent vessel is rarely affected by occlusion of its sidebranch; retrograde propagation of dissection from sidebranch to parent vessel is rare.[9]

7.   **Myocardial Infarction, Emergency CABG and Death.** Myocardial infarction is uncommon after sidebranch occlusion.[4-6,9] Of 167 patients with sidebranch occlusion after PTCA, chest pain occurred in 13% and Q-wave MI in 8%; septal perforator occlusion, which comprised 27% of all branch closures, was not associated with MI. Among patients with branch occlusion in the 1985-1986 NHLBI PTCA Registry, emergency CABG was required in 11% and death occurred in 3%.[37] When data from several large retrospective series are complied, the overall incidence of death is < 1%.

* * * * *

REFERENCES

1. Pinkerton CA, Slack JD. Complex Coronary Angioplasty: A technique for dilatation of bifurcation stenosis. Angiology 1985:543-548.
2. Renkin J, Wijns W, Hanet C, et al. Angioplasty of coronary bifurcation stenoses. Cathet Cardiovasc Diagn 1991;22:167-173.
3. George BS, Myler RK, Stertzer SH, et al. Balloon angioplasty of coronary bifurcation lesions. Cathet Cardiovasc Diagn 1986;12:124-138.
4. Ciampricutti R, El-Gamol M, Van Golder B, et al. Coronary angioplasty of bifurcation lesions without protection of large sidebranches. Cathet Cardiovasc Diagn 1992;27:191-196.
5. Myler RK, Shaw RE, Stertzer SH, et al. Lesion morphology and coronary angioplasty: current experience and analysis. J Am Coll Cardiol 1992. In press.
6. Meier B, Gruentzig AR, King SB III, et al. Risk of side branch occlusion during coronary angioplasty. Am J Cardiol 1984;53:10-14.
7. Boxt LM, Meyeruvitz MF, Taus RH, et al. Sidebranch occlusion complicating percutanous transluminal coronary angioplasty. Radiology 1986;161:681-683.
8. Weinstein JS, Baim DS, Sipperly ME, et al. Salvage of branch vessels during bifurcation lesion angioplasty. Cathet Cardiovasc Diagn 1991;22:1-6.
9. Vetrovec GW, Cowley MJ, Wolfgang TC, et al. Effects of percutaneous transluminal coronary angioplasty in lesion associated branches. Am Heart J 1985;109:921-925.
10. Arora RR, Raymond RE, Dimas AP, et al. Side branch occlusion during coronary angioplasty: incidence, angiographic characteristics, and outcome. Cathet Cardiovasc Diagn 1989;18:210-212.
11. Thomas TS, Williams DO, Most AS. Efficacy of coronary angioplasty of bifurcation lesions: immediate and late outcome. Circulation 1988;78(4):II-632.
12. Shiu MF, Singh A. Spontaneous recanalization of sidebranches occluded during percutaneous transluminal coronary angioplasty. Brit Heart J 1985;54:215-217.
13. Eisenhauer AC, Clugston RA, Ruiz CE. Sequential directional atherectomy of coronary bifurcation lesions. Cathet Cardiovasc Diagn 1993;Suppl 1:54-60.
14. Hinohara T, Rowe MH, Robertson GC, et al. Effect of lesion characteristics on outcome of directional coronary atherectomy. J Am Coll Cardiol 1991;17:1112-20.
15. Grassman ED, Leya FS, Lewis BE, Johnson SA, et al. Examination of common PTCA guidewires used for sidebranch protection during directional coronary atherectomy of bifurcation lesions performed in vivo and in vitro. Cathet Cardiovasc Diagn 1993; Suppl 1:48-53.
16. Safian R, Schreiber T, Baim D. Specific indications for directional coronary atherectomy: Origin left anterior descending coronary artery and bifurcating lesions. Am J Cardiol 1993;72:35E-41E.
17. Mansour M, Fishman RF, Kuntz RE, Carrozza JP. Feasibility of directional atherectomy for the treatment of bifurcation lesions. Cor Art Dis 1992;3:761-765.
18. Lewis B, Leya F, Johnson S, et al. Acute procedural results in the treatment of 30 coronary artery bifurcation lesions with a double-wire atherectomy technique for side-branch protection. Am Heart J 1994;127:1600-1607.
19. Lewis B, Leya F, Johnson S, et al. Outcome of angioplasty (PTCA) and atherectomy (DCA) for bifurcation and non-bifurcation lesions in CAVEAT. Circulation 1993;88:I-601.
20. Campos-Esteve M, Laird J, Kufs W, Wortham CD. Side-branch occlusion with directional coronary atherectomy: Incidence and risk factors. Am Heart J 1994;128:686-690.
21. Kaufmann UP, Garratt KN, Vlietstra RE, Menke KK. Coronary atherectomy: First 50 patients at the Mayo Clinic. Mayo Clin Proc 1989;64:747-752.
22. Safian R, Gelbfish J, Erny R, Schnitt S, Schmidt D, Baim D. Coronary atherectomy. Clinical, angiographic, and histological findings and observations regarding potential mechanisms. Circulation 1990;82:69-79.
23. Rowe MH, Hinohara T, White NW, Robertson GC. Comparison of dissection rates and angiographic results following directional coronary atherectomy and coronary angioplasty. Am J Cardiol 1990;66:49-53.
24. Garratt K, Holmes D, Bell M, et al. Results of directional atherectomy of primary atheromatous and restenosis lesions in coronary arteries and saphenous vein grafts. Am J Cardiol 1992;70:449-454.
25. Fishman R, Kuntz R, Carrozza J, et al. Long-term results of directional coronary atherectomy: Predictors of restenosis.

J Am Coll Cardiol 1992;20:1101-1110.

26. Baim D, Tomoaki H, Holmes D, et al. Results of directional coronary atherectomy during multicenter preapproval testing. Am J Cardiol 1993;72:6E-11E.

27. Cowley M, DiSciascio G. Experience with directional coronary atherectomy since pre-market approval. Am J Cardiol 1993;72:12E-20E.

28. Popma J, Mintz G, Satler L, et al. Clinical and angiographic outcome after directional coronary atherectomy: A qualitative and quantitative analysis using coronary arteriography and intravascular ultrasound. Am J Cardiol 1993;72:55E-64E.

29. Umans V, de Feyter P, Deckers J, et al. Acute and long-term outcome of directional coronary atherectomy for stable and unstable angina. Am J Cardiol 1993;74:641-646.

30. Guarneri E, Sklar M, Russo R, Claire D, Schatz R, Teirstein P. Escape from Stent Jail: An in vitro model. Circulation 1995;92:I-688.

31. Nakamura S, Hall P, Maiello L, Colombo A. Techniques of Palmaz-Schatz stent deployment in lesions with a large side branch. Cathet Cardiovas Diagn 1995;34:353-361.

32. Colombo A, Gaglione A, Nakamura S. "Kissing" stents for bifurcational coronary lesion. Cathet Cardiovas Diag. 1993;30:327-330.

33. Iniguez A, Macaya C, Alfonso F, Goicolea J. Early angiographic changes of side branches arising from a Palmaz-Schatz Stented coronary segment: Results and clinical implications. J Am Coll Cardiol 1994;23:911-915.

34. Mazur W, Grinstead C, Hakim A, et al. Fate of side branches after intracoronary implantation of the Gianturco-Roubin flex-stent for acute or threatened closure after percutaneous transluminal coronary angioplasty. Am J Cardiol 1994;74:1207-1210.

35. Guarneri E, Sklar M, Russo R, Claire D, Schatz R, Teirstein P. Escape from Stent Jail: An in vitro model. Circulation 1995;92:I-688.

36. Bittl JA, Sanborn TA, Tcheng JE, et al. Clinical success, complications and restenosis rates with excimer laser coronary angioplasty: The PELCA Registry. Am J Cardiol 1992;70:1533-1539.

37. Holmes DR JR, Holubkov R, Vlietstra RE, et al. Comparison of complications during percutaneous transluminal coronary angioplasty from 1977 to 1981 and from 1985 to 1986. The National Heart, Lung, and Blood Institute Percutaneous Transluminal Coronary Angioplasty Registry. J Am Coll Cardiol 1988;12:1149-1155.

38. Fischman DL, Savage MP, Leon MB, et al. Fate of lesion-related sidebranches after coronary artery stenting. J Am Coll Cardiol 1993;22:1641-6.

39. Pan M, Medina A, de Lezo JS, et al. Follow-up patency of sidebranches covered by intracoronary Palmaz-Schatz stent. Am Heart J 1995;129:436-440.

40. Whitlow PL, Cowley M, Bass T, et al. Risk of high speed rotational atherectomy in bifurcation lesions. J Am Coll Cardiol 1993;21:445A.

41. Warth DC, Leon MB, O'Neill WW, et al. Rotational atherectomy multicenter registry: Acute results, complications and 6-month angiographic follow-up in 709 patients. J Am Coll Cardiol 1994;24:641-8.

42. Tan Kim, Sulke N, Taub N, Sowton E. Clinical and lesion morphologic determinants of coronary angioplasty success and complications: Current experience. J Am Coll Cardiol 1995;25:855-865.

43. Colombo A, Maiello L, Itoh A, et al. Coronary stenting of bifurcation lesions: Immediate and follow-up results. J Am Coll Cardio;March Special Issue.

44. Mehta S, Popma J, Margolis JR, et al. Complications with new angioplasty devices. Are these device specific? J Am Coll Cardio;March Special Issue.

45. Caputo RP, Chafizedeh ER, Stoler RC, et al. "Stent Jail" — A minimum security prison. J Invas Cardiol 1996;8.

11 PROXIMAL VESSEL TORTUOSITY & ANGULATED LESIONS

Mark Freed, M.D.
Robert D. Safian, M.D.

PROXIMAL VESSEL TORTUOSITY

A. DEFINITION. No single definition of proximal vessel tortuosity has gained widespread acceptance. Different definitions include the presence of two or more bends ≥ 75° proximal to the target lesion; at least one proximal bend ≥ 90°; or the presence of "significant" vessel curvature proximal to the target lesion (without being more specific). Others grade proximal tortuosity according to the number of 45° bends (no/moderate = 0-1 bend, moderate = 2 bends, severe = 3 or more bends).

B. PROCEDURAL OUTCOME

1. **PTCA.** When balloon angioplasty is performed in vessels with proximal tortuosity, there appears to be an increased incidence of procedural failure (inability to cross the lesion with a guidewire, inadequate guiding catheter support) and more acute complications (Table 11.1).[1,2,4,5] However, different results in different studies may be due to varying definitions of tortuosity.

2. **New Interventional Devices.** Severe proximal vessel tortuosity is problematic for successful use of all atherectomy devices, stents, and lasers, which are more bulky, less flexible, and less trackable than conventional balloon catheters. The Rotablator is the most flexible of these devices; activation of the burr may reduce friction and enhance burr movement through moderate-to-severe bends. In one report, Rotablator success was independent of proximal vessel tortuosity,[6] although only 28 such lesions were present. TEC and ELCA are somewhat flexible and may track around moderate bends, but attempts to negotiate extreme tortuosity is potentially dangerous. DCA has long been

Table 11.1. Effect of Proximal Tortuosity on Acute PTCA Outcome

Series	N	Anatomic Subgroup	Success (%)	Other (%)	
Tan[1]	965	No tortuosity	93	Acute closure:	3
(1995)	142	Moderate	93		4.2
	50	Severe	84		6
Ellis[2]	189	Type A	92	Acute complications:	2
(1990)	65	Proximal tortuosity	72		15
Gossman[3]	53	No Shepherd's Crook	98	Difficulty crossing lesion:	13
(1988)	51	Shepherd's Crook	86		33

contraindicated in the setting of extreme tortuosity due to the risk of failure and complications;[5,7,8] however, the recent availability of small housing devices (5 mm) and AtheroCaths with enhanced torque (GTO device) may facilitate passage into tortuous vessels. Virtually all stents are less trackable than most balloon catheters, and in general, slotted tubular (e.g., Palmaz-Schatz) stents are less trackable than coiled wire (e.g., Gianturco-Roubin) stents. Among 623 patients receiving Palmaz-Schatz stents, severe tortuosity favored device failure.[9] The AVE Microstent appears to be the most trackable stent, and is the preferred stent in tortuous vessels (not available in the United States). However, the availability of numerous heavy-duty and extra-support guidewires has permitted the use of even stainless steel slotted stents (e.g., Palmaz-Schatz stent) in vessels with moderate-to-severe tortuosity

C. TECHNICAL CONSIDERATIONS AND APPROACH

1. **Equipment.** The proper combination of guiding catheter, guidewire, and balloon catheter is critical to the success and safety of PTCA of tortuous vessels.

   a. **Guiding Catheter.** The optimal guiding catheter provides stable position, coaxial alignment, easy torque control, kink-resistance, a soft tip, and a stiff shaft to maximize "back-up" support (Figure 11.1). As shown in Table 11.2, the choice of guiding catheter is usually determined by the orientation (take-off) of the target vessel and size of the aortic root.

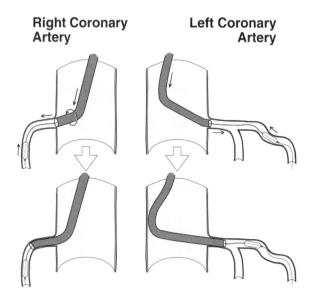

Right Coronary Artery   **Left Coronary Artery**

Figure 11.1 Deep-Seating Maneuver

This maneuver can be used to increase guiding catheter support. To perform this technique, the balloon is retracted as the guide is advanced and gently rotated clockwise. The balloon is then re-advanced while maintaining gentle forward pressure on the guide. Extreme care must be taken to maintain distal guidewire position and to avoid vessel trauma. Once the balloon has reached the stenosis, the guide is withdrawn to its original position.

Table 11.2. Guide Catheter Selection Based on Target Vessel Orientation

Orientation	Tip Configuration
Right Coronary Artery	
Superior take-off	We prefer left Amplatz, Arani-75°, Hockey Stick, IMA, or right Voda; best "back-up" may be with a left Amplatz from the left brachial approach.
Marked inferior take-off	A multipurpose or left Amplatz catheter is chosen. If a Judkins right catheter is used, deep vessel engagement may be required to improve back-up (Figure 11.1).
Horizontal take-off	JR4, Hockey Stick
Left Coronary System	A left Amplatz or left Voda catheter is initially chosen. On occasion, a Judkins left guide can be converted into an Amplatz-like catheter to improve back-up support (Figure 11.1).
Inability to track despite proper guide tip configuration	Choices include the use of large diameter guides (9F), deep-seating maneuver (Figure 11.1), or brachial approach (Chapter 2).

    b. Guidewires. The choice of guidewires is largely based on operator preference. Virtually all guidewire manufactures use a lubricious coating on their guidewires to enhance guidewire movement. Although 0.018" guidewires have superior performance in terms of flexibility, steerability, and support, the choices for low-profile and highly trackable balloon catheters is more limited than with 0.014" guidewires. For tortuous vessels, conventional 0.014" floppy guidewires may be sufficient, but in situations where the guidewire tip prolapses away from the target lesion, a tapered-core guidewire may be better. In some situations, steerability and tip-response are lost as the wire passes through multiple curves — partial advancement of the balloon catheter (or any other suitable transport catheter) may improve guidewire support, torque control, and steerability. If this maneuver fails, other options include the use of stiffer tip guidewires, which may further improve handing characteristics; extra-support guidewires (in which the shaft rather than the tip is stiffer), to straighten vessel curves and ease guidewire movement; and hydrophilic guidewires, some of which are made of Nitinol and are extremely flexible and kink-resistant. Although heavy-duty guidewires (e.g., Platinum-Plus) are generally not well-suited as primary guidewires because of their stiffness and poor torque control, they provide excellent support and will enhance tracking of balloons when other guidewires fail. Although a 0.010" wire may occasionally negotiate proximal tortuosity when other wires fail, most have been removed from the market.

    c. Balloon Dilatation Catheters. As with guidewires, the choice of balloon catheters is largely dependent on operator preference. Important characteristics for negotiating tortuous vessels include deflated profile, trackability, pushability, and guidewire movement. Unfortunately, although deflated balloon profile is perhaps the easiest to measure (and is highly marketed by balloon manufacturers), it is probably the least important variable. Trackability and pushability have more clinical relevance but are difficult to measure.

Technical specifications of balloon products derived from in-vitro testing are less important than how the balloon performs in the hands of the operator; nevertheless, certain design features are worthy of consideration. In general, over-the-wire systems are more trackable and pushable, and are easier to perform guidewire exchanges with than monorail designs. Monorail catheters, on the other hand, have lower profiles than over-the-wire systems. Fixed-wire (balloon-on-a-wire) systems have the lowest profile, but guidewire tip response and steerability are usually inferior to movable guidewires. Generally speaking, if the operator can successfully negotiate a tortuous vessel with a guidewire, numerous different balloon catheters can be used to successfully complete the intervention.

2. **Approach.** A 30-cm long introducing sheath should be placed in the femoral artery to minimize iliac artery tortuosity and enhance guiding catheter support.
    *   Choose a guide catheter that maximizes stable coaxial alignment and back-up support. Further back-up support can be obtained by using larger guides; 8- and 9-F guides usually provide better back-up than 6- or 7-F guides.

    *   Use a 0.014" tapered-core flexible guidewire or hydrophilic wire to cross the lesion. Added support (and ease of guidewire exchange) may be achieved by trailing a transport catheter or over-the-wire balloon several centimeters behind the guidewire tip. (Care must be taken when stiffening the wire in this manner to avoid vessel trauma.) Be sure to advance the guidewire as far beyond the lesion as possible so the balloon tracks over the stiffer portion of the wire. If the guidewire crosses the lesion, but the balloon will not negotiate the bends, exchange your guidewire for an extra-support or Platinum-plus guidewire and try again.

    *   Have the patient take in a deep breath — this will occasionally straighten proximal tortuosity and facilitate guidewire and balloon advancement.

    *   Try a balloon on-the-wire system when an over-the-wire or monorail system fails.

    *   When PTCA fails from the femoral approach, superselective guide catheter intubation from the left brachial approach may increase procedural success (Chapter 2).

ANGULATED LESIONS

A. **BALLOON ANGIOPLASTY (Table 11.3).** PTCA of angulated (> 45-60°) stenoses is associated with increased incidence of procedural failure,[2] major ischemic complications,[2,12,13,22,23] and restenosis. Nevertheless, high procedural success (85-95%) and low complication rates (< 3%) are often reported. Complications are usually due to dissections and abrupt closure, possibly from straightening the vessel during balloon inflation. Noncompliant (PET or thin-walled polyethylene) balloons[10,14] and long balloons may result in less "straightening force,"[15,16] although a recent study found no difference in lumen enlargement or complications between compliant and noncompliant balloons. Angled balloons, which conform to natural bends and purportedly minimize vessel straightening, have also been associated with high success and low complication rates,[12] but their production has been halted due to infrequent use.

B. **NEW INTERVENTIONAL DEVICES.** Virtually all atherectomy and laser devices should be avoided in severely angulated lesions because of the risk of dissection or perforation. One study using the Rotablator reported procedural success in 35/41 (85%) moderately angled lesions (45-60°), but

Table 11.3. Effect of Lesion Angulation on Acute PTCA Outcome

Series	N	Angulation (degrees)	Success (%)	Complications** (%)
Tan[1]	991	< 45	94	2.2[†]
(1995)	136	45-90	88	8.8[†]
	30	> 90	83	13[†]
Myler[10]	543	< 45	94	1.3
(1992)	158	45-90	95	2.5
	78	≥ 90	94	2.6
Savas[11]	69*	≥ 45	88	1
(1992)				
Ellis[2]	189	Type A	92	2
(1990)	144	≥ 45	72	13[++]
	32	≥ 60	53	-

Abbreviation: - Not Reported
++   Dissection occurred in 46% of angulated lesionscompared to 8% of non-angulated lesions
*   All lesions ≥ 2 cm in length were treated with long (40 mm) balloons
**   In-hospital death, MI, or emergency CABG unless otherwise indicated
†   Incidence of acute closure

angle > 60° was a powerful predictor of procedural failure, major ischemic complications, and perforation.[6] In a larger report, compared to non-angulated lesions, Rotablator treatment of 123 angulated lesions > 45° resulted in lower success (86% vs 94%), more dissections (36% vs 16%), and a higher mortality rate (2.7% vs 0.3%).[17] DCA has been used with high success (91%) and low complications (3.6%) in lesions with mild angulation (~ 30°),[7] but angulation ≥ 45° was an independent predictor of procedural failure (relative risk 4.8) and major ischemic complications (relative risk 2.7).[8] Likewise, TEC and ELCA should not be used on severely angulated lesions due to the high risk of complications.[6,18,19] Stents can be used to treat mild-moderately angulated lesions, but the value of stenting highly angulated lesions is uncertain. With coiled wire stents, atheroma may prolapse through the coils leading to suboptimal results and the occasional need for multiple stents. Slotted tubular stents may provide better lumen enlargement but may be difficult to negotiate acute bends. All considered, new device angioplasty of angulated lesions has been associated with an increased incidence of acute closure[20] and perforation.[21]

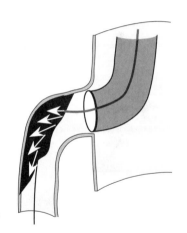
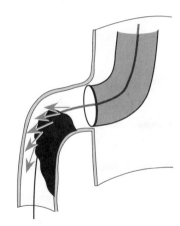

Lesion on Outer Curve:
Device directed into lesion

Lesion on Inner Curve:
Device deflected into disease-free wall

Figure 11.2 Angulated Lesions: Impact of Lesion Location

Angulated lesions with plaque situated along the outer curve may sometimes be considered for ELCA, TEC, or Rotablator. In contrast, when plaque is situated along the inner curve, these devices may deflect away from the plaque and into the disease-free wall, increasing the risk of dissection or perforation.

C.   **APPROACH.** The easiest and safest approach to percutaneous revascularization of highly angulated lesions is PTCA with a long balloon. The choice of balloon material is less important because of the high-degree of conformability of 30-40 mm balloons. If possible, a 0.014" guidewire is preferred since larger guidewires result in more vessel straightening. Inflation pressures ≤ 6 atm. are desirable to minimize the risk of dissection. Fixed wire-balloon systems are also quite conformable (due to the lack of a catheter shaft) and can be used to dilate angulated lesions.

The decision to perform new device angioplasty on angled lesions < 45-60° is based on associated lesion morphology. Severe angulation is a contraindication to the use of laser and atherectomy devices, particularly when the bulk of atherectomy is situated on the inner curve of the angled vessel segment (Figure 11.2). When severe dissections occur in severely angulated lesions, coil stents may track through the lesion; however, atheroma may prolapse through the coils, mandating the placement of multiple stents (Figure 11.3). Slotted tubular stents may provide more resistance to recoil and tissue prolapse, but may be more difficult to insert in angulated segments. Patients with severely angulated stenoses that supply large myocardial territories should be considered for bypass surgery, particularly in the presence of other lesion complexity or mutlivessel disease.

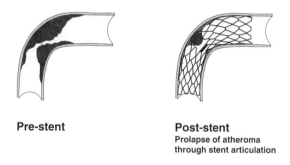

Pre-stent   **Post-stent**
                                 Prolapse of atheroma
                                 through stent articulation

Figure 11.3 Angulated Lesions: Stent Technique

Stenting of angulated lesions may be associated with prolapse of atheroma through the articulation (Palmaz-Schatz stents) or wire coils (Gianturco-Roubin stent). This problem can sometimes be treated by inserting another overlapping stent.

* * * * *

REFERENCES

1. Tan K, Sulke N, Taub N, Sowton E. Clinical and lesion morphologic determinants of coronary angioplasty success and complications: Current experience. J Am Coll Cardiol 1995;25:855-65.

2. Ellis SG, Vandormael MG, Cowley MJ, et al. Coronary morphologic and clinical determinants of procedural outcome with angioplasty for multivessel coronary disease. Implications for patient selection. Circulation 1990;82:1193-1202.

3. Gossman DE, Tuzcu EM, Simpfendorfer C, et al. Percutaneous transluminal angioplasty for Shepherd's Crook right coronary artery stenosis. Cathet Cardiovasc Diagn 1989;15:189-191.

4. Flood RD, Popma JJ, Chuang YC, Salter LF, et al. Incidence, angiographic predictors, and clinical significance of coronary perforation occurring after new device angioplasty. J Am Coll Cardiol 1994;23:301A.

5. Holmes DR, Berdan L, et al. Abrupt closure: The coronary angioplasty versus excisional atherectomy trial (CAVEAT) experience. J Am Coll Cardiol 1994;23:I-585A.

6. Ellis SG, Popma JJ, Buchbinder M, Franco I, et al. Relation of clinical presentation, stenosis morphology, and operator technique to the procedural results of rotational atherectomy and rotational atherectomy-facilitated angioplasty. Circulation 1994;89:882-892.

7. Hinohara T, Rowe MH, Robertson, GC, Selmon MR, et al. Effect of lesion characteristics on outcome of directional coronary atherectomy. J Am Coll Cardiol 1991;17:1112-20.

8. Ellis SG, De Cesare NB, Pinkerton CA, Whitlow P, et al. Relation of stenosis morphology and clinical presentation to the procedural results of directional coronary atherectomy. Circulation 1991;84:644-653.

9. Torre SR, Lai SM, Schatz RA. Relation of clinical presentation and lesion morphology to the procedural results of Palmaz-Schatz stent placement: A new approaches to coronary intervention (NACI) registry report. J Am Coll Cardiol 1994;23:135A.

10. Myler RK, Shaw RE, Stertzer SH, Hecht HS, et al. Lesion morphology and coronary angioplasty: Current experience and analysis. J Am Coll Cardiol 1992;19:1641-52.

11. Savas V, Puchrowicz S, Williams L, et al. Angioplasty outcome using long balloons in high-risk lesions. J Am Coll Cardiol 1992;19(3):34A.

12. Hermans WRM, Foley DP, Rensing BJ, Rutsch W, et al. Usefulness of quantitative and qualitative angiographic lesion morphology, and clinical characteristics in predicting major adverse cardiac events during and after native coronary balloon angioplasty. Am J Cardiol 1993;72:14-20.

13. Tenaglia AN, Zidar JP, Jackman JD, Fortin DF, et al. Treatment of long coronary artery narrowings with long angioplasty balloon catheters. Am J Cardiol 1993;71:1274-1277.

14. Ellis SG and Topol EJ. Results of percutaneous transluminal coronary angioplasty of high-risk angulated stenoses. Am J Cardiol 1990;66:932-937.

15. Barasch E, Conger JL, Janota T, Peters JJ, et al. PTCA of lesions on a bend: Effects of balloon material, balloon length, and inflation sequence. Circulation 1994;90:I-435.

16. Gray WA, Ghazzal ZMB, White HJ. The effects of balloon length and angle severity on the straightening force developed by polyethylene terephthalate (PET) angioplasty balloons. Circulation 1994;90(2):I-587.

17. Chevalier B, Commeau P, Favereau X, Gueri Y, et al. Limitations of rotational atherectomy in angulated coronary lesions. J Am Coll Cardiol 1994;23:285A.

18. Ghazzal ZMB, Hearn JA, Litvack F, Goldenberg T, et al. Morphological predictors of acute complications after percutaneous excimer laser coronary angioplasty. Results of a comprehensive angiographic analysis: Importance of the eccentricity index. Circulation 1992;86:820-827.

19. Bittl JA, Sanborn TA, Tcheng JE, Siegel RM, et al. Clinical success, complications, and restenosis rates with excimer laser coronary angioplasty. Am J Cardiol 1992;70:1533-1539.

20. Hong MK, Popma JJ, Wong SC, Kent KM, et al. Incidence of and factors associated with abrupt closure in patients undergoing elective, new device angioplasty in native coronary arteries. J Am Coll Cardiol 1995;25:122A.

21. Freed M, May M, Lichtenberg A, Strzelecki M, et al. Predictors of angiographic and clinical complications after new device coronary interventions. Circulation 1994;90:I-549.

22. Van Belle E, Bauters C, Lablanche JM, et al. Angiographic determinants of acute closure after coronary angioplasty: A prospective quantitative coronary angiographic study of 3679 procedures. J Am Coll Cardiol 1994;23:222A.

23. Meckel CR, Ahmed W, Ferguson JJ, Strony J, et al. Angiographic predictors of severe dissection during balloon angioplasty: A report from the Hirulog Angioplasty Study. Circulation 1994;90:I-64.

12 CALCIFIED LESIONS

Mark Freed, M.D.
Robert D. Safian, M.D.

In 1988, the American College of Cardiology/American Heart Association Task Force on Assessment of Diagnostic and Therapeutic Cardiovascular Procedures published a report regarding appropriate utilization of PTCA in the treatment of patients with coronary artery disease. In that report, moderate-to-heavy calcification (Type B characteristic) was considered to increase the risk of procedural failure and acute closure. Recent data suggest an improved acute outcome using a multi-device treatment strategy.

A. **LIMITATIONS OF ANGIOGRAPHY.** Intravascular ultrasound (IVUS) has been used to evaluate the depth and extent of coronary artery calcification, and to determine the sensitivity and specificity of coronary angiography for detecting calcium.[1,2] As seen in Table 12.1, the severity of angiographic calcium correlated with increasing arcs and lengths of calcium by IVUS. However, angiography demonstrated poor sensitivity for detecting mild-to-moderate lesion calcium, and only moderate sensitivity for extensive lesion calcium (Table 12.2). In addition, 11% of lesions with angiographic calcium failed to show calcium by IVUS (i.e., false positives). In another report, preinterventional IVUS — used to define the extent and depth of lesion calcium — resulted in a change in therapy in 40% of patients.[2] At the present time, it is unknown whether IVUS-guided therapy improves acute or long-term outcome. However, identification of superficial calcium occupying > 180° arc is associated with poor lumen enlargement after PTCA, but significantly better lumen enlargement after Rotablator. A prospective comparison between IVUS- and angiography-guided therapy suggests that IVUS can be useful for assessment of calcified lesions and for guiding therapy (Chapter 31).

Table 12.1. Assessment of Lesion Calcification By Angiography and IVUS [3]

	Angiographic Assessment of Calcification		
	None/Mild	**Moderate [+]**	**Severe [++]**
No. lesions	715	306	134
IVUS Findings			
lesion calcium (%)	61	90	98
arc of calcium (degrees)	71	165	238
length of calcium (mm)	3.6	7.2	9.7

+   Radiopacities noted during the cardiac cycle
++ Radiopacities noted without cardiac motion generally involving both sides of arterial lumen

Table 12.2. Sensitivity of Angiography for the Detection of Lesion Calcium[3]

IVUS Finding		Sensitivity of Angiography (%)*
Arc of calcium (degrees):	< 90	25
	91 - 180	50
	181 - 270	60
	271 - 360	85
Length of calcium (mm):	≤ 5	42
	6 - 10	63
	≥ 11	61
Location of calcium:	Superficial only	60
	Deep only	54
	Superficial + deep	24

*   Percent of calcified lesions on IVUS with calcium on angiography

B. BALLOON ANGIOPLASTY

1. **Acute Results.** The impact of lesion calcification on PTCA success is variable: One report showed lesion calcium to have an adverse impact on procedural success,[3] while another did not[4] (Table 12.3). In a third report, the presence of lesion calcium independently predicted significant residual stenosis among 3,679 dilated lesions.[5] Mechanisms of suboptimal angiographic outcome include the inability to crack the lesion and elastic recoil (Figure 12.1).

    Likewise, the impact of lesion calcification on major ischemic complications is variable: Some reports showed a correlation between lesion calcium and procedural death, MI, or emergency CABG, while others did not (Table 12.4). Differences in these findings probably reflect the insensitivity of angiography for identifying the depth and extent of lesion calcification, as well as nonuniform selection bias in triaging these lesions to ELCA or Rotablator.

2. **Coronary Artery Dissection.** IVUS has shown that lesion calcium plays a direct role in promoting dissection following PTCA. In a report involving 41 patients undergoing coronary and peripheral angioplasty, both the incidence (88% vs. 53% for non-calcified lesions) and extent of

Table 12.3. Influence of Lesion Calcium on Acute Outcome After PTCA

Series	Morphology	N	Success (%)
Tan[3]	Calcified	81	74
(1995)	Non-calcified	1076	94
Myler[4]	Calcified	140	92
(1992)	Non-calcified	639	95

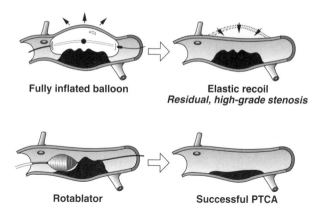

Fully inflated balloon   **Elastic recoil**
                                    Residual, high-grade stenosis

Rotablator   **Successful PTCA**

Figure 12.1 Elastic Recoil After PTCA of Calcified Lesions

Rather than cracking the hard, calcified atheroma, PTCA causes stretching of the contralateral plaque-free wall segment and ineffective dilatation. The Rotablator appears particularly well-suited for this lesion morphology based on its ability to ablate hard, calcified atheroma.

dissection was significantly higher among calcified lesions.[9] When present, the dissection usually originated at the transition point between calcified and noncalcified plaque, presumably due to nonuniform shear forces generated by balloon expansion. In another study of calcified lesions, the incidence of dissection increased from 22% after Rotablator to 77%, after adjunctive PTCA; there was also a shift in the location of dissection from inside to outside the calcified plaque.

3. **Restenosis.** The majority of reports have failed to show any association between lesion calcium and late lumen narrowing after PTCA.

4. **Technical Requirements.** Higher-than-usual inflation pressures are often required to "crack" calcified stenoses, increasing the risk of balloon rupture and vessel trauma. However, in one report, 89% of calcified lesions were successfully dilated with inflation pressures < 10 atm.[6] For heavily calcified lesions that resist dilation despite inflation pressures > 12 atm, use of a parallel guidewire external to the balloon ("force-focused angioplasty.")[10] or Rotablator atherectomy may increase lesion compliance, render the lesion more responsive to PTCA at low inflation pressures, and reduce the incidence of dissection. A 2.7F force-focused angioplasty balloon catheter, which integrates a second eccentric guidewire, is under investigation in Europe.[11] Although ELCA may be used for calcified lesions, the results are less predictable than after Rotablator.

C. **NEW INTERVENTIONAL DEVICES (Table 12.5).** Rotablator atherectomy, and to a lesser extent ELCA, are particularly useful for the management of moderate-to-heavily calcified lesions. In contrast, DCA and TEC have limited ability to resect calcified atheroma and are generally avoided in this

Table 12.4. Lesion Calcium and Ischemic Complications After PTCA

Series	Morphology	N	Complications (%)[+]	Comments
Tan[3] (1995)	Calcified	81	14*	
	Non-calcified	1076	2.5*	
Danchin[6] (1994)	Calcified	285	D / MI / CABG 0.8 / 3.5 / 0	
	Non-calcified	1801	0.7 / 3.0 / 1	
Hermans[7] (1993)	Calcified	69[+]	-	Lesion calcium did not predict major complications
Myler[4] (1992)	Calcified	140	3.6	
	Non-Calcified	639	1.3	
Ellis[8] (1990)	Calcified	46	-	Relative risk = 1.5

Abbreviations: D = death; Q-MI = in-hospital Q-wave myocardial infarction; CABG = emergency coronary artery bypass grafting; - = not reported
+ 69 pts. with a major complication randomly matched to 207 pts. without a major complication
* incidence of acute closure

situation. Although it is tempting to make "head-to-head" comparisons between devices based on the results of nonrandomized data, the substantial interdevice differences in baseline patient characteristics and lesion morphology may lead to improper conclusions and should be avoided unless restricted to carefully matched groups.

1. **Atherectomy**

    a. **Rotablator Atherectomy.** High procedural success (> 90%) and low complication rates (< 5%) can be achieved after Rotablator atherectomy of calcified stenoses.[13,15,26] In fact, Ellis et al[14] found that lesions *without* calcium were at greater risk of procedural complication compared to lesions with calcium. Conclusions regarding the impact of lesion calcium on restenosis have varied: In one report, the incidence of restenosis was no different among calcified and noncalcified lesions (54% vs. 50%),[15] while in another report, restenosis was 2-3 times more likely in calcified lesions.[27] Event-free survival (i.e., freedom from death, MI, CABG, or repeat intervention) was present in ~ 70% of patients at 1-year follow-up. Rotablator atherectomy preferentially ablates calcified atheroma;[28,29] results in a larger and more concentric lumen with fewer dissections in calcified vs. noncalcified lesions;[30] and produces microfractures in calcified deposits, increasing lesion compliance and rendering them more susceptible to PTCA.[29] Among 67 undilatable lesions treated with the Rotablator (73% of which were calcified), overall procedural success was 96%.[17] After atherectomy, 78% of previously undilatable lesions responded to inflation pressures < 6 atm. In an IVUS study of Rotablator followed by PTCA, DCA, or stents, Rotablator + stent achieved the largest lumen

Table 12.5. New Interventional Angioplasty of Calcified Lesions: Acute Outcome

Series	Device	Morphology	N	Success (%)	Complications(%)[++] D / Q-MI / CABG	Comments
Dussaillant[41] (1996)	ROTA/STENT ROTA/DCA ROTA/PTCA	Calcified (vessel ≥ 3mm)	83 120 235	- - -	0 - -	FDS(%): 12 16 24
Mintz[12] (1995)	ROTA/STENT	Calcified (vessel ≥ 3mm)	88	-	-	No subacute thrombosis
Warth[13] (1994)	ROTA	All lesions Calcified	346 107	(85) 95 (92) 97	2.6 1.9	
Ellis[14] (1994)	ROTA	Calcified	232	91	-	
MacIssac[15] (1994)	ROTA	Noncalcified Calcified	1083 1078	95 94	0.5 / 0.5 / 2.4 1.3 / 0.6 / 2.2	RS(%): 50 54
Altmann[16] (1993)	ROTA	No/mild Ca[++] Mod. Ca[++]	182 378	96 96	0.7 / 0 / 1.4 0.7 / 0 / 2.1	EFS(%): 67 75
Reisman[17] (1993)	ROTA	Undilatable stenoses	67	96	0 / 0 / 1.5	RS(%): 36
Popma[18] (1993)	DCA	All lesions Mild-mod Ca[++]	306 60	95 94	- -	EFS(%): 72 80
Hinohara[19] (1991)	DCA	Type A Calcified	105 70	(97) 98 (70) 87	0 5.7	
Ellis[20] (1991)	DCA	Calcified	47	-	-	Relative risk of failure 1.98
TEC[21] database	TEC	Noncalcified Calcified	278 154	(88) 96 (65) 89	- -	
Bittl[22] (1993)	ELCA	Undilatable stenoses	36	92	-	Non Q-MI: 6%
Bittl[23] (1992)	ELCA	Calcified	170	83*	-	RS(%): 43
Levine[24] (1991)	ELCA	Calcified	95	(72) 96	0 / 2 / 2	
deMarchena[25] (1994)	Holmium-laser	All lesions Calcified	365 111	(85) 94 (78) 90	2.7 4.5	

Abbreviations: DCA = Directional Coronary Atherectomy; TEC = Transluminal Extraction Atherectomy; ELCA = Excimer Laser Coronary Angioplasty; EFS = 1-year event-free survival; AC = Abrupt Closure; RS = Restenosis; FDS = Final Diameter Stenosis; - not reported

+   Success is final residual stenosis < 50% (after adjunctive PTCA) without death, Q-wave MI, or emergent CABG; Number in parenthesis is device success before PTCA (for ROTA, TEC & ELCA, success is ≥ 20% reduction in stenosis.

++   Single value denotes overall in-hospital complication rate and smallest residual stenosis (Rota + PTCA = 24%; Rota + DCA = 16%; Rota + stent = 12%, p < 0.0001). At the present time, Rotablator atherectomy is the preferred method of revascularizing moderate-to-heavily calcified stenoses.

b. **Directional Coronary Atherectomy (DCA).** This device has a very limited ability to excise calcified plaque and should be avoided when moderate-to-heavy lesion calcium is present. IVUS studies clearly show that the presence and extent of lesion calcium correlates with ineffective plaque removal after primary DCA.[18,31-34] (DCA may be able to resect calcified plaque after primary Rotablator atherectomy or ELCA.[35]) DCA should also be avoided when there is significant calcification proximal to the target lesion since failure of the device to negotiate rigid calcified vessels and the risk of unroofing proximal plaque are increased. Further improvements in DCA technology and the availability of a special calcium-cutter may increase the application of DCA to calcified lesions.

c. **TEC Atherectomy.** TEC has an extremely limited ability to cut calcium and should not be used on heavily calcified lesions. Because of the excellent flexibility of TEC cutters, vessel calcification proximal to the target lesion is not a contraindication to TEC atherectomy.

2. **Lasers**
   a. **Excimer Laser Coronary Angioplasty (ELCA).** Among 170 calcified lesions treated with ELCA, procedural success (final stenosis < 50% without death, MI, abrupt closure, or emergency CABG) was achieved in 83% — slightly lower than noncalcified stenoses.[23] Improved results may be obtained by starting with small fibers (e.g., 1.3 mm) and lasing with higher fluence (50-60 mJ/mm^2). Although one report found an association between lesion calcification and major complications,[23] two reports did not.[36,37] Restenosis occurs in 40-50% of lesions after ELCA and appears to be independent of lesion calcification.[23] In contrast to Rotablator atherectomy,[29] which actually removes lesion calcium, ELCA increases vessel compliance and renders the lesion more responsive to PTCA by fracturing (rather than removing) intraplaque calcium.[38] Like the Rotablator, ELCA is effective in treating undilatable stenoses. In one report, 33/36 (92%) resistant lesions were successfully treated by ELCA.[22]

   b. **Holmium Laser Angioplasty.** Analysis of the Holmium Laser Coronary Registry revealed lower procedural success and a trend toward more ischemic complications among calcified stenoses. Nevertheless, final results were acceptable and similar to those achieved by ELCA; among 111 calcified stenoses, laser crossing occurred in 78%, procedural success in 90%, and major complications in 4.5%.[25]

3. **Stents.** Heavy lesion calcium increases the risk of incomplete stent expansion[34] and restenosis.[39] Even when heavily calcified plaque is first modified by the Rotablator, final lumen cross-sectional area after stenting may be smaller than in lesions without calcification,[40] but is still larger than the combination of Rotablator followed by PTCA[12,14] or DCA.[14] If a lesion cannot be fully dilated with

a balloon, stent placement is contraindicated since incomplete stent expansion greatly increases the risk of stent thrombosis.

4. **Device Synergy.** Small observational reports suggest that sequential use of Rotablator atherectomy or ELCA (to partially resect or modify lesion calcium) followed by DCA[35] or stenting[40] may facilitate lumen enlargement and improve outcome. Prospective randomized studies will be required to adequately address these issues.

D. TECHNICAL STRATEGY (Figures 12.2, 12.3)

1. Superficial ± Deep Calcium

a. Focal Lesions. If calcification is present on angiography, IVUS should be used to guide therapy based on the depth and extent of lesion calcium (Figure 12.3). For moderate-to-heavily calcified focal stenoses, we recommend Rotablator atherectomy; adjunctive PTCA (using a low-pressure [< 4 atm.] inflation with a noncompliant balloon), DCA, or stenting often results in excellent lumen enlargement without dissection. ELCA is an acceptable alternative; when performed, small initial fibers (1.3 mm), high fluence (50-60 mJ/mm^2), and use of the saline-infusion technique are recommended (Chapter 30). Whether Rotablator or ELCA is chosen, IVUS is used to guide burr (or fiber) sizing, asses the degree of calcium removal, and guide further adjunctive treatment with PTCA, DCA, or stenting. If adjunctive PTCA fails to fully dilate the lesion despite high pressures, "force-focused" angioplasty should be considered: To perform this technique, a *second* guidewire is steered beyond the lesion (after the balloon has been withdrawn into the guide); the balloon is then advanced over the original wire and inflated. The second parallel wire, which acts as a "cutting wire," longitudinally concentrates dilating force and may improve angiographic outcome. The Barath "cutting balloon," a conventional angioplasty balloon with 3-4 longitudinal microtomes, focally incises plaque during balloon inflation and may be advantagous in calcified lesions (Chapter 8).

b. Long Lesions. The ideal treatment of long, calcified lesions is unknown. PTCA may be attempted using a long balloon, but the risk of dissection or suboptimal result may be increased. ELCA is theoretically suited for long lesions; however, its use in hard, calcified lesions may be associated with dissection and incomplete calcium ablation. The Rotablator is effective in treating calcified stenoses up to 10 mm in length; however, its use in longer lesions may be associated with an increased risk of no-reflow, non-Q-wave MI, and restenosis. Slow passes with a small burr (≤ 1.75 mm), with a stepwise increase in burr size not to exceed 0.25 mm, may result in excellent pulverization of calcium, few complications, and good angiographic results.

2. **Deep Calcium Only.** Unlike calcium located at the intimal-lumen interface, deep tissue calcium (at or near the medial-adventitial border) does not usually interfere with PTCA, DCA, or stenting. Initial use of Rotablator or ELCA is not generally required, and device selection can be based on associated lesion morphologies.

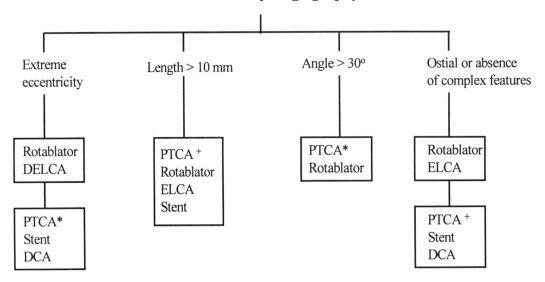

Figure 12.2. Treatment of Calcified Stenoses When IVUS Is <u>NOT</u> Available

Abbreviations: DELCA = directional excimer laser angioplasty; DCA = directional coronary atherectomy

*   High-pressure balloon or longitudinal force-focused PTCA for PTCA failure

+   High-pressure long balloon

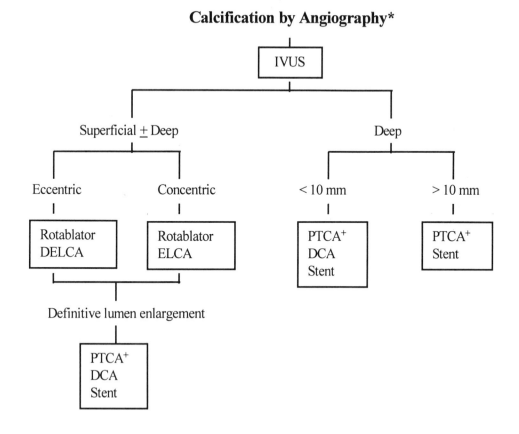

Calcification by Angiography*

Figure 12.3. Treatment of Calcified Stenoses When IVUS is Available

Abbreviations: DELCA = directional excimer laser angioplasty; DCA = directional coroanry atherectomy

* Calcified lesions associated with severe proximal vessel tortuosity or angulation may be unsuitable for all devices except PTCA.

+ High-pressure balloon.

REFERENCES

1. Mintz G, Popma J, et al. Patterns of calcification in coronary artery disease. A statistical analysis of intravascular ultrasound and coronary angiography in 1155 lesions. Circulation 1995;91:1959-1965.
2. Mintz GS, Pichard AD, Kovach JA, et al. Impact of preintervention intravascular ultrasound imaging on transcatheter treatment strategies in coronary artery disease. Am J Cardiol 1994;73:423-430.
3. Tan, K., N. Sulke, et al. Clinical and lesion morphologic determinants of coronary angioplasty success and complications: Current experience. J Am Coll Cardiol 1995;25:855-65.
3b. Braden GA, Herrington DM, Kerensky RA, Kutcher MA, Little WC. Angiography poorly predicts actual lesion eccentricity in severe coronary stenoses: Confirmation by intracoronary ultrasound imaging. J Am Coll Cardiol 1994;March Special Issue:413A.
4. Myler RK, Shaw RE, Stertzer SH, et al. Lesion Morphology and Coronary Angioplasty: Current Experience and Analysis. J Am Coll Cardiol 1992;19:1641-52.
5. Van Belle, E, Bauters C, Lablanche JM, McFadden EP, Quandalle P, Bertrand ME. Angiographic determinants of acute outcome after coronary angioplasty: A prospective quantitaitve coronary angiographic study of 3679 procedures. J Am Coll Cardiol 1994;March Special Issue:222A.
6. Danchin N, Buffet P, Dibon O, et al. Should specific angioplasty techniques be used to treat calcified coronary artery lesions? A retrospective study. Circulation 1994;90:I-436.
7. Hermans WR, Foley D, et al. Usefulness of quantitative and qualitative angiographic lesion morphology, and clinical characteristics in predicting major adverse cardiac events during and after native coronary balloon angioplasty. Am J Cardiol 1993;72:14-20.
8. Ellis SG, Vandormael MG, Cowley MJ, et al. Coronary morphologic and clinical determinants of procedural outcome with angioplasty for multivessel coronary disease. Implications for patient selection. Circulation 1990;82:1193-1202.
9. Fitzgerald P, Ports T, Yock P. Contribution of localized calcium deposits to dissection after angioplasty: An observational study using IVUS. Circulation 1992;86:64-70.
10. Khurana S, Bakalyar D, Schreiber T, et al. Facilitated lumen enlargement by longitudinal force focused angioplasty. J Am Coll Cardiol 1995;March Special Issue:345A.
11. Solar RJ, Meaney DF, Miller RT, et al. Enhanced lumen enlargement with new focused force angioplasty device. Circulation 1995;92:I-147.
12. Mintz GS, Dusaillant GR, Wong SC, Pichard AD, et al. Rotational atherectomy followed by adjunct stents: The preferred therapy for calcified lesions in large vessels? Circulation 1995;92:I-329.
13. Warth D, Leon M, et al. Rotational atherectomy multicenter registry: Acute results, complications and 6-month angiographic follow-up in 709 patients. J Am Coll Cardiol 1994;24:641-648.
14. Ellis S, Popma J, et al. Relation of clinical presentation, stenosis morphology, and operator technique to the procedural results of rotational atherectomy-facilitated angioplasty. Circulation 1994;89:882-892.
15. MacIssac AI, Whitlow PL, Cowley MJ, Buchbinder M. Angiographic predictors of outcome of coronary rotational atherectomy from the completed multicenter registry. J Am Coll Cardiol 1994;March Special Issue:353A.
16. Altmann DB, Popma JJ, Kent KM, et al. Rotational atherectomy effectively treats calcified lesions. J Am Coll Cardiol 1993;21 (Part II):443A.
17. Reisman M, Devlin PG, Melikian J, Fenner J, Buchbinder M. Undilatable noncompliant lesions treated with the rotatblator: Outcome and angiographic follow-up. Circulation 1993;Speical Issue:2949.
18. Popma JJ, Mintz GS, Satler LF, et al. Clinical and angiographic outcome after directional coronary atherectomy. A qualitative and quantitative analysis using coronary arteriography and intravascular ultrasound. Am J Cardiol 1993;72:55E-64E.
19. Hinohara T, Rowe MH, Robertson GC, et al. Effect of lesion characteristics on outcome of directional coronary atherectomy. Circulation 1991;17:1112-1120.
20. Ellis SG, De Cesare NB, Pinkerton CA, et al. Relation of stenosis morphology and clinical presentation to the procedural results of directional coronary atherectomy. Circulation 1991;84:644-653.
21. IVT® Coronary TEC® Atherectomy Clinical Database Investigators Meeting. 1992.
22. Bittl JA, Sanborn TA, Tcheng JE, Watson LE. Excimer laser-facilitated angioplasty for undilatable coronary lesions: Results of a prospective, controlled study. Circulation 1993;March Special Issue:0118.
23. Bittl J, Sanborn T, et al. Clinical success, complications and restenosis rates with excimer laser coronary angioplasty.

Am J Cardiol 1992;70:1533-1539.

24. Levine S, Mehta S, Krauthamer D, et al. Excimer laser coronary angioplasty of calcified lesions. J Am Coll Cardiol 1991;17(2):206A.

25. deMarchena EJ, Mallon SM, et al. Effectiveness of holmium laser-assisted coronary angioplasty. Am J Cardiol 1994;73:117-121.

26. Leon MB, Kent KM, Pichard AD, et al. Percutaneous transluminal coronary rotational angioplasty of calcified lesions. Circulation 1991;84(4):II-521.

27. Leguizamon JH, Chambre DF, Torresani EM, et al. High-speed coronary rotational atherectomy. Are angiographic factors predictive of failure, major complications or restenosis? A multivariate analysis. J Am Coll Cardiol 1995:Special Issue:95A.

28. Mintz G, Potkin B, et al. Intravascular ultrasound evaluation of the effect of rotational atherectomy in obstructive atherosclerotic coronary artery disease. Circulation 1992;86:1383-1393.

29. Kovach J, Mintz G, et al. Sequential intravascular ultrasound characterization of the mechanisms of rotational atherectomy and adjunct balloon angioplasty. J Am Coll Cardiol 1993;22 (4):1024-32.

30. Fitzgerald PJ, Stertzer SH, Hidalgo BO, Myler RK, et al. Plaque characteristics affect lesion and vessel response to coronary rotational atherectomy: An intravascular ultrasound Study. J Am Coll Cardiol 1994;March Special Issue:353A.

31. De Franco AC, Tuzcu EM, Moliterno DJ, et al. "Directional" coronary atherectomy removes atheroma more effectively from concentric than eccentric lesions: Intravascular ultrasound predictors of lesional success. J Am Coll Cardiol 1995;March Special Issue:137A.

32. Matar FA, Mintz GS, Kent KM, et al. Predictors of intravascular ultrasound endpoints after directional coronary atherectomy in 170 patients. J Am Coll Cardiol 1994;March Special Issue:302A.

33. DeLezo JS, Romero M, Medina A, et al. Intraocoronary ultrasound assessment of directional coronary atherectomy: Immediate and follow-up findings. J Am Coll Cardiol 1993;21:298-307.

34. Hong MK, Chuang YC, Prunka N, Satler LF. Predictors of early and late cardiac events in patients undergoing saphenous vein graft angioplasty with PTCA and new device modalities. Circulation 1993;88:I-601.

35. Henson KD, Flood R, Javier SP, et al. Transcatheter device synergy: Use of adjunct directional atherectomy after rotational atherectomy or excimer laser angioplasty. J Am Coll Cardiol 1994;March Special Issue:220A.

36. Ghazzal Z, Hearn J, et al. Morphological predictors of acute complications after percutaneous excimer laser coronary angioplasty. Results of a comprehensive angiographic analysis: Importance of the eccentricity index. Circulation 1992;86:820-827.

37. Baumbach A, Bittl J, Fleck E, et al. Acute complications of excimer laser coronary angioplasty: A detailed analysis of multicenter results. J Am Coll Cardiol 1994;23(6):1305-1313.

38. Mintz GS, Kovach JA, Javier SP, et al. Mechanisms of lumen enlargement after excimer laser angioplasty: An intravascular ultrasound study. Circulation 1995;92:3408-14.

39. Tamura T, Kimura T, Nosaka H, Nobuyoshi M. Predictors of restenosis after Palmaz-Schatz stent implantation. Circulation 1994;90:I-324.

40. Goldberg SL, Hall P, Almagor Y, Maiello L, et al. Intravascular ultrasound guided rotational atherectomy of fibro-calcific plaque prior to intracoronary deployment of Palmaz-Schatz stents. J Am Coll Cardiol 1994;March Special Issue:290A.

41. Dussaillant GR, Mintz GS, Pichard AD, et al. The optimal strategy for treating calcified lesions in large vessels: Comparison of intravascular of intravascular ultrasound results of rotational atherectomy + adjunctive PTCA, DCA, or stents. J Am Coll Cardiol 1996;March Special Issue.

13 ECCENTRIC LESIONS

Mark Freed, M.D.

A. **LIMITATIONS OF ANGIOGRAPHY.** Contrast angiography has poor predictive value for the detection of eccentric plaque morphology. In one report of angiographically-apparent eccentric lesions, only 30/48 (63%) had eccentric plaque morphology by intravascular ultrasound (IVUS), and 21/30 (70%) of angiographically "concentric" lesions were eccentric by IVUS.[1] In a second report, concordance between IVUS and angiography for assessment of lesion eccentricity was only 53%.[2] Eccentric stenoses were found to have greater luminal cross-sectional areas and less calcium than concentric stenoses, suggesting a less advanced form of coronary atherosclerosis. Although eccentricity is usually considered a dichotomous characteristic (i.e., present or absent), more than 2/3 of all coronary stenoses are classified as having some degree of eccentricity.

B. **DEFINITIONS OF ECCENTRIC LESIONS**

Angiographic	Lumen in outer 1/4 of the apparent normal lumen.
IVUS	Ratio of maximal-to-minimal plaque thickness > 2-3, or relative sparing of a portion of the vessel circumference (i.e., minimum plaque thickness < 0.75 mm) .
Pathological	Arc of disease-free vessel wall. (In one report, only 17% of 963 lesions met this definition by IVUS.[2])

C. **BALLOON ANGIOPLASTY (Table 13.1).** High success (> 90%) and low complication rates (< 3-4 %) have been consistently reported for PTCA of most eccentric lesions.[3,4] While originally classified as a "Type B" characteristic (procedural success 60-85%, increased risk of acute closure), most data indicate that lesion eccentricity does not adversely affect procedural success or restenosis.[3-5] Observational reports suggest that compared to concentric lesions, PTCA of eccentric lesions may be associated with more elastic recoil,[6] less effective plaque compression,[7] more vasospasm,[8] and suboptimal lumen enlargement.

D. **NEW INTERVENTIONAL DEVICES (Table 13.1)**
   1. **Directional Atherectomy.** Directional coronary atherectomy (DCA) is highly effective for treating lesions with mild, moderate, and extreme eccentricity.[9] However, when compared to concentric lesions, eccentric lesions required more adjunctive PTCA (13% vs. 3%) and developed more complications (3.2% vs 0%).[10] Greater degrees of eccentricity also correlated with higher rates of restenosis after LAD atherectomy (eccentricity of 0-5%, 51-75%, and 76-99% yielded restenosis

Table 13.1. Percutaneous Revascularization of Eccentric Stenoses

Series	Modality	Morphology	N	Success[+] (%)	Complications[*] (%)
Tan[3] (1995)	PTCA	Concentric	491	93	AC: 2.6
		Eccentric	666	92	3.8
Myler[4] (1992)	PTCA	Concentric	304	92	2.6
		Eccentric	475	96	1.1
Popma[12] (1993)	DCA	Concentric	71	96	-
		Eccentric	235	94	-
Hinohara[13] (1991)	DCA	Concentric	116	92	CABG: 1.73.3
		Eccentric (mild-mod)	122	86	2.4
		Eccentric (extreme)	85	95	
Warth[14] (1994)	Rotablator	Concentric	141	98	0
		Eccentric	205	93	4.4
Multicenter Registry[15] (1992)	TEC	Concentric	207	96	-
		Eccentric	316	92	-
AIS[16] Database (1992)	ELCA	Concentric	135	92	-
		Eccentric	174	89	-
Leon[17] (1993)	DELCA	Concentric	22	90% overall	Death: 0.9
		Eccentric	110		Q-MI: 0.9
					CABG: 3.8
					AC: 3.8
Ghazzal[18] (1993)	DELCA	62/150 (41%) with extreme eccentricity	-	91% overall	-
Resar[19] (1993)	DELCA	Eccentric	66	95	3

Abbreviations: DCA = Directional Coronary Atherectomy; TEC = Transluminal Extraction Atherectomy; ELCA = Excimer Laser Coronary Angioplasty; DELCA = Direction ELCA; EFS = event-free survival; D = death; Q-MI = Q-wave myocardial infarction; CABG = emergency coronary artery bypass grafting; AC = abrupt closure; - = not reported
+   < 50% residual stenosis after device (and adjunctive PTCA) without death, MI, or emergency CABG
*   Single value represents combined incidence of in-hospital death, Q-MI, or emergency CABG, unless otherwise stated

rates of 36%, 43%, and 67%, respectively).[11] Importantly, DCA outcome is highly dependent on associated lesion morphology: DCA success occurred in 95% of eccentric lesions with irregular contour, 86% of eccentric lesions that were long, and only 64% of eccentric lesions that were calcified.[10]   In another report of eccentric lesions, DCA success was 94% and 1-year event-free survival was 72%.[12] Contrary to popular belief, IVUS imaging revealed less plaque resection after

DCA (19% for eccentric vs. 30% for concentric lesions, p=0.02). However, new DCA catheters with the capability of simultaneous ultrasound imaging and tissue excision may improve lumen enlargement and decrease complications.

2. **Rotablator.** For rigid or calcified eccentric stenoses, Rotablator may be useful because of its ability to selectively pulverize hard tissue (principle of differential cutting). Although Rotablator can be used to treat other types of eccentric lesions,[20,21] it may not have any advantage over conventional PTCA. Lesion eccentricity (in addition to tortuousity and lesion length > 10mm) was shown to predict of coronary perforation[22] and intralesional spasm after Rotablator.[23]

3. **TEC Atherectomy.** TEC has no special value in native coronary arteries with eccentric lesions.[15] However, it may be a useful adjunct for eccentric lesions with associated thrombus in saphenous vein bypass grafts (Chapter 17).

4. **Excimer Laser.** Although data from the ELCA registry suggest that lesion eccentricity does not adversely affect procedural success, major complications,[24] or restenosis,[25] angiographic analysis of 220 lesions suggested that lesion eccentricity is a risk factor for the development of emergency CABG, perforation, acute closure, or Q-wave MI.[26] For lesions with extreme eccentricity, particularly in vessels < 3 mm in diameter, directional ELCA may be preferable to conventional ELCA. This excimer system is comprised of an array of eccentrically-arranged fibers that can be directed toward eccentric plaque and away from angiographically normal vessel wall (Figure 13.1). Directional ELCA can successfully treat > 90% of highly eccentric lesions,[27] with significant reduction in plaque mass[17] and only 11% elastic recoil.[18] Final diameter stenosis following directional laser + adjunctive PTCA was 24%, but longterm results are lacking.

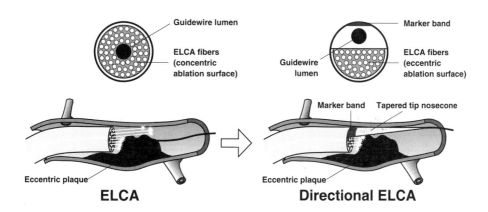

Figure 13.1 Directional ELCA of Eccentric Lesions

When using conventional ELCA for eccentric lesions, part of the concentric ablation surface does not make contact with the plaque. In contrast, the eccentric plaque is fully exposed to the eccentric ablation surface when using directional ELCA.

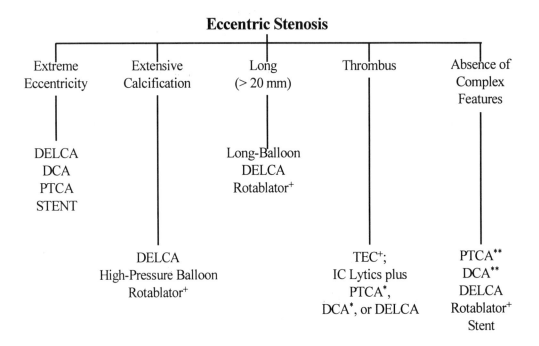

Figure 13.2 Percutaneous Management of Eccentric Stenoses: A Multi-Device Approach

ELCA	Excimer Laser Coronary Angioplasty
DCA	Directional Coronary Atherectomy
TEC	Transluminal Extraction Catheter Atherectomy
+	Mild-moderate eccentricity
*	Should be avoided if a large amount of clot is present
**	Economical approach: TEC, ELCA, Rotablator frequently require adjunctive PTCA

5. **Stents.** Virtually all stent designs are capable of treating lesions with all types of abnormal contour, including eccentric lesions. Stents are unmatched in their ability to enlarge lumen dimensions, resist elastic recoil, and decrease dissection, all of which are important consideration when treating eccentric lesions. Although there is some experience in vessels < 3 mm in diameter, stents are best suited for native vessels or bypass grafts ≥ 3 mm in diameter. The favorable results of simplified anticoagulation regimens (i.e., without warfarin) may make stents the treatment of choice for a wide range of lesions, including those with eccentric morphology. There are insufficient data comparing different stents, but the Palmaz-Schatz stent appears to have the most radial strength and least elastic recoil of all currently available stent designs. In the STRESS trial, late loss was greater in concentric lesions compared to eccentric lesions.[27]

E. **TECHNICAL STRATEGY (Figure 13.2)**

REFERENCES

1. Braden GA, Herrington DM, Kerensky RA, et al. Angiography poorly predicts actual lesion eccentricity in severe coronary stenoses: Confirmation by intracoronary ultrasound imaging. J Am Coll Cardiol 1994;Special Issue:413A.

2. Mintz GS, Popma JJ, Pichard AD, Kent KM, et al. Comparison of intravascular ultrasound and coronary angiography in the assessment of target lesion plaque distribution in coronary artery disease. TCT Meeting (Washington DC), February, 1995; Abstract.

3. Tan K, Sulke N, et al. Clinical and lesion morphologic determinants of coronary angioplasty success and complications: Current experience. J Am Coll Cardiol 1995;25:855-65.

4. Myler RK, Shaw RE, Stertzer SH, et al. Lesion morphology and coronary angioplasty: current experience and analysis. J Am Coll Cardiol 1992;19:1641-52.

5. Ellis SG, Vandormael MG, Cowley MJ, et al. Coronary morphologic and clinical determinants of procedural outcome with angioplasty for multivessel coronary disease. Implications for patient selection. Circulation 1990;82:1193-1202.

6. Kimball BP, Eric SB, Cohen EA, et al. Comparison of acute elastic recoil after directional coronary atherectomy versus standard balloon angioplasty. Am Heart J 1992;124:1459.

7. Baptista J, diMario C, Ozaki Y, de Feyter P, deJaegere P, Roelandt J, Serruys PW. Deterinants of lumen and plaque changes after balloon angioplasty: A quantitative ultrasound study. J Am Coll Cardiol 1994;March Special Issue:414A.

8. Fiscell TA, Bausback KN. Effects of luminal eccentricity on spontaneous coronary vasoconstriction after successful percutaneous transluminal coronary angioplasty. Am J Cardiol 1991;68:530.

9. Matar FA, Mintz GS, Kent KM, Pinnow E, et al. Predictors of intravascular ultrasound endpoints after directional coronary atherectomy in 170 patients. J Am Coll Cardiol 1994;March Special Issue:302A.

10. Ellis S, Popma J, et al. Relation of clinical presentation, stenosis morphology, and operator technique to the procedural results of rotational atherectomy-facilitated angioplasty. Circulation 1994;89:882-892.

11. Schiele TM, Marx R, Vogt M, Leschke M, et al. Eccentricity of coronary arteries is a predictor of chronic restenosis after directional coronary atherectomy. Circulation 1995;92:I-328.

12. Popma JJ, Mintz GS, Satler LF, et al. Clinical and angiographic outcome after directional coronary atherectomy. A qualitative and quantitative analysis using coronary arteriography and intravascular ultrasound. Am J Cardiol 1993;72:55E-64E.

13. Hinohara T, Vetter JW, Selmon MR, et al. Directional coronary atherectomy is effective treatment for extremely eccentric lesions. Circulation 1991;84(4):II-520.

14. Warth D, Leon M, et al. Rotational atherectomy multicenter registry: Acute results, complications and 6-month angiographic follow-up in 709 patients. J Am Coll Cardiol 1994;24:641-648.

15. IVT® Coronary TEC® Atherectomy Clinical Database Investigators Meeting. 1992.

16. Advanced Interventional Systems Coronary Excimer Laser Database. Goldenberg T. 1992.

17. Leon MB, Henson KD, Lavier SP, et al. Early results with directional laser angioplasty is unfavorable coronary lesions. Circulation 1993;88(4);I-23.

18. Ghazzal ZMB, Litvack F, Rothbaum DA, Shefer A, King SB. The directional laser catheter: Quantitative angiographic core lab analysis from the first five centers. Circulation 1993;Special Issue:0113.

19. Fitzgerald PJ. Lesion composition impacts size and symmetry of stent expansion: Initial report from the STRUT Registry. J Am Coll Cardiol 1995;March Special Issue;49A.

20. MacIssac AI, Whitlow PL, Cowley MJ, Buchbinder M. Angiographic predictors of outcome of coronary rotational atherectomy from the completed multicenter registry. J Am Coll Cardiol 1994;March Special Issue:353A.

21. Leguizamon JH, Chambre DF, Torresani EM, et al. High-speed coronary rotational atherectomy. Are angiographic factors predictive of failure, major complications or restenosis? A multivariate analysis. J Am Coll Cardiol 1995:March Special Issue:95A.

22. Hong MK, Chuang YC, Prunka N, Satler LF. Predictors of early and late cardiac events in patients undergoing saphenous vein graft angioplasty with PTCA and new device modalities. Circulation 1993;88:I-601.

23. Fitzgerald PJ, Stertzer SH, Hidalgo BO, Myler RK, Shaw RE, Yock PG. Plaque characteristics affect lesion and vessel response to coronary rotational atherectomy: An intravascular ultrasound study. J Am Coll Cardiol 1994;March Special Issue:353A.

24. Baumbach A, Bittl J, Fleck E, et al. Acute complications of excimer laser coronary angioplasty: A detailed analysis of multicenter results. J Am Coll Cardiol 1994;23(6):1305-1313.

25. Bittl J, Sanborn T, et al. Clinical success, complications and restenosis rates with excimer laser coronary angioplasty. Am J Cardiol 1992;70:1533-1539.

26. Ghazzal Z, Hearn J, et al. Morphological predictors of acute complications after percutaneous excimer laser coronary angioplasty. Results of a comprehensive angiographic analysis: Importance of the eccentricity index. Circulation 1992;86:820-827.

27. Rechavia E, Federman J, Shefer A, et al. Usefulness of a prototype directional excimer laser coronary angioplasty catheter in narrowings unfavorable for conventional excimer of balloon angioplasty. Am J Cardiol 1995;76:1144-46.

14 OSTIAL LESIONS

Mark Freed, M.D.

The presence of an ostial stenosis poses a special management problem for the interventional cardiologist. Of all lesions considered for PTCA, ostial lesions are the most likely to be associated with suboptimal angiographic results due to lesion rigidity and elastic recoil. Aggressive efforts to improve lumen dimensions frequently result in further elastic recoil, dissection, and a high incidence of restenosis. In contrast to non-ostial lesions, the successful treatment of ostial lesions is most dependent on the use of new interventional devices.

A. DEFINITIONS

1. **Aorto-Ostial Stenosis.** A lesion that involves the junction between the aorta and the orifice of the RCA, left main, or a saphenous vein graft.

2. **Branch-Ostial Stenosis**. A lesion that involves the junction between a large epicardial vessel and the orifice of a major branch. In some studies, these are referred to as "origin" lesions.

3. **Other.** Some reports define an ostial lesion as one that is located within 3-5 mm of the vessel orifice, but does not necessarily involve the ostium. The subtleties of these various definitions are important when considering safety and efficacy data reported in studies of ostial lesions.

B. RESULTS

1. **Balloon Angioplasty (Table 14.1).** The earliest study of PTCA of ostial RCA stenoses reported procedural success in 79% and emergency CABG in 9%.[9] These poor results were attributed to inadequate guide support, the frequency of rigid lesions and elastic recoil, and ostial trauma due to high inflation pressures and guiding catheter injury. Since that time, procedural success and complication rates have improved, primarily because of enormous technical advances in PTCA hardware (balloons, guidewires, guiding catheters) and increased operator experience. More recent data indicate that highly-selected ostial lesions can be revascularized almost as effectively as nonostial stenoses.[1,2,8] Nevertheless, even though PTCA success and complication rates have improved, careful quantitative angiographic studies report final residual stenoses of 40-50% for ostial lesions, compared to 25-35% for nonostial lesions.[8] In addition, elastic recoil — accounting for up to a 50% loss in acute luminal gain — is commonly encountered in ostial lesions, even in the absence of other complex characteristics such as calcification, ulceration, and eccentricity. These suboptimal angiographic results may not manifest as acute ischemic complications, but certainly account for the high incidence of restenosis and the need for repeat intervention. It is the poor immediate angiographic result after PTCA of ostial lesions that has generated so much interest and enthusiasm for other new interventional devices.

Table 14.1. PTCA of Ostial Stenoses: Acute Outcome

Series	Lesion	N	Success* (%)	Complications**(%) D/Q-MI/CABG	Other
Tan[1] (1995)	Nonostial AO + BO	1080 77	93 94	- -	Acute closure: 0% 3.5%
Tan[2] (1994)	Nonostial AO BO	48 34 116	90 85 87	6 6 7	Residual stenosis, no. of inflations, and max. inflation pres. highest for AO lesions.
Boehrer[3] (CAVEAT; 1995)	LAD	33	87	0 / 0 / 3	Restenosis (46%)
Sawada[4] (1994)	LAD/LCX	80	90	-	Restenosis (61%) TLR (58%)
Brown[5] (1993)	Ostial LAD Nonostial LAD	40 40	100 98	0 / - / 0 0 / - / 0	-
Myler[6] (1992)	AO + BO	14	93	0	-
Bedotto[7] (1991)	AO	60	85	0	-
Mathias[8] (1991)	BO	106	74	13	-
Topol[9] (1987)	AO	53	79	9.4	Restenosis (38%)

Abbreviations: AO = aorto-ostial; BO = branch-ostial; EFS = event-free survival (freedom from death, MI, CABG, repeat PTCA); D = death; Q-MI = Q-wave myocardial infarction; CABG = emergency coronary artery bypass grafting; LAD = left anterior descending coronary artery; LCX = left circumflex coronary artery; TLR = target lesion revascularization; - = not reported
*   ≤ 50% residual stenosis
**   Single number denotes overall in-hospital complication rate
***   Includes 19 coronary lesions and 22 saphenous vein graft lesions
+   Undersized balloon followed by optimal size balloon
++   Includes 24 ostial lesions in saphenous vein grafts
+++   Includes 48 saphenous vein graft lesions

2. **New Interventional Devices.** Nonrandomized data have been collected on more than 1000 ostial lesions treated with atherectomy, lasers, and stents (Table 14.2). Despite unfavorable lesion characteristics, procedural success rates > 90% and low complications can be achieved. Stenting,

DCA, Rotablator, ELCA and TEC (with adjunctive PTCA as needed) may lead to more effective lumen enlargement than balloon angioplasty alone.[4,20-22] (While PTCA usually leaves a 35-45% residual stenosis, in two stent reports, the final diameter stenosis was only 1%[22] and minus 9%.[26]) Putative mechanisms for these favorable results include the resection (DCA), pulverization (Rotablator), and ablation (ELCA) of plaque, and the elimination of elastic recoil (stent). Despite excellent acute results, restenosis rates are 40-55% for atherectomy[3,4,15] and lasers,[4,25] and 23-35% for stents.[4,22,26] In the CAVEAT-I trial, acute and longterm outcomes were similar for ostial LAD lesions randomized to DCA or balloon angioplasty (Chapter 28).[15]

C. TECHNICAL CONSIDERATIONS

1. Balloon Angioplasty

a. **Guiding Catheter Selection.** Most ostial RCA lesions can be successfully approached with a right Judkins, left Amplatz, or Hockey Stick guide, depending on the vessel takeoff and the degree of coaxial alignment. For ostial LAD, circumflex, and branch ostial lesions, a left Judkins guide will usually suffice unless better support is needed due to vessel tortuosity. If pressure damping occurs, a side-hole catheter or larger diameter guide should be used: smaller diameter guides may have a tendency to engage aorto-ostial lesions more deeply and exacerbate pressure damping, whereas larger diameter guides will tend to sit outside the ostium and result in less pressure damping. In general, coaxial alignment — not aggressive vessel intubation — will minimize ostial injury, permit proper positioning of interventional devices, and facilitate angiographic assessment of the ostium. As long as coaxial alignment is maintained, it is usually possible to advance and center the balloon with the guiding catheter positioned just outside the ostium. Once the balloon is properly positioned, the guiding catheter can be gently retracted 1-2 cm into the aorta (Figure 14.1); gentle forward pressure on the balloon catheter or low-pressure balloon inflation (1-2 atm) may help maintain proper balloon position while the guide is retracted. The balloon should not be fully inflated if partially inside the guiding catheter due to the risk of balloon rupture, dissection, or air embolism. To ensure that the stenosis is not due to transient spasm prior to intervention, it is helpful to administer intracoronary nitroglycerin or perform a subselective injection in the Sinus of Valsalva.

b. **Balloon Dilatation**

1. **Aorto-Ostial Stenosis.** For calcified and non-calcified lesions, a long (30-40 mm) high-pressure balloon may be preferable since high-pressure inflations may be needed. Balloon on-the-wire systems are not routinely chosen as first-line catheters because of the frequent need to upsize balloons or exchange devices. While most interventionalists have been frustrated by the "watermelon seed" effect — proximal or distal balloon migration during inflation (Figure 14.2) — this problem is less common with long balloons, and may also respond to slower-than-usual inflation times or changing to a new device (Rotablator, DCA, ELCA).

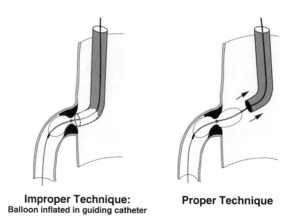

Improper Technique:
Balloon inflated in guiding catheter

Proper Technique

Figure 14.1 Aorto-Ostial Lesions: PTCA Technique

Proper technique requires gentle retraction of the guiding catheter 1-2cm into the aorta prior to balloon inflation. Otherwise, part of the balloon is inflated in the guide, increasing the risk of balloon rupture and ostial trauma.

> 2. **Branch-Ostial Stenosis.** When dilating a branch-ostial lesion (especially ostial LAD or circumflex lesions), the balloon should be positioned to avoid obstructing blood flow down the uninvolved limb of the bifurcation whenever possible. Proper placement can be confirmed by a small (1-2cc) test injection. Generally, the balloon diameter should match the diameter of the branch vessel and not the parent vessel. Other important technical considerations are detailed in Chapter 10.

2. **New Interventional Devices.** The principles of guiding catheters engagement are similar to those of PTCA (see above), and coaxial alignment is an absolute requirement for all new devices approaches to ostial lesions. Maximal visualization of the ostial lesion is essential for positioning the device properly, optimizing angiographic results, minimizing ischemia, and avoiding complications. Aggressive guiding catheter engagements should be avoided because of the danger of guide-induced injury, and the inability to properly position the device and image the ostium. If possible, other fluoroscopic landmarks (ostial calcification, rib margins, vertebral bodies, shaft of the guiding catheter, pacemaker, pulmonary artery catheter, etc.) may be valuable to ensure proper guide position and device placement. It is usually possible to advance and retract the device with the guiding catheter positioned just outside the ostium. Frequent test injections are required to verify that the tip of the guide does not inadvertently engage beyond the ostium. When DCA is performed on aorto-ostial lesions, the housing will partially extend into the aorta (Figure 14.3). When performing TEC, Rotablator, or ELCA, the initial device should be small (device/artery ratio = 0.5); further increases in device size are guided by subsequent angiography to a final

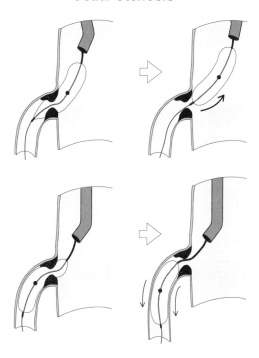

Figure 14.2 "Watermelon-Seed" Effect Complicating Aorto-Ostial PTCA

When dilating ostial lesions, the balloon may prolapse into the aorta or distal vessel, leaving a high-grade residual stenosis. Long balloons (30-40 mm) may be useful in this situation.

device/artery ratio to ≤ 0.8. This approach facilitates passage of the device, and reduces the risk of distal embolization and dissection. Detailed descriptions of atherectomy and laser system techniques are reviewed in Chapters 27-30. Stenting of aorto-ostial lesions is technically demanding and should only be performed by experienced stent operators. In contrast to predilation of non-ostial lesions, predilation of ostial lesions should be performed with full-sized (as compared to undersized) balloons. The proximal 1-2 mm of the stent should extend into the aorta to ensure complete coverage of the lesion. In general, slotted tubular (e.g., Palmaz-Schatz) stents are preferable to coil (e.g., Gianturco-Roubin) stents because of greater radial strength, less stent distortion, and lower chance of guiding catheter damage to the stent. Optimal stent technique should be employed using high-pressure balloons, and the proximal end of the stent should be flared to ensure stent apposition (see also Chapter 26) (Figure 14.4).

D. **CASE SELECTION: LESION SPECIFIC, MULTI-DEVICE THERAPY.** Because of the suboptimal results of PTCA alone, multi-device therapy is recommended. As shown in Table 14.3, associated lesion morphology weighs heavily in selecting the optimal method of revascularization. DCA is well-suited for noncalcified ostial stenoses in vessels ≥ 3 mm. The presence of eccentric or

Table 14.2. New Device Angioplasty of Ostial Stenoses: Acute Outcome

Series	Device	Lesion	N	Success* (%)	Complications (%)** D / Q-MI / CABG	Other
Waksman[10] (1995)	All devices	AO native AO SVG	184 122	89 94	3 2	TLR: 33% 39%
Ellis[11] (1994)	ROTA	-	68	91	-	-
Cowley[12] (1995)	ROTA	Nonost. RCA Ostial RCA	251 109	96 93	1.6 / 0.4 / 0.4 2.8 / 0 / 1.8	AC/RS (%): 4.4 / 48 1.8 / 52
Commeau[13] (1994)	ROTA	AO BO	32 110	97 94	3 / 3 / 3 0.9 / 0.9 / 0.9	-
Koller[14] (1994)	ROTA TEC	AO + BO AO + BO++	29 72	93 90	3 / 3 / 3 1.3 / 0 / 4.1	AC/RS (%): 7 / 39 6 / 59
Stephan[15] (1995)	DCA	AO BO	30 73	70 92	0 / 0 / 3 0 / 0 / 0	RS: 36% 37%
Boehrer[3] (CAVEAT; 1995)	PTCA DCA	Ostial LAD Ostial LAD	33 41	87 86	0 / 0 / 3 0 / 2 / 5	RS: 46% 48%
Popma[16] (1993)	DCA	AO + BO	81	98	-	3 mo. EFS: 66%
Robertson[17] (1991)	DCA	AO BO	41 75	78 92	4.9 0	RS: 46% 54%
Litvack[18] (1994)	ELCA	-	280	89	7	-
deMarchena[19] (1994)	ILCA	-	23	91	4	-
Sabri[20] (1994)	PTCA, Devices†	AO AO	15 31	93 91	0 / 0 / 0 / 0 0 / 6 / 0 / 0	Greater acute gain with devices

Series	Device	Lesion	N	Success* (%)	Complications (%)** D / Q-MI / CABG	Other	
Sawada[4] (1994)	PTCA	Ostial LAD, LCX	80	90	-	RS (%): 61	TLR (%): 58
	ELCA		24	88	-	59	47
	DCA		29	90	-	33	25
	Stent		22	100	-	33	18
Brogan[21] (1993)	ROTA	AO + BO+++	101	97	0 / 0 / 2	Overall 1-year EFS: 64%	
	ELCA		16	94	0 / 0 / 1		
	DCA		58	97	0 / 0 / 1		
	TEC		16	95	0 / 0 / 0		
	Stent		11	91	0 / 0 / 0		
Colombo[26] (1996)	Stent	AO	35	100	0	Post-stent diameter stenosis: -9% RS: 23%	
DeCesare[27] (1996)	Stent	Ostial LAD	23	100	0	Post-stent diameter stenosis: 3% RS: 22%	
Rocha-Singh[22] (1995)	Stent	AO + BO	41***	93	5 / 0 / 0	SAT: 5% RS: 28%	
Zampieri[23] (1993)	Stent	AO	7	100	0	-	
Tierstein[24] (1991)	Stent	AO + BO	28	89	7	RS: 35%	

Abbreviations: D = death; Q-MI = Q-wave myocardial infarction; CABG = emergency coronary artery bypass grafting; AC = acute closure; AO = aorto-ostial; BO = branch-ostial, EFS = event-free survival (freedom from death, MI, CABG, repeat PTCA); DCA = directional coronary atherectomy; ROTA = rotablator; ELCA = excimer laser coronary angioplasty; ILCA = infrared laser coronary angioplasty; TEC = translumunal extraction catheter; TLR = target lesion revascularization; RS = restenosis; SAT = subacute thrombosis; - not reported

* ≤ 40% residual stenosis
** Single number denotes overall in-hospital complication rate
*** Includes 19 coronary lesions and 22 saphenous vein graft lesions
\+ Undersized balloon followed by optimal size balloon
\++ Includes 24 ostial lesions in saphenous vein grafts
\+++ Includes 48 saphenous vein graft lesions

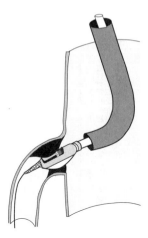

Figure 14.3 Aorto-Ostial Lesions: DCA Technique

Proper technique requires gentle retraction of the guiding catheter 2-3 cm into the aorta prior to cutter activation. It is important to establish other landmarks (rib margins, catheter shaft) to ensure precise positioning of the AtheroCath. Failure to retract the guide may result in partial excision of the tip of the guide during cutter activation.

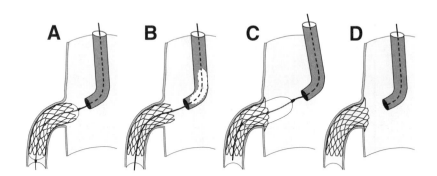

Figure 14.4 Aorto-Ostial Lesions: Stent Technique

A. Position the stent-delivery balloon so 1-2 mm of stent extends into the aorta. The guide must be retracted 1-2 cm before deploying the stent.

B. Remove the delivery balloon while maintaining backward tension on the guide, to prevent it from advancing into the ostium and damaging the stent.

C. Perform adjunctive PTCA with a high pressure balloon to ensure full stent expansion and apposition. Flaring the proximal end of the stent with a slightly larger balloon is useful.

D. Final result.

ulcerated lesions, or small-to-moderate amounts of thrombus are also suitable for DCA. However, other devices should be considered in the presence of moderate-to-heavy calcification, large amounts of clot, diffuse disease, vessel diameter < 3.0 mm, or severe angulation. TEC may be useful for ostial vein graft lesions with thrombus, but is contraindicated in the presence of significant calcification, marked eccentricity, extreme angulation, or dissection. The Rotablator may be of particular benefit for ostial lesions with or without calcification, but should be avoided when either a dissection, thrombus, or severe angulation is present. ELCA may be useful for noncalcified ostial lesions, particularly those with long (>30 mm) segments of disease, and directional ELCA may be useful for eccentric ostial lesions. However, all lasers should be avoided in severely angulated lesions or in the presence of a dissection. Rotablator is preferred for heavily calcified lesions since the results with ELCA are unpredictable. Stents can be used ostial lesions in the absence of fibrocalcific lesions that

Table 14.3. Ostial Lesion Morphology and New Interventional Device Selection

Morphology	DCA	TEC	Rotablator	ELCA	Stent
Type A	+	-	+	+	+
Thrombus	+[a]	+	-	+	+[b]
Calcification (mod-heavy)	±[c]	-	+	±	+[b]
Long segment of disease	-	-	±	±	±
Marked eccentricity	+	-	+	+[d]	+
Angulation (severe)	-	-	-	-	-
Dissection (focal)	±	-	-	-	+
Ulcerated	+	-	+	+	+
Restenosis lesion	+	-	+	+	+

Abbreviations: DCA = Directional Coronary Angioplasty, TEC = Transluminal Extraction Atherectomy, ELCA = Excimer Laser Coronary Angioplasty

+	Favorable
-	Unfavorable
a	Lesions with a large amount of clot should probably not be attempted
b	May be considered after Rotablator (calcified lesions) or TEC (thrombus-containing lesion)
c	New calcium cutter may be useful; may be considered after Rotablator
d	Directional ELCA may have a role

cannot be fully expanded with a balloon. Adjunctive balloon angioplasty is frequently required after DCA, and virtually always after TEC, Rotablator, and ELCA of ostial lesions. Some studies demonstrate that compared to PTCA alone, a further 22% gain in lumen diameter is possible when PTCA is preceded by TEC or ELCA, and a 44% incremental gain when PTCA is preceded by Rotablator ("facilitated angioplasty"). There is also growing optimism for using combinations of new devices for ostial lesions ("device synergy"), including Rotablator + stents, Rotablator + DCA, and DCA + stents. These concepts are discussed in greater detail in Chapter 8.

* * * * *

REFERENCES

1. Tan K, Sulke N, Taub N, Sowton E. Clinical and lesion morphologic determinants of coronary angioplasty success and complications: Current experience. J Am Coll Cardiol 1995;25: 855-65.
2. Tan K, Sulke N, Taub N, Karani S, Sowton E. Percutaneous transluminal coronary angioplasty of aorta ostial, non-aorta ostial, and branch ostial stenoses. J Am Coll Cardiol 1994;March Special Issue:351A.
3. Boehrer JD, Ellis SG, Pieper K, Holmes DR, Keeler GP, et al. Directional atherectomy versus balloon angioplasty for coronary ostial and nonostial left anterior descending coronary artery lesions: Results from a randomized multicenter trial. J Am Coll Cardiol 1995;25:1380-6.
4. Sawada Y, Kimura T, Shinoda E, Sato Y, Nosaka H, Nobuyoshi M. Poor outcome of balloon angioplasty (BA) for ostial left anterior descending and circumflex: Impact of new angioplasty devices. Circulation 1994;90 (Part II):I-436.
5. Brown R, Kochar G, et al. Effects of coronary angioplasty using progressive dilation on ostial stenosis of left anterior descending artery. Am J Cardiol 1993;71:245-247.
6. Myler R, Shaw R, et al. Lesion morphology and coronary angioplasty: Current experience and analysis. J Am Coll Cardiol 1992;19:1641-1652.
7. Bedotto JB, McConahay DR, Rutherford BD. Balloon angioplasty of aorta coronary ostial stenoses revisited. Circulation 1991;84(4):II-251.
8. Mathias DW, Fishman-Mooney J, Lange HW, et al. Frequency of success and complications of coronary angioplasty of a stenosis at the ostium of a branch vessel. Am J Cardiol 1991;67:491-495.
9. Topol EJ, Ellis SG, Fishman J, et al. Multicenter study of percutaneous transluminal angioplasty for right coronary artery ostial stenosis. J Am Coll Cardiol 1987;9:1214-1218.
10. Waksman R, Ghazzal ZMB, Kennard ED, et al. Acute outcome and follow-up of ostial versus proximal lesions treated with new devices: Report of the NACI Registry. Circulation 1995;92:I-73.
11. Ellis S, Popma J, et al. Relation of clinical presentation, stenosis morphology, and operator technique to the procedural results of rotational atherectomy-facilitated angioplasty. Circulation 1994;89:882-892.
12. Cowley CA, Patterson PE, Kipperman RM, Chuang YC, Pacera JH, Popma JJ. Multicenter rotational coronary atherectomy registry experience in coronary artery ostial stenoses. TCT Course (Washington DC), February, 1995.
13. Commeau P, Zimarino M, Lancelin B, et al. Rotational coronary atherectomy for the treatment of aorto-ostial and branch-ostial lesions. Circulation 1994;90 (Part II):I-213.
14. Koller P, Freed M, et al. Success, complications, and restenosis following rotational and transluminal extraction atherectomy of ostial stenoses. Cath Cardiovasc Diagn. 1994;31:255-260.
15. Stephen WJ, Bates ER, Garratt KN, Hinohara T, Muller DWM. Directional atherectomy in coronary and saphenous vein graft ostial stenoses. Am J Cardiol 1995;75:1015-1018.
16. Popma J, Mintz G, et al. Clinical and angiographic outcome after directional coronary atherectomy: A qualitative and quantitative analysis using coronary arteriography and intravascular ultrasound. Am J Cardiol 1993;72:55E-64E.
17. Robertson GC, Simpson JB, Vetter JW. Directional coronary atherectomy for ostial lesions. Circulation 1991;84(4):II-

251.

18. Litvack F, Eigler N, Margolis J, et al. Percutaneous excimer laser coronary angioplasty: results in the first consecutive 3,000 patients. J Am Coll Cardiol 1994;23:323-9.

19. deMarchena EJ, Mallon SM, et al. Effectiveness of holmium laser-assisted coronary angioplasty. Am J Cardiol 1994;73:117-121.

20. Sabri M, Cowley, et al. Immediate results of interventional devices for coronary ostial narrowing with angina pectoris. Amer J Cardiol 1994;73:122-125.

21. Brogan WC, Popma JJ, Pichard AD, et al. A lesion-specific approach to new device therapy in ostial lesions. J Am Coll Cardiol 1993;21(No. 2):233A.

22. Rocha-Singh K, Morris N, et al. Coronary stenting for treatment of ostial stenoses of native coronary arteries or aortocoronary saphenous venous grafts. Am J Cardiol 1995;75: 26-29.

23. Zampieri PA, Colombo A, et al. Results of coronary stenting of ostial lesions. Am J Cardiol 1994;73:901-903.

24. Tierstein P, Stratienko AA, Schatz RA. Coronary stenting for ostial stenosis: Initial results and six month follow-up. Circulation 1991;84(4):II-250.

25. Wong SC, Pompa JJ, Chuang YC, et al. Angiographic and clinical outcomes in saphenous vein graft (SVG) versus native coronary aorto-ostial lesions. J Am Coll Cardiol 1994;March Special Issue:302A.

26. Colombo A, Itoh A, Maiello L, et al. Coronary stent implantation in aorto-ostial lesions: Immediate and follow-up results. J Am Coll Cardiol 1996;March Special Issue.

27. De Cesare NB, Galli S, Loaldi A, et al. Palmaz-Schatz stent for the treatment of left anterior descending ostial stenosis: Acute and long-term results. J Invas. Cardiol 1996;8.

15 LONG LESIONS

Mark Freed, M.D.

A. BALLOON ANGIOPLASTY (Table 15.1)

1. Standard-Length (20 mm) Balloons

a. Success. Although angioplasty success declines as lesion length increases,[1,5,6] procedural success can still be achieved in 87% (range: 74-97%) of lesions > 20 mm in length (Table 15.1). These nonrandomized data, however, may overestimate success rates since long lesions with other complex features (e.g, calcium, angulation) are often treated with long-balloons (30-40 mm) or new devices. In the randomized Amsterdam Rotterdam (AMRO) trial of ELCA vs. PTCA for long coronary lesions,[9] PTCA success was only 79%. Furthermore, intravascular ultrasound has shown that the actual residual stenosis is frequently underestimated by contrast angioplasty since the "normal" reference segment used to measure stenosis severity is often diseased itself (Chapter 31). It may be important to distinguish "long lesions" from "diffuse disease," which are often used interchangeably. We and others consider long lesions to be > 10 mm in length, and diffuse disease as the presence of three or more 50% stenoses in at least one-third of the vessel.

b. Complications. The impact of lesion length on major complications is controversial. Several reports indicate that PTCA of long lesions is associated with an increased risk of coronary artery dissection[6,10,11] and abrupt closure[1,6,12-14] In these studies, the incidence of abrupt closure was 1-6% for lesions <10 mm and 9-14% for lesions > 10 mm. In contrast, other studies reported no relationship between lesion length and acute closure[15] or major complications.[5,16,18,19] These divergent results may be due to differences in patient characteristics, the presence of multivessel disease, associated lesion morphologies, and the use of long (30 - 40 mm) balloons and new devices.

c. Restenosis. The influence of lesion length on restenosis risk is controversial. The Multi-Hospital Eastern Atlantic Restenosis Trial (M-HEART) demonstrated a direct relationship between lesion length and restenosis (lesion lengths of 0.3-2.9 mm, 3.0-4.6 mm, 4.7-7.0 mm, and 7.1-28.0 mm showed restenosis rates of 32%, 33%, 42%, and 49%, respectively).[20] Other reports failed to demonstrate an association.[21,22] Although long lesions may result in a greater loss in lumen diameter at 6-months, these observations do not necessarily correlate with clinical restenosis.[23]

2. Long (30-40 mm) Balloons.

Considerable clinical experience suggests that long (30-40 mm) balloons might improve acute results by distributing inflation pressure more evenly across the diseased vessel segment and atheroma/vessel junction, which is frequently the site of dissection (Figure 15.1). Zidar and associates[6] reported their results with standard-length and long-balloons (Table 15.1). Compared to 20-mm balloons, long-balloons resulted in increased success, fewer

Table 15.1. Balloon Angioplasty of Long Lesions: Acute Outcome

Series	Balloon Length	Lesion Length (mm)	N	Success* (%)	Complications (%)[†] D / Q-MI / CABG	DISS (%)	AC (%)
Appelman[9] (1996)	-	>10	157	79 [††]	0/1.3/1.9	55	0.6
Tan[1] (1995)	20-40	< 10	959	95	-	-	1.5
		10 - 20	153	85	-	-	11
		> 20	45	74	-	-	16
Kaul[2] (1995)	20-40	11 - 20	112	96	1 / 1 / 1	24	3
		> 20	29	97	0 / 3 / 0	32	3
Cates[3] (1994)	80	> 40	54	91	- / - / 4	-	-
Mooney[4] (1993)	-	> 10	327	93	0 / 1 / 1.5	29	5
Myler[5] (1992)	-	≤ 10	365	95	2.1	-	-
		11 - 20	278	91	0	-	-
		> 20	136	89	0	-	-
Zidar[6] (1992)	20	< 10	579	95**	1.2 / - / 4.8	6.6	5.9
	20	> 10	149	90	0.7 / - / 8.1	18.1	14.1
	≥ 30	> 10	90	98	1.1 / - / 3.3	8.9	5.6
Savas[7] (1992)	40	> 20	109	90	2	35	7
	40	> 20 (bend ≥ 45°)	69	88	1	20	7
Goudreau[8] (1991)	20	> 20	39	97	2.5	-	-

Abbreviations: AC = acute closure; DISS = dissection; D = in-hospital death; Q-MI = in- hospital Q-wave myocardial infarction; - = not reported
CABG = emergency coronary artery bypass grafting
*   < 50 % residual stenosis without death, Q-MI, or emergent CABG
**   < 50 % residual stenosis
†   Single number denotes overall in-hospital complications rate.
††   Intention-to-treat analysis (success = guidewire crossing + PTCA success)

dissections, and less acute closure. In fact, long-balloon angioplasty of long lesions results in success and complication rates similar to those of standard-length balloon angioplasty of focal stenoses. Another observational study of 69 long (53 mm) and angulated (>45°) lesions treated with long balloons reported procedural success in 88%, acute closure in 7%, and major ischemic complications in < 1%.[7] In a small (n = 44) randomized trial comparing long- and standard-length balloons, long balloons resulted in fewer dissections, (18% vs. 55%) and required few inflations.[24] Collectively, these data suggest that compared to standard balloons, long balloons are associated with higher procedural success and lower dissection rates.

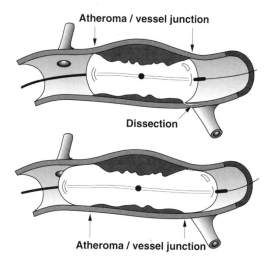

Figure 15.1 Long Lesions: PTCA Technique

When faced with lesion lengths ≥ 20 mm, long (30-40 mm) balloons may be employed to more evenly distribute inflation pressure throughout the diseased vessel segment and atheroma/vessel junction.

3. **Tapered Balloons.** Most branching coronary arteries taper in diameter by at least 0.5 mm over 20 mm of vessel length (average taper = 0.22 mm per 10 mm of arterial length).[25] Significant tapering often poses a problem for optimal balloon sizing, especially for long lesions (Figure 15.2). To address this problem, Banka et al.[25] performed PTCA with a tapered balloon (0.5 mm decrement in balloon diameter over 25 mm of balloon length) to achieve procedural success in 80% and angiographic dissection in only 2% of 104 tapered lesions. Tapered balloons may also be used for high-pressure (12 atm.) balloon inflations to optimize stenting of tapering vessels. It is currently unknown whether tapered balloons offer an advantage over balloons with uniform diameter.

B. **NEW INTERVENTIONAL DEVICES (Table 15.2).** Atherectomy devices, lasers, and stents are used to revascularize long lesions, but interdevice comparisons have been hampered by marked differences in baseline clinical and lesion characteristics. Long lesion length appears to independently predict acute closure[39] and coronary perforation[40] following new devices, emphasizing the need to determine the optimal mode of revascularization.

1. **Atherectomy (Table 15.2)**

   a. **Rotablator Atherectomy.** Although early Rotablator success was possible in only 70% of long lesions,[29] more recent studies have reported success in more than 90% of lesions 16-25 mm in length.[26-28] However, increasing lesion length has been associated with an increased risk of MI,[26,28,29] coronary artery perforation,[41] and restenosis.[42] Despite these complications, many

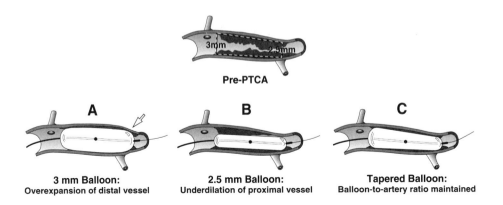

Figure 15.2 Long Lesions in Tapered Vessels: PTCA Technique

Balloon sizing is problematic when faced with a long lesion in a tapered vessel:
A. Sizing the balloon to match the proximal segment results in overdilating the distal segment, increasing the risk of dissection.
B. Sizing the balloon to match the distal segment results in underdilating the proximal segment, leaving a significant residual stenosis.
C. A tapered balloon ensures better matching of balloon and vessel size.

interventionalists believe that Rotablator atherectomy (with adjunctive PTCA as needed) is the preferred method of revascularizing long lesions, especially those with calcium. In such lesions, it is important to use slow passes with a small burr to minimize microcavitation and the generation of large particulate debris, which can result in slow-flow and ischemic complications.

b. **Directional Coronary Atherectomy (DCA).** In an early report by Robertson et al,[30] DCA of long lesions resulted in lower success, more emergency CABG, and higher restenosis rates compared to DCA of focal stenoses. In another early report, lesion length independently predicted abrupt closure, which occurred in 3%, 4%, and 7% of lesions < 10 mm, 10-20 mm, and ≥ 20 mm in length, respectively.[43] In the CAVEAT trial, lesion length (in addition to calcification) predicted DCA failure.[44] More recently, Mooney et al.[4] demonstrated procedural success in 97% of long lesions by making a series of longitudinal cuts through the entire length of the lesion; this allowed better DCA positioning (and less ischemia) during remaining circumferential cuts. Lesions were highly selected for favorable morphology; highly calcified or angulated lesion, and vessels < 3 mm in diameter were excluded.

    c.   **TEC Atherectomy.** Although TEC atherectomy may be used to treat native coronary artery lesions, it may not have an advantage over PTCA except in the presence of thrombus. In small numbers of select long lesions, procedural success for TEC and adjunctive PTCA exceeds 90%.

2.   **Lasers (Table 15.2)**

    a.   **Excimer Laser Coronary Angioplasty (ELCA).** Data from the first 3000 patients enrolled into the ELCA Registry found procedural success rates of 90% for short and long lesions.[34] Importantly, procedural success was independent of lesion length and was achieved in 89% and 87% of lesions > 20 mm and > 30 mm in length, respectively. Although dissections were more common in long lesions,[45] major ischemic complications occurred with equal frequency among short and long lesions.[34,45,46] Randomized device trials comparing ELCA vs. PTCA (AMRO trial), and ELCA vs. PTCA vs. Rotablator (ERBAC trial) for long lesions are now complete. In the **AM**sterdam **RO**tterdam (ARMO) trial, 308 patients with 325 lesions ≥ 10 mm were randomized to ELCA (without saline infusion) or balloon angioplasty. No difference in procedural success, late clinical events, or functional status were observed (Table 15.2).[9,32] There was, however, more acute closure (8% vs. 0.8%, p = 0.005)and a trend towards more restenosis in the ELCA group (52% vs 41%, p = 0.13).[9] ELCA was also associated with additional costs of $4476 per treated segment.[47] In the **E**xcimer-**L**aser **R**otablator **B**alloon **A**ngioplasty **C**omparison (ERBAC) trial, both ELCA and ROTA resulted in better immediate lumen enlargement, but no difference in restenosis at 6 months. The efficacy of ELCA for long lesions with heavy calcification, marked angulation, or thrombus awaits further study.

    b.   **Holmium Laser Angioplasty.** Results from the Holmium Laser Coronary Registry indicate that high procedural success (≥ 90%) and low complication rates (≤ 3%) can be achieved for lesions > 10 mm in length, although success rates were lower for lesions > 20 mm.[35]

3.   **Stents (Table 15.2).** Lesion lengths > 10-20 mm were excluded from the early stent experience since the use of multiple stents increased the risk of subacute stent thrombosis. Recent data are much more favorable. Maiello et al.[36] implanted 274 stents on an elective basis in 89 patients with 108 lesions > 20 mm in length (using IVUS to optimize stent deployment). Procedural success was achieved in 93% of patients, while periprocedural MI, emergency CABG, and stent thrombosis occurred in 3%, 3%, and 1.5% of cases, respectively. Ninety-three percent of successfully stented patients were treated with antiplatelet therapy alone without warfarin. Follow-up angiography was performed on 71% of eligible lesions and revealed a restenosis rate of 35%. In another report, 90-day clinical event rate after emergent or elective implantation of the Gianturco-Roubin stent was associated with vessel diameter and stent expansion, but not lesion length. Excellent results were also obtained by Shaknovich et al.[48] after implanting ≥ 3 Palmaz-Schatz stents in 54 long lesions or dissections (mean length = 50 ± 17 mm) (Table 15.2). Restenosis, however, may be more common in long compared to focal lesions.[49,50]

Table 15.2. New Device Angioplasty of Long Lesions

Series	Device	Lesion Length (mm)	N	Success (%)	D / Q-MI / CABG*** (%)	Other 6 mo (%): D/MI/CABG/PTCA/RS
AMRO Trial[9,32,33] (1996)	ELCA	>10	151	80	0 / 1.3 / 4.5	0 / 1.3 / 6 / 20 / 52
	PTCA	>10	157	79	0 / 1.3 / 1.9	0 / 0.6 / 7 / 17 / 41
Litvack[34] (1994)	ELCA**	<10	1832	91	6	
		10 - 19	1042	92	4.6	
		20 - 29	467	89	6.6	
		≥ 30	251	87	7.3	
Warth[26] (1994)	Rotablator	≤ 10	588	-	- / 0.2 / -	Any complication:* 20%
		11 - 25	195	-	- / 2.1 / -	28%
Ellis[27] (1994)	Rotablator	0 - 4	286	-	4.2	
		5 - 8	69		10.1	
		9 - 12	27		18.5	
		13 - 16	6		50	
Reisman[28] (1993)	Rotablator	<10	953	95	0.6 / 0.7 / 2.6	Non-Q MI: 4%
		11 - 15	180	97	0.6 / 0 / 1.1	5.5%
		15 - 25	143	92	2.1 / 2.8 / 1.4	6.2%
Tierstein[29] (1992)	Rotablator	≤ 10	12	92	-	RS: 22%
		>10	30	70	-	75%
Mooney[4] (1993)	DCA	>10	88	97	0 / 1 / 1	Acute closure: 4.6% Dissection: 19%
Robertson[30] (1990)	DCA	<10	250	93	- / - / 2	RS: 33%
		10 - 19	59	90	- / - / 5	53%
		≥ 20	19	79	- / - / 10	62%
TEC[31] Registry	TEC	< 10	266	93	-	
		10 - 20	220	93	-	
		> 20	38	95	-	

Series	Device	Lesion Length (mm)	N	Success (%)	D / Q-MI / CABG*** (%)	Other
deMarchena[35] (1994)	Holmium-laser	≤ 10	123	97	2.7	
		11 - 20	193	94	3.1	
		> 20	49	90	0	
Maiello[36] (1995)	Elective Stent (IVUS-guided)	> 20	108	93	0/3/3	Stent thrombosis: 1% RS: 35%
Shaknovich[48] (1995)	≥ 3 PSS	50†††	54	-	1.8 / 0 / 1.8	Stent thrombosis: 3.7% vascular complications: 3.7%
Akira[37] (1995)	PSS	> 20	62	-	-	RS: 39%
	GRS		26	-	-	35%
	Wiktor		21	-	-	24%
Sutton[38] (1994)	GRS	-	415†	-	90-day: 20	No correlation between lesion length and complications
		-	224††	-	9	

Abbreviations: D = in- hospital death; Q-MI = in-hospital Q-wave myocardial infarction; CABG = emergency coronary artery bypass grafting; TEC = Transluminal Extraction Catheter; ELCA = Excimer Laser Coronary Angioplasty; GRS = Gianturco-Roubin stent; PSS = Palmaz-Schatz stent; RS = restenosis; - = not reported

* Death, any MI, emergency CABG, dissection, thrombus formation, no-reflow, loss of sidebranch, transfusion or vascular surgery

** Includes saphenous vein graft lesions, (16%)

*** Single number denotes overall in-hospital complication rate

\+ No relation between lesion length and procedural success.

\+\+ Acute procedural + in-hospital complications unless otherwise stated.

† Emergency stents

†† Elective stents

††† Long lesions and dissections (mean length = 50 mm)

C. **APPROACH TO LONG LESIONS.** We currently determine the optimal revascularization modality based on the presence of associated lesion characteristics (Figure 15.3).

1. **Extreme Length.** For lesions > 40 mm, single or multiple long-balloons are preferred. Although Rotablator and ELCA (with adjunctive angioplasty) are acceptable alternatives, no studies have demonstrated superiority to angioplasty alone. For vessels ≥ 3.0 mm, multiple stents may be implanted, but the risk of stent thrombosis, restenosis, and cost may be increased.

2. **Marked Angulation.** Long lesions with on severely angulated vessel segments (>60°) are treated best by long-balloons. Because long balloons conform nicely to vessel contour, contemporary studies do not show advantages of PET over other balloon materials (Chapter 20). ELCA, TEC, Rotablator, and DCA should be avoided because of the risk of dissection and perforation.

3. **Thrombus.** The ideal treatment of long lesions with thrombus is unknown since all devices increase the risk of distal embolization and no-reflow. Although TEC atherectomy may be useful for aspirating thrombus, studies in vein grafts suggest lower success rates and more complications when clot is present (Chapter 17). Intracoronary thrombolytics, either as a prolonged superselective overnight infusion, or as a shorter intracoronary infusion during TEC or long-balloon PTCA, may improve procedural outcome (Chapter 9). For small thrombi, PTCA, DCA, or ELCA may be considered, but the Rotablator is contraindicated due to the risk of no-reflow. CABG may be a reasonable alternative when a large amount of clot is present in a large vessel, especially when multivessel disease and/or poor LV function is present. Other devices such as the Hydrolyzer and Angiojet are currently under investigation in Europe (Chapters 8, 9).

4. **Extensive Calcification.** Long lesions with significant calcification are best treated with Rotablator atherectomy, particularly if IVUS demonstrates the presence of superficial calcification. Rotablator technique involves the use of small burrs (≤ 1.75 mm), slow passes, and incremental upsizing in burr diameter by 0.25 mm to avoid distal embolization and no-reflow. ELCA may also be used for lesions > 30 mm; when performed, the saline infusion technique is recommended to reduce the risk of severe dissection (Chapter 30). When stand-alone or adjunctive PTCA is performed, a high-pressure long-balloon is preferred; a parallel guidewire external to the balloon ("force-focused angioplasty," Chapter 12) may improve angiographic outcome when the lesion resists high-pressure inflations. The use of stents is of uncertain value, and DCA and TEC atherectomy should be avoided.

5. **Marked Eccentricity.** When marked lesion eccentricity is present, long-balloon PTCA is preferred. Directional ELCA may be a reasonable alternative, but TEC atherectomy should be avoided. Long, eccentric lesions can be treated with DCA, but the procedure is arduous and technically demanding. In the absence of calcium, multiple stents may be considered in vessels > 3 mm.

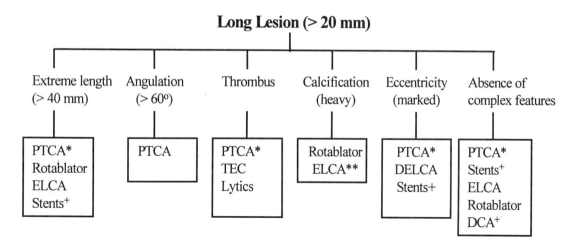

Figure 15.3. Management of Long Lesions

* Long-balloon PTCA is the most economical approach. Other devices invariably require adjunctive PTCA
** Saline-infusion technique
+ Vessel diameter $\geq$ 3 mm

6. **Absence of Complex Features.** In the absence of other complex features, percutaneous options include PTCA, ELCA, Rotablator, DCA, or multiple stents. An economical approach favors stand-alone PTCA since virtually all other devices require adjunctive PTCA.

D. **CONCLUSIONS.** Balloon angioplasty of long lesions may be performed with acceptable procedural success rates, although the risk of acute closure and restenosis appears to be increased when compared to focal stenoses. Other laser and atherectomy devices, with or without adjunctive PTCA, have not been shown to be superior to PTCA alone, and the value of stents for long lesions awaits further definition. For long lesions with other complex features, a lesion-specific, multi-device approach seems appropriate.

* * * * *

REFERENCES

1. Tan K, Sulke N, Taub N, Sowton E. Clinical and lesion morphologic determinants of coronary angioplasty success and complications: Current experience. J Am Coll Cardiol 1995;25: 855-65.
2. Kaul U, Upasani PT, Agarwal R, Bahl VK, Wasir HS. In-hospital outcome of percutaneous transluminal coronary angioplasty for long lesions and diffuse coronary artery disease. Cathet Cardiol Diagn 1995;35:294-300.
3. Cates WU, Knopf WD, Lembo NJ, Bernstein C, et al. The 80 mm balloon: The first 95 vessel cumulative experience. J Am Coll Cardiol 1994;23:58A.
4. Mooney, M., J. Mooney-Fishman, et al. Directional atherectomy for long lesions: Improved results. Cath Cardiovasc Diagn. 1993;1:26-30.
5. Myler R, Shaw R, et al. Lesion morphology and coronary angioplasty: Current experience and analysis. J Am Coll Cardiol 1992;19:1641-1652.
6. Zidar JP, Tenaglia AN, Jackman JD, et al. Improved acute results for PTCA of long coronary lesions using long angioplasty balloon catheters. J Am Coll Cardiol 1992;19(3):34A Abstract.
7. Savas V, Puchrowicz S, Williams L, et al. Angioplasty outcome using long balloons in high-risk lesions. J Am Coll Cardiol 1992;19(3):34A Abstract.
8. Goudreau E, DiSciascio G, Kelly K, et al. Coronary angioplasty of diffuse coronary artery disease. Am Heart J 1991;121:12-19.
9. Appleman YEA, Piek JJ, Strikwerda S, et al. Randomized trial of excimer laser angioplasty vs. balloon angioplasty for treatment of obstructive coronary artery disease. Lancet 1996;347:79-84.
10. Raymenants E, Bhandari S, Stammen F, De Scheerder ID, Desmet W, Piessens J. Effects of angioplasty balloon material and lesion characteristics on the incidence of coronary dissection in 2150 dilated lesions. J Am Coll Cardiol 1993;21 (Part II):291A.
11. Raymenants E, Bhandari S, Stammen F, De Scheerder I, et al. Effects of angioplasty balloon material and lesion characteristics on the incidence of coronary dissection in 2150 dilated lesions. J Am Coll Cardiol 1993;21:291A.
12. Ellis SG, Roubin GS, King SB III, et al. Angiographic and clinical predictors of acute closure after native vessel coronary angioplasty. Circulation 1988;77:372-379.
13. Detre KM, Holmes DR Jr, Holubkov R, et al. Incidence and consequences of periprocedural occlusion. The 1985-1986 National Heart, Lung and Blood Institute Percutaneous Transluminal Coronary Angioplasty Registry. Circulation 1990;82:739-750.
14. Tenaglia AN, Fortin DF, Califf RM, et al. Predicting the risk of abrupt vessel closure after angioplasty in an individual patient. J Am Coll Cardiol 1994;23:1004-1011.
15. de Feyter PJ, van den Brand M, Jaarman G, et al. Acute coronary artery occlusion during and after percutaneous transluminal coronary angioplasty. Frequency, prediction, clinical course, management, and follow-up. Circulation 1991;83:927-936.
16. Hermans WR, Foley D, et al. Usefulness of quantitative and qualitative angiographic lesion morphology, and clinical characteristics in predicting major adverse cardiac events during and after native coronary balloon angioplasty. Am J Cardiol 1993;72:14-20.
17. Ellis SG, Vandormael MG, Cowley MJ, et al, and the Multivessel Angioplasty Prognosis Study Group. Coronary morphologic and clinical determinants of procedural outcome with angioplasty for multivessel coronary disease. Circulation 1990;82:1193-202.
18. Savage MP, Goldberg S, Hirshfeld JW, et al, for the M-Heart Investigators. Clinical and angiographic determinants of primary coronary angioplasty success. J Am Coll Cardiol 1991;17:22-8.
20. Hirshfeld JW Jr, Schwartz JS, Jugo R, et al. Restenosis after coronary angioplasty: A multivariate statistical model to relate lesion and procedure variables to restenosis. J Am Coll Cardiol 1991;18:647-656.
21. Ellis SG, Roubin GS, King SB III, et al. Importance of stenosis morphology in the estimation of restenosis risk after elective percutaneous transluminal coronary angioplasty. Am J Cardiol 1989;63:30-34.
22. Leimgruber PP, Roubin GS, Hollman J, et al. Restenosis after successful coronary angioplasty in patients with single-vessel disease. Circulation 1986;73:710-717.
23. Foley DP, Meilkert R, Umans VA, et al. Is the relationship between luminal increase and subsequent renarrowing linear or non-linear in patients undergoing coronary interventions? J Am Coll Cardiol 1994;Special Issue:302A.
24. Brymer JF, Khaja F, and Kraft L. Angioplasty of long or tandem coronary artery lesions using a new longer balloon dilatation catheter: A comparative study. Cathet and Cardiovasc Diagn 1991;23:84-88.

25. Banka V, et al. Effectiveness of decremental diameter balloon catheters (Tapered balloon). Am J Cardiol 1992;69:188.

26. Warth D, Leon MB, O'Neill W, Zacca N, Polissar NL, Buchbinder M. Rotational atherectomy multicenter registry: Acute results, complications and 6-month angiographic follow-up in 709 patients. J Am Coll Cardiol 1994;24: 641-648.

27. Ellis, S., J. Popma, et al. Relation of clinical presentation, stenosis morphology, and operator technique to the procedural results of rotational atherectomy-facilitated angioplasty. Circulation 1994;89:882-892.

28. Reisman M, Cohen B, Warth D, Fenner J, Gocka IT, Buchbinder M. Outcome of long lesions treated with high speed rotational ablation. J Am Coll Cardiol 1993;21 (Part II):443A.

29. Tierstein PS, Warth DC, Haq N, et al. High speed rotational coronary atherectomy for patients with diffuse coronary artery disease. J Am Coll Cardiol 1991;18:1694-1701.

30. Robertson GC, Selmon MR, Hinohara T, et al. The effect of lesion length on outcome of directional coronary atherectomy. Circulation 1990;82(4):III-623 Abstract.

31. IVT™ Coronary TEC™ Clinical Database. Investigators Meeting 1992.

32. Appelman YE, Piek J, Redekop WK, de Feyter PJ, et al. Excimer laser angioplasty versus balloon angioplasty in longer coronary lesions: A multivariate analysis. Circulation 1995;92:I-74.

33. Foley DP, Appleman YE, Piek JJ. Comparison of angiographic restenosis propensity of excimer laser coronary angioplasty (ELCA) and balloon angioplasty (BA) in the AMsterdam ROtterdam (AMRO) trial. Circulation 1995;92:I-477.

34. Litvack F, Eigler N, Margolis J, et al. Percutaneous excimer laser coronary angioplasty: Results in the first consecutive 3,000 patients. J Am Coll Cardiol 1994;23:323-9.

35. deMarchena EJ, Mallon SM, et al. Effectiveness of holmium laser-assisted coronary angioplasty. Am J Cardiol 1994;73:117-121.

36. Maiello L, Hall P, Nakamura S, et al. Results of stent implantation of diffuse coronary disease assisted by intravascular ultrasound. J Am Coll Cardiol 1995;March Special Issue:156A.

37. Skira I, Hall P, Maiello L, Blengino S, et al. Coronary stenting of long lesions (greater than 20 mm) — a matched comparison of different stents. Circulation 1995;92:I-688.

38. Sutton JM, Ellis SG, Roubin GS, et al. Major clinical events after coronary stenting. The multicenter registry of acute and elective Gianturco-Roubin stent placement. Circulation 1994;89:1126-1137.

39. Hong MK, Popma JJ, Wong SC, Kent KM, et al. Incidence of and factors associated with abrupt closure in patients undergoing elective, new device angioplasty in native coronary arteries. J Am Coll Cardiol 1995;March Special Issue: 122A.

40. Flood RD, Popma JJ, Chuang YC, et al. Incidence angiographic predictors, and clinical significance of coronary perforation occurring after new device angioplasty. J Am Coll Cardiol 1994;March Special Issue:301A.

41. Cohen BM, Weber VJ, Bass TA, et al. Coronary perforation during rotational ablation: Angiographic determinants and clinical outcome. J Am Coll Cardiol 1994;March Special Issue:354A.

42. Leguizamón JH, Chambre DF, Torresani EM, et al. High-speed coronary rotational atherectomy. Are angiographic factors predictive of failure, major complications or restenosis? A multivariate analysis. J Am Coll Cardiol 1995;March Special Issue:95A.

43. Popma J, Topol E, et al. Abrupt vessel closure after directional coronary atherectomy. J Am Coll Cardiol 1992;19:1372-1379.

44. Lincolff AM, Ellis SG, Leya F, Masden RR, et al. Are clinical and angiographic correlates of success the same during directional coronary atherectomy and balloon angioplasty? The CAVEAT Experience. Circulation 1993;88:I-601.

45. Baumbach A, Bittl J, Fleck E, et al. Acute complications of excimer laser coronary angioplasty: A detailed analysis of multicenter results. J Am Coll Cardiol 1994;23(6):1305-1313.

46. Ghazzal, Z., J. Hearn, et al. Morphological predictors of acute complications after percutaneous excimer laser coronary angioplasty. Results of a comprehensive angiographic analysis: Importance of the eccentricity index. Circulation 1992;86:820-827.

47. Appleman YE, Birnie E, Piek JJ, de Feyter PJ, et al. Excimer laser angioplasty versus balloon angioplasty in longer coronary lesions: A cost-effectiveness analysis. Circulation 1995;92:I-512.

48. Shaknovich A, Moses JW, Undemir C, Cohen NT, et al. Procedural and short-term clinical outcomes in multiple Palmaz-Schatz stents (PSSs) in very long lesions/dissections. Circulation 1995;92:I-535.

49. Hall P, Nakamura S, Maiello L, Blengino S, et al. Factors associated with late angiographic outcome after intravascular ultrasound guided Palmaz-Schatz coronary stent implantation: A multivariate analysis. J Am Coll Cardiol 1995;Special Issue:36A.

50. Tamura T, Kimura T, Nosaka H, Nobuyoshi M. Predictors of restenosis after Palmaz-Schatz stent implantation. Circulation 1994;90 (Part II):I-324.

16 CHRONIC TOTAL OCCLUSION

Mark Freed, M.D.

CORONARY ARTERY OCCLUSION

PTCA of chronic total occlusions now comprises 10-20% of all angioplasty procedures and poses a management dilemma for the interventional cardiologist. Although well-developed collaterals are often present and maintain myocardial viability under resting conditions, these intra-and intercoronary networks are often inadequate during periods of increased oxygen demand, resulting in lifestyle-limiting angina. While successful PTCA improves anginal status, increases exercise capacity, and reduces the need for late bypass surgery, it is associated with low success rates, high equipment costs, increased radiation exposure, and a high incidence of restenosis. Improved guidelines for case selection, and new interventional devices and adjunctive pharmacotherapy may favorably impact the management of these patients.

A. **PATHOLOGY (Table 16.1).** Prior to total coronary occlusion, the underlying pathological process is the principal determinant of clinical presentation, presence of collaterals, myocardial viability, and the nature of the coronary obstruction.

- **Acute Occlusion of a Mild-to-Moderately Stenotic Vessel:** In the majority of cases, these patients present with acute myocardial infarction. Collaterals are usually absent or poorly developed. Unless restoration of coronary flow is achieved within 4-6 hrs, myocardial injury is permanent. Pathologically, the obstructed lumen typically consists of ruptured plaque and fresh clot. These types of acute occlusions are readily crossed with conventional guidewires, accounting for procedural success rates > 90%. The likelihood of successful recanalization decreases over the ensuing months as fresh thrombus undergoes organization, fibrosis, and calcification.

- **Total Occlusion of a Long-Standing, Highly-Diseased Vessel:** These patients frequently present with a change in anginal status rather than acute MI. A well-developed collateral network, which may provide flow equivalent to a 90-95% stenosis, is often present and helps maintain myocardial viability and prevent resting myocardial ischemia.[1] Overall contractile function may be normal, or a regional wall motion abnormality may be present due to hibernating myocardium or subendocardial infarction. Pathologically, the major constituent of a chronic occlusion is calcified, atherosclerotic plaque. These obstructions are often resistant to guidewire crossing, accounting for PTCA success rates of only 50-70%.

Table 16.1. Total Coronary Occlusion: Clinical and Pathological Features

	Acute Occlusion	Chronic Occlusion
Presentation	Acute MI	Change in anginal status. Angina is usually exertional (collateral insufficiency).
Histopathology	Ruptured fibrous cap overlies soft atheroma; Acute occlusive thrombus is common.	Complex fibrocalcific atherosclerosis. Layered, chronic organized thrombus.
Spontaneous recanalization	Occasional	Rare

Collaterals
   Intracoronary
   Intercoronary
	
	Rare
	Less common
		
		Occasional (bridging collaterals)
		Common

Myocardial viability	Uncommon unless collaterals present.	Common; collaterals sustain viability. May have normal wall motion.
PTCA success	High	Variable; depends on duration and morphology.

B. PERCUTANEOUS REVASCULARIZATION: INDICATIONS AND BENEFITS

Indications:
- Medically refractory angina
- Large area of ischemia by noninvasive studies
- Favorable angiographic appearance

Proven Benefits:
- Relief of exertional angina
- Improvement in left ventricular function and exercise capacity
- Reduction in the need for late CABG by 50%

Possible Benefits:
- Potential source of collaterals to other vessels
- Improvement in left ventricular remodeling following MI
- Improvement in event-free survival

C. BALLOON ANGIOPLASTY

1. **Procedural Outcome.** Compared to PTCA of nontotal occlusions, revascularization rates for chronic total occlusions remain disappointingly low (Table 16.2). Reported series comprising more than 4400 total coronary occlusions indicate an overall success rate of 69% (range 47-81%) (Table 16.3). The most common reasons for procedural failure include the inability to cross the occlusion with a guidewire (80%), failure to cross the occlusion with a balloon (15%), and the inability to dilate the stenosis (5%).

Table 16.2. PTCA of Nontotal vs. Chronic Total Coronary Occlusion: Acute Outcome

Series	Group	N	Success (%)	Complications (%)* D / MI / CABG	Acute Closure (%)
Berger[82]** (1996)	Nontotal	1295	--	0/.14/0	
	Total	139	--	0/1.5/0.3	
Favereau[2] (1995)	Nontotal	2065	96	1.4	1.8
	Total	292	67	1.7	8
Tan[3] (1995)	Nontotal	1157	93	0.4 / 0.7 / 2.1	3.3
	Total	91	66	0 / 0 / 0	0
Ruocco[4] (1992)	Nontotal	1429	82	0.7 / 4.8 / 3.5	1.5
	Total	271	59	1.8 / 3.6 / 3.3	4.1
Myler[5] (1992)	Nontotal	779	94	1.7	-
	Total	122[†]	76	1.6	-
Plante[6] (1991)	Nontotal				
	Stable Angina	637	-	4[††]	-
	Unstable Angina	442	-	8[††]	-
	Total				
	Stable Angina	44	48	2.5[††]	-
	Unstable Angina	46	65	2.0[††]	-
Stone[7] (1990)	Nontotal	6950	96	0.9 / 1.5 / 1.7	-
	Total	905	72	0.8 / 0.6 / 0.8	-
Safian[8] (1988)	Nontotal	711	90	0.4 / 3 / 2	-
	Functional	102	78	1 / 3 / 3	-
	Total	169	63	0 / 0 / 2	-

Abbreviations: D = in-hospital death, MI = in-hospital myocardial infarction, CABG = emergency coronary artery bypass grafting; Nontotal occlusion = 51-99% stenosis (TIMI flow ≥ 2); Functional total occlusion = 99% stenosis (TIMI flow = 1); Total occlusion = 100% stenosis (TIMI flow = 0); - = not reported

†   Excludes 99 occlusions < 1 week old

††   Death, MI, CABG, or repeat PTCA

*   Single number represents overall complication rate

**   In-hospital complication rate among successfully dilated occlusions

Table 16.3. PTCA of Chronic Total Coronary Occlusion: Acute Outcome

Series	N	Success (%)	Complications* (%) D / Q-MI / CABG	Other
Berger[30]** (1996)	139		0/1.4/2.9	
Favereau[2] (1995)	367	67	1.7	
Kinoshita[9] (1995)	433	81	0.3 / 0 / 0	Cardiac tamponade (1%)
Tan[3] (1995)	91	66	0 / 0 / 0	Acute closure (0%)
Ishizaku[10] (1994)	111	62	0 / 1.6 / 0	Non-Q-MI (5%)
Tan[11] (1993)	312	61	0.3 / - / 1.6	
Shimizu[12] (1993)	468	75	- / - / -	
Stewart[13] (1993)	100	47+	1 / 0 / -	Non-Q-MI (5%)
Maiello[14] (1992)	365	64	0 / 0.6 / 0.3	Perforation (0.6%)
Myler[5] (1992)	122++	76	1.6	
Ivanhoe[15] (1992)	480	66	1 / 2 / -	
Ruocco[4] (1992)	271	59	2 / 1 / 2	Acute closure (4%)
Bell[16] (1991)	354	66	0.3 / 1.7 / 2.5	
Stone[7] (1990)	971	72	0.8 / 0.6 / 0.8	
TOTAL	**4450**	**69%**	-	

Abbreviations: D = death, Q-MI = Q-wave myocardial infarction, CABG = emergency coronary artery bypass grafting; - = not reported
+   RCA success: 27%
++ excludes 99 occlusions < 1 week old
*   Single number represents overall complication rate
**   In-hospital compliation rate successfully dilated occlusions

2. **Predictors of Success.** Case selection remains the single most important predictor of PTCA success. Depending on the presence of certain clinical and angiographic variables, recanalization rates range from 18-87% (Tables 16.4, 16.5, 16.6, Figure 16.1):

- **Complete vs. Functional Occlusion.** Pooled data indicate that functional occlusions (99% stenosis with delayed incomplete opacification of the distal vessel segment) are more often recanalized than complete occlusions (76% vs. 67%). It is essential to differentiate the "intra"-lesional channel of a functional occlusion from the "peri"-lesional channel of a bridging collateral; the former is a predictor of PTCA success, while the latter is a predictor of PTCA failure (see Intracoronary Bridging Collaterals, below).

- **Duration of Occlusion.** The duration of occlusion may be estimated by time interval between a major ischemic event (Q-wave myocardial infarction, new onset angina, or abrupt worsening in anginal status) and PTCA. Successful revascularization is highest for occlusions < 1 week, intermediate for occlusions 2-12 weeks, and lowest for those > 3 months. Occlusion duration alone should not preclude revascularization since procedural success for occlusions > 6 months old may be as high as 50-75%.[8,12]

- **Length of Occlusion.** While it is generally felt that occlusions lengths > 15 mm are associated with lower success rates, this characteristic alone should not preclude PTCA attempts.

Table 16.4. Chronic Total Coronary Occlusions: Predictors of PTCA Outcome

Procedural Success	Procedural Failure
Functional Occlusion	Total Occlusion
Occlusion age < 12 weeks	Occlusion age > 12 weeks
Length < 15 mm	Length > 15 mm
Tapered Stump	Abrupt Cut-off
No Sidebranch at Point of Occlusion	Sidebranch Present
No Intracoronary Bridging Collaterals	Extensive Bridging Collaterals ("Caput Medusa")

- **Sidebranch at Point of Occlusion.** This occlusion characteristic is associated with reduced success due to the tendency of the guidewire to pass, deflect or prolapse into the sidebranch.

- **Presence of a Tapered Stump.** Funnel-shaped occlusions (i.e., tapered stump) are associated with higher recanalization rates than occlusions with an abrupt cutoff. Tapered occlusions frequently contain small recanalized channels (200 microns in diameter) that escape detection by angiography but provide a potential route for successful PTCA.[80] However, when the stump is eccentrically oriented, the risk of subintimal wire passage and vessel perforation are increased.

- **Intracoronary "Bridging" Collaterals.** Small angioplasty series suggested that bridging collaterals was the most important determinant of successful PTCA of chronic total occlusions. However, in a recent large study, Kinoshita et al [9] reported equally high success rates among 109 total occlusions with bridging collaterals and 324 occlusions without bridging collaterals (75% vs. 83%, p = 0.07). The authors attributed the high success rate to operator experience and aggressive use of stiff wires. Our own experience suggests that when minimal bridging and one or more favorable characteristics are evident (e.g., tapered stump, short segment of occlusion), success rates may exceed 50%. However, occlusions that manifest extensive intracoronary collateralization ("caput medusa") are generally considered unsuitable for PTCA due to their extremely low success rate (< 20%). These immature networks of vessels consist

Table 16.5. The Impact of Occlusion Duration on PTCA Outcome

Series	Occlusion Duration	N	Success (%)
Tan[3] (1995)	< 3 mos	42	76
	> 3 mos	49	57
Ishizaku[10] (1994)	< 1 mo	11	91
	> 1 mo	100	56
Myler[5] (1992)	< 1 week	99	87
	1-12 wks	73	88
	> 3 mos	49	59
Bell[16] (1992)	< 1 week	60	74
	1-4 wks	15	93
	1-3 mos	243	67
	> 3 mos	45	64
Maiello[14] (1992)	< 1 mo	73	89
	1-3 mos	77	87
	> 3 mos	110	45
Stone[7] (1990)	< 12 wks	29	90
	> 12 wks	39	74

of dilated vasa vasorum and neovascular channels and are very fragile and susceptible to perforation during crossing attempts.

- **Other Factors**. Other factors variably associated with lower success rates including lesion calcification, proximal vessel tortuosity, distal location, RCA or circumflex occlusion, diffuse proximal disease, multivessel disease, unstable angina, and inexperienced operators.[7,14,15,18,19]

3. **Complications.** Although PTCA of a chronic total occlusion is generally considered a "low-risk" procedure, *it is not risk-free!* Several reports have found that the overall incidence of major complications occur with equal frequency among total and nontotal occlusions, and the presence of a chronic total occlusion is an independent predictor of acute closure.[20,21] Major complications include acute closure (5-10%), MI (0-2%), emergency CABG (0-3%), and death (0-1%) (Table 16.3). In one report,[2] 8% of successfully dilated total occlusions reoccluded within 24 hours, compared to only 1.8% of nontotal occlusions; in all, reocclusion was silent in 87%. In another study of chronic total occlusion,

Table 16.6. The Impact of Occlusion Characteristics on PTCA Outcome

Series	Success (%)			
	Length Short/Long	Occlusion Type Functional[†]/ Total[††]	Tapered Stump Yes / No	Bridging Collaterals Yes / No
Kinoshita[9] (1995)	-	-	-	75 / 83
Tan[11] (1993)	-	-	69 / 43	70 / 20
Maiello[14]** (1992)	71 / 60[+]	68 / 69	83 / 51	67 / 29
Ivanhoe[15] (1992)	-	78 / 60	73 / 60	-
Stone[7] (1990)	85 / 69[++]	83 / 74	88 / 59	18 / 85

Abbreviation: - = not reported
* Success rate: single vs. multivessel disease (75% vs 53%), in vessels $\geq$ 3 mm vs < 3 mm (73% vs 48%), with/without sidebranches (53% vs 69%)
** Success rate with/without sidebranch at occlusion site (61% vs. 69%)
† Functional occlusion = faint, late antegrade filling beyond the lesion
†† Total occlusion = absence of antegrade filling beyond the lesion
+ Short ($\leq$ 15 mm); Long (> 15 mm)
++ Short ($\leq$ 10 mm); Long (> 20 mm)

complications occurred in 20% of patients who presented with unstable angina compared to 2.5% in those with stable angina.[6] Ischemic complications are usually due to dissection or thrombus, proximal vessel injury, sidebranch occlusion, distal embolization, or damage to collaterals. Additional complications include coronary artery perforation (relative risk 3.1,[13] reperfusion arrhythmias (including rare delayed ventricular fibrillation[23]), guidewire entrapment and fracture, and contrast nephropathy. Acute reocclusion may cause profound clinical instability and hemodynamic deterioration, possibly related to a phase-lag in the recruitment of previously functioning collaterals.

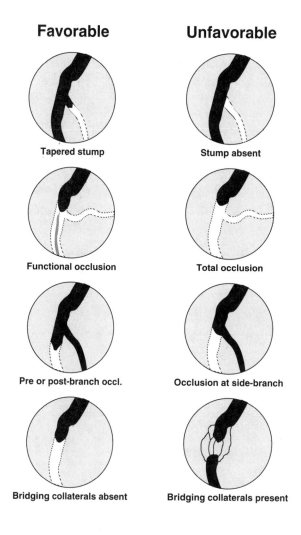

Figure 16.1 Chronic Total Occlusion: Anatomic Descriptors of Procedural Success

Table 16.7. PTCA of Chronic Total Occlusions: Symptoms Status at Follow-up

Series	Successful PTCA (n)	Follow-Up (months)	Asymptomatic (%)
Berger[82] (1996)	139	6	87*
Stewart[13] (1993)	45	12	68*
Ivanhoe[15]** (1992)	264	36	69
Ruocco[4]† (1992)	160	24	69
Bell[16]†† (1991)	234	32	76

*   Asymptomatic or Class I
**   Improvement by ≥ 1 anginal class without further intervention.
**   Successful vs unsuccessful PTCA: 4-yr freedom from death (99% vs 96%), death or MI (93% vs 89%), CABG (87% vs 64%).
†   2-yr death rate in successful vs. unsuccessful PTCA group: 1.2% vs 14.3%.
††   Less need for CABG after successful PTCA. No differences in MI, death, or severe angina between successful and unsuccessful PTCA.

4.   **Late Outcome**

   a.   **Anginal Status and Exercise Capacity (Table 16.7).** The majority of patients with successful PTCA are asymptomatic at follow-up. In the three largest reports, 76%, 69%, and 66% of patients were asymptomatic 1 year,[24] 2 years,[4] and 4 years after PTCA.[15] Absence of symptoms does not exclude restenosis since 40% of patients with restenosis may be free of chest pain.[25]

   b.   **Ventricular Function.** Although data are limited, successful PTCA may improve ventricular relaxation and regional wall motion.[19,26] Global ejection fraction improved in one study,[27] but not in another.[28] Among patients with successfully recanalized occlusions, those with persistent patency and normal flow had better global function and less ventricular dilatation than patients without patent vessels.[29]

   c.   **Death, MI, CABG (Tables 16.8, 16.9).** Most studies indicate that successful recanalization of a chronic total occlusion reduces the need for CABG by 50-75%. However, PTCA does not appear to improve survival or reduce the incidence of late MI.

Table 16.8. PTCA of Nontotal and Chronic Total Coronary Occlusion: Long-Term Outcome

Series	Occlusion Type	F/U (mos)	Death (%)	MI (%)	CABG (%)	PTCA (%)	Combined Event (%)
Berger[30]	Total	6	1.4	2.9	-	-	21[+]
(1996)	Nontotal		0.5	2.4	-	-	18
Violaris[31]	Total	6	0	3.6	3.6	21	29[++,*]
(1995)	Nontotal		0.2	2.8	2.4	17	22
Ruocco[4]	Total	2	-[b]	5	19	9*	25[+]
(1992)	Nontotal		-	9	15	20	30
Safian[8]	Total	2	-	-	14*	-	41[++]
(1988)	Nontotal		-	-	8	-	28

Abbreviations: CABG = emergency coronary artery bypass grafting; MI = in-hospital myocardial infarction; PTCA = percutaneous transluminal coronary angioplasty; F/U = follow-up; - = not reported

[b]   Relative risk 4.39 (1.80 - 10.74) after adjustments for comorbidities; late death for successful vs. failed PTCA 91% vs. 14%, $p < 0.05$)

* $p < 0.05$

+   CABG or PTCA

++   Any death, MI, CABG, or PTCA

Table 16.9. PTCA Success and Chronic Total Coronary Occlusions: Long-Term Outcome

Series	Immediate Result	F/U (mos)	Death (%)	MI (%)	CABG (%)	PTCA (%)	Combined Event (%)
Stewart[13]	Successful	12	2.2	-	16	13	64[++]
(1993)	Unsuccessful		4.1	-	45*	16	31*
Ivanhoe[15]	Successful	4	-	-	13	-	7[+++]
(1992)	Unsuccessful		-	-	36*	-	11*
Bell[16]	Successful	5-7	18	11	18	-	-
(1991)	Unsuccessful		25	5	58*	-	-
Finci[33]	Successful	2	5	-	7	-	33[++]
(1990)	Unsuccessful		3	-	37*	-	41*

Abbreviations: CABG = emergency coronary artery bypass grafting; MI = in-hospital myocardial infarction; PTCA = percutaneous transluminal coronary angioplasty; F/U = follow-up; - = not reported

* $p < 0.05$

++   Any death, MI, CABG, or PTCA

+++   Death or MI

Table 16.10. Restenosis After PTCA of Chronic Total Coronary Occlusion

Series	Occlusion	N	Restenosis[†] (%)	Reocclusion (%)
Berger[30] (1996)	Total	139	49	19
	Nontotal	1295	42	7
Kinoshita[9] (1995)	Total*	433	55	15
Violaris[31]* (1995)	Total	266	45**	19**
	Nontotal	3317	34	5
	Absolute	109	45	24
	Functional	157	45	16
Ishizaku[10] (1995)	Total	62	55	18
Bell[16] (1992)	Total	69	59	14
Ivanhoe[15] (1992)	Total	175	54	16
Anderson[27] (1991)	Total	70	71	34

*   Includes: Absolute occlusion = 100% stenosis, TIMI flow = 0; functional occlusion = 99% stenosis, TIMI flow = 1
†   Restenosis = follow-up stenosis > 50% (≥ 4 months)
** $p < 0.001$ vs. nontotal occlusion

D. EQUIPMENT SELECTION AND PTCA TECHNIQUE. PTCA of a chronic total occlusion is one of the most technically challenging procedures facing the interventionalist. Compared to nontotal occlusions, PTCA of chronic total occlusions is associated with more procedural time; increased cost due to the use of more guiding catheters, guidewires, and balloons; and more radiation exposure to the patient and operator (Table 16.11). Improvements in equipment and technique have improved success and reduced complications.

1. **Guiding Catheter.** It is essential to use a guiding catheter that provides maximal back-up support for guidewire and balloon advancement (Chapter 11). For chronic total occlusions in the left coronary system, a left Voda or left Amplatz will provide maximum support; for total occlusions in the RCA, a left Amplatz or right Voda catheter is preferred. If a Judkins or Multipurpose guiding catheter is used, the "deep-seating" maneuver may be employed to provide extra back-up (Chapter 11). Deep catheter intubation from the left brachial approach (Chapter 2) may enhance support when PTCA from the femoral approach proves unsuccessful.

Table 16.11. Chronic Total Coronary Occlusion: Time, Equipment, and Cost

Series	Occlusion Type	Procedure Time (min)	Radiation Time (min)	Equipment Guides / Wires / Balloons	Cost ($)
Stewart[13]	Total	73	30	-	-
(1993)	Nontotal	59	18	-	-
Bell[16]	Total	74	31	2.0 / 2.7 / 1.8	1947
(1992)	Nontotal	59	18	1.5 / 1.5 / 1.3	1398

Abbreviations: - = not reported

2. **Guidewires**

    a. **Conventional Angioplasty Wires.** Serial use of floppy, intermediate, and standard wires is the most popular approach to crossing a chronic total occlusion, but some operators begin with stiff wires or glidewires. Soft floppy wires will successfully cross 30-50% of recent occlusions (< 6 months), and stiffer wires an additional 25% of cases. However, 25% of occlusions cannot be crossed with any guidewire. Although a 0.014" wire may be initially chosen, we frequently begin with a more pushable 0.016" or 0.018" wire. While 0.035" and 0.038" guidewires have been used to cross total occlusions, their routine use is not recommended due to the risk of subintimal passage and vessel perforation.

        If collaterals are present, a late freeze-frame image can be used to estimate the length of the occlusion, identify the distal vessel, and help direct the guidewire through the expected lumen.[35] Extra back-up support for the guidewire can be achieved by trailing the balloon catheter or a less expensive transport catheter 1-2 cm behind the tip of the guidewire. While attempting to cross the occlusion, excessive rotation (>180°) should be avoided to prevent tip fracture. If the guidewire buckles, it should be retracted and reoriented, rather than forced into the occlusion. Once the wire crosses the occlusion, intraluminal position should be confirmed prior to balloon inflation. Clues to proper guidewire position include free guidewire rotation and easy advancement and retraction of the guidewire. Confirmation of intraluminal positioning is aided by contrast injection through the guiding catheter, central lumen of the balloon, or transport catheter positioned with the occlusion. Clues to improper guidewire position include loss of free rotation, inability to advance the guidwire beyond the occlusion, or inability to advance a balloon or transport catheter through the occlusion. If any of these clues are present, the wire may be subintimal or in a small bridging collateral outside the lumen. In any case, balloon inflation should not be performed because of the risk of dissection and vessel perforation.

    b. **Glidewire (Mansfield/SciMed).** The Glidewire has been successfully employed for peripheral angioplasty and stent placement, and coronary angioplasty and atherectomy. It is comprised of titanium-nickel alloy (Nitinol) core and a hydrophilic polyurethane coating which impart flexibility, kink-resistance, and lubriciousness. The 3-cm tip is soft and flexible to facilitate atraumatic passage. Small series suggest that the Glidewire may successfully cross 30-60% of occlusions that cannot be crossed with conventional guidewires (Table 16.12).[36-38] The Glidewire is commercially available in diameters of 0.016", 0.018", 0.025"; in lengths of 150 cm and 180 cm; and in straight and angled (45° and 70°) tips. All 0.016" and some 0.018"

Table 16.12. Treatment of Occlusions Resistant To Crossing with PTCA Guidwire

Series	N	Device* Success (%)	Final* Success (%)	Other
Glidewire				
Freed[36] (1993)	59	54	39	No perforations.
Rees[37] (1991)	33	58	52	Non-flow-limiting dissections (52%).
Hosney[38] (1990)	8	-	88	0.025" and 0.035" glidewires.
Magnum Wire				
Pande[39] (1992)	28	45	39	See Table 16.13
Haerer[25] (1991)	102	32	32	See Table 16.13
Laserwire				
Serruys[82] (1996)	252[†]	58	-	Coronary perfortion (21%); tamponade (0.8%); non-Q-wave MI (1.6%).
Ultrasound Wire				
Rees[42] (1995)	18	89	78	
ROTACS				
Danchin[43] (1995)	50	-	66	See Table 16.13
Kaltenbach[44] (1991)	152	-	65	Left main dissection (1.5%); no deaths or perforations; restenosis (54%).

Abbreviations: ROTACS = Rotational Angioplasty Catheter System; - = not reported
† Visible entry port and visualization of distal vessel via collaterals required. PTCA guidewire crossing not attempted prior to laserwire.
* Device success = cross occlusion with device; final success = procedural success after, adjunctive PTCA

wires have a radiopaque gold tip. Disadvantages include poor visibility and inability to shape the tip or extend the wire. Accordingly, either a transport catheter or over-the-wire balloon should be advanced over the Glidewire before crossing the occlusion, or a monorail system can be used. If necessary, the Glidewire can be exchanged for a conventional 300-cm angioplasty wire to allow use of larger over-the-wire balloons or a new device.

c. **Magnum-Meier™ Recanalization Wire.** This ball-tipped guidewire (Schneider-USA) consists of a 0.014", 0.018", or 0.021" solid-steel wire shaft; a flexible distal spring wire comprised of Teflonized® tungsten; and a 1-mm olive-shaped tip (Figure 16.2). The wire has been designed to increase pushability and reduce subintimal wire passage. The Magnarail balloon (monorail design) and Magnum-Meier over-the-wire balloon (Schneider-USA) are currently the only commercially available balloons able to accommodate the 0.021" wire. Results from randomized trials have varied: In one study, the Magnum-Meier™ wire outperformed conventional PTCA guidewires,[39] while in another report, lower primary success rates were achieved with the Magnum wire compared to either a conventional guidewire or Omniflex balloon-on-the-wire system (Table 16.13).[25]

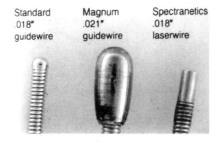

Standard .018" guidewire   Magnum .021" guidewire   Spectranetics .018" laserwire

Figure 16.2 The Magnum-Meier™ Recanalization Wire

3. **Balloon Dilatation Catheter**
   a. **Over-The-Wire Systems.** Although a variety of low-profile on-the-wire and monorail balloon catheters are available, an over-the-wire system is preferred because it allows guidewire exchanges and balloon upsizing, and enhances "push." If difficulty is encountered advancing the balloon into the occlusion, maneuvers that increase guiding catheter support may be of value (e.g., use of deep-seating maneuver [Chapter 11], brachial approach [Chapter 2] and/or larger [9 or 10F] guiding catheters). Constant forward pressure on the balloon is generally more successful than aggressive tapping of the balloon against the occlusion ("jack-hammering"), which usually does not transmit additional torque. If the reference vessel diameter cannot be estimated, the vessel should be predilated with a 1.5 or 2.0 mm balloon, followed by larger balloons if necessary. If the reference vessel diameter is easily estimated (because of collateral filling of the distal vessel), a full-sized balloon may be initially used. For

Table 16.13. Randomized Trials of Chronic Total Coronary Occlusions

Trial	N	Design	1⁰ Success (%)	Comments
Magnum Wire				
Pande[39] (1992)	100	Magnum PTCA	45 67	Magnum success after PTCA failure (39%); PTCA success after Magnum failure (12%). No difference in number of guiding or balloon catheters, or fluoroscopy time.
Haerer[25] (1991)	102	Magnum PTCA Omniflex	32 68 59	Magnum failures salvaged by other systems in 48%.
ELCA				
AMRO Trial[45] (1995)	103	ELCA PTCA	65 61	No difference in 6-month clinical end-points or reocclusion.
ROTACS				
Danchin[43] (1995)	100	ROTACS PTCA	66 60	
STENTS				
Sato[46] (1996)	60†	Stent PTCA	100 -	No subacute stent thrombosis; bailout stenting in PTCA group at 24 hrs (39%). Stent vs. PTCA; MLD past 1) MLD at 24 hrs. 2) 2 ram vs. 1.63 mm), MLD at 3-6 mons (1.6 mm vs. 1.6 mm).
Lytic Infusion				
Kaplan[47] (1995)	60	Intracoronary Urokinase (0.8 MU, 1.6 MU, 3.2 MU)		PTCA success after all lytic regimens (52-56%, p = NS). More bleeding, vascular complications at higher doses. Clinical improvement (76%); reocclusion (9%); restenosis (59%); target vessel revascularization (36%); No MI or death during 2-year follow-up.

Abbreviations: ELCA = Excimer Laser Coronary Angioplasty; ROTACS = Rotational Angioplasty Catheter System; MU = million units (given over 8 hours); - = not reported.
† After successful filation with a 1.5 mm balloon

heavily calcified occlusions, high-pressure balloons may be preferred, but there is otherwise no specific advantage to any balloon material. Procedural success is also independent of inflation technique, speed, duration, or number

b. **On-The-Wire Systems.** Balloon-on-the-wire catheters are generally not considered first-line systems due to their lack of pushability, trackability, and steerability. However, because of their extremely low profile, they may occasionally cross total occlusions when over-the-wire balloons fail.[48] When a fixed balloon-wire system is used, a bare guidewire should be steered beyond the stenosis to maintain coronary access in the event acute closure occurs or balloon upsizing is required. The Probing Catheter (USCI) is a design modification that may improve back-up support and pushability compared to conventional on-the-wire systems. It consists of an inner catheter, which provides back-up for a 0.018" guidewire, and an outer catheter, which is used to deliver a fixed wire-balloon (Probe) to the point of occlusion. A primary success rate of 75% (94% for occlusions < 12 weeks old) has been reported.[49] The Omniflex balloon dilatation catheter (Medtronic) is a modified on-the-wire system with a reinforced wire and an external tip-deflecting handle designed to increase pushability and torqueability. Up to 50% of occlusions resistant to conventional PTCA guidewire crossing have been recanalized using this system.[50]

4. **Adjunctive Thrombolytic Therapy.** Data from small reports (using different lytic agents and infusion regimens) suggest that prolonged intracoronary thrombolytic infusions may improve the recanalization rate of chronic total coronary occlusions. Among 56 resistant occlusions (combined data from 3 studies), a post-lytic improvement in coronary flow and PTCA success was achieved in 63% and 73% of cases, respectively (Table 16.14). These finding were corroborated by Kaplan et al.[47] in a small randomized trial (Table 16.13). The method of prolonged intracoronary thrombolysis is detailed in Chapter 9.

Table 16.14. Intracoronary Thrombolysis for Occlusions Resistant to Guidewire Crossing

Series	N	Lytic	Results	Other
Ajluni[52] (1995)	25	UK (100,000-240,000 U/hour x 8-25 hr) via infusion wire + guide catheter	↑ coronary flow (28%); PTCA success (52%).	MI (8%); significant bleeding (8%); length of stay (5.1 days).
Kaplan[47] (1995)	60	UK (1.6-3.2 MU x 8 hrs) via infusion wire + guide catheter	PTCA success 52-56% for all doses	More bleeding and vascular complications at higher doses.
Cecena[53] (1993)	20	UK bolus (120,000 U i.c.) + up to 200,000 U/hr x 24 hrs via infusion wire + guide catheter	↑ coronary flow (90%); PTCA success (94%).	No MI or emergent CABG; blood transfusion (10%).
Vaska[54] (1991)	11	tPA (5-10 mg/hr x 6 hrs) via infusion wire	↑ coronary flow (91%); PTCA success (82%).	No death, MI, or emergent CABG; acute closure (10%).

Abbreviations: UK = Urokinase; MI = in-hospital Q-wave myocardial infarction; CABG = emergency coronary artery bypass grafting; MU = million units

E. NEW INTERVENTIONAL TECHNOLOGIES. Failure to cross a chronic total occlusion with a guidewire accounts for >50% of unsuccessful procedures. This is extremely important because all currently available devices (balloon, atherectomy, laser, or stent) require initial crossing of the occlusion with a guidewire. Preliminary data suggest that several experimental rotational, laser, ultrasound devices may be capable of recanalizing 30-50% of angioplasty failures (Table 16.12). Once the occlusion is crossed, conventional atherectomy, laser, and stent systems are used to improve lesion contour and luminal geometry (Table 16.15), although the risk of perforation may be increased.[51]

1. Devices for Occlusions Resistant to PTCA Guidewire Crossing (Table 16.12)

    a. Laserwire. An 0.018" excimer laser guidewire (Spectranetics) has been developed to recanalize chronic total occlusions that cannot be crossed with conventional guidewires (Figure 16.2). Use of this guidewire requires meticulous technique and careful patient selection to avoid severe dissection and perforation. Only a small fraction of total occlusions may be suitable for the laserwire since its use must be limited to short segments of occlusion in straight vessels, and the operator must also be able to visualize the proximal and distal extent of the occlusion throughout the ablation procedure. To perform this technique safely, frequent use of orthogonal views or biplane angiography are required to insure that the laser wire is directed along the major axis of the vessel. If contralateral collaterals are present, the donor vessel should be engaged with a second guiding catheter from the contralateral femoral artery to identify the distal end of the occlusion. Even partial penetration of the occlusion may allow successful crossing with a conventional wire. Once a channel is formed, the lesion is treated with PTCA or another device. In the European and US Registries, successful crossing was achieved in 148/252 (58%); perforation occurred in 21% and tamponade in 0.8%.[83] Use of the laserwire, however, is not without its cost: in the European Multicenter Total Surveillance Study, mean procedural time was 110 ± 54 min.[41] A randomized trial (Total Occlusion Trial with Angioplasty assisted by the Laserguide; TOTAL) is underway.

    b. Ultrasound Probe (Figure 8.3). Therapeutic ultrasound catheters that transmit vibrational energy via ball-tipped guidewires are now being used to recanalize total occlusions. Ongoing studies, including the multicenter European CRUSADE trial hope to clarify the mechanism of action and define acute and long-term outcomes.

    c. Vibrational Angioplasty. This technique involves the use of a guidewire attached to a motor. When activated, the motor causes rapid oscillation of the advancing guidewire. In one report, vibrational angioplasty was successful in 14/18 (78%) occlusions resistant to conventional wires and techniques.[42] Severe dissection requiring stenting occurred in 2 cases.

    d. ROTACS: Low-Speed Rotational Angioplasty Catheter System (Figure 8.8). This battery-driven, over-the-wire catheter is comprised of several helical stainless-steel coils, a moveable polyethylene or polyolefin sheath, and a 1.3-1.8 mm olive-shaped ball-tip (Chapter 16). Using an 8F guiding catheter, the ROTACS is advanced over a conventional angioplasty guidewire until it abuts the occlusion. After removing the guidewire, the electric motor is activated, and continuous forward pressure is applied to the catheter while it rotates at 200 rpm. The central lumen of the catheter is used to deliver contrast injections and assess progress. If unsuccessful, the sheath can be advanced to increase support. If the catheter crosses the occlusion, the guidewire should be is reinserted and the ROTACS system exchanged for a conventional balloon catheter. ROTACS was used to successfully recanalize 83/152 (55%) resistant occlusions, including 52% of occlusions 6-12 months old.[44] Due to the occurrence of two left main dissections, ostial LAD lesions emerged as a contraindication to this procedure. The BAROCCO trial, a randomized study of ROTACS vs. PTCA in 100 chronic total coronary occlusions, revealed ROTACS success in 40% and PTCA success in 52% of lesions (p = NS).[43] PTCA was able to salvage 59% of ROTACS failures, whereas only 17% of PTCA failures could be salvaged by ROTACS. The investigators concluded that initial use of ROTACS does not offer an advantage over PTCA, but could be reserved for PTCA failures. At the present time, this device is being used only rarely.

2. **Devices Used For Wire-Crossable Occlusions (Table 16.15)**

   a. **Lasers.** In the multicenter AMRO trial, 103 patients with total occlusions were randomized to excimer laser angioplasty (ELCA) or PTCA. No differences were observed in procedural success (65%), late reocclusion (ELCA 33%, PTCA 23%), or 6-month event-free survival.[45] Most procedural failures were due to inability to cross the occlusion with a guidewire, but if the occlusion was crossed, success rates were 90%.[59,63,71] Major complications were infrequent, although restenosis rates approached 50%.[63]

   b. **Atherectomy** (Chapters 27-29). Among 145 total occlusions crossed with a guidewire in multicenter Rotablator Registry, procedural success was achieved in 91%.[57] Acute closure occurred in 7.2%, half of which developed after the patient left the cath lab. Few data are available regarding the ability of DCA or TEC to recanalize chronic total occlusions. In one report, DCA was successful in 15 of 17 occlusions (88%) after crossing the occlusion with a guidewire.[55,56]

   c. **Stents.** Although the presence of a chronic total occlusion was once a relative contraindication to stenting, recent data suggest a promising role: After successful predilatation of 53 chronic total occlusions with a 1.5 mm balloon, Sato et al[46] randomized patients to PTCA (n = 30) or stent (n= 30). Bailout stenting was required in 36% of the PTCA group, and at 24 hours, minimum lumen diameter was greater in the stent group (2.23 mm vs. 1.63 mm, p < 0.001); there was no difference in the incidence of restenosis (~ 35%) or repeat intervention (~ 30%). In a single observational report of 65 chronic total occlusions (vessel diameter ≥ 3 mm), stents were successfully deployed in 97%, with major complication and restenosis rates of only 3% and 24%, respectively. At 8 months, 85% of patients were asymptomatic and had a negative or improved stress test.[69] Two smaller studies reported 3- and 6-month restenosis rates of only 5%.[68,72] In another observational report by Ooka et al, [67]stenting after successful PTCA reduced reocclusion and restenosis rates compared to PTCA alone. If larger studies confirm these favorable acute and longterm results, primary stenting (or PTCA supported by bailout stenting) may become the preferred method of revascularizing chronic total occlusions.

Table 16.15. Devices For Chronic Total Coronary Occlusions

Device	N	Success[†] (%)	Complications* (%) D / Q-MI / CABG	Other
DCA				
Dick[55] (1991)	7	86	0	Occlusion duration 41 day; (range 5-105 days)
Hinohara[56] (1991)	10	90	0	
ROTABLATOR				
Omoigui[57] (1995)	145	91	1.4 / - / 0	Non-Q-MI (4.3%); dissection (18%); AC (7.2%)
Stertzer[58] (1993)1993)	23	87	0	
ELCA				
Klein[59] (1994)	172 (>3 mos) 107 (<3 mos)	85 90	1 / 0 / 1	AC (4.5%); no perf AC (2.7%); perf (0.9%)
Litvack[60] (1994)	10	93	2.4	
Baumbach[61] (1993)	212	-	-	Total occlusion predictive of perforation
Holmes[62] (1993)	172	90	0.6 / 1.9 / 1.2	
Buchwald[63] (1992)	42	93	-	AC (2.6%); RS (51%)
Bittl[64] (1992)	127	84	-	
HOLMIUM LASER				
deMarchena[65] (1994)	25	100	0	
STENT				
Sato[46] (1995)	53	100	-	
Torre[66] (1994)	27	-	-	Total occlusion predictive of device failure
Ooka[67] (1995)	47 stent 65 PTCA	-[+]	-	RS (44%; reocclusion 10%) RS (68%; reocclusion 35%)

Device	N	Success[†] (%)	Complications* (%) D / Q-MI / CABG	Other
STENT				
Hsu[68] (1994)	36	-[+]	-	Reocclusion at 3 mos. (5%)
Almagor[69] (1993)	65	97	1.5 / 1.5 / -	Asymptomatic at 8 mos. (85%); RS (24%)
Bilodeau[70] (1993)	37**	-	-	SAT (16%); RS (57%; including reocclusion in 20%).

Abbreviations: D = in-hospital death; MI = in-hospital Q-wave myocardial infarction;
CABG = emergency coronary artery bypass grafting; ELCA = Excimer Laser Coronary Angioplasty; DCA = Directional
Coronary Atherectomy; AC = acute closure; SAT = subacute thrombosis; RS = restenosis; - = not reported
†   Device + adjunctive PTCA when needed
*   Single value represents overall in-hospital complications
+   Only successful procedures followed
**   Threatened closure after PTCA

SAPHENOUS VEIN GRAFT OCCLUSION

Of the more than 600,000 saphenous vein bypass grafts placed each year approximately 60-90,000 (10-15%) will be occluded at one year and 300,000 (50%) by 10 years after operation. Among the 10-20% of patients who require re-operation within 10 years, repeat bypass surgery is technically more difficult and has been associated with increased morbidity and mortality compared to the initial operation.

A. **PATHOLOGY.** The etiology of saphenous vein graft occlusion is dependent on the time interval following bypass surgery.[73,74] In the first month, graft occlusions is almost always due to graft thrombosis from poor surgical technique (suture line stenosis, intraoperative vein trauma) or poor distal run-off. Between 1-12 months, initial hyperplasia is the most common cause. After 1 year, occlusion is caused by graft atherosclerosis, which is indistinguishable from coronary arteriosclerosis. Once graft occlusion occurs, retrograde thrombosis to the aorto-ostial junction is common.

B. **PTCA RESULTS.** Although PTCA can successfully revascularize approximately 70% of occluded vein grafts, there is a high incidence of distal embolization (11%), late graft occlusion (40-50%), and late cardiac events (event-free survival of 54% and 34% at 1- and 3-years).[75]

When distal embolization occurs, ~ 50% are associated with vessel closure and/or CK elevation ≥ 2 times normal.[75] Embolization may present as abrupt cutoff of distal vessels (amenable to repeat dilation or lytics), or may be inferred on the basis of myocardial staining ("blush phenomenon") or no-reflow. This latter manifestation was evident in 29% of occluded vein grafts treated with PTCA, of which 55% had subsequent MI.

C. **NEW DEVICES.** TEC atherectomy was used in 68 occluded saphenous vein grafts with procedural success in 75%, significantly lower than the 96% success rate reported for nontotal occlusions. In another report, 27/33 patients (82%) with vein graft occlusions (3d-4wks in age were successfully treated with TEC ± adjunctive lytics and/or PTCA; 4/5 with distal embolization developed MI.[76] Other commercially available devices have not been evaluated in this setting.

D. **PROLONGED INTRAGRAFT THROMBOLYSIS.** Hartmann and associates[77] was the first to systematically study the use of a prolonged infusion of low-dose urokinase (Chapter 9) prior to PTCA of chronically occluded aortocoronary saphenous vein grafts in the hopes of reducing distal embolization, reocclusion, and restenosis. In the multicenter ROBUST trial,[78] 107 patients with one occluded vein graft initially received intracoronary urokinase (100,000 units/hr; half through the guide catheter and half through an infusion wire embedded at least 2 cm in the occlusion). The UK infusion was continued for at least 24 hrs. and could be increased 250,000 - 360,000 units/hr if the angiogram at either 4-8 hrs. or 22-26 hrs. failed to demonstrate recanalization. Full anticoagulation with heparin was maintained during the urokinase infusion, and after the case until therapeutic anticoagulation was achieved with warfarin. Thrombolytic therapy was discontinued when flow was reestablished (at which time PTCA was performed) or no further improvement was seen. All successfully treated patients received warfarin and aspirin for at least 6 months. Successful recanalization was achieved in 69% of patients, with death in 6.5%, MI in 5%, CK-MB elevation in 17%, emergency CABG in 4%, and stroke in 3%. Six-month angiography revealed sustained vessel patency in 40%; angina was present in 22% and 71% of patients with successful and unsuccessful procedures, respectively. Investigators concluded that a prolonged, low-dose infusion of urokinase: 1) can preserve the life of some occluded vein grafts; 2) the procedure should only be attempted in patients < 75 years of age, refractory angina, one occluded graft, and no other reasonable option for therapy. Patients should be excluded in those with a contraindication to lytics, aspirin, or warfarin; a "flush" occlusion; inability to advance the guidewire at least 1 cm into the occlusion; serum creatinine > 2 mg/dL or a history of atrial fibrillation; and 3) PTCA should be avoided if TIMI 0 flow persists after lytics. To avoid washout of the thrombolytic agent into the aorta, Busch et al[79] infused lytic through the central lumen of an inflated balloon (Balloon-Occlusive-Intravascular-Lysis-Enhanced-Recanalization; BOILER) at 10,000 IU/min up to 30 min. Procedural success was achieved in 5/6 (83%) grafts.

CONCLUSIONS

Successful recanalization of chronic total coronary occlusions often results in marked improvements in long-term symptomatic status and exercise capacity, and reduces the need for late CABG by 50%. Despite these benefits, PTCA remains associated with extremely low recanalization rates, high equipment costs, long periods of radiation exposure, and long-term results characterized by a high incidence of reocclusion and restenosis. Although the incidence of major procedural complications is low, MI, emergency CABG, and death have all been reported. Procedural success rates — which may be optimized by proper case selection, equipment selection, and procedural technique — vary between 20-80% depending on the presence of certain clinical and angiographic features including complete vs. functional occlusion, abrupt cutoff vs. tapered stump, length and duration of occlusion, a sidebranch at the point of occlusion, and intracoronary bridging collaterals. The management of totally occluded saphenous vein bypass grafts remains even more problematic. PTCA is associated with a high incidence of acute distal embolization and late revascularization including repeat CABG, which carries an increased risk of perioperative death, MI, and mediastinal bleeding. Preliminary data suggest that one or more new devices may be able to salvage 30-50% of occlusions that cannot be crossed by a conventional angioplasty guidewire. In addition, stenting holds promise as a means of reducing late reocclusion and restenosis. Adjunctive pharmacotherapy may also play an increasingly important role during primary revascularization attempts (prolonged thrombolytic infusions) and for the prevention of reocclusion and restenosis (potent new antiplatelet and antithrombin agents). The role of these various mechanical and pharmacologic strategies will ultimately require prospective, randomized evaluation. Our approach to the patient with chronic total occlusion is summarized in Figures 16.3 and 16.4.

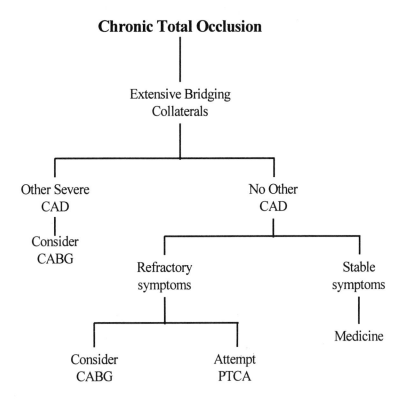

Figure 16.3. Management of Patients with Total Coronary Occlusion & Bridging Collaterals

Abbrevations: CAD = coronary artery disease

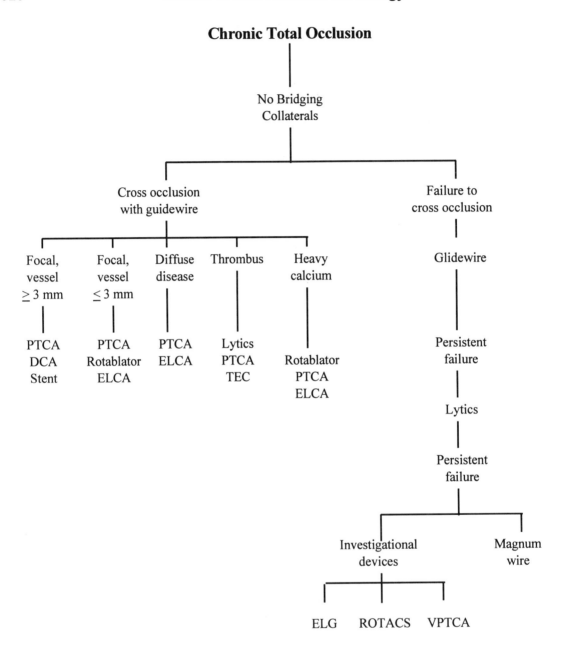

Figure 16.4. Management of Patients with Total Coronary Occlusion Without Bridging Collaterals

Abbrevations: DCA = directional coronary atherectomy; ELCA = excimer laser coronary angioplasty; ELG = excimer laser guidewire; TEC = transluminal extraction catheter; ROTACS = rotational angioplasty catheter system; VPTCA = vibrational angioplasty

REFERENCES

1. Flameng W, Schwarz F, and Hehrlein FW. Intraoperative evaluation of the functional significance of coronary collateral vessels in patients with coronary artery disease. Am J Cardiol 1978;42:187-192.
2. Favereau X, Corcos T, Guerin Y, et al. Early reocclusion after successful coronary angioplasty of chronic total occlusions. J Am Coll Cardiol 1995;25:139A.
3. Tan K, Sulke N, Taub N, Sowton E. Clinical and lesion morphologic determinants of coronary angioplasty success and complications: Current experience. J Am Coll Cardiol 1995;25:855-65.
4. Ruocco NA Jr, Ring ME, Holubkov R, et al. Results of coronary angioplasty of chronic total occlusions (the National Heart, Lung, and Blood Institute 1985-1986 Percutaneous Transluminal Angioplasty Registry). Am J Cardiol 1992;69:69-76.
5. Myler R, Shaw R, Stertzer S, et al. Lesion morphology and coronary angioplasty: Current experience and analysis. J Am Coll Cardiol 1992;19:1641-1652.
6. Plante S. Laarman GJ, de Feyter PJ, et al. Acute complications of percutaneous transluminal coronary angioplasty for total occlusion. Am Heart J 1991;121:417.
7. Stone GW, Rutherford BD, McConahay DR, et al. Procedural outcome of angioplasty for total coronary artery occlusion: An analysis of 971 lesions in 905 patients. J Am Coll Cardiol 1990;15:849-856.
8. Safian RD, McCabe CH, Sipperly ME, et al. Initial success and long-term follow-up of percutaneous transluminal coronary angioplasty in chronic total occlusions versus conventional stenoses. Am J Cardiol 1988;61:23G-28G.
9. Kinoshitaw I, Katoh O, Nariyama J, Otsuji S, et al. Coronary angioplasty of chronic total occlusions with bridging collateral vessels: Immediate and follow-up outcome from a large single-center experience. J Am Coll Cardiol 1995;26:409-15.
10. Ishizaka N, Issiki T, Saeki F, et al. Angiographic follow-up after successful percutaneous coronary angioplasty for chronic total coronary occlusion: Experience in 110 consecutive patients. Am Heart J 1994;127:8.
11. Tan KH, Sulke AN, Taub NA, Watts E, Sowton E. Coronary angioplasty of chronic total occlusions: Determinants of procedural success. J Am Coll Cardiol 1993;21:76A.
12. Shimizu M, Kato O, Otsuji S, et al. Progress in initial outcome of PTCA for complete occlusion. Circulation 1993;88:I-504.
13. Stewart J, Denne L, Bowker T, et al. Percutaneous transluminal coronary angioplasty in chronic coronary artery occlusion. J Am Coll Cardiol 1993;21:1371-1376.
14. Maiello L, Colombo A, Gianrossi R, et al. Coronary angioplasty of chronic occlusions: Factors predictive of procedural success. Am Heart J 1992;124:581-584.
15. Ivanhoe RJ, Weintraub WS, Douglas JS Jr, et al. Percutaneous transluminal coronary angioplasty of chronic total occlusions. Primary success, restenosis, and long-term clinical follow-up. Circulation 1992;85:106-115.
16. Bell MR, Berger PB, Reeder GS, et al. Successful PTCA of chronic total coronary occlusions reduces the need for coronary artery bypass surgery. Circulation 1991;84(4)II-250.
17. Shimizu M, Kato O, Otsuji S, et al. Progress in initial outcome of PTCA for complete occlusion. J Am Coll Cardiol 1993;88(4):I-504.
18. Bell MR, Berger PB, Reeder GS, et al. Initial and long-term outcome of 354 patients after coronary balloon angioplasty of total coronary artery occlusions. Circulation 1992;85:1003.
19. Melchior JP, Meier B, Urban P, et al. Percutaneous transluminal coronary angioplasty for chronic total coronary arterial occlusion. Am J Cardiol 1987;59:535-538.
20. Tenaglia A, Fortin D, Califf R. Predicting the risk of abrupt closure after angioplasty in an individual patient. J Am Coll Cardiol 1994;24(4):1004-1011.
21. Ruocco NA, Ring ME, Holubkov R, Jacobs AK. Results of coronary angioplasty of chronic total occlusions (the National Heart, Lung, and Blood Institute 1985-1986 Percutaneous Transluminal Angioplasty Registry). Am J Cardiol 1992;69:69-76.
22. Stone GW, Rutherford BD, McConahay DR, et al. Procedural outcome of angioplasty for total coronary artery occlusion: An analysis of 971 lesions in 905 patients. J Am Coll Cardiol 1990;15:849-856.
23. Burger W, Kadel C, Keul H, Vallbracht C, Kaltenbach M. A word of caution: Reopening chronic coronary occlusions. Cathet Cardiovasc Diagn 1992;27:35-39.
24. Bell MR, Berger PB, Bresnahan JF, Reeder GS. Initial and long-term outcome of 354 patients after coronary balloon angioplasty of total coronary artery occlusions. Circulation 1992;85:1003-1011.

25. Haerer W, Schmidt A, Eggeling T, et al. Angioplasty of chronic total coronary occlusions. Results of a controlled randomized trial. J Am Coll Cardiol 1991;17(2):113A.

26. Meier B. Total coronary occlusion: A different animal? J Am Coll Cardiol 1991;17:50B.

27. Anderson TJ, Knudtson ML, Roth DL, et al. Improvement in left ventricular function following PTCA of chronic totally occluded arteries. Circulation 1991;84(4):II-519.

28. Serruys PW, Umans V, Heyndrickx GR, et al. Elective PTCA of totally occluded coronary arteries not associated with acute myocardial infarction; short-term and long-term results. Eur Heart J 1985;6:2-12.

29. Danchin N, Angiol M, Beurrie D, et al. Late recanalization of chronic total coronary occlusion: Maintained vessel patency improves global and regional left ventricular function and avoids remodeling. J Am Coll Cardiol 195;25:345A.

30. Berger PB, Holmes DR, Ohman M, et al. Restenosis, reocclusion and adverse cardiovascular events after successful balloon angioplasty of occluded versus nonoccluded coronary arteries. Results from the Multicenter American Research Trial with Cilazapril after Angioplasty to Prevent Transluminal Coronary Obstruction and Restenosis (MARCATOR). J Am Coll Cardiol 1996;27:1-7.

31. Violaris A, Melkert R, Serruys P. Long-term luminal renarrowing after successful elective coronary angioplasty of total occlusions. A quantitative angiographic analysis. Circulation 1995;91:2140-2150.

32. Kadel C, Burger W, Hartmann A, et al. Long-term follow-up in 686 patients with attempted reopening of chronic coronary occlusions. Circulation 1993;88:I-505.

33. Finci L, Meier B, Fayre J et al. Long-term results of successful and failed angioplasty for chronic total coronary arterial occlusion. Am J Cardiol 1990;66:660.

34. Mintz G, Popma J, Pichard A, et al. Increased plaque burden affects procedural outcomes of total occlusions: An intravascular ultrasound study. J Am Coll Cardiol 1995;25:61A.

35. Sherman CT, Sheehan D and Simpson JB. Simultaneous cannulation: A technique for percutaneous transluminal coronary angioplasty of chronic total occlusions. Cathet Cardiovasc Diagn 1987;13:333-336.

36. Freed M, Boatman JE, Siegel N, Safian RD, Grines CL, O'Neill WW. Glidewire treatment of resistant coronary occlusions. Cathet Cardiovasc Diagn 1993;30:201-204.

37. Rees MR, Sivananthan MV, Verma SP. The use of hydrophilic terumo glidewires in the treatment of chronic coronary artery occlusions. Circulation 1991;84(4):II-519.

38. Hosny A, Lai D, Mancherje C, Lee G. Successful recanalization using a hydrophilic-coated guidewire in total coronary occlusions after unsuccessful PTCA attempts with standard steerable guidewires. J Interven Cardiol 1990;3(4):225-230.

39. Pande AK, Meier B, Urban P, de la Serna F. Magnum/magnarail versus conventional systems for recanalization of chronic total coronary occlusions: A randomized comparison. Am Heart J 1992;123:1182-1186.

40. Haerer W, Schmidt A, Eggeling T, et al. Angioplasty of chronic total coronary occlusions. Results of a controlled randomized trial. J Cardiol 1991;17:113A.

41. Serruys PW, Hamburger J, Fleck E, Koolen JJ, et al. Laser guidewire: A powerful tool in recanalization of chronic total coronary occlusion. Circulation 1995;92:I-76.

42. Rees M, Michalis L. Vibrational coronary angioplasty: Challenging chronic total occlusions. Preliminary clinical data. J Am Coll Cardiol 1995;25:368A.

43. Danchin N, Cassagnes J, Juilliere Y, Machescourt J. Balloon angioplasty versus rotational angioplasty in chronic coronary occlusions (the BAROCCO study). Am J Cardiol 1995;75:330-334.

44. Kaltenbach M, Vallbracht C, and Hartmann A. Recanalization of Chronic Coronary Occlusions by Low Speed Rotational Angioplasty (ROTACS). J Interven Cardiol 1991;4:155-165.

45. Appleman Y, Koolen J, deFeyter P, et al. Longterm outcome of excimer laser angioplasty versus balloon angioplasty in functional and total coronary occlusions. J Am Coll Cardiol 1995;25:330A.

46. Sato Y, Nosaka H, Kimura T, Nobuyoshi M. Randomized comparison of balloon angioplasty versus coronary stent implantation for total occlusion. J Am Coll Cardiol 1996;March Special Issue: 742-04.

47. Kaplan BM, Jonse D, Zidar F, Schreiber T, et al. Clinical and angiographic follow-up to a randomized trial of prolonged urokinase infusion for chronic total occlusion in native coronary arteries. Circulation 1995;92:I-784.

48. Höpp HW, Franzen D, Deutsch HJ, et al. New option for balloon recanalization of total coronary occlusions. Cathet Cardiovasc Diagn 1991;24:226-230.

49. Little T, Rosenberg J, Seides S, et al. Probe ™ angioplasty of total coronary occlusion using the probing catheter ™ technique. Cathet Cardiovasc Diagn. 1990;21:124.

50. Hamm CW, Jupper W, Kuck K, et al. Recanalization of chronic total occluded coronary arteries by new angioplasty systems. Am J Cardiol 1990;66:1459.

51. Flood RD, Popma JJ, Chuang YC, Salter LF, et al. Incidence, angiographic predictors, and clinical significance of coronary perforation occurring after new device angioplasty. J Am Coll Cardiol 1994;23:301A.

52. Ajluni S, Jones D, Zidar F, Puchrowicz S, Margulis A. Prolonged urokinase infusion for chronic total native coronary occlusions: Clinical, angiographic, and treatment observations. Cath Cardiovas Diagn. 1995;34:106-110.

53. Cecena FA. Urokinase infusion after unsuccessful angioplasty in patients with chronic total occlusion of native coronary arteries. Cath Cardiovasc Diagn. 1993;28:214-218.

54. Vaska KJ, Whitlow PL. Selective tissue plasminogen activator infusion for chronic total occlusions of native coronary arteries failing angioplasty. Circulation 1991;84:II-250.

55. Dick R, Haudenschild C, Popma J, et al. Directional atherectomy for total coronary occlusions. Coronary Artery Disease 1991;2:189-199.

56. Hinohara T, Rowe M, Robertson G, et al. Effect of lesion characteristics on outcome of directional coronary atherectomy. J Am Coll Cardiol 1991;17:1112-1120.

57. Omoigui N, Reisman M, Franco I, Whitlow P. Rotational atherectomy in chronic total occlusions. J Am Coll Cardiol 1995;25:97A.

58. Stertzer SH, Rosenblum J, Shaw RE, et al. Coronary rotational ablation: Initial experience in 302 procedures. J Am Coll Cardiol 1993;21:287-95.

59. Klein L, Litvack F, Holmes D, et al. Prospective multicenter analysis of excimer laser coronary angioplasty (ELCA) in stenosis with complex morphology. J Am Coll Cardiol 1994:448A.

60. Litvack F, Eigler N, Margolis J, et al. Percutaneous excimer laser coronary angioplasty: Results in the first consecutive 3,000 patients. J Am Coll Cardiol 1994;23:323-329.

61. Baumbach A, Bittl J, Fleck E, Geschwind H, Sanborn T. Acute complications of excimer laser coronary angioplasty: A detailed analysis of multicenter results. J Am Coll Cardiol 1994;23:(6):1305-1313.

62. Holmes DR, Forrester JS, Litvack F, Reeder GS, et al. Chronic total obstruction and short-term outcome: The excimer laser coronary angioplasty registry experience. Mayo Clin Proc 1993;68:5-10.

63. Buchwald AB, Werner GS, Unterberg C, Voth E, Kreuzer H, Wiegand V. Restenosis after excimer laser angioplasty of coronary stenoses and chronic total occlusions. Am Heart J 1992;123:878-885.

65. deMarchena EJ, Mallon SM, Knopf WD, et al. Effectiveness of holmium laser-assisted coronary angioplasty. Am J Cardiol 1994;73:117-121.

66. Torre SR, Lai SM, Schatz RA. Relation of clinical presentation and lesion morphology to the procedural results of Palmaz-Schatz stent placement: A new approaches to coronary intervention (NACI) registry report. J Am Coll Cardiol 1994;23:135A.

67. Ooka M, Suzuki T, Yokoya K, Hayase M, et al. Stenting after revascularization of chronic total occlusion. Circulation 1995;92:I-94.

68. Hsu Y-S, Tamai H, Ueda K, et al. Clinical efficacy of coronary stenting in chronic total occlusions. Circulation 1994;90:I-613.

69. Almagor Y, Borrione M, Maiello L, Khalt B, Finci L, Colombo A. Coronary stenting after recanalization of chronic total coronary occlusions. Circulation 1993;88:I-504.

70. Bilodeau L, Iyer S, Cannon A, et al. Stenting as an adjunct to balloon angioplasty for recanalization of totally occluded coronary arteries: Clinical and angiographic follow-up. J Am Coll Cardiol 1993;21:292A.

71. Rothbaum DA, Linnemeier TJ, Krauthamer D, et al. Excimer laser angioplasty in total coronary occlusions: A registry report. Circulation 1991;84(4)II-744.

72. Ooka M, Suzuki T, Kosokawa H, et al. Stenting vs. non-stenting after revascularization of chronic total occlusion. Circulation 1994;90:I-613.

73. Saber RS, Edwards WD, Holmes DR Jr, et al. Balloon angioplasty of aortocoronary saphenous vein bypass grafts: A histopathologic study of six grafts from five patients, with emphasis on restenosis and embolic complications. J Am Coll Cardiol 1988;12:1501-1509.

74. Waller BF, Rothbaum DA, Gorfinkel HJ, et al. Morphologic observations after percutaneous transluminal balloon angioplasty of early and late aortocoronary saphenous vein bypass grafts. J Am Coll Cardiol 1984;4:784-792.

75. Kahn J, Rutherford B, McConahay D, et al. Initial and long-term outcome of 83 patients after balloon angioplasty of totally occluded bypass grafts. J Am Coll Cardiol 1994;23:1038-1042.

76. Margolis JR, Mehta S, Kramer B, et al. Extraction atherectomy for the treatment of recent totally occluded saphenous vein grafts. J Am Coll Cardiol 1994;23:405A.

77. Hartmann JR, McKeever LS, Stamato NJ, et al. Recanalization of chronically occluded aortocoronary saphenous vein

bypass grafts by extended infusion of urokinase: Initial results and short-term clinical follow-up. J Am Coll Cardiol 1991;18:1517-1523.

78. Hartmann JR, McKeever LS, O'Neill WW, White CJ, et al. Recanalization of chronically occluded aortocoronary saphenous vein bypass grafts with long-term, low dose direct infusion of urokinase (ROBUST): A serial trial. J Am Coll Cardiol 1996;27:60-6.

79. Busch UW, Weingartner F, Renner U, Neumann FJ, et al. Balloon-occlusive-intravascular-lysis-enhanced-recanalization (B-O-I-L-E-R) of thrombotic saphenous vein graft occlusions: A new technique of selective intravascular thrombolysis. J Am Coll Cardiol 1993;21:451A.

80. Katsuragawa M, Fujiwara H, Miyamae M, Sasayama S. Histologic studies in percutaneous transluminal coronary angioplasty for chronic total occlusion: comparison of tapering and abrupt types of occlusion and short and long occluded segments. J Am Coll Cardiol 1993;21:604-611.

81. Jaup T, Allemann Y, Urban P, et al. The Magnum wire for percutaneous coronary balloon angioplasty in 723 patients. J Invas Cardiol 1995;7:259-64.

82. Serruys PW, Leon M, Hamburger JN, et al. Recanalization of chronic total coronary occlusions using a laser guide wire: The Eu and US total experience. J Am Coll Cardiol 1996;March Special Issue.

83. Moussa I, DiMario C, Blengino S, et al. Coronary stenting of chronic total occlusions without anticoagulation: Immediate and long-term outcome. J Invas. Cardiol 1996;8.

84. Mehta S, Margolis JR, Bittl JA, Tcheng JE, et al. Finally, treatment of chronic total occlusions-ablation with excimer laser angioplasty. J Invas. Cardiol 1996;8.

85. Sharma SK, Duvvuri S, Cocke T, et al. Directional coronary atherectomy (DCA) of chronic total occlusions. J Invas. Cardiol 1996;8.

17 CORONARY ARTERY BYPASS GRAFTS

Mark Dooris, M.B.B.S.
Robert D. Safian, M.D.

SAPHENOUS VEIN GRAFTS

Coronary artery bypass surgery (CABG) is a well-established form of revascularization. Despite its ability to relieve angina, and in some patients, prolong survival, deficiencies exist:

- **Recurrent Ischemia.** Ischemia recurs in 17% and 63% of patients at 1- and 10-years, respectively, which may be due to new disease in vessels not previously bypassed, progressive disease in native vessels beyond the graft anastomosis, or disease in the bypass conduits themselves.
- **Vein Graft Failure.** The rate of saphenous vein graft failure is 8% at 1-year, 38% at 5-years and 75% at 10-years.[1] In asymptomatic patients, silent occlusion occurs in 28%, 32%, and 35% of vein grafts at 1-3, 4-6, and 7-11 years after CABG, respectively.[3]
- **Repeat Revascularization.** Repeat CABG or PTCA is required in 4% of patients at 5-years, 19% of patients 10-years, and 31% of patients 12-years after initial CABG.

A. TREATMENT OPTIONS FOR VEIN GRAFT DISEASE

1. **Repeat CABG.** The risks of repeat CABG are 2- to 4-fold higher than initial CABG, with periprocedural death and MI in 2-5% and 2-8% of patients, respectively.[4-10] Five- and 10-year survival rates are 84-94% and 75%, respectively,[11-18] but 5-year event-free survival (freedom from death, MI, PTCA, or CABG) and angina-free survival are only 64% and 50%, respectively.[12,13] These immediate and longterm results reflect the technical difficulty of reoperation and the frequency of unfavorable patient characteristics. Risk factors for perioperative morbidity and mortality after repeat surgery include left main disease, anginal class III or IV, age > 60 years, diabetes mellitus, ejection fraction < 40%, and incomplete revascularization.[9] Some patients are not suitable candidates for reoperation because of small target vessels, poor LV function, serious comorbid medical problems, or limited availability of suitable conduits. In addition, the risk of injury to a patent internal mammary graft is 5-38% at less experienced surgical centers.[19-22]

2. **PTCA.** The technique of PTCA in vein grafts is similar to that in native coronary arteries. Proper guiding catheter selection — important for back-up support during advancement of interventional hardware — depends on target vessel takeoff from the ascending aorta (Figures 17.1, 17.2); the size of the curve depends on the diameter of the aorta. For lesions involving the distal body of the graft, distal anastomosis, or native vessel beyond the anastomosis (Figure 17.3), short (90 cm) guiding catheters and/or PTCA balloon catheters with long shafts (140-150 cm) may be useful (See Chapter 1).

a. **Success and Major Complication Rates.** PTCA of saphenous vein grafts can be performed with procedural success rates of 78-97% and in-hospital complication rates of 0-12% (Table 17.1).[23-42] Contemporary series indicate that despite higher risk patients (i.e., advanced age, LV dysfunction, and multivessel coronary disease), PTCA can be performed without an increased risk of major ischemic complications compared to earlier studies.[43] These clinical complications are usually associated with one or more of the angiographic complications described below.

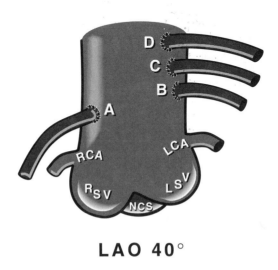

LAO 40°

Figure 17.1 Usual Arrangement of Saphenous Vein Bypass Grafts From the Ascending Aorta

From proximal to distal:
A. Grafts to the distal RCA or distal LCx (L-dominant).
B. Grafts to the LAD.
C. Grafts to the diagonal branches.
D. Grafts to the OM or ramus.

b. **Angiographic Complications**
   1. **Distal Embolization.** Distal embolization causing abrupt vessel cutoff during PTCA occurs in 2-15% of vein grafts > 3 years old, especially in those with soft, friable intraluminal material ("rat-bite" appearance by angiography).[1,32,33,44,46] Independent predictors of distal embolization include diffuse degeneration and large plaque volume, but not thrombus or ulceration.[45] An angioscopy study also found that vein graft friability rather than thrombus was the strongest predictor of distal embolization and no-reflow.[47] When elevated CK-MB is used as a "marker" for distal embolization, rates up to 20% have been reported for PTCA, DCA, TEC, and stents; independent predictors included angiographic thrombus and large vessel diameter, not device type.[46] Preliminary data suggest that c7E3 (ReoPro) may lead to 7-fold and 5-fold reductions in distal embolization

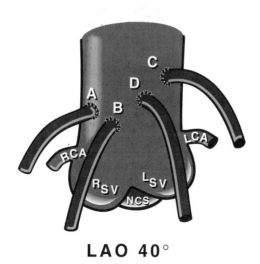

LAO 40°

Figure 17.2 Origin of Saphenous Vein Grafts: Guiding Catheter Selection

A.   Usual orientation of vein grafts to the distal RCA from the lateral wall of the aorta above the right Sinus of Valsalva (RSV).

B.   More anterior origin of vein grafts to the distal RCA.

C.   Usual orientation of vein grafts to the left coronary artery from the anterior wall of the aorta above the left Sinus of Valsalva (LSV).

D.   More anterior orientation of the vein grafts to the left coronary artery.

Guiding Catheter Selection:		**Primary**	**Alternate**
	A.	Multipurpose	JR, AL
	B.	AL	JR, Multipurpose, Hockey Stick
	C.	JR, Hockey Stick	AL, left bypass, Multipurpose
	D.	AL, Hockey Stick	JR, left bypass, Multipurpose

and non-Q-wave MI during vein graft intervention, respectively; in contrast to native vessels, there was no impact on 6-month cardiac event rate.[48] It is important to distinguish distal embolization leading to abrupt cutoff of a distal branch from no-reflow (see below); the former is more readily treated by gentle guidewire manipulation, repeat PTCA, infusion of thrombolytic drugs, or in refractory cases, by emergency CABG; the latter is more responsive to intracoronary calcium blockers (Chapter 21).

2.   **No-Reflow.**   The etiology of no-reflow is uncertain, but may be secondary to microvascular embolization and/or spasm (Chapter 21).   True no-reflow rarely responds to lytic therapy, repeat PTCA, or CABG, but may respond to intracoronary calcium antagonists.[49] The incidence of no-reflow following vein graft intervention is 5-15%, and is more frequent in old (> 3 years) and degenerated grafts.[33,44,50]

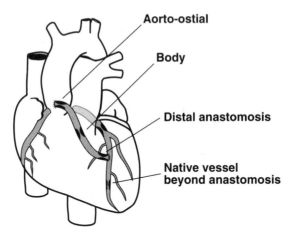

Figure 17.3 Target Lesion Location in Post-CABG Patients

3.   **Abrupt Closure.** Abrupt closure complicates 1-2% of vein graft interventions, which is lower than the 2-12% incidence following native vessel intervention.[23-42] Abrupt closure is usually caused by severe dissection, and is best managed by prolonged balloon inflations, stenting, or directional atherectomy (Chapter 20). Emergency redo bypass surgery is also feasible, but is associated with mortality rates up to 15% due to poor clinical profile, technical difficulties in harvesting conduits, and potential delays in achieving satisfactory cardiopulmonary bypass.[49,51,53]

4.   **Perforation.** Although coronary artery perforation is a rare complication of balloon angioplasty, the incidence is higher following atherectomy or laser angioplasty.[54,55] Cardiac tamponade is unusual after vein graft perforation due to the extrapericardial course of vein grafts and post-pericardiotomy fibrosis. The management of vein graft perforation is similar to that of native vessel perforation (Chapter 22).

c.   **Restenosis.** The major limitation of PTCA in saphenous vein grafts is restenosis, which occurs in 23-73% of patients within 6 months (Table 17.1). Clinical recognition is often difficult because of coexistent multivessel disease and collaterals, which limit the interpretation of myocardial perfusion studies and recurrent symptoms. Independent predictors of restenosis include proximal, ostial, or diffuse disease; vein grafts > 3 years of age; small vessels; and chronic total occlusions. The presence of diabetes, shown to adversely effect longterm outcome after multivessel PTCA (Chapter 3), has also been associated with reduced longterm event-free survival after vein graft angioplasty.[56]

Table 17.1. Results of PTCA in Saphenous Vein Grafts

Series	N (Lesions)	Graft Age (months)	Success (%)	Complications (%) D / MI / CABG	Restenosis (%)
Tan[23] (1994)	50	50	86	- / - / -	39
Morrison[24] (1994)	89	98	93	3 / 3 / 1	51
Unterberg[25] (1992)	55	46	89	- / - / -	-
Miranda[26] (1992)	409	>12	94	- / - / -	-
Meester[27] (1991)	59	56	86	1.2 / 8.3 / 2.4	-
Plokkor[28] (1991)	454*	67	90	0.7 / 2.8 / 1.3	-
Douglas[29] (1991)	672	≤ 120	90	1.2 / 2.3 / 3.5	-
Jost[30] (1991)	49	40	94	0.00	-
Webb[31] (1990)	168	66	85	0.00	50
Dorros (1989) [32]	241	-	91	2.3 / 5.2 / 1.4	-
Platko[33] (1989)	107	50	92	2 / 5.9 / 2	61
Pinkerton[34] (1988)	100	60	93	- / - / -	-
Cote[35] (1987)	83	51	86	0.00	23
Ernst[36] (1987)	33	-	97	0.00	31
Douglas[37] (1986)	235	-	92	0.00	-
Reeder[38] (1986)	19	38	84	5.3 / 5.3 / 0	73

Abbreviations: D = death; MI = myocardial infarction; CABG = emergency coronary artery bypass surgery; - not reported * number of patients

3. **New Interventional Devices.** In busy interventional practices, new devices are used to treat 25-35% of vein grafts undergoing catheter-based intervention. New device angioplasty has allowed more patients with advanced age, LV dysfunction, and extensive coronary disease to undergo percutaneous revascularization, without increasing the incidence of major complications.[43]

a. **Transluminal Extraction Catheter (TEC) (Chapter 29)**

1. **Overall Results.** TEC was approved by the Food and Drug Administration in 1993, and has been advocated as a potential treatment for degenerated vein grafts. As shown in Table 17.2, procedural success rates of 80-90% for nonoccluded vessels and 60-75% for occluded vessels.[57-60] The frequent development of angiographic complications, including distal embolization (2-17%),[57-62] no-reflow (8.8%),[57] and abrupt closure (2.0-5.0%)[57-60] reflect the application of TEC to complex lesions, many of which are poorly suited for other devices. Major clinical complications, including Q-wave MI (0.7-3.7%) and death (0-10.3%) have not been reduced by TEC. Angiographic follow-up suggests restenosis in 60-70%, including late vessel occlusion in 30% in one study.[57] Because TEC relies on cutting and aspiration, it should be well suited for thrombus-containing lesions; angioscopy studies demonstrate partial or complete thrombus removal in 75%,[63,64] although intimal flaps occur in virtually 100% of lesions.[65]

2. **Thrombotic Vein Grafts.** Compared to vein grafts without thrombus treated by TEC, the presence of thrombus increased the risk of angiographic failure (25% vs. 11%), clinical failure (31% vs. 12%), angiographic complications (27% vs 11%), and clinical complications (13.3% vs 2.4%).[66,67] Using CK-MB as a biochemical marker of distal embolization, one study reported a lower incidence of distal embolization after TEC compared to PTCA (7% versus

Table 17.2. In-hospital Results of TEC Atherectomy in Saphenous Vein Grafts

	Meany[59] (1995)	Twidale[60] (1994)	Safian[57] (1992)	Popma[58] (1992)
No. lesions	650	88	158	29
Adjunctive PTCA	74	95	91	86
Success (%)	89	86	84	82
Complications (%)				
Myocardial infarction	0.7	3.4	2.0	3.7
Death	3.2	0	2.0	10.3
Acute closure	2.0	5.0	5.0	-
Distal embolization	2.0	4.5	11.9	17
No-reflow	-	-	8.8	-

Abbreviation: - = not reported

22%, p < 0.02).[68] In the multicenter NACI Registry, distal embolization occurred in 7.4% of lesions, was associated with a 6-fold increase in-hospital mortality and a 5-fold increase in MI, and correlated with myocardial infarction, "stand-alone" TEC, vein graft thrombus, and large vessel diameter.[69] Several studies have suggested a synergistic role ("device synergy") for TEC followed by stenting for degenerated and/or thrombotic vein grafts;[64,70,71] preliminary data suggest that stent deferral (i.e., 1-2 months after TEC) may reduce distal embolization and major clinical complications, although the incidence of silent graft occlusion during the waiting period was 15%;[70] ongoing studies will help clarify the role of an immediate vs. deferred stent strategy.

b. **Directional Coronary Atherectomy (DCA) (Chapter 28).** Morphologic characteristics favorable for vein graft DCA include large caliber, lack of tortuosity, and absence of heavy calcification. When used in focal complex lesions in large grafts, procedural success was 85-97% (lower in ostial and long [> 20 mm] lesions)[72] with major complications in 0-7% (Table 17.3).[72-78] Restenosis after DCA has been reported in 31-63%,[72-75,77] and was lower in de novo (38%) compared to restenotic lesions (75%).[76,79] In the Coronary Angioplasty versus Excisional Atherectomy Trial (CAVEAT II), DCA had higher procedural success rates and better luminal enlargement compared to PTCA, but there was a higher incidence of complications, mostly related to non-Q-wave MI (Table 17.4).[80] At 6 months, there was no difference in angiographic restenosis, but a trend toward less target lesion revascularization after DCA (Table 17.4).[80]

c. **Excimer Laser Angioplasty (ELCA) (Chapter 30).** Although saphenous vein grafts represent up to 15% of vessels treated with ELCA, there are relatively few published data about the immediate and longterm results (Table 17.5).[81-84] In a study of 545 vein graft lesions, procedural success was 92%; adjunctive PTCA was required in 91% of lesions.[82] Angiographic complications included acute vessel closure (4%), distal embolization (3.3%), and perforation (1.3%). At least one major complication occurred in 6.1% of patients including death (1%), Q-wave MI (2.4%), non-Q-wave MI (2.2%), and CABG (0.6%). Lesion length > 10 mm was an independent predictor of procedural failure, major complications and restenosis, while ostial location and vessel diameter < 3 mm were associated with fewer major complications.[82] Angiographic and clinical follow-up reveal a high incidence of late cardiac events, including angiographic restenosis in 52% (including late vessel occlusion in 24%) and a 1-year event-free survival of only 48%.[81] Results using the infrared Holmium laser appear similar.[84]

d. **Stents (Chapter 26).** The randomized Study of Stent vs. Angioplasty for Vein Graft Disease (e.g., SAVED trial) have only recently completed patient enrollment. Preliminary results indicate that stenting results in superior lumen enlargement, higher procedural success, and less need for emergency CABG;[87] however, there were no differences in recurrent cardial events at 1-month.[190] Numerous observational studies show that a variety of stents can be deployed in vein grafts with high success rates (95-100%), a low incidence of stent thrombosis (0-8%) and major clinical complications (0-4%), and a possible reduction in restenosis compared to other devices (Table 17.6).[88-101] Restenosis rates appear higher for ostial and restenotic lesions (30-60%) compared to

Table 17.3. In-hospital Results of DCA in Saphenous Vein Grafts

Series	No. Lesions	Success (%)	Major Complications(%)*
CAVEAT II[80] (1995)	149	89	4.7
Stephan[127] (1995)	57[†]	86	0
Cowley[72] (1993)	363	85	2.5**
Garratt[76] (1992)	26	96	3.8
Pomerantz[75] (1992)	35	94	0
DiScasio[74] (1992)	96	97	1.4
Ghazzal[78] (1991)	286	87	2.1
Selmon[77] (1991)	87	91	2.6
Kaufmann[73] (1990)	14	93	7

*   Major complications = death, myocardial infarction, or emergency coronary artery bypass surgery
** US DCA Registry: Vascular repair (3.5%); non-Q-wave MI 3%; restenosis rate 57% (38% for de novo lesions, 75% for restenotic lesions)

other vein graft sites and de novo lesions (17-39%). Compared to DCA of aorto-ostial vein graft lesions, stenting resulted in better immediate angiographic results and less late target lesion revascularization; event-free survival at 1 year, however, was only 42% for DCA and 53% for stents.[102] Intragraft urokinase has been used in conjunction with stenting for thrombotic vein grafts: In a study of 30 patients, procedural success was achieved in 93.3% using 2.2 million units of urokinase over 20.5 hours.[91] Clinical complications included Q-wave MI (3.3%), non-Q-wave MI (16.7%), and vascular injury (16.7%). In a subgroup of 13 patients with total occlusions, procedural success was achieved in 100% without major complications.[91] An important disadvantage of stenting is the perceived need for vigorous antiplatelet and anticoagulant therapy, which increases bleeding and vascular complications, length of hospital stay, and cost. However, optimal stent techniques, advanced stent designs, and reduced anticoagulation regimens hold promise for improved outcomes and lower costs.[103] Unfortunately, vein graft stenting has been associated with significant attrition in late outcome; event-free survival was 75% at 6 months, 67% at 12 months, and only 55% at 24 months, mostly due to progressive disease in nonstented

Table 17.4. Results of DCA vs. PTCA in Saphaneous Vein Grafts (CAVEAT II)[80]

	DCA No. (%)	PTCA No. (%)
No.	149 (100)	156 (100)
Graft age (years)	9.5	9.9
Lesion location		
aorto-ostial	22 (14.8)	14 (9.0)
proximal body	42 (28.2)	57 (36.5)
mid-body	57 (38.3)	52 (33.3)
distal body	28 (18.8)	43 (27.6)
distal anastamosis	8 (5.4)	7 (4.5)
Lesion length (mm)	10.9	11.0
In-hospital results (%)		
success	89.2	79.0*
final diameter stenosis	31.5	37.6**
acute closure	7 (4.7)	4 (2.6)
distal embolization	20 (13.4)	8 (5.1)[+]
perforation	1 (0.7)	0
Q-wave-MI	2 (1.3)	3 (1.9)
nono-Q-MI	24 (16.1)	15 (9.6)[++]
CABG	1 (0.7)	2 (1.3)
death	3 (2.0)	3 (1.9)
composite endpoint	30 (20.1)	19 (12.2)[++]
Follow-up results (%)		
restenosis	47 (45.6)	48 (50.5)
late cardiac event	(49.3)	(44.3)
target lesion revascularization	(18.6)	(26.2)[++]

Abbreviations: CABG = emergency coronary artery bypass grafting; DCA = directional coronary atherectomy; MI = myocardial infarction

*	$p < 0.05$	+	$p < 0.01$
**	$p < 0.001$	++	$p < 0.10$

Table 17.5. In-hospital Results of ELCA in Saphaneous Vein Grafts

Series	No. Lesions	PTCA (%)	Success (%)	Major Complications (%)*
Strauss[81] (1995)	125	83	89	3.7
Marchena[84†] (1994)	34	-	100	0
Bittl[82] (1994)	545	91	92	6.1
Litvack[83] (1994)	480	-	92	-

Abbreviations: PTCA = adjunctive balloon angioplasty; - = not reported
*   Major complications = death, myocardial infarction, or emergency coronary artery bypass surgery
†   Holmium Laser

vessels.[104] The use of TEC atherectomy or ELCA for debulking vein graft lesions immediately before stenting is under investigation; preliminary data suggest high success rates (>90%) and few major complications (5-6%), but further follow-up data are needed.[189]

e. **Rotablator Atherectomy (Chapter 27).** Rotablator is contraindicated in degenerated vein grafts and thrombus-containing lesions due to the risk of distal embolization, no-reflow, abrupt closure, and myocardial infarction. Rotablator has been used successfully in some aorto-ostial and distal anastomotic vein graft lesions.[105,106]

f. **Other Atherectomy Devices.** New hydrodynamic atherectomy devices are under investigation which rely on the Venturi principle for aspiration of thrombus and debris (Cordis Hydrolyzer, POSSIS Angiojet) (Chapter 8).[107,108,188] Preliminary clinical experience suggest a potential role for these devices, and further studies are underway.

g. **Prolonged Low-Dose Intra-Graft Urokinase Infusion for Chronically Occluded Saphenous Vein Grafts (Chapter 16).** PTCA may be performed on totally occluded vein grafts, but angiographic success is only 70% and 3-year event-free survival only 34%.[109] Small studies suggest that intracoronary urokinase may be a useful adjunct to balloon angioplasty,[110,111] directional atherectomy[112] and stenting[91,113] for occluded vein grafts. Although lytic therapy may increase the chance of immediate success, early complications include MI,[110,114,115] bleeding,[110,116] and hematoma formation;[110] 6-month patency was only 25% for occlusions at the distal anastomosis and 50% for occlusions in the body of the graft.[117] An alternative approach to prolonged infusions is the use of a "pulse-spray" mini-urokinase infusion, which may decrease the dose and duration of urokinase, and minimize bleeding and vascular complications.[118]

Table 17.6. Results of Stents in Saphenous Vein Grafts

Series	Stent	Lesions (N)	Succ. (%)	SAT (%)	Complications (%) D / MI / CABG	VSR/XF (%)	RS (%)
Wong[88] (1995)	PSS	624	98.8	1.4	1.7 / 0.3 / 0.9	8.0/6.3	30
Rechavia[89] (1995)	PSS,B	29	100	0	0 / 0 / 0	3.4/6.8	-
Wong[90] (1995)	PSS,B	309	95.3	1.7	1.3 / 0.9 / 0.4	8.4/25	-
Denardo[91]* (1995)	PSS,B	300	93.3	6.7	0 / 20 / 0	(16.7)	-
Piana[92] (1994)	PSS,B	200	98.5	0.6	- / 0.6 / 0	8.5/14.0	0
Eeckhout[93] (1994)	Wall, Wik	58	100	2	0 / 2 / 2	(14)	33
Keane[94] (1994)	Wall	29	97	3.4	0 / 0 / 0	3.4/6.8	32
Fenton[95] (1994)	PSS	209	98.5	0.5	0.4 / 0 / 0	17.2/12	34
Leon[96] (1993)	PSS	589	97	1.4	1.7 / 0.3 / 0.9	7.5/15.5	30
Fortuna[97] (1993)	Wik	101	95	2	1 / 3 / 1	-	-
Pomerantz[75] (1992)	PSS	84	99	0	0 / 0 / 0	(5)	25
Bilodeau[98] (1992)	GRS	37	-	-	0 / 2.5 / 0	-	35
Strauss[999] (1992)	Wall	145	-	8	- / - / -	-	39
deScheerder[100] (1992)	NWall	95	100	10	1.4 / 4.3 / 2.8	(33)	47
Urban[101] (1989)	Wall	14	100	0	0 / 0 / 0	7.7/7.7	20

Abbreviations: Succ. = procedural success; RS = restenosis; SAT = subacute thrombus; MI = in-hospital q-wave myocardial infarction; CABG = emergency coronary artery bypass surgery; VSR/XF = vascular surgery repair/blood transfusion (number of parentheses indicates combined vascular and bleeding complications if not identified separetely); Wall = Wallstent; Nwall = New Wallstent; Wik = Wiktor stent; PSS = Palmaz-Schatz stent; B = biliary stent; GRS = Gianturco-Roubin stent; - = not reported
*   Thrombotic vein grafts; adjunctive urokinase infusion for 20.5 hrs.

B. **APPROACH TO THE PATIENT WITH PREVIOUS BYPASS SURGERY**. For patients in whom percutaneous revascularization seems warranted, available data suggest that a lesion-specific, multi-device approach may be preferred (Table 17.7). Graft age, lesion location, and lesion morphology may influence immediate and longterm results (Figure 17.4).

1. **Graft Age.** The cause of postoperative graft failure is influenced by the time interval from operation: acute thrombosis within the first month (PTCA within 30 days has been associated with higher restenosis rates[121,122]); fibrointimal hyperplasia between 1-12 months; and varying degrees of complex atherosclerosis after 12 months.[119] Many interventionalists believe that older grafts greatly increase the risk of procedural failure and complications; however, several studies suggest that lesion morphology and the presence of degeneration are more important than graft age per se: A recent study of PTCA in grafts > 3 years old reported success in 94%, major complications in 5%, and death in 1.4% — similar to results in grafts < 3 years old.[120] Preliminary studies also suggest that immediate results and complications after DCA or stents are independent of graft age.[123] In contrast, graft age >36 months was associated with lower procedural success, increased complications, and more late cardiac events after TEC.[124] The optimal strategy for old degenerated vein graft lesions is unknown; repeat bypass surgery may be the preferred treatment in some patients.

2. **Lesion Location**
   a. **Proximal and Aorto-Ostial Lesions.** Balloon angioplasty of proximal and ostial lesions appear to have lower success rates (86% vs. 93%) and higher restenosis rates (up to 80%)

Table 17.7. Lesion-Specific Indications in Vein Grafts

Lesion	PTCA	STENT	DCA	ROTA	TEC	ELCA
Concentric	++	+++	++	±	++	++
Eccentric	++	+++	+++	±	++	++
Ulcerated	++	+++	+++	-	+	++
Ostial	+	+++	++	++	++	++
Total Occlusion	+	++	+	-	++	+
Thrombus	±	-	-	-	++	+
Diffuse Degeneration	-	-	-	-	+	±

Abbreviations: DCA = directional coronary atherectomy; ROTA = rotablator; TEC = transluminal extraction catheter; ELCA = excimer laser coronary angioplasty
+ limited value - should be avoided
++ reasonable alternative +++ first line treatment
± limited value, may be associated with higher incidence of complications than other devices

compared to PTCA of other vein graft sites. All atherectomy devices (DCA, TEC, Rotablator) can be applied to aorto-ostial vein graft lesions with high success and acceptable complication rates, but adjunctive angioplasty is frequently required for definitive lumen enlargement; there are no data to suggest lower restenosis rates compared to PTCA alone.[126] For DCA and stenting of aorto-ostial vein grafts, procedural success occurred in 95%, but at 1 year, target lesion revascularization was required in 20-30% and event-free survival was only 58-74%.[102] In another study of DCA in ostial vein graft lesions, angiographic restenosis occurred in 47% of de novo lesions and 93% of restenotic lesions.[127] Independent predictors of restenosis have been shown to include final lumen diameter and ostial location, but not device type; restenosis occurred in 42% of ostial lesions but only 17% of nonostial lesions.[128]

b. **Lesions in the Body of the Graft.** Interventional strategy depends largely on lesion morphology: Focal stenoses can be treated with PTCA or Palmaz-Schatz stenting with success rates > 90% and complication rates <5%; stenting is frequently chosen over PTCA because restenosis rates appear to be lower (20-35% vs. 42-63%). DCA is also effective, but the incidence of non-Q-wave MI appears to be higher compared to PTCA; restenosis rates are similar.[102]

c. **Distal Anastomotic Lesions.** Distal anastomotic stenoses can be safely and effectively treated with PTCA, which is probably the device of choice for lesions at this location.

3. **Lesion Morphology**
    a. **Vein grafts > 3 mm.** Because of the favorable impact of stents on restenosis, we believe that stenting is the treatment of choice for vein grafts ≥ 3 mm in diameter. At our institution, single or multiple coronary stents (vessel diameter 3.0-4.5 mm) or biliary stents (vessel diameter 4.0-7.0 mm) are used for focal or tubular lesions in the body or ostium of vein grafts. If clot is suspected on clinical or angiographic grounds, useful adjuncts include TEC atherectomy (to excise and aspirate atherothrombotic debris), angioscopy (to confirm the initial presence and subsequent removal of thrombus),[64] and local delivery of urokinase with drug-delivery balloons.[129]

    b. **Vein grafts < 3 mm.** For focal or tubular lesions in vein grafts < 3 mm, no devices have been shown to be superior to PTCA.

    c. **Degenerated Grafts and Chronic Total Occlusions.** Diffusely degenerated vein grafts and chronic total occlusions remain problematic for all catheter-based interventions. In selected cases, multiple biliary or coronary stents can be implanted with acceptable short-term outcome,[130] but longterm data on graft patency are not available. An interventional strategy gaining popularity involves intragraft infusion of urokinase (to establish patency)[91] followed by TEC atherectomy (to debulk residual thrombus), a 3-4 week course of warfarin (to "clean up" the graft), and stenting within 4-6 weeks (for definitive lumen enlargement) (Chapter 26). As previously described, this deferred stent strategy reduced distal embolization and

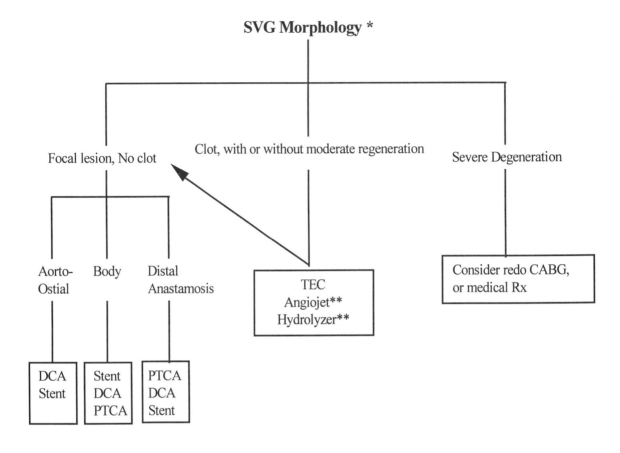

Figure 17.4. Approach to Saphaneous Vein Graft Intervention

*   extent of degeneration is estimated by angiography; angioscopy may be useful for identification of thrombus and friability

**   investigational devices; not available in the U.S.

major clinical complications, but resulted in silent interim occlusion in 15%.[70,131] Recently, Fajadet et al[108] described successful vein graft thrombectomy using the Cordis Hydrolyser; preliminary experience with the POSSIS angiojet also suggests potential benefit (Chapter 8). New local drug delivery systems also show promise and are under active investigation (Chapter 35).

4. **Acute Myocardial Infarction.** There are limited data on percutaneous revascularization of vein grafts in the setting of acute myocardial infarction.[136,137] These studies suggest a larger burden of thrombus in culprit vein grafts (compared to coronary arteries), which is commonly refractory to intravenous thrombolytic therapy; more effective reperfusion may be achieved by percutaneous techniques (PTCA, TEC, Hydrolyzer, Angiojet) with or without intragraft thrombolytic therapy.[135]

INTERNAL MAMMARY ARTERY

The internal mammary artery (IMA) is the conduit of choice for CABG.[136,137] Compared to saphenous vein grafts, IMA grafts demonstrate better flow, less atherosclerosis, and higher 10-year patency rates (95% vs. 25-30%). Despite excellent longterm patency, recurrent ischemia may occur secondary to stenosis in either the IMA or native vessel beyond the anastomosis. PTCA of the left IMA can be performed with success rates of 80-100% and a low incidence of abrupt closure, distal embolization, acute MI, and emergency surgery (Table 17.8).[138-147] Procedural failures and largely due to failure to cross the lesion with the guidewire or balloon, or inability to reach the stenosis due to vessel tortuosity. Restenosis rates are < 20% and generally lower for lesions at the distal anastomosis compared to the body of the graft.[138] PTCA of the right IMA[148,149] and stenting of both IMA's have also been reported.[150-152]

Table 17.8. Results of PTCA of the Internal Mammary Artery

Series	No. Lesions	Success(%)	Restenosis (%)
Hearne[138] (1995)	68	88	19
Sketch[139] (1992)	14	93	8
Popma[140] (1992)	20	80	-
Dimas[141] (1991)	31	90	14
Bell[142] (1989)	7	100	0.00
Hill[143] (1989)	11	82	-
Shimshak[144] (1988)	26	92	13
Pinkerton[145] (1988)	13	92	-

- Not reported

A. **TECHNICAL CONSIDERATIONS.** When IMA angioplasty is indicated, certain technical factors should be considered:

- **Subclavian Artery Tortuosity.** Difficulty may be encountered in cannulating the subclavian artery due to vessel tortuosity. When this occurs, it is easier to enter the left subclavian artery (or brachiocephalic artery) in the 60° LAO projection, which elongates the aortic arch and allows excellent visualization of the great vessels. If the subclavian artery cannot be entered with a preformed IMA guiding catheter, a right Judkins catheter may be used and later exchanged for an IMA catheter. If tortuosity of the subclavian artery precludes tracking of the guiding catheter into the IMA, an ipsilateral brachial approach may be used.[153,154]

- **IMA Engagement.** Caution should be taken to avoid forceful engagement with the guiding catheter since the IMA is prone to catheter-induced dissection and vasospasm. If the IMA is small, a 7F guiding catheter (with or without sideholes) may provide adequate support without pressure damping. Patients should be adequately pretreated with nitroglycerin and calcium channel blockers; selective injections of nitroglycerin (100-300 mcg boluses) should be used liberally.

- **Equipment Selection.** The IMA is frequently very tortuous, and low profile balloons are usually necessary. Equipment selection and technical approaches to PTCA of tortuous vessels are discussed in Chapter 11. Due to the extreme length and redundancy of this conduit, a balloon with a long shaft (150 cm) may be required. Alternatively, short (90 cm) guiding catheters may be used or fashioned (by cutting 10-15 cm from the proximal end of the guide catheter and replacing the hub with an appropriately sized introducing sheath).

B. **CORONARY STEAL AND THE IMA.** After IMA grafting, myocardial perfusion depends on blood flow through the subclavian artery. The coronary-subclavian steal syndrome results from stenosis in the subclavian artery proximal to the IMA, which compromises myocardial blood flow.[155-164] Clinical manifestations include angina or myocardial infarction, usually associated with signs and symptoms of subclavian artery stenosis, such as arm claudication, vertebrobasilar insufficiency, blood pressure difference between arms, a supraclavicular bruit, or diminished brachial and radial pulses. Potential treatment strategies include carotid-subclavian bypass,[164-166] PTCA,[164,167-171] directional atherectomy,[172] and stenting (Chapter 36).[164-173] Occasionally, coronary steal may be due to an unligated internal mammary artery sidebranch;[174-176] in this situation, coil embolization can relieve signs and symptoms of myocardial ischemia.[174-176]

GASTROEPIPLOIC ARTERY

The gastroepiploic artery, which may be used as an *in-situ* graft (i.e., gastroduodenal-to-coronary artery) or as a free arterial graft,[177-181] has longterm patency rates similar to the left internal mammary artery.[179] The *in-situ* conduit poses a number of technical challenges for imaging and percutaneous revascularization due to complex anatomy and tortuosity.[182,183] In this regard, the celiac axis gives rise to the common hepatic artery, which gives rise to the gastroduodenal artery, which in 80-90% of cases ultimately gives rise to the gastroepiploic artery. Selective cannulation of the gastroduodenal artery is required to adequately opacify the conduit. In 10-20% of cases, the gastroepiploic artery arises from the superior mesenteric artery, which increases the length and tortuosity of the conduit.[183] Adequate opacification can be achieved in only 50% of *in-situ* conduits, thereby limiting the sucecss of percutaneous intervention. Among gastroepiploic artery grafts that can be cannulated and adequately opacified, PTCA success is 70-80%;[184-186] vasospasm is common, so pretreatment with nitrates and/or calcium antagonists is recommended.

APPROACH TO PTCA OF NATIVE VESSELS VIA BYPASS GRAFTS

Following CABG, recurrent ischemia may be due to new disease in native vessels distal to the graft anastomosis. The approach to PTCA of these lesions is similar to that of the bypass graft itself; PTCA may be performed via vein grafts or IMA grafts as clinically indicated. In one study, successful PTCA of a native vessel via an SVG was achieved in 90% of patients;[187] immediate results and complications are similar to PTCA of native coronary arteries.

* * * * *

REFERENCES

1. Campeau L, Enjalbert M, Lesperance J, et al. The relation of risk factors to the development of atherosclerosis in saphenous-vein bypass grafts and the progression of disease in the native circulation. N Engl J of Med 1984;311:1329-1332.

2. Weintraub WS, Jones EL, Craver JM, Guyton RA. Frequency of repeat coronary bypass or coronary angioplasty after coronary artery bypass surgery using saphenous venous grafts. Am J Cardiol 1994;73:103-112.

3. White C, Campeau L, Knatterud G, Probstfield J, Investigators atPCCT. Patency of saphaneous vein bypass grafts following elective angiography: Preliminary results from the POST CABG Clinical Trial. J Am Coll Cardiol 1993;21:18A.

4. Reul GJ, Cooley DA, Ott DA, et al. Reoperation for recurrent coronary artery disease. Arch Surg 1979;114:1269-1275.

5. Schaff HV, Orszulak TA, Gersh BJ, et al. The morbidity and mortality of reoperation for coronary artery disease and analysis of late results with use of actuarial estimate of event-free interval. J Thorac Cardiovasc Surg 1983;85:508-515.

6. Foster ED, Fisher LD, Kaiser GC, et al. Comparison of operative mortality and morbidity for initial and repeat coronary artery bypass grafting: The coronary artery surgery study (CASS) registry experience. Ann of Thoracic Surg 1984;38:563-570.

7. Pidgeon J, Brooks N, Magee P, et al. Reoperation for Angina After Previous Aortocoronary Bypass Surgery. Br Heart J 1985;53:269-75.

8. Laird-Meeter K, VanDomBurg R, Vanden Brand MJBM, et al. Incidence, risk, and outcome of reintervention after aortocoronary bypass surgery. Br Heart J 1987;57:427-35.

9. Lytle BW, Loop FD, Cosgrove DM, et al. Fifteen hundred coronary reoperations: results and determinants of early and late survival. J Thorac Cardiovasc Surg 1987;93:847-859.

10. Verheul HA, Moulign AC, Hondema S, et al. Late results of 200 repeat coronary artery bypass operations. Am J of Cardiol 1991;67:24-30.

11. Noyez L, van der Werf T, Janssen D, Klinkenberg T. Early results with bilateral internal mammary artery grafting in coronary reoperations. Am J Cardiol 1992;70:1113-1116.

12. Verheul H, Moulijn A, Hondema S, Schouwink M. Late results of 200 repeat coronary artery bypass operations. Am J Cardiol 1991;67:24-30.

13. Lytle B, Loop F, Cosgrove D, Taylor P. Fifteen hundred coronary reoperations. J Thorac Cardiovasc Surg. 1987;93:847-859.

14. Loop F, Lytle B, Cosgrove D, et al. Reoperation for coronary atherosclerosis. Changing practice in 2509 consecutive patients. Ann Surg 1990;212:378-386.

15. Lamas G, Mudge G, Collins J, et al. Clinical response to coronary artery operation. J Am Coll Cardiol 1986;8:274-279.

16. Pidgeon J, Brook N, MaGee P, Pepper JR. Repoperation of angina after previous aortocoronary bypass surgery. Br Heart J 1985;53:269-275.

17 Foster E, Fisher L, Kaiser G, Meyers W, CASS atPIo. Comparison of operative mortality and morbidity for initial and repeat coronary artery bypass grafting: The CASS Registry Experience. Ann Thorac Surg 1984;38:563-570.

18. Schaff H, Orszulak T, Gersh B, Piehler J. The morbidity and mortality of reoperation for coronary artery disease and analysis of late results with use of actuarial estimate of event-free interval. J Thorac Cardiovasc Surg. 1983;85:508-515.

19. Lytle BW, McElroy D, McCarthy P, Loop FD, et al. Influence of arterial coronary bypass grafts on the mortality in coronary reoperations. J Thorac Cardiovasc Surg 1994;107:675-82

20. Ivert TS, Ekestrom S, Petriffy A, Weiti R. Coronary artery reoperations. Early and late results in 101 patients. Scand J Thoracic Cardiovasc Surg 1988;22:111-8

21. Perrault L, Carrier M, Cartier R, Leclerc Y, Hebert Y, Diaz OS, Pelletier C. Morbidity and mortality of reoperation for coronary artery bypass grafting: signficance of atheromatous vein grafts. Can J Cardiol 1991;7:427-30

22. Gonzalez-Santos JM, Ennabli K, Grondin C. Repeat coronary artery bypass grafting in patients with patent atherosclerotic grafts: a special challenge. Thorac Cardiovasc Surg (West Germany) 1984;32:346-9.

23. Tan K, Henderson R, Sulke N, Cooke R. Percutaneous transluminal coronary angioplasty in patients with prior coronary artery bypass grafting: ten years' experience. Cath Cardiovasc Diagn 1994;31:11-17.

24. Morrison D, Crowley S, Veerakul G, Barbire C, Grover F, Sacks J. Percutaneous transluminal angioplasty of saphenous vein grafts for medically refractory unstable angina. J Am Coll Cardiol 1994;23:1066-1070.

25. Unterberg C, Buchwald A, Wiegand V, Kreuzer H. Coronary angioplasty in patients with previous coronary artery

bypass grafting. J Vasc Dis 1992:653-659.

26. Miranda CP, Rutherford BD, McConahay DR, et al. Angioplasty of older saphenous vein grafts continues to be a sound therapeutic option. J Am Coll Cardiol 1992;19, 3:350A.

27. Meester BJ, Samson M, Suryapranata H, et al. Long-term follow-up after attempted angioplasty of saphenous vein grafts: The Thoraxcenter Experience 1981-1988. Eur Heart J 1991;12:648-653.

28. Plokker HWT, Meester BH, Serruys PW. The Dutch experience in percutaneous transluminal angioplasty of narrowed saphenous veins used for aortocoronary arterial bypass. Am J Cardiol 1991;67:361-366.

29. Douglas JS, Weintraub WS, Liberman HA, et al. Update of saphenous graft (SVG) angioplasty: Restenosis and long-term outcome. Circulation 1991; 84: II-249.

30. Jost S, Gulba D, Daniel WG, Amende I. Percutaneous transluminal angioplasty of aortocoronary venous bypass grafts and effect of the caliber of the grafted coronary artery on graft stenosis. Am J Cardiol 1991;68:27-30.

31. Webb JG, Myler RK, Shaw RE, et al. Coronary angioplasty after coronary bypass surgery: Initial results and late outcome in 422 patients. J Am Coll Cardiol 1990;16:812-820.

32. Dorros G, Lewin RF, Mathiak LM. Coronary angioplasty in patients with prior coronary artery bypass surgery: all prior coronary artery bypass surgery patients and patients more than 5 years after coronary bypass surgery. Cardiol Clin 1989;7:791-803.

33. Platko WP, Hollman J, Whitlow PL, et al. Percutaneous transluminal angioplasty of saphenous vein graft stenosis: long-term follow-up. J Am Coll Cardiol 1989;14:1645-1650.

34. Pinkerton CA, Slack JD, Orr CM, et al. Percutaneous transluminal angioplasty in patients with prior myocardial revascularization surgery. Am J Cardiol 1988;61:15G-22G.

35. Cote GC, Myler RK, Stertzer SH, et al. Percutaneous transluminal angioplasty of stenotic coronary artery bypass grafts: 5 years' experience. J Am Coll Cardiol 1987;9:8-17.

36. Ernst S, van der Feltz T, Ascoop C, et al. Percutaneous transluminal coronary angioplasty in patients with prior coronary artery bypass grafting. J Thorac Cardiovasc Surg 1987;93:268-275.

37. Douglas J, Robinson K, Schlumpf M. Percutaneous transluminal angioplasty in aortocoronary venous graft stenoses: Immediate results and complications. Circulation 1986;74:II-363.

38. Reeder G, Bresnahan J, Holmes DJ, et al. Angioplasty for aortocoronary bypass graft stenosis. Mayo Clin Proc 1986;61:14-19.

39. Corbelli J, Franco I, Hollman J, et al. Percutaneous transluminal coronary angioplasty after previous coronary artery bypass surgery. Am J Cardiol 1985;56:398-403.

40. Gamal M, Bonnier H, Michels R, Heijman J, Stassen E. Percutaneous transluminal angioplasty of stenosed aortocoronary bypass grafts. Br Heart J 1984;52:617-620.

41. Block P, Cowley M, Kaltenbach M, Kent K, Simpson J. Percutaneous angioplasty of stenoses of bypass grafts or of bypass graft anastomotic sites. Am J Cardiol 1984;53:666-668.

42. Douglas JS, Gruentzig AR, King SB, et al. Percutaneous transluminal coronary angioplasty in patients with prior coronary bypass surgery. J Am Colll Cardiol 1983;2:745-754.

43. Douglas J, Weintraub W, King SI. Changing perspectives in vein graft angioplasty. J Am Coll Cardiol 1995;25:78A.

44. Guzman LA, Villa AE, Whitlow P: New atherectomy devices in the treatment of old saphenous vein grafts: Are the initial results encouraging? Circulation 1992;86:I-780.

45. Liu MW, Douglas JS, Lembo NJ, King SBI. Angiographic predictors of a rise in serum creatine kinase (distal embolization) after balloon angioplasty of saphenous vein coronary artery bypass grafts. Am J Cardiol 1993;72:514-517.

46. Altmann D, Popma J, Hong M, et al. CPK-MB elevation after angioplasty of saphenous vein grafts. J Am Coll Cardiol 1993;21:232A.

47. Tilli FV, Kaplan BM, Safian RD, Grines CL, O'Neill WW. Angioscopic plaque friability: a new risk factor for procedural complications following saphenous vein graft interventions. J Am Coll Cardiol 1996 (in-press).

48. Challapalli RM, Eisenberg MJ, Sigmon K, Lemberger J. Platelet glycoprotein IIb/IIIa monocional antibody (c7E3) reduces distal embolization during percutaneous intervention of saphenous vein grafts. Circulation 1995;92:I-607.

49. Abbo KM, Dooris M, Glazier S, O'Neill WW, et al. No-reflow after percutaneous coronary intervention: Clinical and angiographic characteristics, treatment, and outcome. Am J Cardiol 1995;75:778-782.

50. de Feyter PJ, Serruys PW, van den Brand M, Meester H, Beatt K, Surypanyata H. Percutaneous transluminal angioplasty of totally occluded venous bypass grafts: a challenge that should be resisted. Am J Cardiol 1989;64:88-90.

51. Weintraub WS, Cohen CL, Curling PE, et al. Results of coronary surgery after failed elective coronary angioplasty

in patients with prior coronary surgery. J Am Coll Cardiol 1990;16:1341-1347.

52. Kahn JK, Rutherford BD, McConahay DR, Johnson WL, Giorgi LV, Shimshak TM, Hartzler GO. Outcome following emergency coronary artery bypass grafting for failed elective balloon angioplasty in patients with prior coronary bypass. Am J Cardiol 1990;66:285-8

53. Lemmer JH, Ferguson DW, Rakel BA, Rossi NP. Clinical outcome of emergency repeat coronary artery bypass surgery. J Cardiovasc Surg (Torino) 1990;31:429-7

54. Ellis SG, Ajluni S, Arnold AZ, Popma JJ, Bittl JA, Eigler NL, Cowley MJ, Raymond RE, Safian RD, Whitlow PL. Increased coronary perforation in the new device era: incidence, classification, management and outcome. Circulation 1994;90:2725-2730

55. Ajluni SC, Glazier S, Blankenship L, O'Neill WW, Safian RD. Perforations after percutaneous coronary interventions: Clinical, angiographic, and theapeutic observations. Cathet Cardiovasc Diagn 1994;32:206-212.

56. Douglas J, King SI. Ten year follow-up of patients undergoing vein graft angioplasty. Circulation 1994;90:I-333.

57. Safian RD, Grines CL, May MA, Lichtenberg A, Juran N, Schreiber TL, Pavlides GS, Meany TB, Savas V, O'Neill WW. Clinical and angiographic results of transluminal extraction coronary atherectomy in saphenous vein bypass grafts. Circulation 1994;89:302-312.

58. Popma JJ, Leon MB, MIntz GS, Kent KH, Satler LF, Garrand TJ, Pichard AJ. Results of coronary angioplasty using the Transluminal Extraction Catheter. Am J Cardiol 1992;70:1526-32

59. Meany T, Leon MB, Kramer B, et al. A multicenter experience of atherectomy of transluminal extraction in catheter for for the treatment of diseased of saphenous vein grafts. Cathet Cardiovasc Diagn 1995;34:112-120.

60. Twidale N, Barth CW, Keperman RM, et al. Acute results and long-term outcome of transluminal extraction catheter atherectomy for saphenous vein graft stenoses. Cathet Cardiovasc Diagn 1994;31:187-191.

61. Hong MK, Popma JJ, Pichard AD, Kent KH, Satler LF, Chuang YC, Mintz GS, Keller MB, Leon MB. Clinical significance of distal embolization after Transluminal Extraction Atherectomy in diffusely diseased saphenous vein grafts. Am Heart J 1994;127:1496-503

62. Kramer B. Optimal therapy for degenerated saphenous vein graft disease. J Invas Cardiol 1995;7(Suppl D):14D-20D.

63. Annex B, Larkin T, O'Neill W, Safian R. Evaluation of thrombus removal by transluminal extraction coronary atherectomy by percutaenous coronary angioscopy. Am J Cardiol 1994;74:606-609.

64. Kaplan BM, Safian RD, Grines CL, Goldstein JA, et al. Usefulness of adjunctive angioscopy and extraction atherectomy before stent implantation in high-risk aortocoronary saphenous vein grafts. Am J Cardiol 1995;76:822-826.

65. Moses J, Lieberman S, Knopf W, et al. Mechanism of transluminal extraction catheter (TEC) atherectomy in degenerative saphenaous vein grafts (SVG). An angioscopic observational study. J Am Coll Cardiol 1993;21:442A.

66. Moses J, Tierstein P, Sketch M, et al. Angiographic determinants of risk and outcome of coronary embolus and myocardial infarction (MI) with the transluminal extraction catheter (TEC): A report from the New Approaches to Coronary Intervention (NACI) Registry. J Am Coll Cardiol 1994;23:220A.

67. Dooris M, Hoffmann M, Glazier S, et al. Comparative results of transluminal extraction coronary atherectomy in saphenous vein graft lesions with and without thrombus. J Am Coll Cardiol 1995;25:1700-5.

68. Al-Shaibi, KF, Goods CM, Jain SP, et al. Does transluminal extraction atherectomy reduce distal embolization in saphenous vein grafts? Circualtion 1995;92:I-329.

69. Moses JW, Yeh W, Popma JJ, Sketch MH. Predictors of distal embolization with the TEC catheter: A NACI Registry Report. Circulation 1995;92:I-329.

70. Hong M, Pichard A, Kent K, et al. Assessing a strategy of stand-alone extraction atherectomy followed by staged stnt placement in degenerated saphenous vein graft lesions. J Am Coll Cardiol 1995;25:394A.

71. Parks JM. TEC before stent implantation. J Invas Cardiol 1995;7(Suppl D):10D-13D.

72. Cowley MJ, Whitlow PL, Baim DS, Hinohara T, Hall K, Simpson JB. Directional coronary atherectomy of saphenous vein graft narrowings: mulitcenter investigational experience. Am J Cardiol 1993;72:30E-34E.

73. Kaufmann UP, Garratt KN, Vliestra RE, Holmes DR. Transluminal atherectomy of saphenous vein aortocoronary bypass grafts. Am J Cardiol 1990:65:1430-1433

74. DiSciascio G, Cowley MJ, Vetrovec CW, et al. Directional coronary atherectomy of saphenou vein graft lesions unfavorable for balloon angioplasty: Results of a single-center experience. Cathet Cariovasc Diagn 1992;26:75.

75. Pomerantz RM, Kuntz E, Carozza JP, Fishman RF, Mansour M, Schnitt SJ, Safian RD, Baim DS. Acute and long-term outcome of narrowed saphenous venous grafts treated by endoluminal stenting and directional atherectomy. Am J Cardiol 1992;70:161-167

76. Garratt KN, Holmes DR Jr, Bell MR, Berger PB, Kauffmann UP, Bresnahan JF, Vliestra RE. Results of directional atherectomy of primary atheromatous and restenosis lesions in coronary arteries and saphenous vein grafts. Am J Cardiol 1192;70:449-454

77. Selmon MR, Hinohara T, Robertson GC, Rowe MH, Vetter JW, Bartzokis TC, Braden IJ, Simpson JB. Directional coronary atherectomy for vein graft stenoses. J Am Coll Cardiol 1991;17:23A

78. Ghazzal ZMB, Douglas JS, Holmes DR, Ellis SG, Kereiakes DJ, Simpson JB, KIng SB, and the Directional Atherectomy Multicenter Investigational Group. Directional coronary atherectomy of saphenous vein grafts: recent multicenter experience. J An Coll Cardiol 1991;17:219A

79. Hinohara T, Robertson GC, Selmon MR, Vetter JW, Rowe MH, Braden LJ, McAuley BJ, Sheehan DJ, Simpson JB. Restenosis after directional coronary atherectomy. J Am Coll Cardiol 1992;20:623-632

80. Holmes D, Topol e, Califf R, et al. A multicenter, randomized trial of coronary angioplasty versus directional atherectomy for patients with saphenous vein bypass graft lesions. Circulation 1995;91:1966-1974.

81. Strauss BH, Natarajan MK, Batchelor WB, Yardley DE, et al. Early and late quantitative angiographic results of vein graft lesions treated by excimer laser with adjunctive balloon angioplasty. Circulation 1995;92:348-356.

82. Bittl JA, Sanborn TA, Yardley DE, Tcheng JE, Isner JM, Choksi SK, Strauss BH, Abela GS, Walter PD, Scmidhofer M, Power JA for the Percutaneous Excimer Laser Coronary Angioplasty Registry. Predictors of outcome of percutaneous excimer laser coronary angioplasty of saphenous vein bypass graft lesions. Am J Cardiol 1994;74:144-148

83. Litvack F, Eigler N, Margolis J, Rothbaum, D, et al. Percutaneous excimer laser coronary angioplasty: Results in the first consecutive 3,000 patients. J Am Coll Cardiol 1994;23:323-329.

84. De Marchena EJ, Mallon SM, Knopf WD, et al. Effectiveness of Holmium laser-assisted coronary angioplasty. Am J Cardiol 1994;73:117-121.

85. Serruys PW, de Jaegere P, Kiemeneij F, et al. A comparison of balloon-expandable stent implantation with balloon angioplasty in patients with coronary artery disease. N Engl J Med 1994;331: 489-95

86. Fischman DL, Leon MB, Baim DS et al. A randomized comparison of coronary -stent placement and balloon angioplasty in the treatment of coronary artery disease. N Engl J Med 1994;331:496-501.

87. Savage M, Douglas J, Fischman D, et al. Coronary stents versus balloon angioplasty for aorto-coronary saphenous vein bypass graft disease: Interim results of a randomized trial. J Am Coll Cardiol 1995;25:79A.

88. Wong SC, Baim D, Schatz R, et al. Immediate results and late outcomes after stent implantation in saphenous vein graft lesions: The multicenter US Palmaz-Schatz Stent experience. J Am Coll Cardiol 1995;26:704-712.

89. Rechavia E, Litvack F, Macko G, Eigler N. Stent implantation of saphenous vein graft aorto-ostial lesions in patients with unstable ischemic syndromes: Immediate angiographic results and long-term clinical outcome. J Am Coll Cardiol 1995;25:866-870.

90. Wong SC, Popma J, Pichard A, Kent K. Comparison of clinical and angiographic outcomes after saphenous vein grafts angioplasty using coronary versus "biliary" tubular slotted stents. Circulation 1995;91:339-350.

91. Denardo SJ, Morris NB, Rocha-Singh, KJ, et al. Safety and efficacy of extended urokinase infusion plus stent deployment for treatment of o bstructed, older saphenous vein grafts. Am J Cardiol 1995;76:776-780.

92. Piana RN, Moscucci M, Cohen DJ, Kugelmass AD, Senerchia C, Kuntz RE, Baim DS, Carozza JP Jr. Palmaz-Schatz stenting for treatment of focal vein graft stenosis: immediate results and long-term outcome. J Am Coll Cardiol 1994;23:1296-30.

93. Eeckhout E, Goy JJ, Stauffer JC, Vogt P, Kappenberger L. Endoluminal stenting of narrowed saphenous vein grafts: long-term clinical and angiographic follow-up. Cathet Cardiovasc Diagn 1994;32:139-46

94. Keane D, Buis B, Reifart N, Plokker TH. Clinical and angiographic outcome following implantation of the new less shortening wallstent in aortocoronary vein grafts: Introduction of a second gerneration stent in the clinical arena. J Interven Cardiol 1994;7(6):557-564.

95. Fenton S, Fischman D, Savage M, et al. Long-term angiographic and clinical outcome after implantation of balloon-expandable stents in aortocoronary saphenous vein grafts. Am J Cardiol 1994;74:1187-1191.

96. Leon MB, Wong SC, Pichard A. Balloon expandable stent implantation in saphenous vein grafts. In Hermann HC, Hirschfeld JW (Eds). Clinical use of the Palmaz Schatz Intracoronary Stent. Futura Publishing Company Inc. 1993; 111-121.

97. Fortuna R, Heuser R, Garratt K, Schwartz R, Buchbinder M. Wiktor intracoronary stent: Experience in the first 101 vein graft patients. Circulation 1993;88:I-309.

98. Bilodeau L, Iyer S, Cannon A, et al. Flexible coil stent (Cook, Inc.) in saphenous vein grafts: clinical and angiographic

follow-up. J Am Coll Cardiol 1992;19:264A.

99. Strauss B, Serruys P, Bertrand M, Puel J. Quantitative angiographic follow-up of the coronary wallstent in native vessel and bypass grafts European experience-March 1986 to March 1990). Am J Cardiol 1992;69:475-481.

100. deScheerder I, Strauss B, deFeyter P, Beatt K. Stenting of venous bypass grafts: a new treatment modality for patients who are poor candidates for reintervention. Am Heart J 1992;123:1046-1054.

101. Urban P, Sigwart U, Golf S, Kaufmann U, Sadeghi H, Kappenberger L. Intravascular stenting for stenosis of aortocoronary venous bypass grafts. J Am Coll Cardiol 1989;13:1085-1091.

102. Wong SC, Popma J, Hong M, et al. Procedural results and longterm clinical outcomes in aorto-osital saphenous vein graft lesions after new device angioplasty. J Am Coll Cardiol 1995;25:394A.

103. Wong C, Popma J, Chuang Y, et al. Economic impact of reduced anticoagulation after saphenous vein graft stent placement. J Am Coll Cardiol 1995;25:80A.

104. Sketch M, Wong C, Chuang Y, et al. Progressive deterioration in late (2-year) clinical outcomes after stent implantation in saphenous vein grafts: The Multicenter JJIS experience. J Am Coll Cardiol 1995;25:79A.

105. Bass T, Gilmore P, Buchbinder M. Coronary rotational atherectomy (PTCRA) in patients with prior coronary revascularization: A registry report. Circulation 1992;86:I-653.

106. Freed M, Niazi K, O'Neill W. Percutaneous coronary rotational atherectomy: The William Beaumont Hospital experience. p.297. In Restenosis After Intervention With New Mechanical Devices. ed. Dordrecht, The Netherlands: Kluwer Academic, 1992.

107. van Ommen V, Veen Mat Daemen E, Habets J, Wellens H. In vivo evaluation of the safety to the vessel wall of the hydrolyser (a hydrodynamic thrombectomy catheter). J Am Coll Cardiol 1994;23:406A.

108. Fajadet J, Bar O, Jordan C, Robert G, Laurent J, Callard J, Cassagneau B, Marco J. Human percutaneous thrombectomy using the new Hydrolyser catheter: preliminary results in saphenous vein grafts. J Am Coll Cardiol 1994;220A

109. Kahn J, Rutherfors B, McConahay D, et al. Initial and long-term outcome of 83 patients after balloon angioplasty of totally occluded bypass grafts. J Am Coll Cardiol 1994;23:1038-1042.

110. Hartmann JR, McKeever LS, Stamato NJ, et al. Recanalization of Chronically Occluded aortocoronary Saphenous Vein Bypass Grafts by Extended Infusion of Urokinase: Initial Results and Short-term Clinical Follow-up. J Am Coll Cardiol 1991;18, 6:1517-1523.

111. Hartmann J, McKeever L, Teran J. Prolonged infusion of urokinase for recanalization of chronically occluded aortocoronary bypass grafts. Am J Cardiol 1988;61:189-191.

112. Sabri MN, Johnson D, Warner M, Cowley MJ. Intracoronary thrombolysis followed by directional coronary atherectomy: a combined approach for thrombotic vein graft lesions considered unsuitable for angioplasty. Cathet Cardiovasc Diagn 1992;26:15-18

113. Eagan J, Strumpf R, Heuser R. New treatment approach for chronic total occlusions of saphenous vein grafts: thrombolysis and intravascular stents. Cathet Cardiovasc Diagn 1993;29:62-69101.

114. Blankenship JC, Modesto TA, Madigan NP. Acute myocardial infarction complicating urokinase infusion for total saphenous vein graft occlusion. Cath Cardiovasc Diagn 1993;28:39-43.

115. Gurley JC, MacPhail BS. Acute myocardial infarction due to thrombolytic reperfusion of chronically occluded saphenous vein coronary bypass grafts. Am J Cardiol 1991;68:274-276.

116. Taylor MA, Santoran EC, Aji J, Eldredge WJ, Cha SD, Dennis CA. Intracerebral hemorrhage complicating urokinase infusion into an occluded aortocoronary bypass graft. Cathet Cardiovasc Diagn 1994;31:206-210.

117. Hartmann J, McKeever L, O'Neill W, White C, Whitlow P, Enger E. Recanalization of chronically occluded bypass grafts: The effect of angioplasty site following extended urokinase infusion on 6-month patency. J Am Coll Cardiol 1995;25:149A.

118. Torre S, Marotta C, Blum M, Banas J. "Pulse Spray" mini-urokinase infusion for recanalization of recently occluded saphenous vein grafts. J Am Coll Cardiol 1995;25:94A.

119. de Feyter PJ, van Suylen RJ, de Jaegere PPT, Topol EJ, Serruys PW. Balloon angioplasty for the treatment of saphenous vein bypass grafts. J Am Coll Cardiol 1993;21:1539-49.

120. Bredlau CE, Roubin GS, Leimgbruber PP, et Al. In-hospital morbidity and mortality in patients undergoing elective coronary angioplasty. Circulation 72;5:1044-1052.

121. Dorogy ME, Highfill WT, Davis RC. Use of angioplasty in the management of complicated perioperative infarction following bypass surgery. Cathet Cardiovasc Diagn 1993;29:279-82.

122. Kahn JK, Rutherford BD, McConahay DR, Giorgi LV, Johnson WL, Shimshak TM, Hartzler GO. Early postoperative

balloon coronary angioplasty for failed coronary artery bypass grafting. Am J Cardiol 1990;66:943-6

123. Abdelmeguid A, Ellis S, Whitlow P, et al. Lack of graft age dependency for success of directional coronary atherectomy and Palmaz-Schatz stenting. J Am Coll Cardiol 1993;21:31A.

124. Abdelmeguid A, Ellis S, Whitlow P, et al. Discordant results of extraction atherectomy in old and young saphenous vein grafts: The NACI Experience. J Am Coll Cardiol 1993;21:442A.

125. Koller PT, Freed M, Grines CL, O'Neill WW. Success, complications and restenosis following rotational and transluminal extraction atherectomy of ostial stenoses. Cathet Cardiovasc Diagn 1994;31:255-260.

126. Abdelmeguid AE, Whitlow PL, Simpfendorfer C, Sapp SK, et al. Percutaneous revascularization of ostial saphenous vein graft stenoses. J Am Coll Cardiol 1995;26:955-960.

127. Stephan W, Bates E, Garratt K, Hinohara T, Muller D. Directional atherectomy of coronary and saphenous vein graft ostial stenoses. Am J Cardiol 1995;75:1015-1018.

128. Hong M, Popma J, Chuang Y, et al. Predictive model of target-lesion revascularization after balloon and new device saphenous vein graft angioplasty. J Am Coll Cardiol 1994;23:139A.

129. Glazier, Keiman FJ, Bauer JF, Mitchel DB, et al. Treatment of thrombotic saphenous vein graft stenoses/occlusions with local urokinase delivery with the dispatch catheter-initial results. Circulation 1995;92:I-671.

130. Kaul U, Agarwal R, Mathur A, Wasir HS. Intracoronary stent placement in thrombus containing vein graft lesions. J Invas Cardiol 1995;7:248-250.

131. Heuser R. Treatment alternatives for chronically occluded saphenous vein grafts. J Invas Cardiol 1995;7:94-96.

132. Grines CL, Booth DC, Nissen SE, Gurley JC, Bennett KA, O,Connor WN, De Maria AN. Mechanisms of acute myocardial infarction in patients with prior coronary artery bypass grafting and therapeutic implications. Am J Cardiol 1990;66:1292-6

133. Santiago P, Vacek JL, Rosamond TL, Kramer KH, Crouse LJ, Beauchamp GD. Comparison of results of coronary angioplasty during acute myocardial infarction with and without prior coronary bypass surgery. Am J Cardiol 1993;72:1348-1351

134. Kahn JK, Rutherford BD, McConahay DR, Johnson W, Giorgi VL, LIgon R, Hartzler GO. Usefulness of angioplasty for acute myocardial infarction in patients with prior coronary artery bypass grafting. Am J Cardiol 1990;65: 698-702

135. Kaplan BM, Larkin T, Safian RD, O'Neill WW, et al. A propsective study of extraction atherectomy in patients with acute myocardial infarction. J Am Coll Cardiol 1996 (in-press).

136. Spencer FC. The internal mammary artery: The ideal coronary bypass graft? N Engl J Med 1986;314:50-51.

137. Loop FD, Lytle BW, Cosgrove DM, et al. Influence of internal mammary-artery graft on 10 year survival and other cardiac events. N Engl J Med 1986;314:1-6.

138. Hearne S, Wilson J, Harrington J, et al. Angiographic and clinical follow-up after internal mammary artery graft angioplasty: A 9-year experience. J Am Coll Cardiol 1995;25:139A.

139. Sketch MH Jr., Quigley PJ, Perez JA et al. Angiographic follow up after internal mammary artery angioplasty. Am J Cardiol 1992;70:401.

140. Popma JJ, Cooke RH, Leon MB et al. Immediate procedural and long-term clinical results in internal mammary artery angioplasty. Am J Cardiol 1992;69:1237

141. Dimas AP, Arora RR, Whitlow PL, et al. Percutaneous transluminal angioplasty involving internal mammary artery grafts. Am Heart J 1991;122:423

142. Bell MR, Vliestra RE, et al. Percutaneous transluminal angioplasty of left internal mammary artery grafts: Two years experience with a femoral approach. Br Heart J 1989;61:417

143. Hill DM, McAuley BJ, Sheehan DJ et al. Percutaneous transluminal angioplasty of left internal mammary artery bypass grafts. J Am Coll Cardiol 1989;13:221A

144. Shimshak TM, Giorgi LV, Johnson WL et al. Application of percutaneous transluminal coronary angioplasty to the internal mammary artery graft. J Am Coll Cardiol 1988;12:1205

145. Pinkerton CA, Slack JD, Orr CM, Van Tassel JW. Percutaneous transluminal angioplasty involving internal mammary artery bypass grafts: a femoral approach. Cathet Cardiovasc Diagn 1987;13:414

146. Cote G, Myler RK, Stertzer SH et al. Percutaneous transluminal angioplasty of stenotic coronary artery bypass grafts. J Am Coll Cardiol 1987;9:8

147. Singh S,. Coronary angioplasty of internal mammary artery graft. Am J Med 1987,82:361

148. Steffenin o G, Meier B. Finci L, von Segesser L, Velebit V. Percutaneous transluminal angioplasty of right and left internal mammary artery grafts. Chest 1986;90:849-51

149. Brown RI, Galligan L, Penn IM, Weinstein L. Right internal mammary artery graft angioplasty through a right brachial

approach using a new custom guide catheter: a case report. Cathet Cardiovasc Diagn 1992;25:42-5

150. Almagor Y, Thomas J, Colombo A. A balloon expandable stent ath the origin of the left internal mammary artery graft: a case report. Cathet Cardiovasc Diagn 1991;24:256-258

151. Bajaj RK, Roubin GS. Intravascular stenting of the right internal mammary artery. Cathet Cardiovasc Diagn 1991; 24:252-255

152. Hadjimiltiades S, Gourassas J, Louridas G, Tsifodimos D. Stenting the distal anastomotic site of the left internal mammary artery graft: a case report. Cathet Cardiovasc Diagn 1994;32:157-161

153. Dorros G, Lewin RF. The brachial artery method to transluminal internal mammary artery angioplasty. Cathet Cardiovasc Diagn 1986;12:341-346

154. Salinger M, Drummer B, Furey K, Bott-Silverman C, Franco I. Percutaneous angiplasty of internal mammary artery graft stenosis using the brachial approach: a case report. Cathet Cardiovasc Diagn 1986;12:261-5

155. Ishi K, Hirota Y, Kawamura K, Suma H, Takeuchi A. Coronary-subclavian steal corrected with percutaneous transluminal angioplasty. J Cardiovasc Surg (Torino) 1191;32:275-7

156. Laub GW, Muralidharan S, Naidech H, Fernandez H, Adkins M, McGrath LB. Percutaneous transluminal subclavian angioplasty in a patient with postoperative angina. Ann Thorac Surg 1991;52:850-1

157. Belz M, Marshall JJ, Cowley MJ, Vetrovec GW. Subclavian balloon angioplasty in the management of the coronary-subclavian steal syndrome. Cathet Cardiovasc Diagn 1992;25:161-3

158. Soulen MC, Sullivan KL. Subclavian artery angioplasty proximal to a left internal mammary coronary artery bypass graft: case report. Cardiovasc Intervent Radiol 1991;14:355-7

159. Feld H, Nathan P, Raninga D, Shani J. Symptomatic angina secondary to coronary-subclavian steal syndrome treated successfully by percutaneous transluminal angioplasty of the subclavian artery. Cathet Cardiovasc Diagn 1992;26:12-4

160. Holmes JR, Crane R. Coronary steal through a patent internal mammary artery graft: treatment by subclavian angioplasty. Am Heart J 1993;125:1166-7

161. Shapira S, Braun SD, Puram B, Patel G, Rotman H. Percutaneous transluminal angioplasty of proximal subclavian artery stenosis after left internal mammary to left anterior descending artery bypass surgery. J Am Coll Cardiol 1991;18:1120-3

162. Perrault LP, Carrier M, Hudon G, Lemarbre L, Hebert Y, Pelletier LC. Transluminal angioplasty of the subclavian artery in patients with internal mammary artery grafts. Ann Thorac Surg 1993,56:927-30

163. Motarjeme A, Gordon GI. Percutaneous transluminal angioplasty of the brachiocephalic vessels: guidelines for therapy. Int Angiol 1993;12:260-9

164. Rabah MM, Gangadharan V, Brodsky M, Safian RD. Unstable coronary ischemic syndromes due to coronary subclavian steal: Case reports and review of the literature. Am Heart J 1996 (in-press).

165. Ziomek S, Quinones-Baldrich WJ, Busuttil RW. The superiority of synthetic arterial grafts over autologous veins in carotid-subclavian bypass. J Vasc Surg 1986;3:140-5.

166. McIvor ME, Williams GM, Brinker J. Subclavian coronary steal through a LIMIA-to LAD bypass graft. Cathet Cardiovasc Diagn 1988;14:100-104.

167. Ishii K, Hirota Y, Kitz Y, Kawamura K, et al. Coronary-subclavian steal corrected with percutaneous transluminal angioplasty. J Cardiovasc Surg 1991;32:275-277.

168. Benzuly K, Kaplan B, Bowers T, Safian RD. Coronary-subclavian steal due to fishulae from the left internal mammary artery to the pulmonary artery: Treatment by coil embolization. Cathet Cardiovasc Diagn (in-press).

169. Laub GW, Muraldharan S, McGrath LB. Percutaneous transluminal subclavian angioplasty in a patient with postoperative angina. Ann Thorac Surg 1991;52:850-1.

170. Perrault LP, Carrier M, Hudon G, Pelletier LC. Transluminal angioplasty of the subclavian artery in patients with internal mammary grafts. Ann Thorac Surg 1993;56:927-930.

171. Dorros G, Lewin RF, Jamnadas P, Mathiak LM. Peripheral transluminal angioplasty of the subclavian and innominate arteries utilizing the brachial approach: acute outcome and follow-up. Cathet Cardiovasc Diagn 1990;19:71-76.

172. Breall JA, Grossman W, Stillman IE, Gianturco LE, Kim D. Atherectomy of the subclavian artery for patients with symptomatic coronary-subclavian steal syndrome. J Am Coll Cadiol 1993;21:1564-1570.

173. Breall JA, Kim D, Baim DS, Skillman JJ, Grossman W. Coronary-subclavian steal; and unusual cause of angina pectoris after successful internal mammary-coronary artery bypass grafting. Cathet Cardiovasc Diagn 1991;24:274-276.

174. Sbarouni E, Corr L, Fenech A. Microcoil embolization of large intercostal branches of internal mammary artery grafts. Cathet Cardiovasc Diagn 1994;31:334-336

175. Mishkel GJ, Willinsky R. Combined PTCA and microcoil embolization of a left internal mammary artery graft. Cathet

Cardiovasc Diagn 1192;27:141-6

176. Benzuly K, Kaplan B, Bowers T, Safian RD. Coronary-subclavian steal due to fishulae from the left internal mammary artery to the pulmonary artery: Treatment by coil embolization. Cathet Cardiovasc Diagn (in-press).

177. Lytle BW, Cosgrove DM, Ratliff NB, Loop F. Coronary artery bypass grafting with the right gastroepiploic artery. J Thorac Cardiovasc Surg 1989;97(6):826-31

178. Verkkala K, Jarvinen A, Keto P, Virtanen K, Lehtola A, Pellinen T. Right gastroepiploic artery as a coronary bypass graft. Ann Thorac Surg 1989, 47:719-9

179. Grandjean JG, Boonstra PW, den Heyer P, Ebels T. Arterial revascularization with the right gastroepiploic artery and internal mammary arteries in 300 patients. J Thorac Surg 1994,107:1309-1315

180. Perrault LP, Carrier M, Hebert Y, Hudon G, Cartier R, Leclerc Y, Pelletier LC. Clinical experience with the right gastroepiploic artery in coronary bypass grafting. Ann Thorac Surg 1993;56:1082-4

181. Suma H, Wanibuchi Y, Terada Y, Fukuda S, Takayama T, Furuta S. The right gastroepiploic artery graft. Clinical and angiographic midterm results in 200 patients.

182. Tanimoto Y, Matsuda Y, Fujii B, Kobayashi Y, Hatashi K, Takashiba K, Hamada Y, Hanazono S, Ando K, Hashimoto T. Angiography of the right gastroepiploic artery for coronary artery bypass graft. Cathet Cardiovasc Diagn 1989;16:35-8

183. Ishiki T, Yamaguchi T, Nakamura M, et al. Postoperative angiographic evaluation of gastroepiploic artery grafts: technical considerations and short-term patency. Cathet Cardiovasc Diagn 1991;21:233-8

184. Komiyama N, Nakanishi S, Yanagashita Y, Nishiyama S, Seki A, Watanabe Y, Konishi T, Fuse K. Percutaneous transluminal coronary angioplasty of gastroepiploic artery graft. Cathet Cardiovasc Diagn 1990;21:177-9

185. Watson LE, Schoolar EJ. PTCA of Gastroepiploic Bypass. Cathet Cardiovasc Diagn 1991;22:193-196.

186. Ishiki T, Yamaguchi T, Tamura T, Saeki F, Furuta Y, Ikari Y, Chiku N, Suma H. Percutaneous angioplasty of stenosed gastroepiploic artery grafts. J Am Coll Cardiol 1993, 22:727-32

187. Bartlett JC, Tuzcu M, Simpfendorfer C, Dorosti K. Percutaneous transluminal coronary angioplasty of native coronary arteries via saphenous vein grafts. J Invas Cardiol 1991;3:62-65.

188. Ramee S, Kuntz R, Schatz R, et al. Preliminary experience with the POSSIS coronary angiojet rheolytic thrombectomy catheter in the VeGAS 1 pilot study. J Am Coll Cardial 1996; March Special Issue.

189. Hong M, Wong S, Popma J, et al. Favorable results of debulking followed by immediate adjunct stent therapy for high risk saphenous vein graft lesions. J Am Coll Cardial 1996; March Special Issue.

190. Douglas J, Savage M, Bailey S, et al. Randomized trial of coronary stent and balloon angioplasty in the treatment of saphenous vein graft stenosis. J Am Coll Cardial 1996; March Special Issue.

18 PTCA EXOTICA: UNUSUAL PROBLEMS IN THE INVASIVE LABORATORY

Cindy L. Grines, M.D.
Robert D. Safian, M.D.

The vast majority of invasive procedures can be performed in an efficient, routine manner based on well-established techniques. Part of the attraction to the field however, is the unforseen and often problematic situations that can arise requiring ingenuity, skill, and creativity. This section will focus on these types of situations and illustrate possible solutions.

A. LARGE VESSEL CORONARY ANGIOPLASTY

1. **Hugging Balloon Technique.** Although larger coronary balloons are under- going clinical testing, currently available coronary angioplasty equipment permits selection of a maximum of 4.0mm balloons. Mechanical characteristics of deflation time, flexibility, and profile have presented difficulties in the production of larger balloons. Occasionally, oversized vessels (coronary arteries or vein grafts) require a larger balloon to achieve a balloon to artery ratio of 1:1. This problem was initially overcome by instrumenting both femoral arteries and engaging the vessel with two separate guiding catheters. Side by side "hugging" balloons were simultaneously inflated to achieve a larger area of dilatation. More recently, larger lumen guiding catheters have made two separate access sites unnecessary (see Chapter 1)[1]. Simultaneous inflation of both balloons will yield a slightly smaller combined diameter than the sum of each balloon alone. For example, the area occupied by two side by side 2mm balloons ($7.14mm^2$) approximates the area of a single 3.0mm balloon ($7.07mm^2$) and is much smaller than a single 3.5mm balloon ($9.6mm^2$). Also, the cross-section of two balloons is oval rather than round. Feld et al. has suggested that the altered geometric configuration may be useful in lesions which fail to dilate with a single balloon at high pressures.[2]

2. **Peripheral Angioplasty Balloon.** Peripheral angioplasty balloons have been used to dilate large coronary arteries.[3] Contemporary balloons with lower profiles now allow peripheral balloon passage through large lumen coronary guiding catheters (see Chapter 1).

B. RETROGRADE NATIVE VESSEL ANGIOPLASTY.

Angioplasty of native coronary vessels via both internal mammary and saphenous vein bypass grafts can frequently be performed using standard techniques. The natural tendency of the guidewire is to advance from the graft antegrade into the distal native vessel. Occasionally, the lesion is located proximal to the graft insertion point and the wire must travel retrograde to the proximal native vessel. The wire frequently must make a very sharp bend in a direction that may prove difficult to maneuver. Using a single core guidewire (see Chapter 1) will help prevent prolapse in the wrong direction; the curve on the tip must be severely angled. It may be useful to advance the balloon to the anastomosis and then reshape the wire tip to negotiate the severe angle. The balloon itself must be as flexible as possible with a small nose tip. If these techniques fail, a second wire may be passed antegrade into the native vessel and a balloon is inflated just distal to the graft insertion. This balloon is then used to deflect a second wire in the desired retrograde direction (Figure 18.1).

C. **INABILITY TO REACH LESION THROUGH A BYPASS GRAFT.** Rarely, when performing PTCA of native vessels through bypass grafts the standard 135cm balloon shaft will not extend far enough to cross the lesion. Multiple are now available with shaft lengths 135-150 cm; 90 cm guides may also be used (see Chapter 1).

D. **GUIDEWIRE TECHNIQUES**
    1. **Guiding Catheter Exchange Over Guidewire.** During angioplasty it is possible to cross a complex lesion with a guidewire only to find that the guiding catheter does not offer sufficient support to cross with the balloon. This can be easily accomplished using heavy-duty 0.014-inch or 0.018-inch guides, which permit complete exchange of balloons, guiding catheters, and vascular sheaths, without relinquishing guidewire position (see Chapter 1). Another novel approach is to use the Relay catheter; this is a modified monorail catheter which provides an excellent platform for exchanging vascular sheaths and guiding catheters, without relinquishing guidewire position (see Table 1.16).

    2. **Lost Guidewire Technique.** When exchanging out one balloon over-a-wire system for another over a guidewire which has been extended, occasionally the guidewire may come apart at the point where it was extended. If this happens inside the balloon catheter, one is left with a guidewire still across the lesion but no longer extending out the hub of the balloon catheter. To avoid lasing guidewire position attach a 5cc syringe of heparinized saline to the central lumen of the balloon catheter and make forceful injections. This will move the guidewire forward; as the balloon is withdrawn slowly, repeated injections will maintain guidewire position. To successfully accomplish this exchange, there must be no friction at the Y-connector and no traction must on the catheter; straightening the catheter is mandatory.

    3. **Use of Guidewire to Engage LIMA.** Sometimes diagnostic catheters are unable to engage the ostium of the left internal mammary artery (LIMA). After placing a LIMA catheter in the left subclavian artery just proximal to the origin of the mammary artery, a .014" floppy guidewire can be used to enter the vessel, facilitating diagnostic angiography.[8]

E. **GUIDING CATHETER TECHNIQUES**
    1. **Guiding Catheter Exchange Over Guidewire** (described in Section E, guidewire techniques).

    2. **Techniques to Improve Torque Control and engage the guiding catheter.** A tortuous aorto-femoral system may make torquing of catheters very difficult. A long sheath (23cm) or an 8F Mullins sheath (used for transseptal technique commonly) may be used to aid in torque control. A .038' J-wire or Amplatz wire will provide more support. If a giant lumen guiding catheter is being used, .063" wires are available.

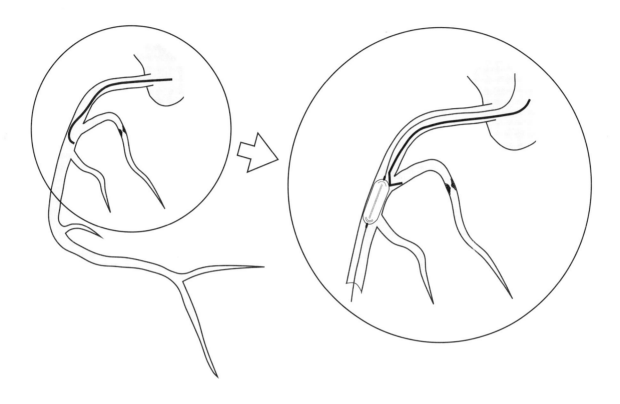

Figure 18.1 Deflection Technique

An angled branch which cannot be engaged with the guidewire. Wire is deflected off the balloon allowing passage into the target branch.

3. **High Coronary Flow.** Guiding catheters are useful in cases involving high coronary flow such as aortic valve disease, left ventricular hypertrophy, or circumflex dominant systems.

4. **Thrombus Aspiration.** Several reports have described the use of guiding catheters to remove intracoronary thrombus.[13-16] This can be accomplished with 6-8 FR multipurpose or right Judkins catheters, by attaching a 50cc to the hub of the guide. The guide should be advanced own a guidewire and balloon catheter, before aspirating, to minimize injury to the vessel.

5. **Intracoronary Balloon Thrombectomy.** Kipperman et al. reported a somewhat different method of intracoronary thrombectomy using an inflated balloon in a manner similar to a Fogarty catheter.[17] The balloon was inflated to 2atm and slowly withdrawn into the guide catheter; with inflated balloon catheter held well within its lumen, the guiding catheter was removed under continuous suction. A large organized thrombus was found within the guiding catheter. Several major risks must be considered when performing this procedure. Systemic or local embolization may be

reduced by maintaining constant suction as the guiding catheter is withdrawn but still is a concern. Withdrawing an inflated balloon may create intimal damage and dissection. These risks must be weighed against the outcome if the vessel remains totally occluded. If the balloon is to be withdrawn while inflated, the authors recommend doing so only in relatively short, straight sections of artery. Proximal coronary artery occlusion may lead to shock and cardiac arrest before surgical intervention can occur. Aspiration is a quick, simple technique which may be successful in a limited number of patients who appear moribund.

6. **Air Aspiration.** Aspiration of a large air embolus has been reported[18] using a balloon catheter passed distally down a bypass graft.

F. **PERCUTANEOUS REMOVAL OF EMBOLIZED FRAGMENTS.** Complications of retained fragments following intravascular catheterization include thromboembolism perforation, embolization, infection, and arrhythmias. In one review of 68 cases of centrally embolized fragments, 17 died of related cardiopulmonary complications.[19] The three most frequent risks of retained intracoronary guidewire fragments are coronary artery occlusion, thromboembolism, and embolization of the fragment itself. Fragments extending into the aorta also pose the risk of cerebral or systemic embolization of the foreign body or thrombus. The incidence of complications increases with increasing length of time between embolization and retrieval. Some recent reports, however, suggest that short guidewire fragments retained in totally occluded coronary arteries may have a benign prognosis when left in situ.[20] Intravascular foreign bodies that are long standing (>1 week duration) should not be removed percutaneously since they may become incorporated into the surrounding fibrous tissue and injure the vessel with removal. One series of 5400 consecutive PTCA procedures reported 12 (.2%) patients who had complications resulting in retention of PTCA equipment components.[20] The incidence may be lower now. A number of instruments have been used to retrieve intravascular foreign bodies (Table 18.1). The most commonly used devices by interventional cardiologists is the preformed Snare (Figure 18.2, 18.3, 18.4).

G. **EMBOLIZATION OF CORONARY FISTULAS.** Coronary artery fistulas are the most common hemodynamically significant coronary anomaly. Fistulas arising from either the left or right coronary arteries are common and over 90% drain into the venous circulation (RV, RA, PA). The majority are asymptomatic until the fifth or sixth decade when symptoms of left ventricular failure occur secondary to the left-to-right shunt. Other complications include angina (resulting from a coronary "steal" syndrome), endocarditis, fistula rupture, and progressive dilatation. Indications for

Table 18.1 Instruments for Retrieval of Intravascular Foreign Bodies

• Snares	• Preshaped Catheters
• Baskets (Dormia, Dotter)	• Platinum-Cobalt Magnet
• Forceps	• Fogarty Balloon Catheter
• Cardiac Biotome	• Guidewires

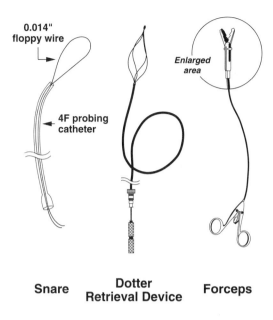

**0.014"
floppy wire**

**4F probing
catheter**

*Enlarged
area*

| Snare | Dotter
Retrieval Device | Forceps |

Figure 18.2   Retrieval Devices

Multiple different types of retrieval devices are available.

closure include a significant left-to-right shunt (QP/QS >1.5), signs of heart failure, or ischemia. While previously this required a surgical procedure, selected cases may now be done percutaneously by using detachable balloons, microcoil embolization, or microparticle embolization.

H.   **ENTRAPPED GUIDEWIRE REMOVAL.** Occasionally guidewires can become firmly caught in the coronary vessels. The wire tip may unwind and lengthen with forceful retraction. Initial management includes the administration of large doses of intracoronary nitroglycerin, or verapamil (100 micrograms I.C.) to alleviate spasm. Next, the balloon should be advanced toward the distal end of the wire; the more coaxial that it is to the distal wire the better the traction will be transmitted to the wire. Vigorous traction should be avoided since the wire may break where the spring coil joins the core. Some recommend balloon dilatation in the area of the wire, or balloon inflation just distal to the trapped wire; both measures should be used with Preformed snares may be employed to remove wire fragments.

I.   **ENTRAPPED BALLOON REMOVAL.** Entrapment of the balloon is a rare; it may be associated with balloon rupture in hard, calcified lesions. Initial efforts should include intracoronary vasodilators, attempts to re-inflate the balloon to free the torn edges from the vessel wall, or inflating another balloons side-by-side. If these efforts prove unsuccessful, the patient should have the balloon surgically removed and bypass grafting performed (Figure 18.5).

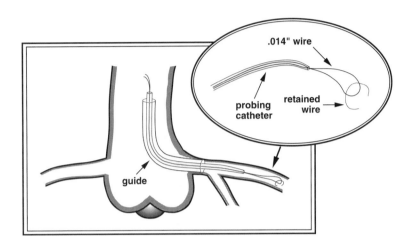

Figure 18.3   Snare

A probing catheter with a guidewire. Snare is advanced through the engaged guiding catheter. Once the snare is looped around the fragment, the probing catheter is advanced to entrap the fragment.

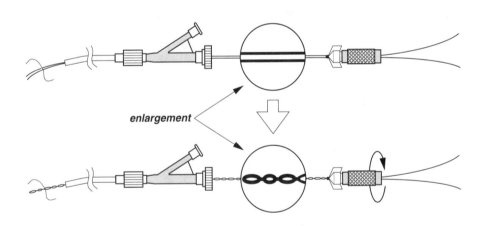

Figure 18.4   Fragment Catcher

Both guidewires are first advanced past the fragment. Multiple rotations using a torque tool are used to entrap the fragment.

Retained Hardware

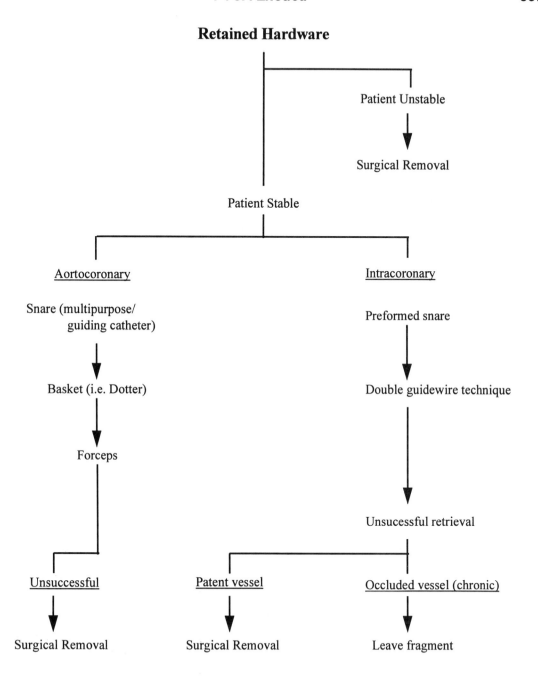

Figure 18.5 Retrieval of Retained Fragment

A clinical approach to fragment removal taking into account the patient's condition and location of the fragment.

REFERENCES

1. Krucoff MW, Smith JE, Jackman JD Jr, et al. "Hugging balloons" through a single 8-french guide: salvage angioplasty with lytic therapy in the infarct vessel of a 40-year-old man. Cathet Cardiovasc Diagn 1991;24:45-50.

2. Feld H, Valerio L and Shani J. Two hugging balloons at high pressures successfully dilate a lesion refractory to routine coronary angioplasty. Cathet Cardiovasc Diagn 1991;24:105-107.

3. Arafah M, Aldridge HE and Schwartz L. Percutaneous transluminal angioplasty of stenotic saphenous vein right coronary bypass grafts utilizing a peripheral balloon dilatation catheter without a guiding catheter. Cathet Cardiovasc Diagn 1989;17:92-96.

4. Villavicencio R, Urban P, Muller T., et al. Coronary balloon angioplasty through diagnostic 6 french catheters. Cathet Cardiovasc Diagn 1991;22:56-59.

5. Feldman R, Glemser E, Kaizer J, et al. Coronary angioplasty using new 6 french guiding catheters. Cathet Cardiovasc Diagn 1991;23:93-99.

6. Moles VP, Meier B, Urban P, et al. Percutaneous transluminal coronary angioplasty through 4 french diagnostic catheters. Cathet Cardiovasc Diagn 1992;25:98-100.

7. Warren SG and Barnett JC. Guiding catheter exchange during coronary angioplasty. Cathet Cardiovasc Diagn 1990;20:212-215.

8. Schreiber TL, Gangadharan V and O'Neill W. Guidewire facilitation of internal mammary artery cannulation. J Interven Cardiol 1990;3:23-26.

9. Nakhjavan FK. Use of angioplasty guidewire for technically difficult angiography. Cathet Cardiovasc Diagn 1988;14:213.

10. Das GS and Wysham DG. Double wire technique for additional guiding catheter support in anomalous left circumflex coronary artery angioplasty. Catheter Cardiovasc Diagn 1991;24:102-104.

11. Hartzler GO. Three-wire technique. A unique approach to percutaneous transluminal coronary angioplasty of a trifurcation lesion. Cathet Cardiovasc Diagn 1987;13:174-177.

12. Nakhjavan FK and Najmi M. Exit block: a new technique for difficult side branch angioplasty. Cathet Cardiovasc Diagn 1990;20:43-45.

13. Lablanche JM, Fourrier JL, Gommeaux A, et al. Percutaneous aspiration of a coronary thrombus. Cathet Cardiovasc Diagn 1989;17:97-98.

14. Brown SE, Segar DS, Weinberg BA, et al. Transcatheter Aspiration of Intracoronary Thrombus After Myocardial Infarction. Am Heart J 1990;120:688-690.

15. Kahn JK and Hartzler GO. Thrombus Aspiration in Acute Myocardial Infarction. Cathet Cardiovasc Diagn 1990;20:54-57.

16. Holmes, Lapeyre, Schuartz et al. Thrombectomy of occluded coronary arteries: an initial clinical experience. J Am Coll Cardiol 1991;82(4) III-622 Abstract.

17. Kipperman RM, Feit AS, Einhorn AM, et al. Intracoronary thrombectomy: A new approach to total occlusion. Cathet Cardiovasc Diagn 1989;18:244-248.

18. Haraphongse M and Rossall RE. Large air embolus complicating coronary angioplasty. Cathet Cardiovasc Diagn 1989;17:168-171.

19. Burri C, Henkeneyer H, Passler HH. Katheterembolien. Schw Med Wschr 1971:101:1537.

20. Hartzler G, Rutherford B, McConahay D. Retained percutaneous transluminal coronary angioplasty components and their management. Am J Cardiol 1987;60:1260-1264.

21. Bogart DB, Earnest JB, and Miller JT. Foreign body retrieval using a simple snare device. Cathet Cardiovasc Diagn 1990;19:248-250.

22. Mikolich JR and Hanson MW. Transcatheter retrieval of intracoronary detached angioplasty guidewire segment. Cathet Cardiovasc Diagn 1988:15:44-46.

23. Savas V, Schreiber T and O'Neill W. Percutaneous extraction of fractured guidewire from distal right coronary artery. Cathet Cardiovasc Diagn 1991;22:124-126.

24. Serota H, Deligonul U, Lew B, et al. Improved method for transcatheter retrieval of intracoronary detached angioplasty guidewire segments. Cathet Cardiovasc Diagn 1989;17:248-251.

25. Gurley JC, Booth DC, Hixson C., et al. Removal of retained intracoronary percutaneous transluminal coronary angioplasty equipment by a percutaneous twin guidewire method. Cathet Cardiovasc Diagn 1990;19:251-256.

26. Nyuyen K, Myler RK, Hieshima G, et al. Treatment of coronary artery stenosis and coronary arteriovenous fistula by

interventional cardiology techniques. Cathet Cardiovasc Diagn 1989;18:240-243.

27. Doorey AJ, Sullivan KL and Levin DC. Successful percutaneous closure of a complex coronary-to-pulmonary artery fistula using a detachable balloon: benefits of intra-procedural physiologic and angiographic assessment. Cathet Cardiovasc Diagn 1991;23:23-27.

28. Jost S, Simon R, Amende I, et al. Transluminal balloon embolization of an inadvertent aorto-to-coronary venous bypass to the anterior cardiac vein. Cathet Cardiovasc Diagn 1989;17:28-30.

29. Strunk BL, Hieshima GB and Shafton EP. Treatment of congenital coronary arteriovenous malformations with micro-particle embolization. Cathet Cardiovasc Diagn 1991;22:133-136.

30. Jondeau G, Lacombe P, Rocha P, et al. Swan-ganz catheter-induced rupture of the pulmonary artery: successful early management by transcatheter embolization. Cathet Cardiovasc Diagn 1990;19:202-204.

31. Watson LE. Snare loop technique for removal of broken steerable PTCA wire. Cathet Cardiovasc Diagn 1987;13:44-49.

32. Interventional Radiology. Athanasoulis, Pfister, Greene, et al. 1982. W.B. Saunders, Co.

19 CORONARY ARTERY SPASM

Mark Freed, M.D.

A. BALLOON ANGIOPLASTY

1. **Intralesional Spasm.** Coronary artery spasm has been reported to occur in 1-5% of balloon angioplasty procedures.[1,2] Risk factors include noncalcified lesions,[1,3] possibly eccentric lesions [4] and younger patients, but not variant angina.[5,6] Intravascular ultrasound or angioscopy may be useful in cases where it is difficult to distinguish refractory spasm from severe recoil or dissection. Fortunately, most cases can be successfully treated by intracoronary vasodilators (nitrates and/or calcium blockers) ± repeat PTCA at low inflation pressures. Eccentric lesion morphology was associated with vasospasm in one report,[3] but not in another.[4] Finally, variant angina does not appear to independently predict procedure-related spasm.

2. **Distal Epicardial Spasm.** Spasm of the distal vessel is common after PTCA and virtually all percutaneous devices; repeat angiograms taken 15-30 minutes after balloon deflation demonstrate a 16-30% reduction in minimal lumen diameter[7,8] and a 28% reduction in cross-sectional area.[9] In an early report, distal epicardial spasm was immediately reversed by intracoronary nitroglycerin; it could also be prevented by continuous IV nitroglycerin but not by pretreatment with aspirin or oral calcium-channel blockers.[8] More recent data suggest that serotonin — released into the coronary circulation from circulating platelets — plays an important pathogenetic role; in these reports, ketanserin, a selective serotonin$_2$-receptor antagonist, was shown to blunt distal epicardial spasm after PTCA.[9,10] Treatment is pharmacologic and consists of nitrates (sublingual, intravenous, or intracoronary), nifedipine (sublingual), and/or diltiazem or verapamil (intravenous or intracoronary).

3. **Distal Microvascular Spasm.** In contrast to epicardial spasm, spasm of the distal microvascular bed rarely response to nitrates. The incidence, risk factors, and management of this condition are reviewed in the chapter on "No-Reflow" (Chapter 21). Preferred treatment is intracoronary calcium antagonists.

4. **Post-Procedural Spasm.** The PTCA site remains susceptible to spasm for several months after the procedure. Ergonovine[11] and acetylcholine[12] can induce vasospasm after PTCA in 15% and 46% of patients, respectively.[11] Spontaneous episodes of spasm may develop in the weeks or months following PTCA[6,11] and cause rest angina.

B. Pathophysiology.
Balloon dilatation results in coronary endothelial denudation and loss of endothelium-derived relaxing factor (EDRF). Depletion of this potent vasodilator increases sensitivity to local vasoconstrictors (e.g., serotonin from aggregating platelets) and decreases sensitivity to vasodilators such as prostacyclin and prostaglandin E_2.[13] Other putative mechanisms include increased

production or impaired degradation of norepinephrine or platelet-derived vasoconstrictors (thromboxane, serotonin, platelet-activating factor); altered arachidonic acid metabolism, resulting in the overproduction of vasoconstricting prostanoids and leukotrienes; release of endothelium-derived contractile factor (EDCF); local adrenergic nerve dysfunction; and simulation of stretch-dependent myogenic tone.[7-10,14-16] A decrease in forearm bloodflow and an increase in vascular resistance has been observed after coronary angioplasty; these changes were abolished by pretreatment with a regional infusion of phentolamine (α-blocker) or verapamil,[17] suggesting the presence of a generalized neural or hormonal mechanism.[18]

C. **New Devices.** Compared to PTCA, coronary artery spasm after new devices appears to occur with equal or greater frequency.[19-27] Spasm has been reported in 4 - 36% of Rotablator cases;[16,24,28,29,37] in one study, severe spasm resulting in threatened or abrupt occlusion and requiring repeat PTCA or CABG occurred in 12/743 patients (1.6%).[19] Spasm has been reported in 1.2 - 16% of ELCA procedures:[21,22,25-27,30] independent predictors including smoking (relative risk 2.1), no diabetes (relative risk 2.2), and stenosis severity $\leq$ 90% (relative risk 1.6). Spasm has also been reported in 0.8 - 1.6% of DCA and 6.6% of holmium-laser cases.[20,27] Most cases of coronary spasm following new devices respond to intracoronary and intravenous nitrates $\pm$ repeat balloon dilatation.

D. **Management (Figure 19.1)**
   1. **Nitrates.** Coronary artery spasm usually resolves promptly after the administration of intracoronary nitroglycerin (200-300 mcg), but doses may need to be repeated.

   2. **Removal of PTCA Hardware.** Balloon and guiding catheters should be withdrawn from the coronary ostium to minimize mechanical irritation to the vessel. If intralesional spasm is evident, the guidewire should remain across the lesion to maintain vascular access. If spasm occurs distal to the PTCA site, partial or complete removal of the guidewire may be required for the spasm to resolve.

   3. **Calcium Channel Antagonists.** Intracoronary verapamil (100 mcg/min up to 1.0 - 1.5 mg)[31] or intracoronary diltiazem (0.5-2.5 mg over $\geq$1 min.; total: 5-10 mg)[32] may reverse coronary spasm refractory to intracoronary nitroglycerin. A temporary transvenous pacemaker should be readily available, although the risk of AV block, bradycardia, and hypotension are low.

   4. **Repeat Balloon Dilatation.** If intralesional spasm persists despite the use of nitrates, a prolonged (2-5 minute) low-pressure (1-4 atm.) inflation using a balloon matched to the reference segment is frequently successful at "breaking" the spasm. In fact, the vast majority of episodes of spasm respond to nitrates and repeat PTCA. Refractory spasm should prompt placement of an autoperfusion balloon catheter to restore antegrade blood flow, stabilize hemodynamics, and potentially "tack-up" an inapparent dissection.

   5. **Anticholinergics.** Acetylcholine may induce paradoxical vasoconstriction in de-endothelialized arteries,[33] presumably due to a local loss of EDRF. Therefore, if spasm is accompanied by evidence

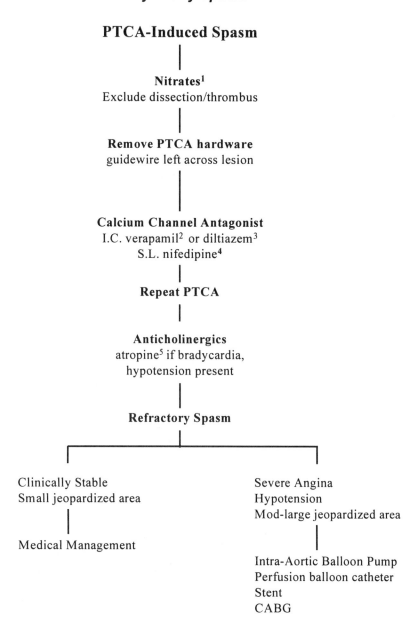

PTCA-Induced Spasm

Nitrates[1]
Exclude dissection/thrombus

Remove PTCA hardware
guidewire left across lesion

Calcium Channel Antagonist
I.C. verapamil[2] or diltiazem[3]
S.L. nifedipine[4]

Repeat PTCA

Anticholinergics
atropine[5] if bradycardia,
hypotension present

Refractory Spasm

Clinically Stable
Small jeopardized area

Medical Management

Severe Angina
Hypotension
Mod-large jeopardized area

Intra-Aortic Balloon Pump
Perfusion balloon catheter
Stent
CABG

Figure 19.1. Management of Intraprocedural Spasm

1. Nitroglycerin 100-300 mcg i.c. bolus; and intravenous infusion (20 mcg/min)
2. Verapamil 100 mcg/min i.c. up to 1.5 mg; temporary pacemaker on standby
3. Diltiazem 0.5 - 2.5 mg i.c. over 1 min; temporary pacemaker on standby
4. Nifedipine 10 mg sublingual
5. Atropine 0.5 mg I.V.; may repeat every 5 min. up to 2.0 mg

of vagal hypertonia (i.e., hypotension and bradycardia), atropine may be carefully administered (0.5 mg IVevery 5 minutes to a total of 2.0 mg).

6. **Systemic Circulatory Support.** A management dilemma may arise when severe spasm is associated with ischemia and hypotension since administration of nitrates and/or calcium channel blockers could exacerbate hypotension and lead to further clinical deterioration. In this setting, it is best to proceed with intracoronary nitrates or calcium antagonists while preparing to support the systemic circulation with IABP or percutaneous cardiopulmonary support (CPS) as required. Alpha-adrenergic drugs may exacerbate vasospasm and should be avoided, but inotropic drugs such as dobutamine can be used if needed.

7. **Stents.** Intracoronary stenting has been used successfully for refractory spasm, but should be reserved for situations in which all other nonoperative alternatives have failed. Most such cases of "refractory" spasm are probably dissections, which should respond to stenting.

8. **Coronary Artery Bypass Grafting.** Emergency bypass surgery should be considered for refractory spasm when there is ongoing ischemia, the vessel is suitable for grafting, and all other approaches have been exhausted.

9. **Superimposed Coronary Dissection and Thrombus.** Multiple angiographic views of the target lesion should be obtained to exclude superimposed dissection and/or thrombus. If present, they should be managed as described in Chapters 20 and 9, respectively. If not already performed, coronary angioscopy or intravascular ultrasound may help clarify the nature of the lesion and guide further therapy.

E. **Prevention.** A continuous intravenous infusion of nitroglycerin (10-50 mcg/min) may prevent distal spasm and is used routinely at our institution for all patients undergoing coronary intervention. Long-acting nitrates and/or calcium blockers are usually started 12-24 hours following the procedure and continued for a minimum of 1 week. A minority of operators also administer a calcium channel antagonist intravenously (verapamil 5 mg over 1-2 minutes) at the start of the case. Some interventionalists withhold β-blockers before Rotablator atherectomy since distal vasospasm (which occurs in 4-36% of cases[16,24,28,29]and may be due to sympathetic stimulation[16]) can be potentiated by β-blockers.

PTCA FOR VARIANT ANGINA

Patients with variant (Prinzmetal's) angina present with unpredictable bouts of effort angina or rest pain and ST-segment changes due to spontaneous of coronary vasospasm. Dynamic obstruction of coronary blood flow may occur in angiographically normal coronary arteries, but more commonly occurs in vessels with moderate or severe fixed stenoses.[34] Although medical management alone is effective in the majority of cases, some patients continue to have disabling symptoms leading to MI sudden death. The prognosis is especially poor when tachy- or bradyarrhythmias occur during episodes of pain, and when spasm is superimposed on fixed lesions.[34] Compared to patients undergoing surgery for classic angina pectoris, coronary artery bypass grafting with or without sympathetic denervation is associated with a higher incidence of post-operative MI, early graft closure, and recurrent angina.[35] PTCA and stenting have occasionally been applied to patients with spasm superimposed on fixed lesions. Small observational reports suggest a number of general conclusions (Table 19.1).[5,6,36]

Table 19.1. PTCA of Organic Stenoses in Variant Angina

1. A high technical success rate can be achieved.

2. Procedural complications, including PTCA-induced coronary artery spasm, are no more frequent than during PTCA for other types of coronary disease.

3. Recurrent spasm and rest angina are not uncommon following PTCA; pharmacologic therapy with high-dose nitrates and calcium channel antagonists may reduce their frequency and severity.

4. Restenosis rates are approximately 50%.

5. Many patients derive symptomatic benefit, although the impact on event-free survival (compared to medical therapy or CABG) has not been evaluated.

6. The role of new interventional devices in this disorder is unknown.

* * * * *

References

1. Cowley M, Dorros G, Kelsey S, Van Raden M, Detre K. Acute coronary events associated with percutaneous transluminal coronary angioplasty. Am J Cardiol 1984;53:12C-16C.
2. Holmes DJ, Holubkov R, Vlietstra R, et al. Comparison of complications during percutaneous transluminal coronary angioplasty from 1977 to 1981 and from 1985 to 1986: The National Heart, Lung, and Blood Institute Percutaneous Transluminal Coronary Angioplasty Registry. J Am Coll Cardiol 1988;12:1149-1155.
3. Fitzgerald PJ, Stertzer SH, Hidalgo BO, et al. Plaque characteristics affect lesion and vessel response to coronary rotational atherectomy: An intravascular ultrasound study. J Am Coll Cardiol 1994:March Special Issue:353A.
4. Fischell T, and Bausback K. Effects of luminal eccentricity on spontaneous coronary vasoconstriction after successful percutaneous transluminal coronary angioplasty. Am J Cardiol 1991;68:530-534.
5. Corcos T, David PR, Bourassa MG, et al. Percutaneous transluminal coronary angioplasty for the treatment of variant angina. J Am Coll Cardiol 1985;5:1046-1054.
6. David PR, Waters DD, Scholl M, et al. Percutaneous coronary angioplasty in patients with variant angina. Circulation 1982;66:695-702.
7. Indolfi C, Piscione F, Esposito G, et al. Mechanisms of coronary vasoconstriction after successful single angioplasty of the left anterior descending artery. J Am Coll Cardiol 1993:March Special Issue:340A.
8. Fischell T, Derby G, Tse T, Stadius M. Coronary artery vasoconstriction routinely occurs after percutaneous transluminal coronary angioplasty. A quantitative arteriographic analysis. Circulation 1988;78:1323-1334.
9. Golino P, Piscione F, Benedict CF, et al. Local effect of serotonin released during coronary angioplasty. N Engl J Med 1994;330:523-8.
10. Tousoulis D, Tentolouris C, Apostolopoulos T, Toutouzas P. Effects of intracoronary ketanserin in proximal and distal segments post angioplasty. J Am Coll Cardiol 1993:March Special Issue:341A.
11. Hollman J, Austin GE, Gruentzig AR, et al. Coronary artery spasm at the site of angioplasty in the first two months after successful percutaneous transluminal coronary angioplasty. J Am Coll Cardiol 1983;2:1039-1045.
12. Kirigaya H, Aizawa T, Ogasaware K, et al. Enhanced vasospastic activity to acetylcholine of the coronary arteries undergoing previous balloon angioplasty. J Am Coll Cardiol 1993:March Special Issue:341A.
13. Cohen RA, Shepherd JT, and Vanhoutte PM. Inhibitory role of endothelium in the response of isolated coronary arteries to platelets. Science 1983;221:273-274.
14. Lam JT, Chesebro JH, Steele PM, et al. Vasospasm related to platelet deposition? Relationship in a porcine preparation of arterial injury in vivo. Circulation 1987;75:243-248.
15. Cohen RA, Zitany KM and Weisbrod RM. Accumulation of 5-hydroxy-tryptamine leads to dysfunction of adrenergic nerves in canine coronary artery following intimal damage in vivo. Circulation 1987;61:829-833.
16. Gregorini L, Marco J, Fajadet J, Brunel, P, et al. Urapidil (α 1-sympathetic blocker) attenuates post-rotational ablation "elastic recoil". Circulation 1995;92:I-94.
17. Ceravolo R, Piscoine F, Malone A, Stingone AM, et al. Reflex forearm vasoconstriction after successful angioplasty of the left anterior descending coronary artery. Circulation 1995;92:I-323.
18. Ceravolo R, Indolfi C, Piscione F, et al. Coronary and limb vascular vasoconstriction after successful single angioplasty of the left anterior descending coronary artery. J Am Coll Cardiol 1995;March Special Issue:108A.
19. Warth D, Leon M, et al. Rotational atherectomy multicenter registry: Acute results, complications and 6-month angiographic follow-up in 709 patients. J Am Coll Cardiol 1994;24:641-648.
20. deMarchena EJ, Mallon SM, et al. Effectiveness of holmium laser-assisted coronary angioplasty. Am J Cardiol 1994;73:117-121.
21. Bittl J, Sanborn T, et al. Clinical success, complications and restenosis rates with excimer laser coronary angioplasty. Am J Cardiol 1992;70:1533-1539.
22. Ghazzal Z, Hearn J, et al. Morphological predictors of acute complications after percutaneous excimer laser coronary angioplasty. Results of a comprehensive angiographic analysis: Importance of the eccentricity index. Circulation 1992;86:820-827.
23. Hinohara T, Rowe M, et al. Effect of lesion characteristics on outcome of directional coronary atherectomy. J Am Coll Cardiol 1991;17:1112-1120.
24. Safian R, Niazi K, et al. Detailed Angiographic Analysis of High-Speed Mechanical Rotational Atherectomy in Human Coronary Arteries. Circulation 1993;88(3):961-968.
25. Litvack F, Eigler N, et al. Percutaneous excimer laser coronary angioplasty: Results in the first consecutive 3,000

patients. J Am Coll Cardiol 1994;23:323-9.

26. Baumback A, Bittl J, Fleck E, et al. Acute complications of excimer laser coronary angioplasty: A detailed analysis of multicenter results. J Am Coll Cardiol 1994;23:1305-1313.

27. Mehta S, Popma JJ, Margolis JR, et al. Angiographic complications after new device angioplasty in native coronary arteries: A NACI Angiographic Core Laboratory Report. TCT Meeting (Washington DC),February, 1995.

28. Bertrand M, Lablanche J, Leroy F, Bauters C. Percutaneous transluminal coronary rotary ablation with Rotablator (European experience). Am J Cardiol 1992;69:470-474.

29. Tierstein PS, Warth DC, Haq N, et al. High-speed rotational coronary atherectomy for patients with diffuse coronary artery disease. J Am Coll Cardiol 1991;18:1694-1701.

30. Initial results of the European Multicenter Registry on Coronary Excimer Laser Angioplasty. European Study Group. Circulation 1991;84(4):II-362.

31. Babbitt DG, Perry JM, and Forman MB. Intracoronary verapamil for reversal of refractory coronary vasospasm during percutaneous transluminal coronary angioplasty. J Am Coll Cardiol 1988;12:1377-1381.

32. McIvor ME, Undemir C, Lawson J, Reddinger J. Clinical effects and utility of intracoronary diltiazem. Cathet Cardiovasc Diagn. 1995;35:287-291.

33. Ludmer PL. Selwyn AP, Shook TL, et al. Paradoxical vasoconstriction induced by acetylcholine in atherosclerotic coronary arteries. N Engl J Med 1988;315:1046-1051.

34. Waters DD, Miller DD, Szlachcic J, et al. Factors influencing the long-term prognosis of treated patients with variant angina. Circulation 1983;63:258-265.

35. Gaasch WH, Lufshanowski R, Leachment RD, et al. Surgical management of prinzmetal's variant angina. Chest 1974;66:614-621.

36. Bertrand ME, LaBlanche JM, Thieuleux FA, et al. Comparative results of percutaneous transluminal coronary angioplasty in patients with dynamic versus fixed coronary stenosis. J Am Coll Cardiol 1986;8:504-508.

37. Mehta S, Popma J, Margolis JR, et al. Complications with new angioplasty devices. Are these device specific? J Am Coll Cardio;March Special Issue.

20 DISSECTION AND ACUTE CLOSURE

Mark Freed, M.D.
William W. O'Neill, M.D.
Robert D. Safian, M.D.

Acute coronary occlusion is the major cause of in-hospital death, MI, and emergency CABG following percutaneous intervention. Awareness of its timing, risk factors, and prognosis allow for prompt recognition and early implementation of remedial measures.

A. **CLASSIFICATION.** Unfortunately, no single classification of acute closure has gained widespread acceptance. The most popular definitions include:

- **Acute Closure:** Acute worsening of stenosis severity accompanied by a reduction in coronary flow (TIMI grade 0-2) as a consequence of coronary intervention. At William Beaumont Hospital, acute closure is subclassified into "imminent closure" (high-grade residual stenosis with TIMI 2 flow) and "established closure" (total occlusion with TIMI 0-1 flow).

- **Threatened Closure:** Angiographic appearance of dissection or thrombus causing > 50% residual stenosis post-intervention with normal coronary flow (TIMI 3).

However, different criteria of acute closure have been used by different investigators (e.g., TIMI 2 flow and > 50% residual stenosis may qualify as acute, threatened, or imminent closure.

B. **INCIDENCE AND TIMING OF ABRUPT CLOSURE.** Acute closure occurs in 2-11% of elective PTCAs, [1-4] 50-80% of which occur while the patient is still in catheterization laboratory. [5,6] (In the BARI trial, in-lab acute closure occurred in 9% of patients.[7]) Episodes developing outside the angioplasty suite usually occur within the first 6 hours and are rare after 24 hours. In one report, 63% of acute closures occurred within 1 hour, and 84% within 6 hours of the procedure.[8] In another report, 54% occurred within 6 hours, 21% within 6-12 hours, 25% within 12-24 hours, and no cases presented later than 24 hours after PTCA.[6] Acute closure does not appear to be reduced after the primary use of atherectomy or laser devices.[9-20,106] In CAVEAT-I,[104] abrupt closure was more common after DCA than PTCA (8% vs. 3.8%, p = 0.005), although in CAVEAT-II and CCAT, there was no difference in acute closure between these devices (Chapter 28). In the Optimal Atherectomy Restenosis Study (OARS), in which IVUS-guided DCA and PTCA were used to achieve a < 10% stenosis after atherectomy, in-lab acute closure occurred in 1%.[107] Although uncommon, acute closure may first present 1-2 days after atherectomy.[14,21] In the AMRO trial (ELCA without saline infusion vs. PTCA for long lesions), ELCA resulted in more actue closure (8% vs. 0.8%, p = 0.005).[38] In contrast to other devices, primary stenting has reduced the incidence of acute closure to < 1%; in the randomized STRESS and BENSTENT trials (Chapter 26), vessel closure was 1.5-2 times higher than PTCA. A recent report from the NACI Registry of 2233 native coronaries treated by new devices revealed an acute closure rate of 0% for stents compared to 1.3-8.3% for atherectomy and 7.4% for excimer laser (devices were not matched for lesion morphology).[106] Unfortunately, subacute stent thrombosis, which occurs between day 2-15 in ~ 2-5% of procedures, offsets some of this early beneficial effect.

C. **CAUSES OF ABRUPT CLOSURE.** The most common causes of acute closure include coronary dissection, thrombus formation, thrombosis and/or spasm. Coronary dissection exposes prothrombogenic constituents of the plaque (e.g., tissue thromboplastin) and vessel wall (fibrillar collagen), initiating a series of platelet-coagulation cascade-vessel wall interactions that may lead to thrombus, spasm, and acute closure. Acute occlusion may also occur after PTCA of a thrombus-containing lesion as mechanical disruption releases thrombin from its fibrin-bound state to stimulate further thrombosis (Chapter 9). While some degree of coronary spasm may contribute to abrupt closure from dissection and/or thrombus, isolated spasm is an infrequent cause of acute total obstruction.

1. **Coronary Artery Dissection**. Small intimal dissections are frequent after balloon angioplasty, but are usually associated with a benign course. In contrast, large complex dissections may cause acute vessel closure, with a high incidence of emergency CABG, myocardial infarction, and death. Patients with abrupt closure virtually always require further intervention; potential treatment options include prolonged balloon inflations (with or without a perfusion balloon), directional atherectomy, stenting, and emergency CABG for refractory cases. The ideal treatment for dissections not associated with vessel closure or impaired flow is unknown; better understanding of the natural history of such dissections may improve the clinical outcome.

Table 20.1. Coronary Artery Dissection: NHLBI Classification System

Dissection Type	Description	Angiographic Appearance
A	Minor radiolucencies within the coronary lumen during contrast injection with minimal or no persistence after dye clearance.	
B	Parallel tracts or double lumen separated by a radiolucent area during contrast injection with minimal or no persistence after dye clearance.	
C	Extraluminal cap with persistence of contrast after dye clearance from the coronary lumen.	
D	Spiral luminal filling defects.	
E+	New persistent filling defects.	
F+	Those non-A-E types that lead to impaired flow or total occlusion.	

+ May represent thrombus

a. **Classification.** Coronary artery dissection is usually defined angiographically; of the various classification schemes; the NHLBI classification is the most popular (Table 20.1). Types A and B are considered "minor" dissections since they do not appear to adversely impact procedural outcome. In contrast, Types C - F are considered "major" dissections and are associated with a 5-fold risk of myocardial infarction, emergency CABG, or death. Dissections that are long (>10mm), impair flow, or result in > 50% residual stenosis also increase the risk of ischemic complications.

b. **Incidence of Dissection**

1. **PTCA.** Following balloon angioplasty, coronary dissection is detected by angiography in 20-40% of cases,[2,23-26] and by intravascular ultrasound (IVUS) or angioscopy in 60-80% of cases.[27,28] Non-flow-limiting dissections should be not necessarily be considered a complication, since the mechanism of lumen enlargement for PTCA involves stretching of the vessel wall and cracking of plaque, which manifest as dissection. In some situations, angiography may suggest the presence of a dissection when none exists; these are important to recognize to avoid unnecessary attempts to repair the "dissection." Simple technical faults, such as weak contrast injections, may cause dye streaming and give the false impression of an intimal tear; these are readily identified by better injections to clearly opacify the lumen. In addition, deep guide catheter intubation may deform the proximal vessel and suggest the presence of a stenosis or dissection, repositioning the guide will often correct this problem, and intracoronary nitroglycerin (100-200 mcg i.c.) may also be used to relive associated spasm. Finally, a common angiographic findings is a pseudolesion, which is a segmental shelf-like deformity due to excessive straightening and invagination of the vessel wall, frequently associated with extra support guidewires. These pseudolesions can be very disturbing and easily confused with vessel injury from balloons or other devices. It is important to consider a pseudolesion when a new stenosis appears remote from the target lesion, particularly when heavy-duty guidewires are employed in tortuous guidewires are employed in tortuous vessels or for tracking new interventional devices. Because of the uncertainly created by these pseudolesions it is generally best to substitute a softer, more flexible guidewire, if possible; if the pseudolesion doe not improve or resolve, it may be necessary to completely remove the guidewire to ensure that a real lesion is not present.

2. **New Devices.** As shown in Table 20.2, angiographic dissection rates vary for different devices; these differences probably reflect differences in the mechanism of lumen enlargement and in the nature of the target lesion. The saline infusion technique has reduced be the incidence of dissection after ELCA; in a randomized trial, patients undergoing ELCA with blood displacement by intracoronary saline (prewarmed; 1-2 cc/min through the guiding catheter) had fewer severe dissections compared to conventional ELCA (7% vs. 24%; p = 0.05).[103] The impact of cutting and tapered balloons on dissection rates await further testing.

c. **Pathophysiology of Dissection.** The mechanism of lumen enlargement after PTCA is plaque fracture, intimal splitting, and localized medial dissection. These simple or "therapeutic" dissections may escape detection by angiography, or give the appearance of minor intraluminal radiolucencies or haziness. Complex dissections are characterized by deep medial tears which may create long or spiral dissections. These "complex" dissections: 1) often give the angiographic appearance of either an extraluminal "cap," contrast staining, and residual stenosis > 50%; 2) may expose collagen and tissue factor, increasing the risk of thrombosis; 3) substantially increase the risk of acute vessel closure and major ischemic complications; and 4) usually require further intervention.

1. **Influence of Lesion Calcium.** Dissections frequently occur at the junction point between calcified and non-calcified plaque, and may be due to the nonuniform transmission of dilating force across vessel segments of differing elastic properties.[35] Among calcified lesions treated by Rotablator atherectomy, IVUS has documented dissection from within the plaque after Rotablator, but at the junction of normal vessel wall and calcified atheroma after adjunctive PTCA.[27]

2. **Laser-Induced Dissection.** Absorption of excimer laser energy produces acoustic shock waves, which may generate a pressure of 100 atm.; this acoustic effect induce vessel trauma, manifested as dissection, abrupt closure, or perforation.[36] Administration of a saline bolus and infusion at time of lasing ("flush and bathe" technique) may attenuate acoustic injury (Chapter 30).[37,103]

Table 20.2. Angiographic Dissection Rates After Percutaneous Intervention

Modality	Incidence (%)
PTCA[2,23-26]	20 - 40
ELCA[13,19,20,29-31] DELCA[20] TEC[13]	20 - 30*
Rotablator[13,16,18,31,32] Cutting balloon[33] Tapered balloon[34]	10 - 30
DCA[13,15]	10 - 15
Stent[13,24]	< 10

Abbreviations: DELCA = directional excimer laser coronary angioplasty; TEC = transluminal extraction catheter; DCA = directional coronary atherectomy
*   10-20% when ELCA is performed with the saline infusion technique

Table 20.3. Angiographic and Clinical Predictors of Dissection after PTCA

Calcified lesions[26,38]

Eccentric lesions[25,38]

Long lesions[26]

Intermediate lesion length[25]

Diffuse disease[26]

Complex lesion morphology (Type B or C)[9]

Vessel curvature[25]

Absence of unstable angina[25]

d. **Risk Factors for Dissection After Balloon Angioplasty.** As summarized in Tables 20.3, 20.4, angiographic, clinical, and procedural variables impact the risk of coronary dissection.

e. **Prognosis After Dissection**
   1. **Ischemic Complications.** Severe coronary artery dissections increase the risk of ischemic complications (death, MI, emergency CABG) more than 5-fold.[16,24,61,62] In the STRESS trial, the presence of a dissection resulted in lower procedural success (75% vs. 92%) and higher in-hospital ischemic events (15% vs. 3%).[24] As shown in Tables 20.5, 20.6, certain clinical and angiographic features increase the risk of ischemic complications once a dissection has occurred.[2,22,60,63,64,65]

Table 20.5. Risk Factors for Major Ischemic Events in the Presence of a Dissection[22,60]

Dissection length > 15 mm

NHLBI dissection types C-F (Table 20.1)

Residual diameter stenosis > 30%

Residual cross-sectional area < 2 mm^2

Transient in-lab occlusion

Unstable angina

Chronic total occlusion

Table 20.4. The Impact of Balloon Angioplasty Technique or Coronary Dissection Rate

Parameter	Effect on Dissection Rate			Comments
	Possible ↑	Possible ↓	None	
Balloon catheter design			✓	Choice of catheter type (over-the-wire, on-the-wire, monorail) based on operator preference.
Balloon material (compliant vs. noncompliant)			✓	Compliant balloons have been associated with higher,[40] equal,[41,42] and lower dissection rates.[25] More recent randomized trials show no difference in clinical outcome.[43,44] High-pressure inflations using compliant balloons for resistant lesions may cause "dog-boning" and increase the risk of dissection.
Balloon sizing	✓			Most reports indicate that balloon oversizing (balloon-to-artery ratio > 1.2) is a powerful independent predictor of dissection.[26] Attempt to match the balloon diameter to the distal reference segment (balloon-to-artery ratio = 1.0).
Inflation pressure (high vs. low)			✓	Studies are small or retrospective. Most operators begin with low-pressure inflations and reserve high-pressure inflations for significant residual stenosis. Inflations exceeding rated burst pressure increase the risk of balloon rupture and vessel dissection. High-pressure inflations using compliant balloons may result in overstretching and dissection.
Duration of inflation (long vs. short)		✓		Randomized studies comparing 3 inflations at 1 min. vs. 4-5 min. demonstrated fewer and less severe dissections with prolonged inflations.[45] Whether multiple short inflations are comparable to fewer long inflations is unknown.
Inflation speed (slow vs. fast)		✓		Two randomized studies reported fewer dissections with gradual inflations,[46,47] while no effect was seen in another.[48] Studies also suggest a benefit for gradual, prolonged inflations.[49,50]
Oscillating inflations		✓		Nonrandomized study reported major dissections in 0.3% of lesions using this technique.[51] When combined with gradual balloon deflation, more dissections occurred.[52]

Parameter	Effect on Dissection Rate			Comments
	Possible ↑	Possible ↓	None	
Deflation speed (slow vs. fast)	✓			Gradual deflation resulted more of major dissections in two randomized trials.[52,53]
Predilatation		✓		Nonrandomized study reported major dissections in only 1.3% of patients,[54] while no effect was seen in a small randomized study.[55] Use of a dual-balloon catheter (distal balloon to predilate, proximal balloon for final dilatation) resulted in a low dissection rate.[56]
Long balloon for long lesions		✓		See Chapter 15
Noncompliant long-balloon for angled lesions		✓		See Chapter 11
Noncompliant balloon for calcified lesions		✓		See Chapter 12
Tapered balloon for tapered lesions		✓		See Chapter 15

2. **Healing and Restenosis (Table 20.6).** The majority of dissections that do not result in acute ischemic complications disappear with time.[57,58] Follow-up angiography indicates that 4-16% of dissections disappear within 24 hours, and 63-93% by 3-6 months.[14,58,59] While small earlier studies suggested a lower incidence of restenosis with dissection, large recent repots indicate that dissection has no impact on restenosis rates.[25,58,59]

D. RISK FACTORS FOR ACUTE CLOSURE

1. **Acute Closure.** Of the many clinical, angiographic, and procedural variables reported to increase the risk of acute closure (Tables 20.7, 20.8), the most powerful predictor is the presence of a complex dissection (relative risk ~ 6). Recently, Stack and colleagues[74] developed a scoring system to predict the risk of acute closure for any lesion in any individual patient: By adding together the points assigned to all adverse lesion characteristics (Table 20.9), a "lesion score" is obtained and used to estimate the risk of acute closure (Figure 20.1). Among 658 patients for whom this scoring system was applied, 20% of patients had ≤ 2.5% risk and 25% of patients had > 10% risk of acute closure.

2. **Cardiac Death After Acute Closure.** Clinical and angiographic variables have been used to identify patients at increased risk of cardiac death after acute closure (Table 20.10). The most powerful predictor is the jeopardy score, which estimates net ventricular dysfunction (Figure 20.2), as well as blood pressure and the risk of death after acute closure (Table 20.11).[80]

E. PREVENTION OF ACUTE CLOSURE

1. **Antiplatelet Agents**
   a. **Aspirin.** Preprocedural aspirin has been shown to reduce the incidence of acute coronary occlusion by 50-75%.[71] Although the optimal dose and timing are unknown, equivalent reductions in ischemic complications were seen for patients randomly assigned to low-dose (80 mg/day) or high-dose (1500 mg/day) therapy.[81] (Since aspirin absorption may be impaired

Table 20.6. Fate of PTCA-Induced Coronary Artery Dissection

Healing[57-59]	The majority of dissections not resulting in acute ischemic complications disappear with time.
Restenosis[25,58,59]	The presence of a dissection has no impact on restenosis.
Ischemic Complications	Depending on clinical and procedural variables (Table 20.6), the risk of an acute ischemic complication is 2-60%.

Table 20.7. Risk Factors for Acute Closure After Elective PTCA

Series	Total Procedures (n)	Acute Closure (%)	Risk Factors	
			Preprocedural	Procedural
Tenaglia[74] (1994)	658	8.1	Thrombus, length > 5mm Branch point stenosis RCA location Total occlusion	
deFeyter[6] (1991)	1423	7.3	Multivessel disease Unstable angina Eccentric or irregular	
Ellis[73] (1988)	4722	4.4	Multivessel disease Length > 2 lumen diameters Angle > 45° Branch-point stenosis Thrombus	Dissection Post-PTCA stenosis > 30% Final pressure gradient >20mmHg Prolonged heparin
Other[71,72,79]			No aspirin	Inadequate heparin Balloon-to-artery ratio > 1.0

Abbreviations: CABG = coronary artery bypass grafting; CAD = coronary artery desease; MI = myocardial infartion

when coadministered with antacids or H_2 blockers, our bias is to avoid low-dose aspirin). Elective angioplasty is postponed if the patient has not received ≥ 325 mg/day of aspirin for at least 1 day prior to PTCA. When angioplasty must be performed urgently, the patient is given 4 baby aspirins (81 mg each) to immediately chew and swallow; intraprocedural dextran, dipyridamole, and/or c7E3 (platelet receptor Iib/IIIa antagonist) may also be administered.

b. **Platelet Receptor IIb/IIIa Inhibitors.** The platelet receptor IIb/IIIa plays an integral role in platelet aggregation and thrombus formation. IIb/IIIa inhibitors have been developed in an effort to improve acute and longterm outcome following coronary intervention. In the EPIC trial, 2099 patients undergoing PTCA for unstable angina, acute MI, or high-risk lesion morphology were randomized to one of 3 treatment arms: bolus and maintenance infusion of ReoPro the monoclonal antibody c7E3 (bolus 0.25 mg/kg; infusion of 10 mcg/min x 12 hrs.); bolus dose only; or placebo. Aspirin and heparin were given in conventional doses. Patients receiving the bolus + infusion had 35% reduction in major ischemic complications (12.8% to 8.3%; p = 0.008); however, major bleeding complications increased from 7% to 14% . In the EPILOG trial, the combined endpoint of death or MI (CPK 3x normal) at 30-days was lower in patients receiving ReoPro plus low-dose heparin compared to those receiving standard-dose heparin without ReoPro (2.6% vs. 8.2%; p < 0.01); this benefit was observed without an increase in major bleeding (1.8% vs. 3.1% for heparin only group; p = NS). The main trial was stopped prematurely in December 1995 due to these results. Likewise, enrollment was stopped in the European CAPTURE trial (ReoPro vs. conventional medical therapy 18-24 hrs.

Table 20.7. Risk Factors For Acute Coronary Occlusion

Clinical	Angiographic	Procedural
Female gender[6,14,38]	Bend > 45 degrees[2,3,23,42,73]	PTCA technique (Table 20.4)
Age[42]	Branch point[73,74]	Dissection[2,23,61,67,73]
Diabetes Mellitus[66]	Multilesion[67,73]	Residual stenosis > 35%[73]
Unstable angina[6,61,64,67]	Long Lesion[2,42,61,73,75]	Prolonged post-PTCA heparin[73]
I.C. Urokinase during PTCA[68]	Thrombus[67,73-75]	Final translesional pressure gradient ≥ 20 mmHg[73]
Dissection or thrombus on 15-min angiogram[69]	Multivessel[6,61,67,73]	Transient in-lab closure
heparin < 24 hrs. prior to PTCA	Eccentric[61,73]	
Myocardial infarction[77]	Vessel supplies collaterals[67]	
High-risk for CABG[67]	Tandem lesions[42]	
Inadequate antiplatelet therapy[71,72]	RCA location[74]	
	LCA location[3]	
	Eccentric or irregular border[6]	
	Severe stenosis[2,3,67]	
	Type B_2 or C lesion[2,66]	
	Chronic total occlusion[72,74,75,78]	
	Calcified lesion[2,61]	
	Inadequate anticoagulation[79]	

Table 20.9. Scoring System for Prediction of Abrupt Closure[74]

Characteristic	Points
For Nontotal Occlusions:	
Branch location	
Yes	13
No	0
Length (mm)	
> 10	10
5 - 10	5
< 5	0
Thrombus score	
2	12
1	6
0	0
RCA	
Yes	6
No	0
For Total Occlusions:	
Total occlusion	19
RCA	
Yes	6
No	0

*   Individual lesion score is sum of points for all adverse characteristics that are present; scores are calculated differently for total and for nontotal occlusions because morphologic characteristics cannot be graded in the presence of a total occlusion.

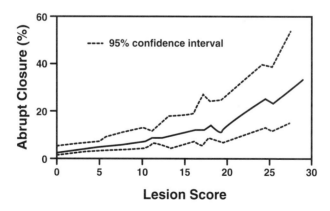

Figure 20.1 Lesion Score

Risk of acute closure based on lesion characteristics (dashed lines indicate 95% confidence intervals). See Table 20.7 for calculation of lesion score.

prior to PTCA for medically-refractory unstable angina) due to a significant reduction in the combined endpoint of in-hospital death, MI, or emergency CABG in the ReoPro group (Chapter 34). The IMPACT trial randomized 150 patients to a 4-hour or 12-hour infusion of Integrelin, a synthetic peptide inhibitor of the IIb/IIIa receptor, versus placebo. Integrelin tended to reduce major ischemic complications after PTCA (5.9% vs. 12.2% for placebo; p = 0.18) without an excess in major bleeding complications. These promising agents are currently the subject of intense investigation (Chapter 34).

    c.   **Ticlopidine, Dipyridamole, Dextran.** Ticlopidine (75 mg orally 4 times/day) and dextran are used as an antiplatelet agents in may stent protocols; however, insufficient data exist to recommend their routine administration during angioplasty. One retrospective report found that patients treated with IV dipyridamole (30 mg over 1 hour) just prior to PTCA had fewer ischemic complications, but a randomized trial (dipyridamole 75 mg orally 4 times/day) failed to demonstrate a beneficial effect. We empirically administer ticlopidine, dextran, and/or dipyridamole to patients with a previous anaphylactic reaction to aspirin, or when urgent PTCA is required and the patient has not been receiving aspirin. Ticlopidine must be given 3-5 days prior to intervention for maximal antiplatelet activity to be present at the time of PTCA.

Table 20.10. Cardiac Death Following Acute Closure[5,80]

Cause of Death	Risk Factors
LV failure	Female gender
	Multivessel disease
	Jeopardy score
	Collaterals originating from target vessel
	PTCA of proximal RCA
RV failure	PTCA of proximal RCA
Left main dissection	None

Abbreviations: LV = left ventricular; RV = right ventricular; RCA = right coronary artery

Table 20.11. Systolic Blood Pressure and Risk of Death Following Acute Closure: Correlation With the Jeopardy Score[80]

Jeopardy Score*	Systolic Blood Pressure (mmHg)		Jeopardy Score*	Mortality (%)
	Men	Women		
≤ 2.0	113 ± 20	109 ± 15	≤ 2.0	2.3
2.5-3.0	117 ± 13	81 ± 24	2.5-3.0	10.0
3.5-4.5	96 ± 7	65 ± 4	3.5-5.0	11.5
5.0-6.0	75 ± 5	68 ± 13	5.5-6.0	33.3

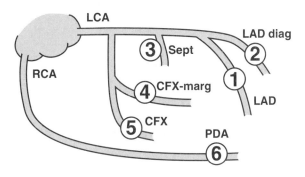

Figure 20.2   Jeopardy Score

Six arterial segments are used to calculate the jeopardy score, which considers the total region of jeopardized myocardium (supplied by the target vessel and providing collaterals to other regions) and the degree of baseline LV dysfunction. Scoring system:

    1 point: for each myocardial region supplied by the target lesion.

    1 point: for each myocardial region supplied by a vessel with diameter stenosis ≥ 70%.

    0.5 point: for each myocardial region that is hypokinetic at baseline and not supplied by a vessel with significant stenosis.

2. **Anticoagulants**

    a. **Heparin.** Conventional bolus dosing of 10,000 units of heparin results in suboptimal prolongation of the activated clotting time (ACT) in 5% of patients with stable angina and 15%

of patients with unstable angina.[82] Since a low intraprocedural ACT is a powerful predictor of acute closure,[79] we employ a weight-adjusted dosing protocol (weight < 180 lbs = 10,000 unit bolus; weight 180-250 lbs = 12,000-15,000 unit bolus; weight > 250 lbs = 18,000 unit bolus). An ACT is obtained 30-60 seconds following the initial bolus of heparin. For low ACT values (i.e., < 300 sec. for PTCA; < 350 sec. for stenting, DCA or ELCA; < 400 sec. for percutaneous cardiopulmonary bypass), an additional 5000-7500 unit bolus is administered. Once a therapeutic ACT is achieved, 5000 unit boluses (followed by repeat ACTs) are administered at 45-60 minute intervals during the procedure. Patients undergoing elective procedures with good angiographic results are usually managed without post-procedural heparin. However, patients who either present with an acute ischemic syndrome or have a suboptimal angiographic outcome (complex dissection, haziness, thrombus, sidebranch occlusion, no-reflow, distal embolization) often receive a prolonged (12-24 hour) heparin infusion to maintain an ACT between 160-200 seconds (or PTT of 2.0 - 2.5 x control) based on blood samples obtained at least twice daily. Since a temporal association between heparin discontinuation and acute coronary occlusion has been suggested,[83] heparin should be discontinued at a time of the day when emergency revascularization is feasible.

    b.   **Hirudin.** Unlike heparin, hirudin is a direct and potent inhibitor of both freely circulating *and* clot-bound thrombin. Hirulog, a synthetic analog of hirudin, was substituted for heparin in 291 patients undergoing elective PTCA (bolus dose of 0.45 - 0.55 mg/kg followed by a continuous infusion of 1.8 - 2.2 mg/kg/hr x 4 hours; an additional 0.2 mg/kg/hr up to 20 hrs. was administered for periprocedural dissection, haziness, thrombus, or clinical signs of ischemia). Hirulog was associated with rapid onset, minimal bleeding complications, and an abrupt closure rate of only 3.9%.[76] Recommendations regarding the use of hirudin and its analogs await further investigation.

3.   **Intra-Aortic Balloon Pump (IABP).** Ohman et. al.[77] randomized 182 patients undergoing PTCA for acute MI to IABP x 48 hours vs. standard care. Patients receiving IABP had less reocclusion on predischarge catheterization (8% vs. 21%), fewer composite in-hospital events rate (death, MI, emergent CABG or PTCA, stroke, or recurrent ischemia; 13% vs. 24%), and no increase in severe bleeding complications. It will be important to determine whether routine prophylactic IABP can reduce periprocedural acute closure in patients with unstable angina or those with high-risk lesion morphology undergoing elective intervention.

4.   **PTCA Technique.** Balloon-to-artery ratios > 1.1 and slow balloon deflation may increase the risk of severe coronary dissection and should be avoided. Long balloons and noncompliant balloons may reduce the risk of acute closure for long lesion and angulated lesions, respectively. There is divergence of opinion regarding other technical considerations including the number of inflations, inflation speed, duration of inflation, and the use of oscillating inflations (Table 20.4).

F. RECOGNITION OF ABRUPT CLOSURE. Acute coronary occlusion typically presents with the sudden onset of chest pain (90%) and ST segment elevation (75%). Less common presentations include hypotension (20%) and sudden death from heart block or ventricular fibrillation (1-10%). The clinical consequences of acute closure depend the myocardial distribution of the target vessel, the presence and adequacy of collaterals, the extent of associated coronary disease, and baseline ventricular function. The ability to triage and manage patients with recurrent chest pain at our institution has been greatly facilitated by comparing 12-lead ECG changes and chest pain characteristics post-intervention to those induced during balloon inflation ("ischemic fingerprint"). As outlined in Figure 20.3, if chest pain develops outside the catheterization laboratory, an ECG is promptly obtained, and nitrates and an IV bolus of heparin (5,000 units if already receiving a heparin infusion; 10,000 units if not) are administered. The patient is immediately returned to the angioplasty suite — or triaged to emergency CABG (Figure 20.4) — for persistent ST elevation or marked depression, hemodynamic instability, or nitrate-resistant symptoms and/or ECG changes that mimic those caused during balloon inflation. Patients with nitrate-responsive pain are managed by increasing the IV nitrate infusion and lengthening the period of heparinization (ACT maintained between 190-230 seconds); the oral dose of calcium channel blockers may be increased. Repeated episodes of nitrate-responsive pain should prompt immediate return to the catheterization laboratory.

G. MANAGEMENT OF ABRUPT CLOSURE. While the ideal combination of device and pharmacotherapy is unknown, all agree that stents represent the most important advance in the mechanical treatment of abrupt closure (Table 20.12).

　1. Initial Management (Figure 20.5). Once abrupt closure is recognized, intracoronary nitroglycerin (100-200 mcg) should be administered and ACT > 300sec should be confirmed. The lesion should be redilated for at least 5 minutes with a balloon matching the diameter of the adjacent reference vessel (balloon/artery ratio = 1.0-1.1); conventional, long, or perfusion balloons may be used depending on the extent of ischemia and the length of dissection. If repeat PTCA establishes vessel patency (TIMI flow = 3), a stable lumen for at least 10 minutes, and a final diameter stenosis ≤30%, it is reasonable to treat the patent conservatively with an overnight heparin infusion (ACT 180-200 sec.) and follow the patient clinically. Adjunctive thrombolytic therapy with intracoronary urokinase (250,000-500,000 units over 5-15 min.) or tPA (20 mg over 1-3 min.) is reserved for situations where definite residual thrombus is identified; routine lytic therapy for abrupt closure caused by dissection may prevent adherence of the intimal flap to the underlying vessel wall and is not recommended.[84]

　2. Poor Results After Repeat PTCA (Figure 20.6)

　　a. Vessels > 3.0 mm. If repeat PTCA results in a suboptimal result (final diameter stenosis >30%, flow limiting dissection, or progressive deterioration in the angiographic result over 10 minutes), further intervention is warranted. If mechanical interventions are contemplated, it is absolutely mandatory that the operator identify the distal extent of dissection. In vessels ≥ 3.0 mm, focal dissections or simple plaque separations are best managed by stenting, which has proven to be more effective than prolonged perfusion balloon inflations (Table 20.13). Ideally, the entire dissection should be covered completely by 1 or 2 stents. The choice of which stent to use is largely dependent on the operator; virtually all stents have been used with high procedural success rates. (In a small report of bailout stenting, the Palmaz-Schatz stent resulted in a larger MLD at follow-up and fewer repeat interventions [44% vs. 15%] compared to the Gianturco-Roubin stent.[108]) Although the Gianturco-Roubin stent might be preferable if important sidebranches are involved, the Palmaz-Schatz stent provides more radial strength and is easier to insert in the presence of tortuous anatomy. Occasionally, multiple overlapping stents may be required if there is severe recoil or if tufts of damaged tissue protrude through the stent struts into the lumen. (See Chapter 26 for bailout stenting technique.) Analysis of patients who required stenting for acute closure (n = 160) in the IMPACT-II trial revealed that treatment with Integrelin was associated with less MI at 30-days compared to placebo (16% vs. 32%, p = 0.017), suggesting the importance of GP IIb/IIIa inhibition in this setting.[105] DCA can be used to treat selected focal dissections,[89-91] but stent implantation is probably easier and more reliable. To minimize the risk of perforation during bailout DCA, a slightly undersized AtheroCath is chosen, oriented away from the angiographically normal vessel wall, and deployed at low inflation pressures (10-20 psi). DCA should be avoided when the dissection is > 10 mm or occurs in a vessel < 3.0 mm; proximal vessels are moderate-severely tortuous or heavily calcified; the dissection has periadventitial dye staining or occurs on a severely angulated vessel segment; or a large amount of untreated clot is present. Extensive spiral dissections (dissection length > 25mm) should be treated with multiple tandem stents;[92] if at all possible, the most distal stent should be implanted first. (Laser balloon angioplasty, which combined heat and pressure to weld intimal-medial separations, was withdrawn from the market due to its infrequent use and restenosis rates of 70%; other thermal devices await testing.) Persistent suboptimal results (flow impairment, > 50% residual stenosis) after stenting or DCA should be treated a bailout catheter, IABP (for TIMI flow < 3, labile hemodynamics, or a large risk territory), and CABG.

b. **Vessels < 3.0 mm.** For abrupt closure in vessels < 3mm, prolonged balloon inflations should be employed for 10-30 minutes, since other mechanical techniques are less effective in such vessels. Although routine use of oversized balloons (balloon/artery ratio > 1.1) is not recommended because of the chance of extending the dissection (and converting a focal dissection to a long, spiral dissection), oversized balloons may be considered in small vessels if conventional balloon sizing fails. In general, DCA is not recommended for abrupt closure in vessels < 3mm. Stenting should be considered if other techniques have failed and may also be used as a bridge to surgery.

3. **Refractory Abrupt Closure.** Emergency CABG is virtually always indicated for refractory abrupt closure. A bailout catheter and IABP will improve coronary blood flow and support the systemic circulation during transfer to the operating room. Medical management (IV heparin ± IABP) without CABG can be considered for vessels with small myocardial territories, especially

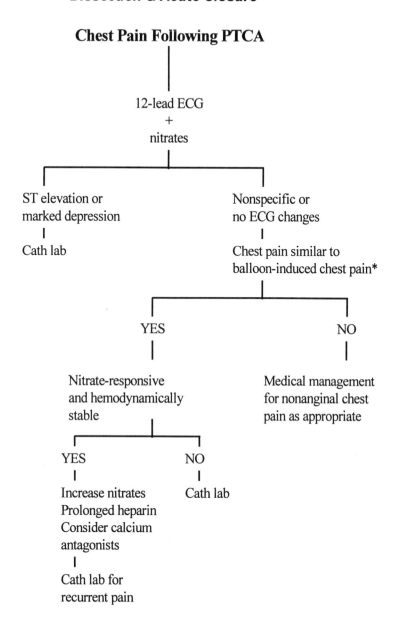

Chest Pain Following PTCA

Figure 20.3. Triage of Patients with Chest Pain Following PTCA

---

*   If PTCA was performed on a chronic total occlusion, these patients should return to the cath lab for repeat angiography.

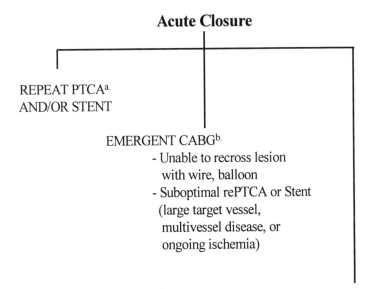

REPEAT PTCA[a.]
AND/OR STENT

EMERGENT CABG[b.]
- Unable to recross lesion
  with wire, balloon
- Suboptimal rePTCA or Stent
  (large target vessel,
  multivessel disease, or
  ongoing ischemia)

MEDICAL MANAGEMENT ALONE
- Vessel supplying small
  amount of viable myocardium
- Well collaterarlized vessel
- Hemodynamically stable
- Unsuccessful rePTCA or Stent
  in poor surgical candidate

Figure 20.4. Patient Triage Following PTCA-Induced Acute Closure

a.   Redilatation is successful in 40-80% of cases.

b.   If possible, we stabilize the patient in the Cath Lab and attempt to restore vessel patency while the operating room is prepared for emergency surgery.

Table 20.12. In-hospital Outcome After "Bail-Out" Stenting.

Series	Stent	No. (pts)	In-hospital Complications (%)	
			Stent Thrombosis	**D / MI / CABG**
Goy[30] (1995)	PSS	32	13	8 / 6.3 / 0
Urban[31] (1995)	PSS	52	4	0 / 10 / 4
Metz[32] (1994)	PSS	88	9	3 / 26 / 8
Schomig[33] (1994)	PSS	339	6.9	1.3 / 4.0 / 9
Kiemeneij[34] (1993)	PSS	52	23	3 / - / 15
Reifart[35] (1992)	PSS	64	32	6 / 3 / 5
Chan[37] (1995)	GRS	42	4.8	0 / 4.8 / 7.1
Sutton[38] (1994)	GRS	415	-	3 / 5 / 12
Agrawal[39] (1994)	GRS	240	7	-
George[40] (1993)	GRS	518	8.7	2.2 / 5.5 / 4.3
Roubin[41] (1992)	GRS	115	7.6	1.7 / 16 / 4.2
Goy[30] (1995)	Wiktor	33	18	9 / 8 / 3
Vrolix[42] (1994)	Wiktor	180	13.3	3.3 / 12 / 16.5
Garratt[43] (1994)	Wiktor	308	3	3.7 / 2.7 / 8.7
Reifart[35] (1992)	Strecker	48	21	10 / 2 / 6
Ozake[44] (1995)	MicroStent	20	0	0 / 10 / 5

Abreviations: D = death; MI = myocardial infarction; CABG = emergency coronary artery bypass surgery; PSS = Palmaz-Schatz stent; GRS - Gianturco-Roubin stent; - = not reported

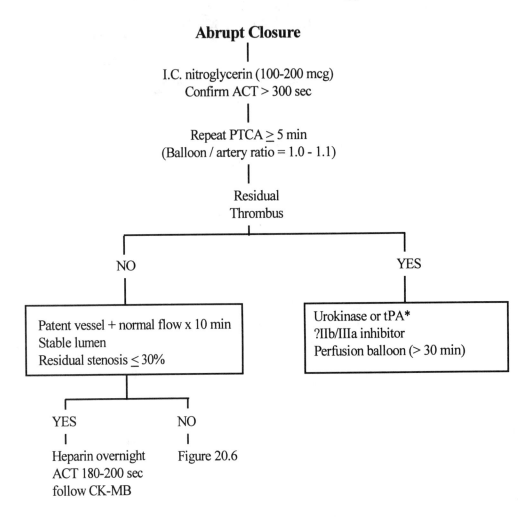

Abrupt Closure

I.C. nitroglycerin (100-200 mcg)
Confirm ACT > 300 sec

Repeat PTCA ≥ 5 min
(Balloon / artery ratio = 1.0 - 1.1)

Residual
Thrombus

NO   YES

Patent vessel + normal flow x 10 min
Stable lumen
Residual stenosis ≤ 30%

Urokinase or tPA*
?IIb/IIIa inhibitor
Perfusion balloon (> 30 min)

YES   NO

Heparin overnight   Figure 20.6
ACT 180-200 sec
follow CK-MB

Figure 20.5. Management of Abrupt Closure

* Urokinase (250,000-500,000 units I.C. over 5-15 min or I.C. infusion 100,000-200,000 U/hr for 12-24 hr) or tPA (20 mg I.C. over 1-2 min)

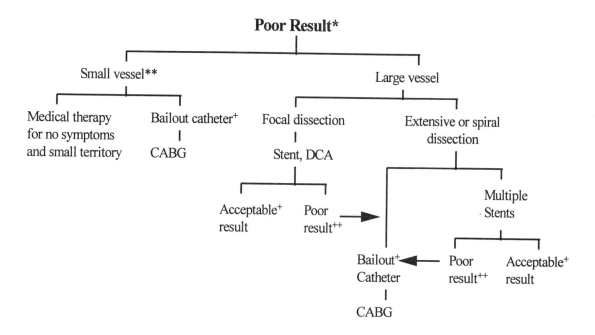

Figure 20.6. Management of Poor Result After Repeat PTCA for Abrupt Closure

* Impaired flow, severe dissection, ongoing ischemia, and/or residual stenosis > 50%
** Consider balloon/artery ratio > 1.1; consider stent
+ IABP for ongoing ischemia, labile hemodynamics, or large myocardial territory
++ Consider stent-in-a-stent for residual filling defect

when the vessel is well-collateralized, and the patient is stable and a poor candidate for CABG.

4. **In-hospital Management After Successful Reversal of Abrupt Closure.** Following successful therapy, the patient is admitted to a monitored unit for further observation and management. Supportive measures required during the procedure (e.g., intra-aortic balloon pump, pulmonary artery catheter) usually remain in place overnight and are discontinued the following day in clinically stable patients. Heparin is continuously administered for a minimum of 24 hours to reduce the risk of recurrent acute closure. Most operators empirically treat patients salvaged by stenting or DCA with warfarin for 2-6 weeks; in these cases, IV heparin is continued until a therapeutic INR is achieved (2.0-3.0). Warfarin should be considered when residual thrombus is evident after salvage PTCA. Patients with an uncomplicated course are usually ready for discharge by the second or third hospital day (or when therapeutically anticoagulated if this management strategy is chosen).

H. OTHER MANAGEMENT ISSUES

1. **Non-Flow-Limiting Dissection.** The majority of small intimal disruptions (residual stenosis <

30%, length < 10 mm, normal flow) do not require further mechanical or drug therapy. The treatment of more extensive non-flow-limiting dissections is controversial. In a matched case-control study, stenting failed to confer a clinical benefit over conventional therapy and resulted in more transfusions and a longer hospital stay.[88] Nevertheless, the majority of interventionalists stent non-flow-limiting dissections with high-risk features (residual stenosis ≥ 30%, dissection length ≥ 15 mm). Our approach to coronary artery dissection is described in Figure 20.7.

2. **Primary Thrombotic Closure.** Compared to vessel dissection, primary thrombosis is a much less common cause of abrupt closure (exception: DCA, where primary thrombosis may account for ≥ 50% of abrupt closures). When present, the most effective form of therapy is repeat balloon dilatation in conjunction with intracoronary thrombolysis.[93,94] Various thrombolytic agents and regimens have been employed (although the optimal agent, dose route, and timing of administration are unknown). These include urokinase (100,000-250,000 units i.c. over 30 min.),[93] streptokinase (0.25-1.5 million units i.c. over 60 min.),[95] and r-tPA (20 mg i.c. over 5 min.[96] or 40-60 mg IV over 60-120 min.[97]). Local drug delivery systems (e.g., Dispatch catheter, LocalMed) show great promise in this setting and are discussed in Chapter 35.

Table 20.13. Prolonged Perfusion Balloon (PPB) Inflations vs. Stenting for Acute Closure

Series	Design	Stent	N	Results
Ray[85] (1995)	Randomized TASC II trial	-	22 PPB 22 Stent	Stent with greater success (91% vs. 46%), able to salvage 83% of PB failures, and lower restenosis (22% vs. 50%). CABG avoided in 91%; stent thrombosis resulting in MI in 11%.
deMuinck[86] (1994)	Retrospective, non-randomized	PSS	61 PPB 36 Stent	Stent with less residual stenosis, better restoration of normal flow (94% vs. 70%), less emergency CABG (0% vs. 21%), and more subacute thrombosis (22% vs. 0%). No difference in acute closure, restenosis, or event-free survival at 3-month.
Barberis[87] (1994)	Retrospective	PSS	36 PPB 37 Stent	Stent with greater success (95% vs. 72%), more subacute thrombosis (13% vs. 0%); able to salvage 90% of PB failures.
Lincoff[88] (1993)	Matched case-control	GRS	61 PPB* 61 Stent	Stent with less residual stenosis (26% vs. 49%), better restoration of TIMI 3 flow (97% vs. 72%), and reduced need for emergency surgery (9% vs. 27%) for patients with acute closure. No clinical benefit for stenting patients with threatened closure (i.e., dissection with normal flow).

Abbreviations: GRS = Gianturco-Roubin Stent, PSS = Palmaz-Schatz Stent; TASC = Trial of Angioplasty versus Stents in Canada; - = Not reported
* Prolonged inflations ± perfusion balloon

For thrombotic closure resistant to PTCA and lytics, new devices and antiplatelet agents may be of value. TEC atherectomy has been used to aspirate thrombus, but is contraindicated in vessels < 3.0 mm and when a dissection is present. When used in conjunction with intracoronary thrombolysis, DCA may effectively excise small amounts of clot. ELCA may desiccate thrombus but is not usually considered a first-line rescue device, and the Rotablator is contraindicated due to the risk of distal embolization. Other devices such as the Hydrolyzer and Angiojet are under investigation in Europe (Chapter 8). Other measures include the use of a continuous overnight superselective infusion of urokinase (80,000 units per hour through an end-hole infusion wire just proximal to the clot, and 40,000 units per hour through the guiding catheter) (Chapter 9).[98] In a small observational report, c7E3 (platelet IIb/IIIa inhibitor; 0.25 mg/kg IV bolus followed by a 12-hr infusion of 10 mcg/min) was given to 16 patients who developed intracoronary thrombus in response to PTCA, 4 of whom failed intracoronary urokinase. ReoPro decreased thrombus, improved flow, and was well-tolerated. All 16 cases underwent successful repeat PTCA without in-hospital ischemic complications.[99] If these promising results are confirmed in larger studies, "rescue ReoPro" may prove to be among the more useful adjunctive therapies for intracoronary thrombus complicating PTCA.

I. **PROGNOSIS.** As shown in Table 20.14, the prognosis of abrupt closure has improved over time.[38] Nevertheless, acute closure remains associated with a 5-fold increase in periprocedural death, and a 10-25 fold increase in periprocedural MI and emergency CABG (Table 20.15). The effect of successfully-treated acute closure on long-term outcome is controversial: Some reports suggest higher restenosis and ischemic complications rates.[70-100] Among 250 patients with uncomplicated reversal of abrupt closure, ischemic events (death, MI, or repeat revascularization) at 6 months occurred in 45% compared to only 20% in patients without abrupt closure (p <0.001).[101] In contrast, among 88 patients with transient in-lab closure responding to additional intervention, there was no adverse effect on longterm prognosis unless associated with a significant elevation in CK-MB.[102]

CLINICAL EVIDENCE OF ACTIVE ISCHEMIA

    - ongoing chest pain
    - ST segment deviation
    - hemodynamic instability

      or

ANGIOGRAPHIC EVIDENCE OF A POOR OUTCOME

    - residual stenosis > 30%
    - spiral dissection > 15 mm
    - pressure gradient >25 mmHg
    - TIMI flow ≤ 2
    - Types C - F dissection

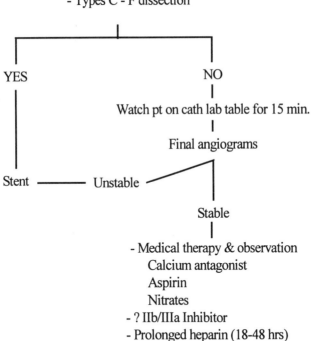

YES   NO

Watch pt on cath lab table for 15 min.

Final angiograms

Stent ——— Unstable

Stable

    - Medical therapy & observation
      Calcium antagonist
      Aspirin
      Nitrates
    - ? IIb/IIIa Inhibitor
    - Prolonged heparin (18-48 hrs)
    - Consider coumadin or SQ heparin x 1 month

Figure 20.7. Management of Coronary Artery Dissection

Table 20.14. Time Period of Acute Closure and Incidence of Complications[99]

Time Period	In-Hospital Complications (%)	
	Q-MI	CABG
1980-84	27	63
1985-88	16	42
1989-92	8	32

Abbrevations: Q-MI = Q-wave mycardial infarction; CABG = emergency coronary bypass grafting

Table 20.15. The Risk of Adverse Events for Patients With and Without Acute Closure*

	Incidence of Ischemic Complications (%)	
Event	Acute Closure	No Acute Closure
Death	50	1
MI	10 - 50	2
Emergency CABG	25 - 60	3
Perioperative death	5 - 10	-
Perioperative MI	40	-

Abbreviation: MI = myocardial infarction; CABG = emergency coronary artery bypass grafting; - = not reported
* Excludes patients who present with acute MI

* * * * *

REFERENCES

1.	Ramee SR, White CJ, Jain A, et al. Percutaneous coronary angioscopy versus angiography in patients undergoing coronary angioplasty. J Am Coll Caridol 1991;17(2):125A.

2.	Tan K, Sulke N, Taub N, Sowton E. Clinical and lesion morphologic determinants of coronary angioplasty success and complications: Current experience. J Am Coll Cardiol 1995;25:855-65.

3.	Van Belle E, Bauters C, Lablanche J-M, McFadden E, Bertrand M. Angiographic determinants of acute outcome after coronary angioplasty: A prospective quantitative coronary angiographic study of 3679 procedures. J Am Coll Cardiol 1994:223A.

4.	Lincoff AM, Popma JJ, Ellis SG, Hacker J. Abrupt vessel closure complicating coronary angioplasty: Clinical, angiographic, and therapeutic profile. J Am Coll Cardiol 1992;19(5):926-935.

5.	Ellis S, Roubin G, King S, et al. In-hospital cardiac mortality after acute closure after coronary angioplasty: Analysis of risk factors from 8,207 procedures. J Am Coll Cardiol 1988;11:211-216.

6.	de Feyter PJ, van den Brand M, Jaarman G, van Domburg R. Acute coronary artery occlusion during and after percutaneous transluminal coronary angioplasty. Frequency, prediction, and clinical course, management, and follow-up. Circulation 1991;83:927-936.

7.	The Bypass Angioplasty Revascularization Investigation (BARI): Five year mortality and morbidity in a randomized study comparing CABG and PTCA in patients with multivessel coronary disease. The BARI Investigators. N Engl J Med (submitted)

8.	Simpfendorfer C, Belardi J, Bellamy G, Galan K. Frequency, management and follow-up of patients with acute coronary occlusions after percutaneous transluminal coronary angioplasty. Am J Cardiol 1987;59:267-269.

9.	Bansal A, Choksi NA, Levine AB, et al. Determinants of arterial dissection during PTCA: Lesion type versus inflation rate. J Am Coll Cardiol 1989;12(2):229A.

10.	Popma JJ, Topol EJ, Pinkerton CA, et al. Abrupt closure following directional coronary atherectomy: Clinical, angiographic and procedural outcome. J Am Coll Cardiol 1991;17(2):23A.

11.	Bertrand M, Lablanche J, Leroy F, Bauters C. Percutaneous transluminal coronary rotary ablation with Rotablator (European experience). Am J Cardiol 1992;69:470-474.

12.	Safian R, Lai S, Buchbinder M, Sanbron T, Sketch M. Incidence and management of abrupt closure after new device interventions. Report from the NACI Registry in 2988 lesions. Circulation 1993;88(Suppl.):I-585.

13.	Mehta S, Popma J, Margolis J, et al. Angiographic complications after new device angioplasty in native coronary arteries: A NACI Angiographic Core Laboratory Report. TCT Meeting (Washington DC), February, 1995.

14.	Popma J, Topol E, Hinohara T, et al. Abrupt vessel closure after directional coronary atherectomy. J Am Coll Cardiol 1992;19:1372-1379.

15.	Hinohara T, Rowe M, Robertson G, et al. Effect of lesion characteristics on outcome of directional coronary atherectomy. J Am Coll Cardiol 1991;17:1112-1120.

16.	Warth D, Leon M, O'Neill W, et al. Rotational atherectomy multicenter registry: Acute results, complications and 6-month angiographic follow-up in 709 patients. J Am Coll Cardiol 1994;24:641-648.

17.	Ellis S, Popma J, Buchbinder M, et al. Relation of clinical presentation, stenosis morphology, and operator technique to the procedural results of rotational atherectomy and rotational atherectomy--facilitated angioplasty. Circulation 1994;89:882-892.

18.	Safian R, Niazi K, et al. Detailed Angiographic Analysis of High-Speed Mechanical Rotational Atherectomy in Human Coronary Arteries. Circulation 1993;88: 961-968.

19.	Litvack F, Eigler N, Margolis J, et al. Percutaneous excimer laser coronary angioplasty: Results in the first consecutive 3,000 patients. J Am Coll Cardiol 1994;23:323-329.

20.	Painter J, Popma J, Pichard A, et al. A comparison of early and late clinical outcomes in patients undergoing concentric and directional laser coronary angioplasty. TCT Meeting (Washington DC), February, 1995.

21.	Chevalier B, Meyer P, Corcos T, et al. Delayed acute closure after rotational atherectomy: A multicenter registry. Circulation 1994;90:I-213.

22.	Huber M, Mooney J, Madison J, Mooney M. Use of a morphologic classification to predict clinical outcome after dissection from coronary angioplasty. Am J Cardiol 1991;68:467-471.

23.	Hermans WR, Foley DP, Rensing BJ, Rutsch W. Usefulness of quantitative and qualitative angiographic lesion morphology, and clinical characteristics in predicting major adverse cardiac events during and after native coronary balloon angioplasty. Am J Cardiol 1993;72:14-20.

24.   Bailey S, Ricci D, Kiesz S, et al. Incidence and clinical impact of dissections after PTCA and stent placement: Results from the Randomized STent REStenosis Study. TCT Meeting (Washington DC), February, 1995.

25.   Hermans WR, Rensing BJ, Foley DP, Deckers JW. Therapeutic dissection after successful coronary balloon angioplasty: No influence on restenosis or on clinical outcome in 693 patients. J Am Coll Cardiol 1992;20:767-780.

26.   Sharma SK, Israel DH, Kamean JL, Bodian CA. Clinical, angiographic, and procedural determinants of major and minor coronary dissection during angioplasty. Am Heart J 1993;126:39-47.

27.   Kovach J, Mintz G, Pichard A, et al. Sequential intravascular ultrasound characterization of the mechanisms of rotational atherectomy and adjunct balloon angioplasty. J Am Coll Cardiol 1993;22:1024-32.

28.   den Heijer P, Foley D, Escaned J, Hillege H. Angioscopic versus angiographic detection of intimal dissection and intracoronary thrombus. J Am Coll Cardiol 1994;24(3):649-654.

29.   Ghazzal Z, Hearn J, Litvack F, et al. Morphological predictors of acute complications after percutaneous excimer laser coronary angioplasty. Results of a comprehensive angiographic analysis: Importance of the eccentricity index. Circulation 1992;86:820-827.

30.   Baumbach A, Bittl J, Fleck E, Geschwind H, Sanborn T. Acute complications of excimer laser coronary angioplasty: A detailed analysis of multicenter results. J Am Coll Cardiol 1994;23(6):1305-1313.

31.   Dussaillant G, Popma J, Pichard A, et al. Rotational atherectomy vs. excimer laser angioplasty: A multivariable analysis of early and late procedural outcome. J Am Coll Cardiol 1995;25:330A.

32.   Brown D, Giordano F, Buchbinder M. Coronary dissection following rotational atherectomy: Clinical characteristics, angiographic predictors and acute outcomes. J Am Coll Cardiol 1995;25:123A.

33.   Popma J, Knopf W, Davidson C, et al. Angiographic outcome after "cutting" balloon angioplasty. J Am Coll Cardiol 1995;25:268A.

34.   Knopf W, Yakubov S, Satler L, et al. Angiographic and procedural outcome after coronary angioplasty using a decremental diameter (tapered) balloon catheter. TCT Meeting (Washington DC), February, 1995.

35.   Fitzgerald PJ, Ports TA, Yock PG. Contribution of localized calcium deposits to dissection after angioplasty. An observational study using intravascular ultrasound. Circulation 1992;86:64-70.

36.   van Leeuwen T, Meertens J, Velema E, Post M, Borst C. Intraluminal vapor bubble induced by excimer laser pulse causes microsecond arterial dilation and invagination leading to extensive wall damage in the rabbit. Circulation 1993;87:1258-.

37.   Tcheng J, Wells L, Phillips H, Deckelbaum L, Golobic R. Development of a new technique for reducing pressure pulse generation during 308-nm excimer laser coronary angioplasty. Cathet Cardiovas Diagn. 1995;34:15-22.

38.   Scott N, Weintraub W, Liberman H, Morris D, Douglas J, King S. Outcome after acute closure syndrome following coronary angioplasty. Circulation 1993;88:I-299.

39.   Popma J, Painter J, Pichard A, et al. Incidence, predictors, prognostic significance of coronary dissections after excimer laser coronary angioplasty (ELCA). TCT Meeting (Washington DC), February, 1995.

40.   Berry K, Drew T, McKendall G, et al. Balloon material as a risk factor for coronary angioplasty procedural complications. Circulation 1991;84:II-130.

41.   Mooney MR, Fishman-Mooney J, Longe TF, Brandenburg RO. Effect of balloon material on coronary angioplasty. Am J Cardiol 1992;69:1481-1482.

42.   Raymenants E, Bhandari S, Stammen F, De Scheerder I, Desmet W, Piessens J. Effects of angioplasty balloon material and lesion characteristics on the incidence of coronary dissection in 2150 dilated lesions. J Am Coll Cardiol 1993;21:291A.

43.   Talley JD, Blankenship S, Spokojny WA, Anderson HV, et al. Does the type of balloon material used in elective PTCA make a difference in clinical complications? Results from the CRAC study. Circulation 1995;92:I-74.

44.   Safian RD, Hoffmann MA, Almany S, et al. Comparison of coronary angioplasty with compliant and noncompliant balloons (The Angioplasty Compliance Trial). Am J Cardiol 1995;76:518-520.

45.   Cribier A, Elchaninoff H, Chan C, et al. Comparative effects of long (> 12 min) versus standard (<3 min) sequential balloon inflations in PTCA. Preliminary results of a prospective randomized study: Immediate results and restenosis rates. J Am Coll Cardiol 1994;23:58A.

46.   Remetz MS, Cabin HS, McConnell S, Cleman M. Gradual balloon inflation protocol reduces arterial damage following percutaneous transluminal coronary angioplasty. J Am Coll Cardiol 1988;11:131A.

47.   Ilia R, Cabin H, McConnell S. et al. Coronary angioplasty with gradual versus rapid balloon inflation. Cathet Cardiol Vasc Diagn 1993;29:199-202.

48.   Bansal A, Choksi N, Levein AB, et al. Determinants of arterial dissection after PTCA: lesion type versus inflation rate. J Am Coll Cardiol 1989;13:229A.

49.   Tenaglia AN, Quigley PJ, Kereiakes DJ, et al. Coronary angioplasty performed with a gradual and prolonged inflation using a perfusion balloon catheter: procedural success and restenosis rate. Am Heart J 1992;124:585-589.

50.   Farcot JC, Berland J, Stix A, et al. Gradual, low-pressure and prolonged (10 minutes) protected inflations decreased complications and improved results of proximal LAD angioplasty. Eur Heart J 1991;12:263.

51.   Shawl F, Dougherty K, Hoff S. Does inflation strategy influence acute outcome and long-term results. Circulation 1993;88:I-587.

52.   Blankenship J, Ford A, Henry S, Frey C. Coronary dissection resulting from angioplasty with slow oscillating vs. rapid inflation and slow vs. rapid deflation. Cath Cardiovasc Diagn. 1995;34:202-209.

53.   Foster C, Teskey R, Kells C, et al. Does the speed of balloon deflation affect the complication rate of coronary angioplasty. J Am Coll Cardiol 1993;21:290A.

54.   Banka V, Kochar G, Maniet A, Voci G. Progressive coronary dilation: An angioplasty technique that creates controlled arterial injury and reduces complications. Am Heart J 1993;125:61-71.

55.   McKeever LS, O'Donnell MJ, Stamato NJ, et al. The effect of predilatation on coronary angioplasty-induced vessel wall injury. Am Heart J 1991;122:1515-1518.

56.   Banka VS, Fail PS, Kochar GS, Maniet AR. Dual-balloon progressive coronary dilatation catheter: design and initial clinical experience. Am Heart J. 1994;127:430-435.

57.   Nobuyhshi M, Kimura T, Nosaka H, et al. Restenosis after successful percutaneous transluminal coronary angioplasty: Serial angiographic follow-up of 229 patients. J Am Coll Cardiol 1988;12:616-623.

58.   Cappelletti A, Margonato A, Berna G, Chierchia S. Spontaneous evolution of nonocclusive coronary dissection after PTCA: A 6-month angiographic follow-up study. J Am Coll Cardiol 1995;25:345A.

59.   Savage M, Dischman D, Bailey S, et al. Vascular remodeling of balloon-induced intimal dissection: Long-term angiographic assessment. J Am Coll Cardiol 1995;25:139A.

60.   Bell M, Berger PB, Reeder GS, et al. Coronary dissection following PTCA: Predictors of major ischemic complications. Circulation 1991;84(4):II-130.

61.   Bredlau CE, Roubin GS, Leimgruber PP, Douglas JS. In-hospital morbidity and mortality in patients undergoing elective coronary angioplasty. Circulation 1985;72(5):1044-1052. 71.

62.   Foley D, Hermans W, Rensing B, Serruys P. Predictability of major adverse cardiac events after balloon angioplasty from clinical data and quantitative and qualitative angiographic analysis. J Am Coll Cardiol 1993;21:339A.

63.   Ellis SG, Gallison L, Grines CL, et al. Incidence and predictors of early recurrent ischemia after successful percutaneous transluminal coronary angioplasty for acute myocardial infarction. Am J Cardiol 1989;63:263-268.

64.   Roubin GS, Lin S, Niederman A, et al. Clinical and anatomic descriptors for a major complication following PTCA. J Am Coll Cardiol 1987;9:20A.

65.   Ferguson J, Bittl J, Strony J, Adelman B. The relationship of dissection and thrombus after PTCA to in-hospital outcome: Results of a prospective multicenter study. Circulation 1993;88:I-217.

66.   Ellis S, Vandormael M, Cowley M, et al. Coronary morphologic and clinical determinants of procedural outcome with angioplasty for multivessel coronary disease. Circulation 1990;82:1193-1202.

67.   Detre KM, Holmes DR, Holubkow R, Cowley MJ. Incidence and consequences of periprocedural occlusion. The 1985-1986 National Heart, Lung, And Blood Institute Percutaneous Transluminal Coronary Angioplasty Registry. Circulation 1990;82:739-750.

68.   Ambrose J, Almeida O, Sharma S, Torre S. Adjunctive thrombolytic therapy during angioplasty for ischemic rest angina. Results of the TAUSA Trial. Circulation 1994;90:69-77.

69.   Ambrose J, Sharma S, Almeida O, et al. Delayed views post PTCA predict acute and in-hospital complications in patients with unstable angina. J Am Coll Cardiol 1995;25:392A.

70.   Tenaglia AN, Fortin DF, Frid DJ, Gardener LH. Long-term outcome following successful reopening of abrupt closure after coronary angioplasty. Am J Cardiol 1993;72:21-25.

71.   Barnathan E, Schwartz J, Taylor L, et al. Aspirin and dipyridamole in the prevention of acute coronary thrombosis complicating coronary angioplasty. Circulation 1987;76:125-134.

72.   Schwartz L, Bourassa MG, Lesperange J, Aldridge HE. Aspirin and dipyridamole in the prevention of restenosis after percutaneous transluminal coronary angioplasty. N Engl J Med 1988;318:1714-1719.

73.   Ellis S, Roubin G, King S, et al. Angiographic and clinical predictors of acute closure after native vessel coronary angioplasty. Circulation 1988;77:372-379.

74. Tenaglia A, Fortin D, Califf R. Predicting the risk of abrupt closure after angioplasty in an individual patient. J Am Coll Cardiol 1994;24:1004-1011.

75. Myler R, Shaw R, Stertzer S, et al. Lesion morphology and coronary angioplasty: Current experience and analysis. J Am Coll Cardiol 1992;19:1641-1652.

76. Topol E, Bonan R, Jewitt D, et al. Use of a direct antithrombin, hirulog, in place of heparin during coronary angioplasty. Circulation 1993;87:1622.

77. Ohman E, George B, White C, et al. Use of aortic counterpulsation to improve sustained coronary artery patency during acute myocardial infarction (Results of a randomized trial). Circulation 1994;90:792-799.

78. Favereau X, Corcos T, Guerin Y, et al. Early reocclusion after successful coronary angioplasty of chronic total occlusions. J Am Coll Cardiol 1995;25:139A.

79. Dougherty KG, Marsh KC, Edelman SK et al. Relationship between procedural activated clotting time and in-hospital post-PTCA outcome. Circulation 1990;82:111-189.

80. Ellis SG, Myler RK, King SB, Douglas JS. Causes and correlates of death after unsupported coronary angioplasty: Implications for use of angioplasty and advanced support techniques in high-risk settings. Am J Cardiol 1991;68:1447-1451.

81. Mufson L, Black A, Roubin G, et al. Randomized trial of aspirin in PTCA: Effect of high versus low dose aspirin on major complications and restenosis. J Am Coll Cardiol 1988;11:236A.

82. Ogilby JD, Kopelman HA, Klein LW, et al. Adequate heparinization during PTCA: Assessment using activated clotting time. J Am Coll Cardiol 1988;11:237A.

83. Gabliani G, Deligonul U, Kern M, Vandermael M. Acute coronary occlusion occurring after successful percutaneous transluminal coronary angioplasty: Temporal relationship to discontinuation of anticoagulation. Am Heart J 1988;116:696-700.

84. Spielberg C, Schnitzer L, Linderer T, et al. Influence of catheter technology and adjunct medication on acute complications in percutaneous coronary angioplasty. Cathet Cardiovasc Diagn 1990;21:72-76.

85. Ricci HR, Ray S, Buller CE, O'Neill B, et al. Six month follow-up of patients randomized to prolonged inflation of stent for abrupt occlusion during PTCA—Clinical and angiographic data: TASC II. Circulation 1995;92:I-475.

86. de Muinck E, den Heijer P, van Dijk R. Autoperfusion balloon versus stent for acute or threatened closure during percutaneous transluminal coronary angioplasty. Am J Cardiol 1994;74:1002-1005.

87. Barberis P, Marsico F, De Servi S, et al. Treatment of failed PTCA with perfusion balloon versus intracoronary stent: A short-term follow-up. J Am Coll Cardiol 1994:136A.

88. Lincoff M, Topol E, Chapekis A, et al. Intracoronary stenting compared with conventional therapy for abrupt vessel closure complicating coronary angioplasty: A matched case-control study. J Am Coll Cardiol 1993;21(4):866-875.

89. Bier J, Cannistra A, Mukherjee S, et al. Histopathologic findings following directional coronary atherectomy performed for failed balloon angioplasty. Circulation 1994;90:I-63.

90. Berdan L, Holmes D, Davidson-Ray L, Lam L, Talley D, Mark D. Economic impact of abrupt closure following percutaneous intervention: The CAVEAT Experience. J Am Coll Cardiol 1994;23:434A.

91. Movsowitz H, Emmi R, Manginas A, et al. Directional coronary atherectomy for failed balloon angioplasty: Outcome depends on the underlying pathology. Circulation 1993;88:I-601.

92. Shaknovich A, Moses JW, Undemir C, Cohen NT, et al. Procedural and short-term clinical outcomes of multiple Palmaz-Schatz stents (PSSs) in very long lesions/dissections. Circulation 1995;92:I-535.

93. Schieman G, Cohen BM, Kozina J, Erickson JS. Intracoronary urokinase for intracoronary thrombus accumulation complicating percutaneous transluminal coronary angioplasty in acute ischemic syndromes. Circulation 1990;82:2052-2060.

94. Pavlides GS, Schreiber TL, Gangadharan V, et al. Safety and efficacy of urokinase during elective coronary angioplasty. Am Heart J 1991;121:731-737.

95. Haft JL, Goldstein JE, Homoud MK, et al. PTCA following myocardial infarction: Use of bailout fibrinolysis to improve results. Am Heart J 1990;120:243-247.

96. Hermann G, Zahorsky R, Meissner A, et al. Effects of acute rt-PA thrombolysis during PTA in patients with impending coronary occlusion. Eur Heart J 1990;11:23 (abstr).

97. Gulba DC, Daniel WG, Simon R, Jost S. Role of thrombolysis and thrombin in patients with acute coronary occlusion during percutaneous transluminal coronary angioplasty. J Am Coll Cardiol 1990;16(3):563-568.

98. Chapekis A, George B, Candela R. Rapid thrombus dissolution by continuous infusion of urokinase through an intracoronary perfusion wire prior to and following PTCA: Results in native coronaries and patent saphenous vein

grafts. Cathet Cardiovasc Diagn 1991;23:89-92.

99. Muhlestein JB, Gomez, MA, Karagounis LA, Anderson JL. "Rescue ReoPro": Acute utilization of abciximab for the dissolution of coronary thrombus developing as a complication of coronary angioplasty. Circulation 1995;92:I-607.

100. Tenaglia AN, Fortin FD, Frid DJ, et al. Restenosis and long-term outcome following successful treatment of abrupt closure during and after angioplasty: Stabilization using a guidewire. Cathet Cardiovasc Diagn 1987;13:391-393.

101. Piana RN, Ahmed WH, Ganz P, Dodge T Jr., et al. The legacy of uncomplicated abrupt vessel closure during coronary angioplasty: Increased ischemic events after hospital discharge. Circulation 1995;92:I-75.

102. Abdelmeguid AE, Whitlow PL, Sapp SK, et al. Long-term outcome of transient, uncomplicated in-laboratory coronary artery closure. Circulation 1995;91:2733-2741.

103. Deckelbaum LI, Natarajan MK, Bittl JA, et al. Effect of intracoronary saline infusion on dissection during excimer laser coronary angioplasty: A randomized trial. J Am Coll Cardiol 1995;26:1264-9.

104. Holmes DR, Simpson JB, Berdan LG, et al. Abrupt closure: The CAVEAT I Experience. J Am Coll Cardiol 1995;26:1494-500.

105. Zidar JP, Kruse KR, Thel MC, et al. Integrelin for emergency coronary artery stenting. J Am Coll Cardiol 1996;March Special Issue.

106. Mehta S, Popma J, Margolis JR, et al. Complications with new angioplasty devices. Are these device specific? J Am Coll Cardiol 1996;March Special Issue.

107. Popma JJ, Baim DS, Kuntz RE, et al. Early and late quantitative angiographic outcomes in the Optimal Atherectomy Restenosis Study (OARS). J Am Coll Cardiol 1996;March Special Issue.

108. Ortiz-Fernandex A, Goicoles MJ, Perex-Vizcayno M, et al. Late clinical and angiographic outcome of bailout coronary stenting. A comparison study between Gianturco-Roubin and Palmaz-Schatz stents. J Am Coll Cardiol 1996;March Special Issue.

109. Appleman YEA, Piek JJ, Strikwerda S, et al. Randomized trial of excimer laser angioplasty versus balloon angioplasty for treatment of obstructive coronary artery disease. Lancet 1996;347:79-84.

21 NO-REFLOW

Katherine M. Abbo, M.D.
Robert D. Safian, M.D.

A. **DEFINITION.** The no-reflow phenomenon was originally observed in experimental models of acute myocardial infarction (MI) and was described as a failure to restore normal myocardial blood flow despite removal of the coronary obstruction.[1,2] Since that time, no-reflow has been shown to complicate thrombolytic therapy and percutaneous revascularization with PTCA and other devices.[3-9] Defined angiographically, no-reflow manifests as an acute reduction in coronary flow (TIMI grade 0-1) in the absence of dissection, thrombus, spasm, or high-grade residual stenosis at the original target lesion. Lesser degrees of flow impairment (TIMI grade 2) are generally referred to as "slow-flow."

B. **ETIOLOGY.** The mechanisms and mediators responsible for no-reflow remain speculative, but the end result appears to be severe microvascular dysfunction. Potential mechanisms of microvascular dysfunction include vasospasm, distal embolization of thrombus or other debris, oxygen free radical-mediated endothelial injury, capillary plugging by erythrocytes and neutrophils, and intracellular/interstitial edema with intramural hemorrhage.[1,2]

C. **INCIDENCE.** The reported incidence of no-reflow or slow-flow after percutaneous intervention ranges from 0.6-12.2%, depending on the definition used and the clinical setting (Table 21.1).[4,5,7,11,12] No-reflow is more common after mechanical revascularization of thrombus-containing lesions (i.e., acute MI not true) and degenerated vein grafts containing friable debris. Among new devices, no-reflow is highest after Rotablator atherectomy (1.2-9.0%) (Table 21.2), correlates with total burr activation time,[13-15] and is reversible in > 60% of episodes; the frequent response to intracoronary calcium antagonists is strongly suggestive of microvascular spasm.[7] In contrast, no-reflow after TEC atherectomy is frequently irreversible,[7] suggesting microembolization with vessel debris and capillary plugging. While the use of TEC correlated with persistent flow impairment,[7] these results may have been biased by its use in situations known to be associated with no-reflow (degenerated vein grafts, salvage revascularization after failed thrombolytic therapy for acute MI).

D. **CLINICAL MANIFESTATIONS AND PROGNOSIS.** In the catheterization laboratory, no-reflow usually manifests as ECG changes and chest pain.[7] However, depending on the myocardial territory, baseline ventricular function, and the presence of other coronary artery disease, no-reflow may be clinically silent, or induce a spectrum of ischemic manifestations including conduction disturbances, hypotension, myocardial infarction, cardiogenic shock, and death.[3,5,7] In one study, no-reflow was associated with a 10-fold higher incidence of death (15%) and myocardial infarction (31%) compared to patients without no-reflow (even after excluding patients who presented with acute MI).[7]

Table 21.1. Incidence and Outcome of No-Reflow After Percutaneous Intervention

Series	Incidence	Definition	Clinical Setting	Treatment & Outcome
Abbo[7] (1995)	66/10,767 (0.6%)	TIMI ≤ 1	All devices; patients with and without acute MI	Best response to verapamil (67%); worst response to urokinase (10%); high rate of adverse outcome (death 15%, MI 31%)
Wyrens[11] (1995)	24/614 (4.0%)	TIMI ≤ 1	All devices	Excellent response to diltiazem (96%)
Piana[5] (1994)	39/1919 (2%)	TIMI ≤ 2	PTCA, DCA	Excellent response to verapmil (95%)
Shani[12] (1992)	11/90 (12.2%)	"slow-flow"	PTCA for acute MI	All 6 patients treated with verampamil had improvement in flow
Wilson[4] (1989)	5/370 (1.3%)	"slow-flow"	PTCA; patients with and without acute MI	No response to NTG, papaverine, or lytics

Abbreviations: MI = myocardial infarction; PTCA = percutaneous transluminal coronary angioplasty; DCA = directional coronary atheterctomy; NTG = nitroglycerin

E. **PROPHYLAXIS.** Prophylaxis against no-reflow has not been systematically studied. However, Rotablator operators frequently insert a temporary transvenous pacemaker for target lesions in a dominant RCA or large LCx, to offset the adverse hemodynamic effects of bradycardia and/or AV block in the event no-reflow occurs. Some operators also add a cocktail of nitroglycerin and either verapamil, diltiazem, or adenosine to the heparinized Rotablator flush solution (Chapter 27). Pretreatment with calcium blockers for high-risk lesions is currently under evaluation.

F. **MANAGEMENT (Figure 21.1).** The optimal treatment of no-reflow is unknown. Since it occurs in a variety of clinical settings and is likely to have more than one mechanism, it is unlikely that a single definitive treatment will be appropriate for all cases. *Remember: No-reflow is a diagnosis of exclusion*!: High-grade residual stenosis due to flow-limiting dissection, thrombus, and spasm should be systematically excluded since their treatment and outcome are generally more favorable than those of no-reflow. Although mild degrees of flow impairment may improve spontaneously, active therapy is always recommended for no-reflow, as summarized in Figure 21.1 and detailed here:

1. **Reverse Superimposed Spasm.** Intracoronary nitroglycerin (200-800 mcg) rarely has any effect on no-reflow but may reverse superimposed spasm.[4,7] Since its use is not associated with unnecessary delay or enhanced risk, it should be used in all cases.

2. **Exclude Coronary Dissection.** Multiple angiographic views should be obtained to exclude a flow-limiting dissection. Even following "successful" PTCA, angioscopy often demonstrates intimal disruptions or frank dissections that are underestimated by angiography.[10,16] If contrast stains at the

Table 21.2. No-Reflow or "Slow-ReFlow" after Rotablator Atherectomy

Series	Type*	Incidence
Ellis[14] (1994)	Slow-flow	28 / 308 (9.1%)
Warth[15] (1994)	No-reflow	9 / 743 (1.2%)
Safian[13] (1993)	No-reflow	7 / 116 (6.1%)

* Slow-flow = TIMI flow = 2; No-reflow = TIMI flow ≤ 1

PTCA site, a flow-limiting dissection and/or thrombus is likely, and repeat balloon inflations should be performed. Caution should be used in stenting lesions with no-reflow since poor distal runoff may increase the likelihood of stent thrombosis.

3. **Administer Intracoronary Calcium Antagonists.** The most recent and important advance in the treatment of no-reflow is the use of intracoronary calcium antagonists. Intracoronary administration of either verapamil (100-200 mcg, total dose up to 1.0-1.5 mg) or diltiazem (0.5-2.5 mg bolus, total dose up to 5-10 mg) has been shown to reverse no-reflow in 65-95% of cases.[7,ref] In one report, resolution of no-reflow was 3-4 times more likely if verapamil was administered.[7] These agents should be administered through the central lumen of the balloon catheter to facilitate drug delivery to the distal vascular bed;[3,4,11] drug administered through the guiding catheter may not reach the distal vessel. Although high-degree AV block is unusual following intracoronary calcium blockers, a temporary pacemaker should be readily available. Hypotension caused by no-reflow is not a contraindication to intracoronary calcium blockers — adjunctive therapy with pressures, inotropes, and IABP should be used as needed to support the systemic circulation while the calcium blocker is administered.

4. **Treat Distal Embolization.** If no-reflow persists despite these measures, especially following coronary intervention of a thrombus-containing lesion, an intracoronary thrombolytic agent may be considered for presumed distal embolization (e.g., urokinase 100,000-500,000 units over 5-30 minutes). However, in several clinical and experimental studies, urokinase alone was ineffective in reversing no-reflow, so its risks should be carefully weighed against its benefits.[4,7,17,18]

5. **Clear Microvascular Plugging.** A rapid and moderately forceful injection of intracoronary saline or contrast may help clear microvascular plugging due to damaged endothelial cells, erythrocytes, neutrophils or thrombus.

6. **Increase Coronary Perfusion Pressure.** Although intra-aortic balloon counterpulsation (IABP) may augment coronary perfusion pressure, promote clearance of vasoactive substances, and limit

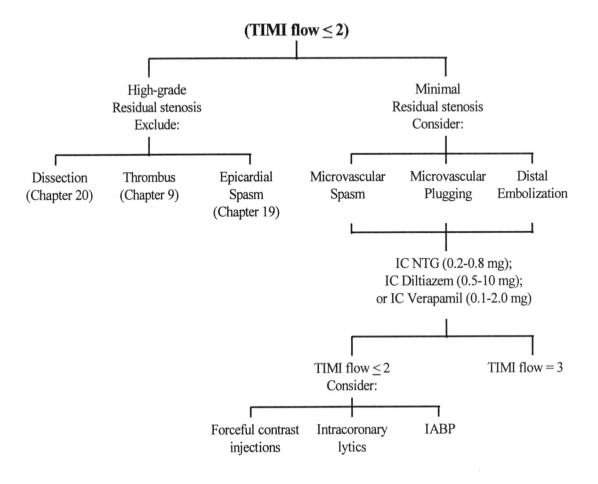

Figure 21.1. Impaired Flow After Intervention

infarct size, it has not been shown to reverse no-reflow. We recommend IABP therapy for patients with ongoing ischemia, hemodynamic compromise, or final TIMI flow < 3. For patients with hemodynamic collapse, percutaneous cardiopulmonary bypass may provide circulatory support during sustained periods of no-reflow.

7. **Coronary Artery Bypass Surgery.** Unfortunately, CABG is not beneficial for no-reflow, since the epicardial coronary artery is widely patent and the obstruction to coronary flow is at the capillary level.

8. **Triage to ICU.** Because of the adverse outcome associated with no-reflow, patients who do not respond immediately to treatment should be monitored in an intensive care unit. Serial cardiac

enzymes should be measured and a noninvasive assessment of LV function should be obtained. If myocardial infarction ensues, routine post-MI care should be administered.

9. **Other Approaches.** Potent coronary vasodilators such as papaverine and adenosine have been used in some cases of no-reflow with success. Intracoronary adenosine (10-20 mcg) is theoretically attractive because it inhibits neutrophil function and decreases neutrophil-mediated free-radical formation and endothelial injury. Antioxidants such as superoxide dismutase and allopurinol (which may decrease reperfusion injury) and mannitol (which may decrease myocardial edema) have been studied in experimental MI, but their value for no-reflow is unknown.

* * * * *

REFERENCES

1. Kloner RA, Ganote CE, Jennings RB. The "no-reflow" phenomenon after temporary coronary occlusion in the dog. J Clin Invest 1974;54:1496-1508.
2. Kloner RA. No-reflow revisited. J Am Coll Cardiol 1989;14:1814-1815.
3. Kitazume H, Iwama T, Kubo H, et al. No-reflow phenomenon during percutaneous transluminal coronary angioplasty. Am Heart J 1988;116:211-215.
4. Wilson RF, Lesser JR, Laxson DD, et al. Intense microvascular constriction after angioplasty of acute thrombotic coronary arterial lesions. Lancet 1989:801-811.
5. Piana RN, Paik GY, Moscucci M, et al. Incidence and treatment of no-reflow after percutaneous coronary intervention. Circulation 1994;89:2514-2518.
6. Ellis SG, Popma JJ, Buchbinder M, et al. Relation of clinical presentation, stenosis morphology, and operator technique to the procedural results of rotational atherectomy and rotational atherectomy-facilitated angioplasty. Circulation 1994;89:882-892.
7. Abbo KM, Dooris M, Glazier S, et al. No-reflow after percutaneous coronary intervention: Clinical and angiographic characteristics, treatment and outcome. Am J Cardiol 1995;75:778-782.
8. Feld H, Schulhoff N, Lichstein E, et al. Direct angioplasty as primary treatment for acute myocardial infarction resulting in the no-reflow phenomenon predicts a high mortality rate. Circulation 1992;86 (suppl);I-135.
9. Pomerantz RM, Kuntz RE, Diver DJ, et al. Intracoronary verapamil for the treatment of distal microvascular spasm following PTCA. Cath and Cardiovasc Diagn 1991;24:283-288.
10. Ritchie JL, Hansen D, Johnson C, et al. Combined mechanical and chemical thrombolysis in an experimental animal model: Evaluation by angiography and angioscopy. Am Heart J 1990;119-164.
11. Weyrens FJ, Mooney J, Lesser J, Mooney MR. Intracoronary diltiazem for microvascular spasm after interventional therapy. Am J Cardiol 1995;75:849-850.
12. Shani J, Feld H, Frankel R, Hollander G. Clinical cardiology: percutaneous transluminal coronary angioplasty in ischemic syndromes. Circulation 1992;86 (suppl):I-852.
13. Safian RD, Niazi KA, Strzelecki M, et al. Detailed angiographic analysis of high-speed mechanical rotational atherectomy in human coronary arteries. Circulation 1993;88:961-968.
14. Ellis SG, Popma JJ, Buchbinder M, et al. Relation of clinical presentation, stenosis morphology, and operator technique to the procedural results of rotational atherectomy and rotational atherectomy-facilitated angioplasty. Circulation 1994;89:882-892.
15. Warth DC, Leon MB, O'Neill W, et al. Rotational atherectomy multicenter registry: Acute results, complications and 6-month angiographic follow-up in 709 patients. J Am Coll Cardiol 1994;24:641-8.
16. Ramee SR, White CJ, Jain A, et al. Percutaneous coronary angioscopy versus intravascular ultrasound in patients

undergoing coronary angioplasty. J Am Coll Cardiol 1991;17(2):125A.

17. Kloner RA, Alker KJ. The effect of streptokinase on intramyocardial hemorrhage, infarct size, and the "no-reflow" phenomenon during coronary reperfusion. Circulation 1984;70:513-521.

18. Kloner RA, Alker K, Campbell C, et al. Does tissue-type plasminogen activator have direct beneficial effects on the myocardium independent of its ability to lyse intracoronary thrombi? Circulation 1989;79:1125-1136.

22 CORONARY ARTERY PERFORATION

Steven C. Ajluni, M.D.
Robert D. Safian, M.D.

A. **INCIDENCE AND CLASSIFICATION.** Coronary artery perforation is a rare but important complication of percutaneous revascularization. Angiographic evidence for perforation has been reported in 0.1% of lesions treated with PTCA and 0.5-3.0% of lesions treated with Rotablator, DCA, TEC, or ELCA (Table 22.1).[1-7] At our institution, perforations are classified angiographically as free perforations (free contrast extravasation into the pericardium), contained perforations (localized rounded crater of contrast outside the contrast-filled lumen), or other unclassified perforations (Figure 22.1). In one report, the relative proportion of these types of perforation was 31%, 50%, and 19%, respectively; perforation was caused by a balloon or new device in 74%, a guidewire in 20%, and an indeterminate cause in 6%.[1]

B. **MECHANISMS AND RISK FACTORS.** During PTCA, perforation may occur as a consequence of guidewire advancement, balloon advancement, balloon inflation, or balloon rupture.[8-14] Since PTCA results in dissection and stretching of the vessel wall, oversized balloons (balloon/artery ratio >1.2) may extend these dissections through the adventitia, resulting in vessel perforation. Balloon rupture, particularly those associated with pinhole leaks (as opposed to longitudinal tears), may create high-pressure jets that increase the risk of dissection and/or perforation. Devices that alter the integrity of the vascular wall may also lead to perforation by tissue removal (TEC, DCA), pulverization

Table 22.1. Incidence of Perforation After Percutaneous Intervention

Series	N	Perforation (%)						
		All devices	PTCA	DCA	ROTA	TEC	ELCA	Stent
Ajluni[1] (1994)	8932	0.4	0.1	0.3	0	1.3	2.0	0
Ellis[2] (1994)	12,900	0.5	0.1	0.7	1.3	2.1	1.9	-
Flood[3] (1994)	2426	0.7	0.6	0.3	0.4	0	1.7	0.2
Lansky[4] (1994)	708	2.0	-	3.2	-	2.0	1.7	1.1

Abbreviations: PTCA = percutaneous transluminal coronary angioplasty; DCA = directional coronary atherectomy; ROTA = Rotablator; TEC = transluminal extraction catheter, ELCA = excimer laser coronary angioplasty; - = not reported

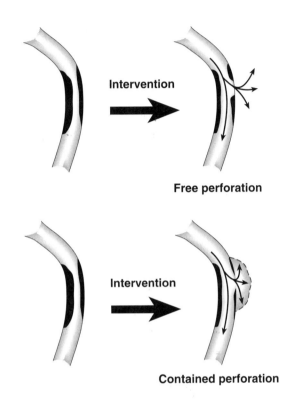

Intervention

Free perforation

Intervention

Contained perforation

Figure 22.1 Types of Coronary Artery Perforation

(Rotablator), or ablation (ELCA).[1-6] Oversized devices, especially when used to treat bifurcation lesions and lesions located in severely angulated vessel segments, substantially increase the risk of perforation. Intracoronary stenting can also lead to perforation from the use of stiff guidewires or oversized compliant (for stent delivery) or high-pressure balloons (for optimal stent expansion), or from subintimal passage of the stent into a vessel with severe dissection.[15] Regardless of the device, the risk of perforation is increased when complex lesion morphology is present (e.g., chronic total occlusion, vessel bifurcation, severe tortuosity or angulation).[15,6]

C. OUTCOME. Coronary artery perforation can result in pericardial hemorrhage and cardiac tamponade (17-24% of patients),[1,2,5] fistulae to the left or right ventricle,[9,10] or coronary arteriovenous fistulae. Clinically, coronary perforation is associated with a high incidence of death (0-9%), MI (4-26%), emergency surgery (24-36%), and blood transfusion (34%) (Table 22.2).[1,2,5,6] Some perforations are angiographically inapparent and may go undetected during the interventional procedure, only to manifest

Table 22.2. Clinical Outcome After Coronary Artery Perforation

Series	Device(s)	No. Perforations (Incidence)	In-hospital Complications (%)		
			CABG	**MI**	**Death**
Ajluni[1] (1994)	All devices* except stent	35 (0.4%)	37	26	5.6
Ellis[2] (1994)	All devices* except stent	62 (0.5%)	24	19	0
Bittl[5] (1993)	ELCA	23 (3.0%)	34.7	4.3	9
Holmes[6] (1994)	ELCA	36 (1.3%)	36.1	16.7	4.8
Cohen[16] (1994)	ROTA	22 (0.7%)	41	45.5	9
Flood[3] (1994)	All devices*	19 (0.7%)	33	5.6	5.9

Abbreviations: PTCA = percutaneous transluminal coronary angioplasty; TEC = transluminal extraction catheter; ELCA = excimer laser coronary angioplasty; ROTA = Rotablator; DCA = directional coronary atherectomy; CABG = emergency coronary artery bypass surgery, MI = myocardial infarction
* All devices = PTCA, TEC, DCA, ROTA, ELCA, Stent

8-24 hours later with the sudden appearance of cardiac tamponade. While bypass graft perforation may result in chest wall or mediastinal hemorrhage, cardiac tamponade is unusual due to partial pericardiectomy during bypass surgery, the subsequent development of pericardial adhesions, and the location of most bypass grafts outside the pericardium.[1,12]

D. PREVENTION

1. **Guidewire Positioning.** During all percutaneous interventions, the tip of the guidewire should advance smoothly beyond the stenosis and retain torque-response. If there is buckling of the guidewire, restricted tip movement, or resistance to guidewire advancement, the wire may be subintimal and should be withdrawn and repositioned. If there is any concern that the balloon catheter may have entered a false lumen, a gentle contrast injection may be delivered through the central lumen of the balloon after removing the guidewire. Persistent contrast staining indicates that a false channel has been entered and requires withdrawal and repositioning of both the guidewire and balloon — balloon inflation within a false lumen may result in coronary artery rupture and rapid clinical deterioration.

2. **Device Sizing.** In some studies, oversized devices (device-to-artery ratio ≥ 0.8 for TEC, ELCA and

Rotablator; balloon-to-artery ratio >1.2 for PTCA) were important correlates of angiographic perforation.[1,5] Therefore, high-risk lesions (e.g., bifurcations, angulated stenoses, severe proximal tortuosity, total occlusion) are best approached using balloon-to-artery ratios of 1.0 for PTCA, and device-to-artery ratio of 0.5-0.6 for lasers, TEC, and Rotablator. When these latter devices are used, it may be prudent to achieve further lumen enlargement by adjunctive PTCA (balloon-to-artery ratio = 1) rather than upsizing to a larger device.

3. **Other Device Considerations.** When DCA is used to excise dissection flaps, the risk of perforation may be reduced by orienting the AtheroCath away from the normal wall, and using an undersized device and inflation pressures < 20 psi. DCA should not be used to treat long or spiral dissections, dissections on severely angulated vessel segments, or dissections associated with periadventital dye staining, due to the risk of perforation. Stent-related perforations may be avoided by meticulous attention to balloon sizing and stent position. Stents should not be used when the distal extent of a dissection cannot be identified angiographically.

E. **MANAGEMENT (Figure 22.2).** In general, guidewire perforations rarely result in adverse sequelae.[1] In contrast, perforations caused by balloons, atherectomy devices, or lasers may result in hemopericardium and hemodynamic collapse.[1,2] Regardless of the cause, initial management should focus on sealing the perforation nonoperatively and stabilizing the patient hemodynamically. The cardiac surgeons should be notified immediately and the operating room prepared for possible emergency surgery.

1. **Nonoperative Management of Coronary Perforation**
   a. **Prolonged Balloon Inflation.** A balloon (balloon-to-artery ratio = 0.9-1.0) should be immediately positioned at the site of contrast extravasation and inflated to 2-6 atm for at least 10 minutes. If sealing is incomplete, a second low-pressure inflation should be performed for 15-45 minutes, using a perfusion balloon catheter whenever possible to prevent distal myocardial ischemia. Additional heparin should not be given. Prolonged balloon inflations (and pericardiocentesis if needed) may avoid the need for surgery in 60-70% of patients who develop coronary perforation during percutaneous intervention.[1,2,5,6] In rare cases, stent-vein allografts have been used to seal perforations and pseudoaneurysms (Figure 26.15), but this technique is technically demanding and is not appropriate for patients with profound hemodynamic collapse.

   b. **Pericardiocentesis.** Echocardiography should be performed at the first sign of perforation, if possible. If pericardial hemorrhage is evident, immediate pericardiocentesis is performed. If hemodynamic collapse occurs secondary to perforation pericardiocentesis should not be delayed for any reason. As nonoperative attempts proceed to treat the perforation, the pericardiocentesis needle should be exchanged for a multiple-side-hole catheter, allowing continuous aspiration and monitoring of pericardial blood volume.

   c. **Reversal of Anticoagulation.** Initial efforts to seal the perforation should occur while the patient remains fully anticoagulated (to prevent vessel thrombosis). However, some

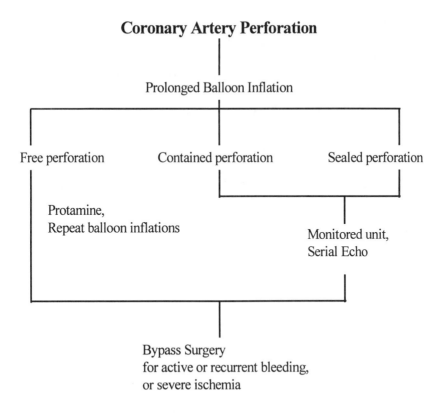

Figure 22.2. Management of Coronary Artery Perforation

interventionalists recommend immediate administration of protamine to reverse the effects of systemic heparinization when free perforation occurs after atherectomy or laser devices. If contrast extravasation persists despite prolonged balloon inflations, incremental doses of protamine should be administered (25-50mg intravenously over 10-30 minutes) while repeat balloon inflations are attempted. Vessel closure may be an acceptable alternative to pericardial hemorrhage if bypass surgery is not feasible or if perforation occurs in a small side branch. Although stent-vein allografts have been used to seal coronary pseudoaneurysms, they may be less useful for acute perforations and hemodynamic collapse due to unreliable delivery to the target lesion.

d. **Monitoring Following Successful Nonoperative Management.** All patients require careful observation in a monitored unit. Continuous monitoring of the right atrial pressure will allow early detection of ongoing pericardial hemorrhage. If pericardiocentesis was performed during PTCA, the drainage catheter should remain in place for 6-24 hrs, and serial echocardiography should be performed every 6-12 hours to detect reaccumulation of pericardial effusion. If bleeding persists or recurs, the patient should be referred for emergency surgery.

2. **Operative Management.** If the perforation is large, associated with severe ischemia, or if hemodynamic instability or perforation persists despite nonoperative measures, emergency surgery should be performed to control hemorrhage, repair the perforation or ligate the vessel, and bypass all vessels containing significant stenoses. If possible, a perfusion balloon catheter should be positioned and inflated at low pressure while the operating room is being prepared; intermittent flushing of the central lumen with heparinized saline will prevent clotting and ensure antegrade blood flow. Operative management may be required in 30-40% of patients who develop perforation.[1,2,5,6]

* * * * *

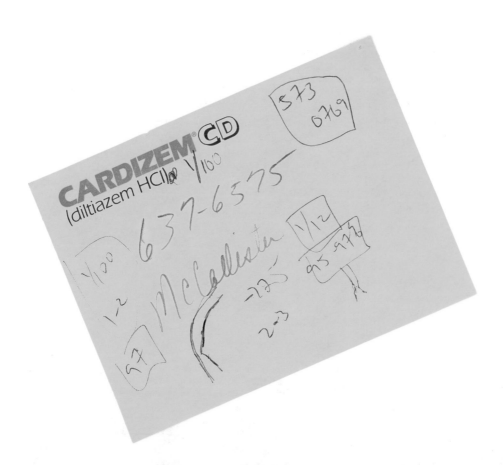

REFERENCES

1. Ajuni SC, Glazier S, Blankenship L, et al. Perforations after percutaneous coronary interventions: clinical, angiographic, and therapeutic observations. Cath Cardiovasc Diagn. 1994;32:206-212.

2. Ellis SG, Ajluni S, Arnold AZ, et al. Increased coronary perforation in the new device era. Incidence, classification, management, and outcome. Circulation 1994;90:2725-2730.

3. Flood RD, Popma JJ, Chuang, Ya Chien, et al. Incidence, angiographic predictors, and clinical significance of coronary perforation occurring after new device angioplasty. J Am Coll Cardiol 1994;23:301A.

4. Lansky A, Popma JJ, Baim DS, et al. Angiographic outcome after new devices saphenous vein graft Angioplasty. Abstract from Transcatheter Cardiovascular Therapeutics, 1995.

5. Bittl JA, Ryan TJ, Keaney JF, et al. Coronary artery perforation during excimer laser coronary angioplasty. J Am Coll Cardiol 1993;21:1158-1165.

6. Holmes DR, Reeder GS, Ghazzai ZM, et al. Coronary perforation after excimer laser coronary angioplasty: the excimer laser coronary angioplasty registry experience. J Am Coll Cardiol 1994;23:330-335.

7. Cowley MJ, Dorros G, and Kelsey SF. Acute coronary events associated with percutaneous transluminal coronary angioplasty. Am J Cardiol 1984;53:12C-16C.

8. Saffitz JE, Rose TE, Oaks JB, et al. Coronary arterial rupture during coronary angioplasty. Am J Cardiol 1983;51:902-904.

9. Kimbiris DM, Iskandrian AS, Goel I, et al. Transluminal coronary angioplasty complicated by coronary artery perforation. Cathet Cardiovasc Diagn 1982;8:481-487.

10. Iannone LA and Iannone DP. Iatrogenic left coronary artery fistula-to-left ventricle following PTCA: A previously unreported complication with nonsurgical treatment. Am Heart J 1990;120:1215-1217.

11. Cherry S and Vandormael M. Rupture of a coronary artery and hemorrhage into the ventricular cavity during coronary angioplasty. Am Heart J 1990;113:386-388.

12. Teirstein PS and Hartzler GO. Nonoperative management of aortocoronary saphenous vein graft rupture during percutaneous transluminal coronary angioplasty. Am J Cardiol 1987;60:377-378.

13. Meier B. Benign coronary perforation during percutaneous transluminal coronary angioplasty. Br Heart J 1985;54:33-35.

14. Grollier G, Bories H, Commeau P, et al. Coronary artery perforation during coronary angioplasty. Clin Cardiol 1986;9:27-29.

15. Benzuly K, Safian RD. Coronary artery perforation: an unreported complication after stenting. Cathet Cardiovasc Diagn (in-press).

16. Cohen BM, Weber VJ, Bass TA, et al. Coronary perforation during rotational ablation: Angiographic determinants and clinical outcome. J Am Coll Cardiol 1994;23:354A.

17. Mehta S, Popma J, Margolis JR, Moore L, et al. Complications with new angioplasty devices. Are these device specific? J Am Coll Cardiol 1996;March, Special Issue.

18. Dorros G, Jain A, Kumar K. Management of coronary artery rupture: Covered stent or microcoil embolization. Cathet Cardiovasc Diagn. 1995;36:148-154.

19. Kaplan BM, Stewart RE, Sakwa MP, et al. Repair of a coronary pseudoaneurysm with percutaneous placement of a saphenous vein allograft attached to a biliary stent. Cathet Cardiovasc Diagn. 1996 (in-press).

EMERGENCY BYPASS SURGERY FOR FAILED PTCA

23

Francis L. Shannon, M.D.
Marc P. Sakwa, M.D.

A. INTRODUCTION. The role of the cardiac surgeon in managing the acute complications of percutaneous coronary procedures continues to evolve as our interventional colleagues expand the scope of their therapy. Most notable is the decreasing need for emergent cardiac surgery as cardiologists gain greater experience with new angioplasty devices and the liberal use of intracoronary stents for unstable dissections. This success has encouraged the employment of percutaneous revascularization for patients who are older, have multivessel coronary disease, and poor left ventricular function. Unfortunately, performing emergent cardiac surgery on this group of relatively high risk patients has yielded greater surgical morbidity and mortality. These changes in the profile of patients with failed or unsatisfactory coronary intervention have produced a more selective approach to performing emergent coronary bypass grafting in our institution.

1. **Levels of Surgical Back-Up for Percutaneous Interventions.** Historically, percutaneous coronary angioplasty has been a "joint venture" between interventional cardiologists and cardiac surgeons. As Andreas Gruntzig related to Joseph Craver at Emory University in 1978: "For a successful coronary angioplasty program, good cardiology is important; but superior cardiac surgery is essential."[1] Since that time, the incidence of emergency coronary bypass grafting for failed PTCA has decreased from 7% to 2%.[2] This operational fact as well as the exponential growth of percutaneous procedures in many centers has produced an array of contingency plans for the surgical treatment of angioplasty failures. In the United States, nearly all interventional cardiology programs have on-site surgical capabilities to perform emergency coronary bypass grafting;[3] however, many European programs rely on off-site cardiac surgical facilities for "back-up."[4-6] Among programs with on-site surgical capability, the degree of support ranges from a strict "stand-by" arrangement, in which an open operating room and surgical team are immediately available, to "back-up," in which emergency cardiac surgery is performed in the next available operating room.[7] The overall procedural mortality rates and average time intervals to surgical revascularization are similar when comparing these two strategies.[8,9] The scheme adopted by any interventional cardiology program depends on the angioplasty risk profile of its patient population, technical expertise of its cardiologists and elective case volume of its cardiac surgical team. For our institution in which 3500 PTCAs and 1200 cardiac surgical procedures are performed each year, we feel that the surgical back-up plan described below is the safest and most cost-effective.

2. **Surgical Consultation Before PTCA.** Our initial surgical involvement with most patients undergoing coronary angioplasty consists of an agreement to be available for evaluating procedural

results and performing emergency cardiac surgery, if indicated. Prior to percutaneous intervention, we perform a more detailed assessment in patients with multiple or complex coronary arterial lesions, poor left ventricular function, severe associated medical problems, previous CABG or lack of adequate bypass conduits. This appraisal is necessary to formulate interventional limits so that patients who would not be expected to benefit from emergency cardiac surgery are identified and informed of their risks. Thus, many high risk PTCAs are identified in which "salvage" cardiac surgery is not a therapeutic option in the event of an unsatisfactory percutaneous result.

For all other cases, a cardiac surgical team and appropriate operating room facilities are made ready for urgent management of specific PTCA complications on a "next available" basis. The timing of this surgical support varies in accordance with the potential for an immediately life-threatening complication of a specific intervention as well as the number of scheduled cardiac surgical procedures. In this arrangement, optimal surgical back-up is facilitated by scheduling high-risk PTCAs during times that the cardiac surgical suites are available. For patients who ultimately require emergency surgical revascularization, use of autoperfusion catheters and intra-aortic balloon pump support attenuates myocardial ischemia while the operating room is being prepared. Interventional complications requiring emergency CABG after hours and on weekends are supported by an off-site "on call" cardiac surgical team that is ready to initiate operation within 60 minutes of notification. We have observed an average delay of 100 minutes between determination of refractory ischemia in the catheterization lab and initial myocardial reperfusion by cardioplegia delivery to the affected zone in the operating room. This period includes an average time of 30 minutes for sterile cardiopulmonary monitoring line placement by anesthesia and internal mammary artery mobilization among patients who are stabilized by autoperfusion catheters and/or intra-aortic balloon pump placement. In catastrophic situations, we have performed definitive surgical revascularization within 30 minutes of the onset of lethal myocardial ischemia. This surgical response time compares favorably with others reported in the literature and is associated with relatively low rates of procedural morbidity and mortality for our high risk interventional population.[10]

B. INCIDENCE. Review of the literature shows that the incidence of PTCA failure requiring emergency cardiac surgery has decreased from 5% to approximately 2% over the last five years.[1,11-13] The majority of these studies include patients who require operation within 24 hours of PTCA. This liberal definition of "emergency surgery" includes many patient who develop a delayed myocardial ischemic syndrome following intervention and therefore are more stable than those who require immediate surgery. For the purposes of this discussion, we define "emergency" as a cardiac surgical procedure required within 6 hours of the percutaneous intervention. This time interval encompasses the majority of patients who are acutely ischemic from abrupt closure or critical re-stenosis that is refractory to further percutaneous intervention and therefore need immediate surgical revascularization.

Despite variations in reporting results, the true incidence of emergent CAB for PTCA failure has decreased in recent years. This trend is due to the following factors: (1) Enhanced skill of interventional cardiologists in avoiding catastrophic complications, (2) Better patient selection on the basis of coronary lesion morphology and location, (3) Liberal use of intracoronary stents for unstable dissections and (4) Medical management of small myocardial infarctions resulting from unsatisfactory interventions. Encouraged by their increasing clinical success and technical prowess, interventional cardiologists have expanded the scope of their percutaneous interventions to include patients with multivessel coronary artery disease, poor left ventricular function, advanced age and evolving myocardial infarction. The net result of these developments is that the current group of patients requiring immediate surgery for failed PTCA is at greater risk for operative morbidity and mortality because surgical reperfusion is often the only hope for survival.

C. **INDICATIONS FOR EMERGENCY CABG.** Once summoned to the cardiac cath lab, the surgeon does an initial evaluation of the patient as a candidate for emergency cardiac surgery. This assessment includes consideration of pertinent co-morbid conditions, current hemodynamic status and coronary anatomy.

1. **Important Associated Conditions**

    a. **Age.** Patients greater than 80 years old in cardiogenic shock have a 90% operative mortality rate when undergoing emergency CABG for failed PTCA in our institution. Octogenarians who require emergency CABG and are not in shock still have the highest mortality of all age subgroups; therefore, we recommend very selective evaluation in this patient population.

    b. **Mental Status.** Patients who have suffered cardiac arrest prior to or during the percutaneous intervention should be examined closely. Recent stroke and prolonged cardiopulmonary arrest causing an unresponsive state are relative contraindications to emergency CABG.

    c. **Conduit Availability.** Patients with prior removal of greater saphenous veins for cosmetic reasons or previous vascular surgical procedures (CABG or femoral-infrapopliteal arterial bypass) are poor candidates; myocardial ischemia time is increased by the time necessary for mobilization of arterial or lesser saphenous venous conduits. Cryopreserved human saphenous veins may be used in these circumstances, but one year patency is less than 50%.[14]

    d. **Previous Cardiac Surgery.** Myocardial ischemia time may be prolonged by the increased difficulty in dissection when trying to obtain access for cannulation and coronary exposure. Risk of graft atheroembolization may be increased by the cardiac manipulation necessary to go on cardiopulmonary bypass urgently.

    e. **Thrombolytic Agents.** Prior infusion of thrombolytic, antithrombin or antiplatelet agents as an adjunct to PTCA increases the tendency for postcardiopulmonary bypass coagulopathy, but is not a contraindication to emergency surgery. Judicious use of clotting factor transfusions (platelet concentrates and cryoprecipitate) usually reduces total blood loss and delayed hemorrhage requiring re-operation.

2. **Indications for Emergency Cardiac Surgery**

   a. **Acute Occlusion** of a major coronary artery that is not amenable to restoration of adequate flow by percutaneous and pharmacologic measures. This complication accounts for 70% of PTCA failure cases requiring emergency surgery. Refractory mechanical occlusion must be differentiated from the "no reflow" phenomenon that has been observed as a consequence of intense distal arterial spasm or microembolism in the absence of an obstructing proximal lesion.[15] We have found that this latter process is best treated medically because there is no intra-arterial occlusion amenable to surgical bypass.

   b. **Unsatisfactory Angioplasty Result with Refractory Myocardial Ischemia.** Persistent proximal coronary stenoses due to atheromatous plaque or dissection that compromises less than 70% of the luminal diameter usually heal over time and can be treated medically. Among those with coronary stenosis exceeding 70% intraluminal diameter, coronary vasodilators and intra-aortic balloon pump frequently relieve myocardial ischemia and permit urgent surgical revascularization (usually within 24 hours). While these measures minimize ischemia, they do not reduce the incidence of abrupt closure that results from intracoronary trauma. Thus, emergency CABG is indicated for patients with unstable dissections and persistent stenosis in a coronary artery as well as patients who are refractory to medical treatment and have large areas of myocardium at risk. Currently, only 25% of our PTCA failures requiring surgery fall into this category because of increasing interventional expertise.

   c. **Coronary Artery Perforations with Pericardial Tamponade.** Previous reviews have considered coronary perforation to be an absolute indication for emergency surgery. Over the past two years, we have managed this problem by initially attempting to seal the perforation with prolonged intra-coronary balloon inflations (up to 30 minutes), on-table echocardiographic assessment of pericardial fluid accumulation, and pigtail catheter drainage of large pericardial effusions. Using this selective approach, we have performed emergency CABG and arterial repair for only 40% of patients with coronary perforations. The primary indications for emergency surgery in this group were hemodynamic compromise secondary to expanding epicardial hematomas and persistent arterial hemorrhage despite prolonged balloon inflations. Recently, we have placed saphenous vein grafts on stents and employed them in the coronary artery to cover the perforation. While we have had some initial success, the use of this technique is in the developmental stages.

   d. **Left Main Coronary Arterial Injury or Occlusion.** Although infrequent, this complication can result from direct mechanical trauma from guiding catheters, intracoronary devices or retrograde propagation of a large dissection. Cardiovascular collapse is usually precipitous and immediate surgery should be undertaken, although one is often unsuccessful in salvaging the patient.

e. **Retained Intracoronary Foreign Bodies With or Without Obstruction.** Fractured fragments of balloon catheters and guidewires that remain trapped in a proximal coronary artery are potential causes of mechanical or thrombotic occlusion. Misplaced or incompletely deployed stents in native coronary arteries or saphenous vein grafts are also a source for mechanical total occlusion and therefore warrant emergency surgery. We usually attempt to extract these foreign bodies to prevent distal embolization and thrombosis of coronary arteries. Regardless, we feel that a bypass placed distal to the site of obstruction is sufficient to avert distal migration of the retained hardware and maintain adequate distal arterial perfusion.

D. **CONTRAINDICATIONS TO EMERGENCY SURGERY.** There are few absolute criteria to deny a dying patient a chance to survive with emergency surgery; the following factors may preclude successful operative outcome:
1. Acute cerebral injury from hypoxia, vascular emboli or cerebrovascular insufficiency.
2. Metastatic or untreated malignancy.
3. Acquired Immunodeficiency Syndrome.
4. End-stage lung disease. (FEV_1 < 1.0 liters/min. or R.A. pO_2 < 45 mm Hg).
5. Inoperable diffuse coronary artery disease.
6. Multiple previous cardiac operations with no available bypass conduits.
7. Irreversible left ventricular.
8. Cardiogenic shock with inability to be weaned from percutaneous cardiopulmonary support (CPS).
9. Advanced age (> 80 years) with cardiogenic shock.

All of these contraindications to emergency CABG are based on consideration of a patient's life expectancy, the systemic and cardiopulmonary reserve necessary to survive the stresses of surgery and our own experience. This is particularly true for our series of 15 patients placed on CPS for cardiogenic shock secondary to a PTCA catastrophe. Unlike reports from other centers,[16] we had only one surgical survivor. Consequently, we insist that the patient on CPS demonstrate sufficient myocardial viability and contractility to eject blood with a pulse pressure of at least 60 mHg before we will perform emergency cardiac surgery. This criterion is based on our observation that percutaneous circulatory support can give a false appearance of cardiovascular integrity in the presence of an irreversibly dilated and damaged heart.

E. **PREPARATION FOR SURGERY.** All possible interventions to minimize systemic and myocardial ischemia should be employed while the operating room is being prepared to receive the patient. These measures fall into the following categories:
1. **Restoration of Adequate Oxygen Delivery to the Heart and Systemic Circulation.** Attention to airway management with endotracheal intubation and ventilation as well as maintenance of adequate systemic perfusion pressure with intra-aortic balloon pump placement and inotropic drug administration are essential, but often overlooked. Reducing the pre-operative oxygen debt of these compromised patients reduces the stress of emergency cardiopulmonary bypass. This is

particularly true for patients who are subclinically hypoxemic from the cumulative effects of sedative drugs, low cardiac output and acute blood loss.

2. **Maintenance of Distal Coronary Blood Flow.** In the presence of acute occlusion, passage of a guidewire across the obstruction usually restores flow and permits placement of an autoperfusion catheter or other device across the occlusion; however, once the decision has been made to perform emergency surgery, further percutaneous manipulations to open the artery should be abandoned if the operating room is ready.

3. **Pharmacologic Coronary Vasodilation.** Once the previously mentioned objectives have been met, coronary perfusion can be further enhanced by administration of intravenous nitrates. It is difficult to titrate drug dosage in the acute setting of angioplasty; therefore, simply maintaining a "background" infusion level may be sufficient to prevent rebound or reactive coronary vasoconstriction.

    Among patients who suffer cardiac arrest, the preparations for surgery are condensed to initiating standard CPR and mobilizing the patient for transport to the operating room. Placement of an intra-aortic balloon pump for augmentation of systemic perfusion during CPR is the best use of femoral arterial access, rather than attempting to traverse the occluded coronary artery. Initiation of percutaneous cardiopulmonary support is considered only if an operating room is not immediately available. Immediate transport to the OR and initiation of cardiopulmonary bypass within 30 minutes of cardiac arrest is our goal and has yielded better than 90% survival at our institution.

F. **SURGICAL TECHNIQUES.** If the patient is hemodynamically stable and without signs of significant myocardial ischemia, we proceed as with elective CABG. Radial arterial and central venous monitoring lines are placed, full sterile prep is applied and the left internal mammary artery is mobilized if needed for LAD bypass. All other patients undergo expeditious anesthetic induction and placement on full cardiopulmonary bypass (CPB) while saphenous veins are harvested for bypass. The immediate goals in surgical resuscitation of the unstable patient are decompression of the left ventricle on full CPB so that global myocardial oxygen demand is reduced and adequate systemic perfusion is restored.

1. **Conduit Selection.** Use of the internal mammary artery for revascularization is primarily determined by the hemodynamic stability of the patient, coronary anatomy, and ability to adequately protect the ischemic zone. Of secondary concern is the suitability of the mammary artery for both reconstruction of an extensive coronary dissection and provision of adequate distal perfusion. We have been able to use the LIMA for emergency revascularization of the left anterior descending coronary artery in over 50% of our recent cases. For all other coronary lesions, we use saphenous vein because of its dependable patency rates, versatility in both patching and bypassing complex coronary injuries, and ease of harvesting in crisis situations. We have not used cryopreserved human saphenous vein extensively, but have considered it as an option in older patients with good LV function and no autologous venous conduits.

2. **Myocardial Protection.** Initial reperfusion of the ischemic zone with blood cardioplegia is a critical component of surgical success in salvaging myocardium. In most circumstances, we use both antegrade cardioplegia delivery (via the aortic root) to assure global cardiac arrest and retrograde delivery (via a catheter in the coronary sinus) to achieve perfusion of myocardial zones supplied by critically narrowed or totally occluded coronary arteries. We have selectively used Buckberg's protocol of "warm induction cardioplegia" without substrate enhancement for patients with cardiogenic shock or large ischemic territories.[17] In theory, induction of diastolic cardiac arrest at an infusion temperature of 36^0 C allows replenishment of depleted myocardial stores of ADP and ATP prior to the absolute ischemic time from aortic cross clamping which is necessary for surgical revascularization. After initial warm induction, we deliver sufficient volumes of cold blood cardioplegia both antegrade and retrograde to achieve a myocardial septal temperature of less than 15^0 C. Throughout the remainder of aortic cross clamp time, we reinfuse cold blood cardioplegia with a lower potassium concentration (15 meq/L) every 15 to 20 minutes. We generally do not deliver a "hot shot" of antegrade cardioplegia before removal of the aortic cross clamp, but allow full cardiac reperfusion on bypass for at least 20 to 30 minutes before attempting to wean the patient from full support. Using this method of myocardial reperfusion and protection, we have been able to separate most patients from cardiopulmonary bypass with a cardiac index of at least 1.8 L/min/meter^2 over the past three years.

3. **Coronary Arterial Repair and Revascularization.** One of the most challenging aspects of emergency CABG involves the need to bypass and repair long spiral arterial dissections. The challenge exists in the delivery of distal perfusion while maintaining some antegrade flow to proximal coronary septal branches. In addition, we have found that inappropriately placed stents cause similar challenges. In this situation, we recommend long patch angioplasty with saphenous veins; first achieving good distal flow and then attempting to re-attach the intima proximally to establish antegrade perfusion. When stents are used, we often try to remove them as long as they are easily accessible from the chosen bypass site. Despite the onion skin appearance of the layers of the damaged coronary arteries in these cases, we have demonstrated salvage of surprisingly long segments of the arterial tree on subsequent coronary angiography. We also use variations of this same saphenous vein patch angioplasty technique for distal perforations. Direct coronary arterial repair is not anatomically feasible for very proximal perforations of the LAD and circumflex; rather, we perform distal coronary bypass and oversew the suspected epicardial region with pledgetted mattress sutures to prevent further bleeding. These approaches to the injured coronary artery are not standardized, but constitute our solutions to the technical problem of restoring as much myocardial perfusion as possible.

4. **Special Considerations.** Once the coronary arterial injury is treated, we address our secondary goal of providing complete myocardial revascularization. Decision-making in this phase of the operation has become more complex because most patients have coexistent multivessel coronary artery disease or previous percutaneous procedures involving other epicardial arteries. In general, the number of emergency bypasses performed depends on the condition of the patient prior to

operation, the adequacy of myocardial protection during surgery and the severity of associated coronary disease. If the patient is stable and operation is proceeding well, we place venous bypass grafts to al coronary arteries greater than 1.5 mm in diameter with proximal stenoses exceeding 70% of the intraluminal diameter. In addition, we often prophylactically bypass coronary arteries without current critical stenosis that were previously diseased, but successfully opened by angioplasty within one month of operation. Our rationale for prophylactic grafting is to prevent post-operative ischemic symptoms from native coronary re-stenosis. Currently, this approach applies to recently opened coronaries that were additionally treated with an intracoronary stent because we are not convinced that stented vessels are "resistant" to re-stenosis.

5. **Operative Adjuncts.** Complex cases of emergency surgery for failed PTCA often require extraordinary measures to separate the patient from cardiopulmonary bypass and sustain cardiovascular integrity for at least 24 to 48 hour in order to permit myocardial recovery from the ischemic insult. Pharmacologic support includes ultra-high dose inotropic and pressor infusions, intravenous levothyroxine and meticulous correction of acidosis. Blood component replacement to maintain optimal oxygen delivery with a hemoglobin level greater than 9 gm/ml and clotting factor administration to reverse the coagulopathy created by cardiopulmonary bypass and pre-operative antiplatelet or thrombolytic therapy is aggressively initiated before the chest is closed. Single or biventricular support devices are considered for patients less than 65 years of age who seem to have suffered massive, but potentially reversible myocardial injury. The chest is left open and the heart is covered with a sterile esmarch barrier when massive cardiac swelling from fluid resuscitation, myocardial edema, and epicardial hematoma preclude sternal closure without extrinsic compression of the heart. Among survivors, these measures are associated with a surprisingly low rate of wound and other infectious complications.

G. RESULTS

1. **Mortality.** Despite dramatic increases in the number of percutaneous interventions done in recent years, there have been few reports of current surgical mortality rates for PTCA failures. The early data came from an era in interventional cardiology in which simple procedures with fewer devices were performed on healthier patients with single and double vessel coronary artery disease. For this period of 1980 to 1987, fifteen studies comprising 548 patients requiring emergency CABG for PTCA failure reported an average operative mortality of 9% (range 0 to 17%).[8,9,18-28] While these studies have little relevance to the current era, they provide benchmark for analyzing our current results with more high-risk patients. For the period of 1985 to 1992, three studies disclose overall operative mortality rates of 5.7% to 12.5% with an even higher average mortality rate of 40% for patients who are in cardiogenic shock at the time of operation.[1,10,12] The best recent data comes from the Society of Thoracic Surgeons' national database in which the operative mortality rate among 3,975 patients requiring emergency CABG within 6 hours PTCA was 5.6% for the period of 1990 to 1993.[29] This compares favorably with the results of our own institution over the last 3 years in which 4 post-operative deaths occurred among 75 patients (5.3%) who were not in shock at the time of operation. Among 34 patients in shock, our operative mortality rate was

38.5%; ten of these thirteen deaths occurred in patients who underwent emergency PTCA for an evolving myocardial infarction and therefore had irreversible myocardial damage prior to intervention that precluded a high rate of salvage even with aggressive reperfusion strategies.

2. **Morbidity**

   a. **Perioperative Myocardial Infarction.** The cumulative perioperative rate of myocardial infarction in the early multicenter studies was 42% (range: 28%-63%).[8,9,18-28] The majority of these patients underwent emergency CABG prior to the widespread use of the perfusion catheter, retrograde coronary sinus cardioplegia administration and use of modified surgical reperfusion described by Buckberg. The full impact of these measures on the incidence of myocardial infarctions as defined by ECG changes and post-operative cardiac enzyme levels remains to be determined. However, a recent review in which pre-procedural platelet inhibition and current surgical techniques were used demonstrated a reduction in the incidence of myocardial infarction to 12.5%.[30] In our own experience, approximately 40% of patients manifested the classic signs of myocardial infarction post-operatively, but show less impressive functional deficits on echocardiographic assessment of the infarct zone and have fewer clinical complications related to the myocardial injury. Clearly, patients with abrupt coronary arterial closure suffer myocardial infarcts; however, the amount of damage seems to be significantly reduced by the measures employed to maintain perfusion and prevent further reperfusion injury.

   b. **Low Cardiac Output State.** During the initial 24 hours following operation, a cardiac index less than 2.0 L/min/m^2 is associated with a higher incidence of multisystem organ dysfunction and death. Nonoliguric renal failure and prolonged mechanical ventilation are the primary non-cardiac complications resulting from poor ventricular function and occur in 5-10% of patients. The majority of patients recover from these complications if they have sufficient systemic reserve and gradual improvement in cardiac function. However, they are very susceptible to recurrent pulmonary edema, ventricular dysrhythmias, pulmonary embolism and sepsis which can result in late death even if they receive meticulous post-operative care.

   c. **Non-Cardiac Morbidity.** Other than post-cardiotomy hemorrhage requiring re-operation and systemic vascular injuries from interventional catheter placement, the incidence of systemic post-CABG complications is similar to that of elective procedure.

* * * * *

REFERENCES

1. Craver JM, Weintraub WS, Jones EL, et. al. Emergency coronary artery bypass surgery for failed percutaneous coronary angioplasty. An Surg 1992; 215:425-433.
2. Vogel JH. Changing trends for surgical standby in patients undergoing percutaneous transluminal coronary angioplasty. Am J Cardiol. 1992; 69:25F-35F.
3. Cameron DE, Stinson DC, Greene PS, et al. Surgical standby for percutaneous coronary angioplasty: "A survey of patterns of practice." An Thoracic Surg 1990;50:35-39.
4. Iniguez A, Macaya C, Hernandez R, et al. Comparison of results of percutaneous Transluminal coronary angioplasty with and without selective requirement of surgical standby. Am J of Cardiology; 1992; 69:1161-1165.
5. Klinke WP and Hui W. Percutaneous transluminal angioplasty without on-site surgical facilities. Am J Cardiology 1992;70:1520-1525.
6. Richardson SG, Morton P, Murtagh JG, et al. Management of acute coronary occlusion during percutaneous coronary angioplasty: "Experience of complications in a hospital without on-site facilities for cardiac surgery." British Med J 1990;300:355-358.
7. Meier B. "Surgical standby for PTCA." Textbook of Interventional Cardiology, E. Topol (Ed) WB Sanders (1994); p. 565-575.
8. Feyter PJ, Jaegere PP, Murphy ES, et al. Abrupt coronary artery occlusion during percutaneous transluminal coronary angioplasty. Am Heart J 1992;123:1633-1642.
9. Scott NA, Weintraub WS, Carlin SF, et al. Recent changes in the management and outcome of acute closure after percutaneous transluminal coronary angioplasty. Am J of Cardiology 1993;71:1159-1163.
10. Lazar HL, Faxon DP, Paone G, et al. Changing profiles of failed coronary angioplasty patients: "Impact on surgical results." Ann Thorac Surg 1992;53:269-273.
11. Greene MA, Gary LA, Slater D, et al. Emergency aortocoronary bypass after failed angioplasty. Ann Thorac Surg 1991;51:194-199.
12. Taylor PC, Boylan MJ, Lytle BW, et al. Emergent coronary bypass for failed PTCA: "A 10-year experience with 253 patients." J Invasive Cardiol :97-98.
13. Carey JA, Davres SW, Balcon R, et al. Emergency surgical revascularization for coronary angioplasty complications. Br. Heart J 1994; 72:428-435.
14. Glick DB, Liddicoat JR, Karp RB. "Alternative conduits for coronary artery bypass grafting." Advances in Cardiac Surgery. RB Karp (Ed) Mosby Year Book(1990) p. 191-201.
15. Piana RN, Paik GY, Moscucci M, et al. Incidence and treatment of no-reflow after percutaneous coronary intervention. Civc 1994;89:2514-2518.
16. Denny TL, Magovern JA, Kao RL, et al. Resuscitation of injured myocardium with adenosine and biventricular assist. Ann Thorac Surg 1993;105:864-884.
17. Allen BS, Buckberg GD, Fontain RM, et al. Superiority of controlled surgical reprfusion versus percutaneous transluminal coronary angioplasty in acute coronary occlusion. J Thorac Cardiovasc Surg; 1993;105:864-884.
18. Lazar HL, Haan CK. Determinants of myocardial infarction following emergency coronary artery bypass for failed percutaneous coronary angioplasty. Ann Thorac Surg 1987;44(56):646-650.
19. Pelletier LC, Pardini A, Renkin J, et al. Myocardial revascularization after failure of percutaneous transluminal coronary angioplasty. J Thorac Cardiovasc Surg 1985;90:265-271.
20. Brediau CE, Roubin GS, Leimgruber PP, et al. In-hospital morbidity and mortality in patients undergoing elective coronary angioplasty. Circulation 1985;72:1044-1052.
21. Acinapura AJ, Cummingham JN Jr, Jacobowitz IJ, et al. Efficacy of percutaneous transluminal coronary angioplasty compared with single-vessel bypass. J Thorac Cardiovasc Surg 1985;89:35-41.
22. Killen DA, Hamaker WR, Reed WA. Coronary artery bypass following percutaneous transluminal coronary angioplasty. Ann Thorac Surg 1985;40:133-138.
23. Golding LA, Loop FD, Hollman JL, et al. Early results of emergency surgery after coronary angioplasty. Circulation 1986;74:(Suppl III), III-26.
24. Parsonnet V, Fisch D, Gielchinsky I, et al. Emergency operation after failed angioplasty. J Thorac Cardiovasc Surg 1988; 96:198-203.

25. Naunheim KS, Fiore AC, Fagan D et al. Emergency coronary artery bypass grafting for failed angioplasty: "Risk factors and outcome." Ann Thorac Surg 1989;47:816-823.
26. Stark KS, Satler LF, Krucoff MW, et al. myocardial salvage after failed coronary angioplasty. J Am Coll Cardiol 1990;15:78-82.
27. Kahn JK, Rutherford BD, McConahy DR, et al. Outcome following emergency coronary artery bypass grafting for failed elective balloon coronary angioplasty in patients with prior coronary bypass. Am J Cardiol 1990; 66: 285-288.
28. Barner HB, LEA IV JW, Naunheim KS, et al. Emergency coronary bypass not associated with pre-operative cardiogenic shock in failed angioplasty, after thrombolysis and for acute myocardial infarction. Civc Suppl. I 1989;79:I152-I159.
29. Clark RE, Acinapura J, Anderson RD, et al. Data analysis of the society of thoracic surgeons. National Cardiac Surgery Database. Tue Third Year-1994, p78.
30. Boerher JD, Kereiakes DJ, Maveita FL, et al. Effects of profound platelet inhibition with c 7E3 before coronary angioplasty an complications of coronary bypass surgery. Am J Cardiol. 1994;74: 1166-1170.

24 RESTENOSIS

Mauro Moscucci, M.D.
David WM Muller, M.B.B.S.

Since the inauguration of PTCA in 1977, advances in catheter technology, operator experience, support systems, imaging modalities, adjunctive pharmacotherapy, and new device techniques have enhanced early outcomes after percutaneous revascularization; high procedural success (> 90%) and low complication rates (< 5%) are readily achieved.[2,3] Despite this achievement, longterm outcome continues to be limited by high restenosis rates: Almost 100,000 patients each year require repeat target lesion revascularization, exposing the patient to additional risks and increasing health care expenditures by $2 billion annually. An improved understanding of the mechanisms of restenosis has led to new mechanical and pharmacological approaches aimed at curbing this vexing problem.

A. **DEFINITIONS.** Restenosis rates are generally reported as "angiographic restenosis," defined according to continuous or binary angiographic variables such as minimal lumen diameter and percent diameter stenosis, and "clinical" restenosis, defined on the basis of clinical variables such as recurrent cardiac events and repeat revascularization.

1. **Angiographic Restenosis**

    a. **Dichotomous Events.** Many definitions view restenosis as a dichotomous event (i.e., either present or absent). The most common definition is diameter stenosis > 50% at follow-up,[8] which was based on early studies showing impaired coronary flow reserve in such lesions.[9] Another common definition is a post-intervention residual stenosis < 50% that increases to > 50% at follow-up; this definition does not necessarily correlate with clinical restenosis, but is often used to compare different treatments or devices. Depending on which definition is chosen (Table 24.1), restenosis rates may vary widely (Figure 24.1).[10]

Table 24.1. Angiographic Definition of Restenosis

EMORY	Diameter stenosis ≥ 50% at follow-up.
NHLBI I	An increase in diameter stenosis ≥ 30% at follow-up (compared to immediately after intervention).
NHLBI II	Residual stenosis < 50% after PTCA increasing to diameter stenosis ≥ 70% at follow-up.
NHLBI III	An increase in diameter stenosis at follow-up to within 10% of the diameter stenosis before PTCA.
NHLBI IV	A > 50% loss of the initial gain achieved after PTCA
THORAXCENTER IIA	≥ 0.72 mm lumen loss at folllow-up.

Abbreviations: NHLBI = National Heart, Lung, and Blood Institute

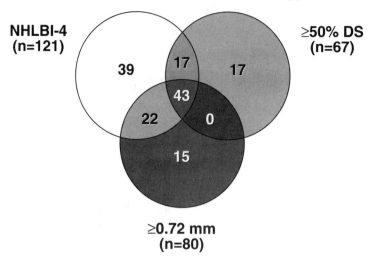

Figure 24.1 Venn Diagram Showing the Number of Lesions with Restenosis Using Three Different Definitions

Adapted from Beatt et al,[10] with permission.

b.   **Continuous outcomes.** "Restenosis" occurs to a variable extent in virtually all lesions,[11] with changes in lumen diameter following a Gaussian distribution.[12] By expressing lumen diameter and diameter stenosis as a cumulative distribution curve, restenosis rates can be determined for any dichotomous definition of restenosis (Figure 24.2). As demonstrated in Figure 24.3, cumulative distribution curves give a better visual estimate of changes in lumen diameter following percutaneous therapy, and allow more effective comparisons between different interventions.

Another important advance in the analysis of restenosis comes from expressing the relationship between lumen diameter at baseline, immediately after intervention, and during follow-up in terms of *acute gain* and *late loss* (Figure 24.4). Acute gain, defined as the difference in lumen diameter before and immediately after intervention, is due to plaque removal and/or arterial expansion. Late loss, defined as the difference in lumen diameter after intervention and at follow-up,[13] reflects the net effects of intimal hyperplasia, elastic recoil, and vascular remodeling.[14] Several studies have shown that the relationship between acute gain and late loss is constant between devices:[15] for every 1 mm of acute gain in lumen diameter, 50% (i.e., 0.5 mm) is lost over 3-6 months.[16,17] However, this relationship has recently been disputed (Chapter 8). The *loss index* is the numerical description of this relationship, and is defined as late loss divided by acute gain;[33] a typical loss index is 0.5.

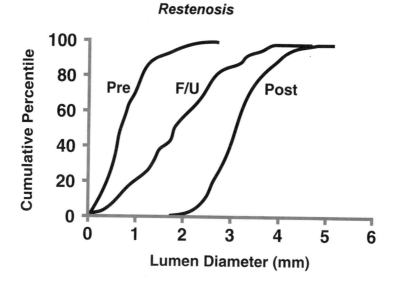

Figure 24.2 Cumulative Frequency Distribution Analysis

Cumulative distribution of baseline minimal lumen diameter (PRE), post intervention minimal lumen diameter (POST), and follow-up minimal lumen diameter (F/U).

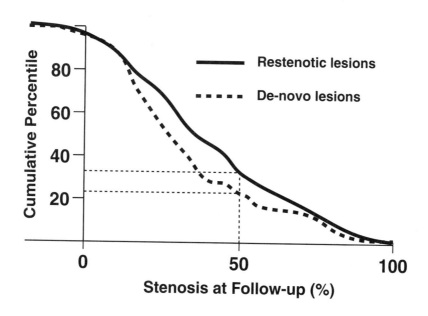

Figure 24.3 Cumulative Frequency Distribution of Diameter Stenosis at Follow-up

If diameter stenosis ≥50% is used as the definition of restenosis, the incidence of restenosis is 24% for de-novo lesions and 37% for restenotic lesions (adapted from Moscucci et al,[54] with permission).

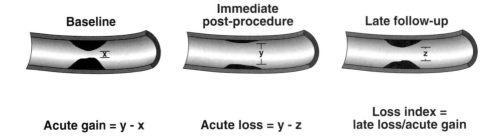

Figure 4.4   Relationship Between Acute Gain, Late Loss, and Loss Index

2. **Clinical Restenosis.** Angiographic analyses offer insight into the mechanisms of restenosis and permit quantitative comparisons between devices. However, the value of an intervention must ultimately be weighed into terms of its impact on clinical outcome, including recurrent angina, objective evidence of ischemia on functional studies, need for repeat revascularization (PTCA or CABG), myocardial infarction and death. The correlation between angiographic findings and clinical symptoms is often poor (Table 24.2). Target lesion revascularization, defined as "clinically-driven" (recurrent symptoms and a positive stress test) revascularization of the original target lesion, has been used as a clinical surrogate for restenosis.[20-22] Repeat revascularization of a residual stenosis > 50% in the absence of objective evidence of ischemia (i.e., "oculostenotic reflex") is *not* considered restenosis by clinical criteria. In the majority of patients, restenosis manifests as recurrent angina; sudden death and myocardial infarction are rare manifestation of restenosis. (Restenotic lesions, which consist primarily of intimal hyperplasia and fibrous tissue, may be less prone to rupture and acute thrombosis.)

Table 24.2.   Correlation Between Angiographic Findings and Clinical Symptoms After Intervention

Presentation	Correlation
Angiographic restenosis	• The stenosis may not be "functionally significant;" patients are often asymptomatic.
No angiographic restenosis	• Single vessel disease: symptoms rare. • Multivessel disease: symptoms may be due to incomplete revascularization and/or progression of underlying atherosclerosis.
Recurrent angina	• Single vessel disease: angiographic restenosis is likely. • Multivessel disease: angiographic restenosis is not necessarily present — symptoms may be due to incomplete revascularization and/or progression of underlying atherosclerosis.[18]
Absence of recurrent symptoms	• Angiographic restenosis is unlikely.[18,19]

B. MECHANISMS OF RESTENOSIS. Restenosis was originally thought to be caused solely by intimal hyperplasia. Data now support the notion that restenosis is a complex process consisting of various degrees of elastic recoil, intimal thickening, and vascular remodeling (Figure 24.5):

1. **Elastic Recoil** is defined as the difference between inflate balloon diameter and minimal lumen diameter upon balloon deflation. The degree of elastic recoil depends on plastic changes in the atherosclerotic plaque and elastic characteristics of the arterial wall. Most elastic recoil occurs within 30 minutes after balloon deflation (but may occur up to 24 hours), can result in a 50% decrease in cross-sectional area,[23] and is more common after PTCA of eccentric and ostial lesions. Elastic recoil is greatest after PTCA, intermediate after DCA, and lowest after stenting. Angiographic analysis suggests that early recoil is associated with a higher incidence of restenosis;[24,25] elimination of elastic recoil may explain the reduction in angiographic restenosis and repeat revascularization after stenting.[22]

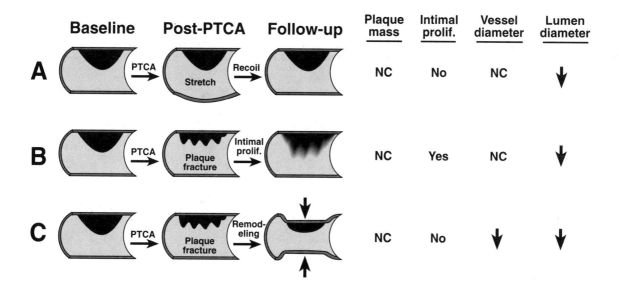

Figure 24.5 Mechanisms of Restenosis

A. Elastic Recoil: After PTCA, there is stretching of the arterial wall, which simply returns to its original dimensions.
B. Intimal Proliferation: After PTCA, there is plaque fracture; the vessel heals by intimal proliferation leading to restenosis.
C. Remodeling: After PTCA, there is plaque fracture; remodeling of the vessel wall leads to a decrease in the normal vessel diameter, and restenosis.
Note: These mechanisms are not mutually exclusive, and may occur together in a given patient.

2. **Intimal Thickening** is a generalized response to vessel injury caused by PTCA and other devices. Activation of the coagulation cascade and inflammatory cells results in the production of chemotactic and growth factors, which lead to thrombus formation, intimal hyperplasia (i.e., smooth muscle cell migration and proliferation), and accumulation of connective tissue matrix. Atherectomy specimens support the proliferative nature of restenosis; de novo lesions are usually hypocellular, whereas restenotic lesions are typically hyperplastic.[26,27] While the angiographic relationship between acute gain and late loss supports a general correlation between the extent of arterial injury and the amount of intimal thickening, some data suggest that the type of injury may be important as well; laser-balloon angioplasty (thermal injury) and possibly DCA may lead to greater intimal hyperplasia than other devices (Section D1, below). Multiple trials using lipid lowering drugs, antimitotics, and other antiproliferative agents have failed to reduce intimal thickening.

3. **Arterial Remodeling.** Experimental studies[28,29] and serial intravascular ultrasound imaging in humans[30] demonstrate a "constriction" or shrinkage of the vessel and loss in luminal diameter after coronary intervention. The ability of stents to virtually eliminate late arterial remodeling is an important factor in the ability of stents to reduce restenosis.

C. **TIME COURSE OF RESTENOSIS.** Restenosis after PTCA is uncommon in the first month, plateaus within 3-6 months, and is unusual after 12 months.[31,32] The time course of restenosis after atherectomy, laser, and stenting is similar to PTCA, but several angiographic studies have shown a further increase in minimal lumen diameter between 6 months and 3 years after stent implantation, suggesting that 6-month angiography may *underestimate* the benefit of stenting.[34,35,36]

D. **PREDICTORS OF RESTENOSIS**
1. **Geometric Factors.** Important studies by Kuntz and colleagues,[13,15,37] and results from the CAVEAT-I[38] and STRESS trials,[20] indicate an inverse relationship between post-procedural lumen diameter and restenosis (i.e., "bigger is better"). These studies found that the device type itself had little if any impact on restenosis. Other studies, however, suggest the contrary: In the ERBAC trial, a trend toward *more* restenosis was observed in the Rotablator and excimer laser groups (vs. PTCA) despite *larger* post-procedural lumen diameters.[39] Very high (> 70%) restenosis rates were also reported after laser balloon angioplasty despite excellent initial lumen enlargement,[40] leading to withdrawal of this device from the market. Another study found that DCA resulted in more late loss than PTCA despite similar acute gains.[41] Collectively, these studies suggest that the final lumen diameter and possibly the device type (i.e., type of vessel injury) impact on late lumen dimensions and restenosis. A final controversy surrounds the impact of deep wall excision during DCA: some studies have shown higher restenosis rates,[42] while other have not.[43]

2. **Biological Factors.** As shown in Table 24.3, certain clinical and angiographic variables have been identified as risk factors for restenosis.

E. PREVENTION OF RESTENOSIS

1. **Pharmacological Interventions.** Over the last decade, there have been numerous clinical trials of fish oil, corticosteroids, cytostatic agents, calcium channel blockers, lipid lowering agents, ACE inhibitors, low molecular weight heparin, high-dose vitamin E, and somatostatin analogues (Figure 24.6); only calcium channel blockers and fish oil appear to have some beneficial effects on restenosis.[59] Two recent randomized trials suggest that c7E3 (platelet GP receptor IIb/IIa inhibitor) and angiopeptin (somatostain analog) significantly decrease clinical restenosis;[60,61] however, follow-up angiography was not performed in the EPIC trial of c7E3, and there was no difference in angiographic restenosis in the angiopeptin trial. This latter trial, in which clinical but not angiographic restenosis was reduced, suggests that plaque stabilization ("passivation") may decrease clinical events without directly impacting intimal proliferation.

2. **Mechanical Interventions.** The Palmaz-Schatz stent is the only device that has been shown to reduce the incidence of restenosis compared to PTCA; randomized trials (STRESS, BENESTENT) have conclusively demonstrated a decrease in restenosis for de novo lesions in native coronary arteries. In addition, multiple observational studies strongly suggest lower restenosis rates in saphenous vein grafts;[66,67] results of the randomized SAVED trial (Stenting or Angioplasty in VE in graft Disease) are expected to confirm these latter studies. The role of other devices in preventing restenosis is uncertain. In the ERBAC trial, despite a lower post-procedural diameter stenoses, restenosis rates were higher after Rotablator and excimer laser compared to PTCA.[39] The impact of optimal debulking technique with the Rotablator (followed by PTCA or stents) is being

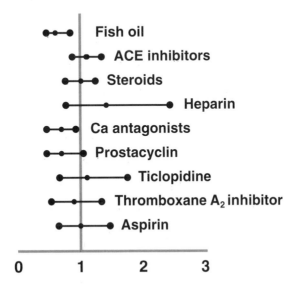

Figure 24.6 Meta-Analysis of Clinical Restenosis Trials

Restenosis is defined as follow-up diameter stenosis $\geq 50\%$ (odds ratio and 95% confidence intervals). Data entries < 1 indicate benefit for restenosis (adapted from Hillegass et al [59]).

Table 24.3 Risk Factors for Primary Restenosis

CLINICAL	YES*	MAYBE	NO**
Variant angina	X		
Recent onset angina (<2-6 mos)	X		
Unstable angina	X		
IDDM	X		
Chronic dialysis	X		
Tobacco use (continued)		X	
Primary PTCA in AMI		X	
Hypercholesterolemia		X	
Male gender		X	
Previous MI			X
Hypertension			X
Age			X
Previous Restenosis			X

ANGIOGRAPHIC			
Long lesion (>20mm)	X		
Multivessel/Multilesional+	X		
SVG (proximal & body lesions)	X		
Chronic total occlusion	X		
Collaterals to dilated vessel	X		
Ostial stenosis	X		
Angulation (>45° angle)	X		
LAD stenosis		X	
Eccentricity			X
Calcification			X
Bifurcation lesion			X
Thrombus			X
Proximal location			X
LIMA			X
SVG (distal anastomosis)			

PROCEDURAL			
Pressure gradient > 20mmHg	X		
Residual stenosis > 30%	X		
No dissection present			X
Balloon inflation variables			
Number of inflations			X
Inflation time			X
Maximum inflation pressure			X
Balloon material			X
Inflation technique			X

*   Majority of studies demonstrate an association

**   Majority of studies fail to find an association

+   Although multivessel/multilesional PTCA leads to an increased probability that at least one lesion will restenose when compared to single lesion PTCA, the overall rate is lower than predicted based on cumulative probabilities.

evaluated in the DART, CARAT, STRATAS, and RotaStent trials (Chapter 27). Ongoing studies of directional atherectomy (OARS, BOAT) will determine whether a reduction in restenosis is possible using "optimal atherectomy" technique (Chapter 27). Ongoing intravascular ultrasound studies will determine whether IVUS-guided stenting further reduces restenosis compared to angiography-guided stenting. Finally, it is unlikely that modifications in PTCA technique or materials will reduce restenosis, although drug-impregnated balloons may emerge as a beneficial technology. Considering the strong correlation between final lumen diameter and restenosis, attempts to optimize lumen dimensions after intervention may be the most practical method to decrease restenosis.

F. DETECTION OF RESTENOSIS

1. **Patients Symptoms.** As previously discussed in Section A2, recurrent symptoms have a low positive predictive value for restenosis; in contrast, absence of symptoms in previously symptomatic patients is good evidence for the absence of restenosis (i.e., good negative predictive value).[72]

2. **Functional Testing (Figure 24.4).** While exercise testing without perfusion imaging can provide useful information about symptomatic status, functional capacity, and the presence of myocardial ischemia, it has low sensitivity for detecting restenosis.[72-74] Stress testing using thallium-201 scintigraphy has better sensitivity (for detection) and specificity (for exclusion) and is often used to evaluate patients with symptoms suggestive of restenosis. Exercise radionuclide angiography has an even better ability to exclude restenosis after a negative test, but only 40% of patients with positive tests have restenosis. Finally, the sensitivity and specificity of exercise and dobutamine echocardiography appear to be similar to thallium-201 scintigraphy.[73]

   It is important to emphasize that functional testing performed within 4 weeks of PTCA is frequently associated with false positive results,[75] which may be due to local vasoconstriction, myocardial stunning, or hibernating myocardium. Therefore, functional testing should be deferred for at least 6 weeks after intervention unless the patient presents with early recurrence of symptoms. Routine serial evaluations after PTCA are usually not recommended,[76] but may be useful in patients with atypical symptoms, silent ischemia, or extensive areas of myocardium at risk.[74,76]

G. CLINICAL FOLLOW-UP OF THE PTCA PATIENT.

The use of noninvasive exercise testing and/or repeat cardiac catheterization in the clinical follow-up of the PTCA patient depends on: 1) the symptomatic status of the patient pre-PTCA; 2) the amount of viable myocardium supplied by the dilated vessel; 3) the extent of associated coronary artery disease; and 4) the adequacy of ventricular function. If the dilated vessel supplies a large amount of viable myocardium, an exercise test is usually performed at 4 weeks; patients are re-cathed for an early or markedly positive test regardless of their symptomatic status. If the dilated vessel supplies a small jeopardized area, asymptomatic individuals are followed clinically; a stress test is recommended if atypical angina develops, and repeat cardiac catheterization is performed for either recurrent typical or atypical angina associated with a positive stress test. Most interventionalists perform an exercise test at 4-6 months after PTCA to screen for restenosis; a possible exception is the individual who is asymptomatic pre-PTCA, is asymptomatic at follow-up, and had a small caliber vessel dilated.

H. MANAGEMENT OF RESTENOSIS. The management of patients with restenosis depends on patient characteristics, myocardium at risk, lesion morphology, extent of coexisting coronary artery disease, and LV function. Repeat PTCA can be performed with high success (> 95%) and low complications rates (< 3-5%),[51-53] and is frequently the procedure of choice for restenosis after PTCA or stenting.[77] Coronary stents have been shown to decrease restenosis in de novo coronary lesions, but are not approved for restenotic lesions. Early registry data suggest higher restenosis rates for stenting of restenotic lesions compared to de novo lesions.[78] More recently, however, a study of 97 restenotic lesions treated with Palmaz-Schatz stenting revealed a restenosis rate of only 19%; compared to patients with restenostic lesions treated by PTCA, those treated by stenting had fewer late cardiac events (4.8% vs. 20%) but more in-hospital complications (6.5% vs. 1.7%).[80] Directional atherectomy can be used to treat restenosis, but restenosis rates tend to be higher for restenotic compared to de novo lesions.[57] In a recent study of 1087 restenotic lesions treated by PTCA, DCA or stents, procedural success was achieved in 94-96%; despite better initial lumen enlargement for DCA and stents, in-hospital complications, recurrent restenosis, and 3-year event-free survival were similar for all 3 devices.[81]

I. RECOMMENDATIONS. The primary prevention of restenosis involves choosing the right device (lesion-specific approach), using techniques to optimize lumen enlargement, and prescribing regimens that aggressively modify risk factors (e.g., HMG CoA reductase inhibitors, antihypertensives, antidiabetes agents, exercise, weight-control, smoking cessation). A good argument can be made for stenting all de novo lesions in vessels > 3.0 mm at moderate-to-high risk for restenosis. Likewise, patients undergoing PTCA or atherectomy for unstable angina, MI, or high-risk lesion morphology as defined in the EPIC trial (Chapter 34) may benefit from a bolus + infusion of ReoPro.

For patients with proven restenosis, repeat percutaneous revascularization (PTCA, DCA, stenting) can be performed with success rates > 95% and sustained clinical benefit in 50-80% of patients. The decision

Table 24.4. Detection of Restenosis

	Positive Predictive Value[†]	Negative Predictive Value[††]
Exercise treadmill		
Without thallium[91-99]	57 ± 2%	75 ± 1%
With thallium[93-97,100-102]	66 ± 2%	81 ± 2%
Radionuclide angiography[91,93,96,103,104]	39 ± 4%	85 ± 2%

† Positive predicte value: The probability of restenosis being present when the test is positive.
†† Negative predictive value: The probability of restenosis being absent when the test is negative.

to perform a third or fourth intervention (as opposed to bypass surgery or medical therapy alone) must taken into account the technical difficulty and angiographic result of the most recent procedure, the time interval to symptom recurrence, the amount of viable myocardium at risk, the extent of associated coronary disease, the adequacy of ventricular function, and the desires of the patient.

J. **FUTURE DIRECTIONS.** Site-specific pharmacological[82] and molecular approaches[83] may prove useful in suppressing intimal hyperplasia and curbing restenosis. Some studies suggest that local drug delivery may be useful for treating thrombus in unstable angina or after coronary interventions,[84] although inhibition of intimal hyperplasia after balloon injury has not been demonstrated. Finally, several experimental studies suggest a role for vascular gene therapy,[89,90] in which a particular gene is overexpressed, and for antisense oligonucleotides,[85-90] which inhibit cell proliferation by preventing gene expression.

* * * * *

REFERENCES

1.   Gruentzig AR. Transluminal dilatation of coronary artery stenoses. Lancet 1978;1:263.

2.   Baim DS (ed): A symposium: Interventional Cardiology-1987. Am J Cardiol 1988;61:1g-117g.

3.   Detre K, Holubkov R, Kelsey S, et al. Percutaneous transluminal coronary angioplasty in 1985-1986 and 1977-1981. The National Heart, Lung and Blood Institute Registry. N Engl J Med 1988;318:265-270

4.   Gruentzig AR, King SB III, Schlumpf M., et al. Long-term follow-up after percutaneous transluminal coronary angioplasty. The early Zurich experience. N Engl J Med. 1987;316:1127-1132.

5.   Parisi AF, Folland ED, Hartigan P. A comparison of angioplasty with medical therapy in the treatment of single vessel coronary disease. Veterans Affairs ACME Investigators. N Engl J Med 1992;326:10-16.

6.   Goy JJ, Eeckhout E, Burnand B et al. Coronary angioplasty versus left internal mammary artery grafting for isolated proximal left anterior descending artery stenosis. Lancet 1994;343:1449-1453.

7.   Coronary angioplasty versus coronary artery bypass surgery: the Randomized Intervention Treatment of Angina (RITA) trial. Lancet 1993;341:573-380.

8.   Roubin G, King SI, Douglas J, JR. Restenosis after percutaneous transluminal coronary angioplasty: The Emory University Hospital experience. Am J Cardiol 1987;60:39B-43B.

9.   Gould K, Lipscomb K, Hamilton G. Physiological basis for assessing critical coronary stenosis: instantaneous flow response and regional distribution during coronary hyperemia as measures of coronary flow reserve. Am J Cardiol 1974;33:87-97.

10. Beatt KJ, Serruys PW, Renseing BJ, Hugenoltz PG. Restenosis after coronary angioplasty: New standards for clinical studies. J Am Coll Cardiol 1990;15:491-498.

11. Beatt KJ, Luijten H, de Feyter P, van den Brand M, Reiber J, Serruys P. Change in diameter of coronary artery segments adjacent to stenosis after percutaneous transluminal coronary angioplasty: Failure of percent diameter stenosis measurement to reflect morphologic changes induced by balloon dilation. J Am Coll Cardiol 1988;12:315-323.

12. Rensing BJ, Hermans WM, Deckers JW, deFeyter PJ. Lumen narrowing after percutaneous transluminal coronary balloon angioplasty follows a near gaussian distribution: A quantitative angiographic study in 1,445 successfully dilated lesions. J Am Coll Cardiol 1992;19:939-945.

13. Kuntz R, Safian R, Levine M, Reis G, Diver D, Baim D. Novel approach to the analysis of restenosis after the use of three new coronary devices. J Am Coll Cardiol 1992;19:1493-1499.

14. Gordon PC, Gibson M, Cohen DJ, Carrozza J, Kuntz R, Baim D. Mechanisms of restenosis and redilation within coronary stents-quantitative angiographic assessment. J Am Coll Cardiol 1993;21:1166-1174.

15. Kuntz RE, Gibson CM, Nobuyoshi M, Baim DS. Generalized model of restenosis after conventional balloon angioplasty, stenting and directional atherectomy. J Am Coll Cardiol 1993;21:15-25.

16. Schwartz R, Huber K, Murphy J, et al. Restenosis and the proportional neointimal response to coronary artery injury: Results in a porcine model. J Am Coll Cardiol 1992;19:267-274.

17. Beatt KJ, Serruys PW, Luijten HE, et al. Restenosis after coronary angioplasty: The paradox of increased lumen diameter and restenosis. J Am Coll Cardiol 1992;19:258-266.

18. Holmes D, Vlietstra R, Smith H, et al. Restenosis after percutaneous transluminal coronary angioplasty (PTCA): a report from the PTCA Registry of the NHLBI. Am J Cardiol 1984;53:77C-81C.

19. Gruentzig AR, King SB III, Schlumpf M, et al. Long term follow-up after percutaneous transluminal coronary angioplasty. The early Zurich experience. N Engl J Med 1987;316:1127-1132.

20. Fishman D, Leon M, Baim D. A randomized comparison of coronary stent placement and balloon angioplasty in the treatment of coronary artery disease. N Engl J Med 1994;331:496-501.

21. Serruys P, deJegere P, Kiemeneij F, et al. A comparison of balloon expandable stent implantation with balloon angioplasty in patients with coronary artery disease. N Engl J Med 1994;331(8):489-495.

22. Rodriguez A, Santaera O, Larribau M, et al. Coronary stenting decreases restenosis in lesions with early loss in luminal diameter 24 hours after successful PTCA. Circulation 1995;91:1397-1402.

23. Rensing BJ, Hermans WRM, Beatt KJ, et al. Quantitative angiographic assessment of elastic recoil after percutaneous transluminal coronary angiography. Am J Cardiol 1990;66:1039-1044.

24. Rodriguez A, Lassileau M, Santaera O, et al. Early decreases in minimal luminal diameter after PTCA are associated with higher incidence of late restenosis. J Am Coll Cardiol 1993;21:34A.

25. LaBlanche Jm on behalf of the FACT. Investigators. Recoil twenty-four hours after coronary angioplasty: A

computerized angiographic study. J Am Coll Cardiol 1993;21:34A.

26. Johnson DE, Hinohara T, Selmon MR, Braden LJ. Primary peripheral arterial stenoses and restenoses excised by transluminal atherectomy: A histopathologic study. J Am Coll Cardiol 1990;15:419-425.

27. Garratt K, Edwards W, Kaufmann U, Vlietstra R, Holmes D. Differential histopathology of primary atherosclerotic and restenotic lesions in coronary arteries and saphenous vein bypass grafts: Analysis of tissue obtained from 73 patients by directional atherectomy. J Am Coll Cardiol 1991;17:442-448.

28. Post M, Borst C, Kuntz R. The relative importance of arterial remodeling compared with intimal hyperplasia in lumen renarrowing after balloon angioplasty (A study in the normal rabbit and the hypercholesterolemic Yucatan micropig). Circulation 1994;89:2816-2821.

29. Lafont A, Guzman L, PL W. Restenosis after experimental angioplasty. Intimal, medial and adventitial changes associated with constrictive remodeling. Circ Res 1995;76:996-1002.

30. Mintz G, Kovach J, Javier S, Ditrano C, Leon M. Geometric remodeling is the predominant mechanism of late lumen loss after coronary angioplasty. Circulation 1993;88:I-654.

31. Serruys PW, Luijten HE, Beatt KJ, et al. Incidence of restenosis after successful coronary angioplasty: a time-related phenomenon. A quantitative angiographic study in 342 consecutive patients at 1, 2, 3, and 4 months. Circulation 1988;77:361-371.

32. Nobuyoshi M, Kimura T, Nosaka H, Mioka S. Restenosis after successful percutaneous transluminal coronary angioplasty: Serial angiographic follow-up of 229 patients. J Am Coll Cardiol 1988;12:616-623.

33. Guidance for the Submission of Research and Marketing Applications for Interventional Cardiology Devices: PTCA Catheters, Atherectomy Catheters, lasers, Intravascular Stents. Interventional Cardiology Devices Branch, Division of Cardiovascular, Respiratory and Neurology Devices, Office of device Evaluation, US Food and Drug Administration, May 1993:29.

34. Kimura T, Yokoi H, Tamura T, Nakagawa Y, Nosaka H, Nobuyoshi M. Three years clinical and quantitative angiographic follow-up after the Palmaz-Schatz coronary stent implantation. J Am Coll Cardiol 1995;25:375A.

35. Hermiller J, Fry E, Peters T, et al. Late lesion regression within the Gianturco-Roubin Flex stent. J Am Coll Cardiol 1995;25`:375A.

36. Kimura T, Nosaka H, Yokoi H, Iwabuchi M. Serial angiographic follow-up after Palmaz-Schatz stent implantation: Comparison with conventional balloon angioplasty. J Am Coll Cardiol 1993;21:1557-1563.

37. Kuntz R, Safian R, Carrozza J, Fishman R, Mansour M, Baim D. The importance of acute luminal diameter in determining restenosis after coronary atherectomy or stenting. Circulation 1992;86:1827-1835.

38. Topol E, Leya F, Pinkerton C, et al. A comparison of directional atherectomy with coronary angioplasty in patients with coronary artery disease. N Engl J Med 1993;329:221-227.

39. Vandormeal M, Reifart N, Preusler W, et al. Comparison of excimer laer angioplasty and rotational atherectomy wtih balloon angioplasty for complex lesions: ERBAC study final results. J Am Coll Cardiol 1994;57A.

40. Spears JR, Reyes VP, Wynne J, et al. Percutaneous coronary laser balloon angioplasty: Initial results of a multicenter experience. J Am Coll Cardiol 1990;16:293-303.

41. Umans VAWM, Keane D, Foley D, et al. Optimal use of directional coronary atherectomy is required to ensure long-term angiographic benefit: A study with matched procedural outcome after atherectomy and angioplasty. J Am Coll Cardiol 1994;24:1652-1659.

42. Garratt KN, Holmes DR, Bell MR, et al. Restenosis after directional coronary atherectomy: differences between primary atheromatous and restenosis lesions and influence of subintimal tissue resection. J Am Coll Cardiol 1990;16:1665-1671.

43. Kuntz RE, Hinohara T, Safian RD, et al. Restenosis after directional coronary atherectomy: effects of luminal diameter and deep wal excision. Circulation 1992;86:1394-1399.

44. Carrozza JR, Kuntz RE, Fishman RF, Baim DS. Restenosis after arterial injury caused by coronary stenting in patients with diabetes mellitus. Ann Intern Med. 1993;118(5):344-349.

45. Simons M, Leclerc G, Safian RD, Isner JM. Relation between activated smooth-muscle cells in coronary artery lesions and restenosis after atherectomy. N Engl J Med 1993;328:608-613.

46. Kuntz RE, Hinohara T, Robertson GC, et al. Influence of vessel selction on the observed restenosis rate after endoluminal stenting or directional coronary atherectomy. Am J Cardiol 1992;70:1101-1108.

47. Hirshfeld JW, Schwartz JS, Jugo R, et al. Restenosis after coronary angioplasty: A multivariate statistical model to relate lesion and procedure variables to restenosis. J Am Coll Cardiol 1991;18:647-656.

48. Hermans WR, Rensing BJ, Kelder JC, et al. Postangioplasty restenosis rate between segments of the major coronary

arteries. Am J Cardiol 1992;194-200.

49.   Violaris A, Melkert R, Serruys P. Influence of serum cholesterol and cholesterol subfractions on restenosis after successful coronary angioplasty. A quantitative angiographic analysis of 3336 lesions. Circulation 1994;90:2267-2279.

50.   Fishman RF, Kuntz RE, Carrozza JP, Miller MJ, et al. Long-term results of directional coronary atherectomy: Predictors of restenosis. J Am Coll Cardiol 1992;20:1101-1110.

51.   Williams DO, Gruentzig A, Kent K, Detre K, Kelsey S, To T. Efficacy of repeat percutaneous transluminal coronary angioplasty for coronary restenosis. Am J Cardiol 1984;53:32C-35C.

52.   Dimas AP, Grigera F, Arora RR, et al. Repeat coronary angioplasty as treatment for restenosis. J Am Coll Cardiol 1992;19:1310-1314.

53.   Meier B, King SBI, Gruentzig AR. Repeat coronary angioplasty. J Am Coll Cardiol 1984;4:463-466.

54.   Moscucci M, Piana R, Kuntz R, Kugelmass A. The effect of prior coronary restenosis on the risk of subsequent restenosis after stent placement or directional atherectomy. Am J Cardiol 1994;73:1147-1153.

55.   Glazier J, Varricchione T, Ryan T. Factors predicting recurrent restenosis after percutaneous transluminal coronary balloon angioplasty. Am J Cardiol 1989;63:902-905.

56.   Quigley P, Hlatky M, Hinohara T. Repeat percutaneous transluminal coronary angioplasty and predictors of recurrent restenosis. Am J Cardiol 1989;63:409-413.

57.   Hinohara T, Robertson G, Selmon M, et al. Restenosis after directional coronary atherectomy. J Am Coll Cardiol 1992;20:623-632.

58.   Teirstein P, Hoover C, Ligon R. Repeat coronary angioplasty: Efficacy of a third angioplasty for a second restenosis. J Am Coll Cardiol 1989;13:291-296.

59.   Hillegass WB, Ohman ME and Califf RM. Restenosis: the clinical issues. In Topol EJ (ed). Textbook of Interventional Cardiology, 2nd Edition, Philadelphia, WB Saunders Company, 1993; 415-435.

60.   Topol E, Califf R, Weisman H, et al. Randomized trial of coronary intervention with antibody against platelet IIb/IIIa integrine for reduction of clinical restenosis: results at six months. Lancet 1994;343:881-86.

61.   Emanuelsson H, Beatt K, Bagger J. Long-term effects of angiopeptine treatment in coronary angioplasty. Reduction of clinical events but not of angiographic restenosis. European Angiopeptin Study Group. Circulation 1995;91:1689-1696.

62.   Safian RD, Hoffmann MA, Almany S, et al. Comparison of coronary angioplasty with compliant and noncomplicqant balloons (The Angioplasty Compliance Trial). Am J Cardiol 1995;76:518-520.

63.   DiSciascio G, Vetrovec GW, Lewis SA, et al. Clinical and angiographic recurrence following PTCA for nonacute total occlusions: comparisons of one versus five minute inflations. Am Heart J 1990;120:529-532.

64.   Ohman EM, Marquis JF, Ricci DR, et al. A randomized comparison of the effects of gradual prolonged versus standard primary balloon inflation on early and late outcome. Results of a multicenter clinical trial. Perfusion Balloon Catheter Study Group. Circulation 1994;89:1118-1125.

65.   Roubin GS, Douglas JS, King SB, et al. Influence of balloon size on initial success rate, acute complications, and restenosis after PTCA. Circulation 1988;78:557-565.

66.   Piana R, Moscucci M, Cohen D, et al. Palmaz-Schatz stenting for treatment of focal vein graft stenosis: Immediate results and long-term outcome. J Am Coll Cardiol 1994;23:1296-304.

67.   Wong SC, Baim DS, Schatz RA, et al. Immediat results and late outcomes after stent implantation in saphenous vein graft lesions: the multicenter U.S. Palmaz-Schatz stent experience. J Am Coll Cardiol 1995;26:704-712.

68.   Simonton CA, Leon MB, Kuntz RE, et al. Acute and late clinical and angiographic results of directional atherectomy in the optimal atherectomy restenosis study (OARS). Circulation 1995;92:I-545.

69.   Baim DS, Kuntz RE, Sharma SK, et al. Acute and late results of phase of the balloon versus optimal atherectomy trial (BOAT). Circulation 1995;92:I-544.

70.   Colombo A, Hall P, Nakamura S, et al. Intracoronary stenting without anticoagluation accomplished with intravascular ultrasound guidance. Circulation 1995;91:167.

71.   Russo RJ, Teirstin PS for the AVID investigators. Angiography versus intravascular ultrasound-directed stent placement. Circulation 1995;92:I-546.

72.   Bengston J, Mark D, Honan M. Detection of restenosis after elective percutaneous transluminal angioplasty using the exercise treadmill test. Am J Cardiol 1990;65:28-34.

73.   Hecht H, DeBord L, Shaw R. Usefulness of supine bicycle stress echocardiography for the detection of restenosis after percutaneous transluminal coronary angioplasty. Am J Cardiol 1993;71:293-296.

74. Pfisterer M, Rickenbacher P, Klowski W, Muller-Brand J. Silent ischemia after percutaneous transluminal coronary angioplasty: Incidence and prognostic significance. J Am Coll Cardiol 1993;22:1446-1454.

75. Manyari D, Knudtson M, Kloiber R. Sequential thallium-201 myocardial perfusion studies after successful percutaneous transluminal coronary angioplasty: delayed resolution of exercise-induced scintigraphic abnormalities. Circulation 1988;77:86-95.

76. Miller D, Verani M. Current status of myocardial perfusion imaging after percutaneous transluminal coronary angioplasty. J Am Coll Cardiol 1994;24:260-266.

77. Baim D, Levine M, Leon M, Levine S, Ellis S, Schatz R. Management of restenosis within the Palmaz-Schatz coronary stent (the U.S. multicenter experience). Am J Cardiol 1993;71:364-366.

78. Ellis SG, Savage M, Fishman D, et al. Restenosis after placemnet of Palmaz-Schatz stents in native coronary arteries. Initial results of a multicenter experience. Circulation 1992;86:1836-1844.

79. Colombo A, Almagor Y, Maiello L, et al. Results of coronary stenting for restenosis. J Am Coll Cardiol 1994;23:118A.

80. Penn I, Ricci D, Almond DG, et al. Stenting results in increased early complications and fewer late reinterventions: Final clinical data from the trial of Angioplasty and Stents in Canada (TASC) I. Circulation 1995;92:I-475.

81. Waksman R, Weintraub WS, Ziyad MB, Douglas JS, Shen Y, King SB. Balloon angioplasty, Palmax-Schatz stent, and directional coronary atherectomy for restenotic lesions: Retrospective comparison in a single center. J Am Coll Cardiol 1995;25;330A.

82. Muller DWM. Restenosis: site-specific therapy. In Topol EJ (ed). Textbook of Interventional Cardiology, 2nd Edition, Philadelphia, WB Saunders Company, 1993; 436-448.

83. Muller DWM. Gene therapy for cardiovascular disease. Br Heart J 1994;71:309-311.

84. Mitchell JR, Arzin MA, Fram DB, et al. Inhibition of platelet deposition and lysis of intracoronary thrombus during balloon angioplasty using urokinase-coated hydrogel balloons. Circulation 1994;90:1979-1988.

85. Ohno T, Gordon D, San H, et al. Gene therapy for vascular smooth muscle cell proliferation after arterial injury. Science 1994;265:781-784.

86. von der Leyen HE, Gibbons GH, Morishita R, et al. Gene therapy inhibiting neointimal vascular lesion: in vivo transfer of endothelial cell nitric oxide synthase gene. Proc Natl Acad Sci USA 1995;92:1137-1141.

87. Change MW, Barr E, Seltzer J, et al. Cytostatic gene therapy for vascular proliferative disorders with a constitutively active form of the retinoblastoma gene product. Science 1995;267:518-522.

88. Asahara T, Bauters C, Pastroe C, et al. Local delivery of vascular endothelial growth factor accelerates reendothelialization and attenuates intimal hyperplasia in balloon-injured rate carotid artery. Circulation 1995;91:2793-2801.

89. Simons M, Edelman ER, Dekeyser JL, et al. Antisense c-myb oligonucleotides inhibit intimal arterial smooth muscle cell accumulation in vivo. Nature 1992;359:67-70.

90. Morhisita R, Gibbons GH, Ellison KE, et al. Initimal hyperplasia after vascular injury is inhibited by antisence cdk2kinase oligonuclerotides. J Clin Invest 1994;93:1458-1464.

91. O'Keefe JH, Lapeyre AC, Holmes DR, et al. Usefulness of early radionuclide angiography for identifying low-risk patients for late restenosis after percutaneous transluminal coronary angioplasty. Am J Cardiol 1988;61:51-54.

92. El-Tamimi H, Davies GJ, Hackett D, et al. Very early prediction of restenosis after successful coronary angioplasty: Anatomic and functional assessment. J Am Coll Cardiol 1990;15:259-264.

93 Wijns W, Serruys P, Reiber J, et al. Early detection of restenosis after successful percutaneous transluminal coronary angioplasty by exercise-redistribution thallium scintigraphy. Am J Cardiol 1985;55:357-361.

94. Wijns W, Serruys PW, Simoons ML, van den Brand M, de Feyter PJ, Reiber JH, Hugenholtz PG. Predictive value of early maximal exercise test and thallium scintigraphy after successful percutaneous transluminal coronary angioplasty. Br Heart J 1985;53:194-200.

95. Scholl JM, Chaitman BR, David PR, et al. Exercise electrocardiography and myocardial scintigraphy in the serial evaluation of the results of percutaneous transluminal coronary angioplasty. Circulation 1982;66:380-390.

96. Ernst SMPG, Hillebrand FA, Kelin B, et al. The value of exercise tests in the follow-up of patients who underwent transluminal coronary angioplasty. Int J Cardiol 1985;7:267-279.

97. Rosing DR, Van Raden MJ, Mincemoyer RM, et al. Exercise, electrocardiographic and functional responses after percutaneous transluminal coronary angioplasty. Am J Cardiol 1984;53:36C-41C.

98. Honan MB, Bengtson JR, Pryor DB, et al. Exercise treadmill testing is a poor predictor of anatomic restenosis after angioplasty for acute myocardial infarction. Circulation 1989;80:1585-94.

99. Hillegass WB, Ancukiewicz M, Bengtson JR, et al. Does follow-up exercise testing predict restenosis after successful balloon angioplasty? Circulation 1992;I-137.

100. Hardoff R, Shefer A, Gips S, et al. Predicting late restenosis after coronary angioplasty by very early (12 to 24 h) thallium-201 scintigraphy: implications with regard to mechanisms of late coronary restenosis. J Am Coll Cardiol 1990;15:1486-1492.

101. Jain A, Mahmarian JJ, Borges-Neto S, et al. Clinical significance of perfusion defects by thallium-201 single photon emission tomography following oral dipyridamole early after coronary angioplasty. J Am Coll Cardiol 1988;11:970-976.

102. Lam JYT, Chaitman BR, Byers S, et al. Can dipyridamole thallium imaging predict restenosis after coronary angioplasty? Circulation 1987;76:373.

103. DePuey EF, Leatherman RD, Dear WE, et al. Restenosis after transluminal coronary angioplasty detected with exercise-gated radionuclide ventriculography. J Am Coll Cardiol 1984;4:1103-1113.

104. DePuey EG, Boskovic D, Krajcer Z, et al. Exercise radionuclide ventriculography in evaluating successful transluminal coronary angioplasty. Cathet Cardiovasc Diagn 1983;9:153-166.

105. Ellis SG, Roubin GS, King SB III, et al. Importance of Stenosis Morphology in the Estimation of Restenosis Risk After Elective Percutaneous Transluminal Coronary Angioplasty. Am J Cardiol 1989;63:30-34.

106. Leimgruber PP, Roubin GS, Hollman J, et al. Restenosis After Successful Coronary Angioplasty in Patients with Single-Vessel Disease. Circulation 1986;73:710-717.

107. Roubin GS, King SB III, Douglas JS Jr. Restenosis After Percutaneous Transluminal Coronary Angioplasty: The Emory University Hospital Experience. Am J Cardiol 1987;60:39B-43B.

108. Kahn JK, Rutherford BD, McConahay DR, et al. Short and Long-Term Outcome of Percutaneous Transluminal Coronary Angioplasty in Chronic Dialysis Patients. Am Heart J 1990;119:484-489.

109. Galan KM, Deligonul U, Kern MJ, et al. Increased Frequency of Restenosis in Patients Continuing to Smoke Cigarettes After Percutaneous Transluminal Coronary Angioplasty. Am J Cardiol 1988;61:260-263.

110. Vandormael MG, Deligonul U, Kern MJ, et al. Multilesion Coronary Angioplasty: clinical and Angiographic Follow-up. J Am Coll Cardiol 1987;10:246-252.

111. Myler RK, Topol EJ, Shaw RE, et al. Multiple Vessel Coronary Angioplasty: Classification, Results and Patterns of Restenosis in 494 Consecutive Patients. Cathet Cardiovasc Diagn 1987;13:1-15.

112. Cowley MJ, Mullin SM, Kelsey SF, et al. Sex Differences in Early and Long-Term Results of Coronary Angioplasty in the NHLBI PTCA Registry. Circulation 1985;71:90-97.

113. Topol EJ, Ellis SG, Fishman J, et al. Multicenter Study of Percutaneous Transluminal Coronary Angioplasty for Right Coronary Artery Ostial Stenosis. J Am coll Cardiol 1987;9:1214-1218.

114. Holmes DR Jr, Vliestra RE, Smith HC, et al. Restenosis After Percutaneous Transluminal Coronary Angioplasty: A Report from the PTCA Registry of the National Heart, Lung, and Blood Institute. Am J Cardiol 1984;53:77C-81C.

115. Jacobs AK, Folan DJ, McSweeney SM, et al. Effect of Plasma Lipids on Restenosis Following Coronary Angioplasty. J Am Coll Cardiol 1987;9:183 Abstract.

116. Melchior JP, Meier B, Urban P, et al. Percutaneous Transluminal Coronary Angioplasty for Chronic Total Coronary Arterial Occlusion. Am J Cardiol 1987;59:535-538.

117. Block PC, Cowley MJ, Kaltenbach M, et al. Percutaneous Angioplasty of Stenoses of Bypass Grafts or of Bypass Graft Anastomotic Sites. Am J Cardiol 1984;53:666-668.

25 MEDICAL AND PERIPHERAL VASCULAR COMPLICATIONS

James W. Kinn, M.D.
Steven C. Ajluni, M.D.
Cindy L. Grines, M.D.

RENAL INSUFFICIENCY

Depending upon the etiology, PTCA-induced renal insufficiency may be transient and quickly respond to medical measures or may progress to oliguric renal failure with volume overload, electrolyte and acid-base disturbances, and frank uremia. The most common manifestations include decreasing urine output and a rising serum creatinine in the may first hours to 3-5 days after PTCA. Early recognition, diagnosis and treatment may prevent progression to frank renal failure.

A. **ETIOLOGY.** Common causes of renal insufficiency in the post-PTCA patient are listed in Table 25.1. The most common cause is dye-induced tubular injury with or without superimposed hypovolemia (NPO status, dye-induced diuresis, procedural blood loss). Less common causes include prerenal azotemia from PTCA-induced myocardial ischemia and LV dysfunction, renal ischemia from angiotensin converting enzyme inhibitors, athero- or thromboembolism, aortic dissection, a malpositioned intra-aortic balloon pump, and post-renal obstruction from prostatism or anticholinergic drug administrations. Dye-induced renal dysfunction is the most common cause of renal insufficiency in the PTCA patient. Defined as a rise in serum creatinine >25% within 48 hrs of exposure, the incidence of dye-induced renal dysfunction varies from <1% in normal patients to approximately 50% in the highest risk groups.[1-3] Proposed mechanisms for renal dysfunction following dye exposure include: a direct reduction in renal perfusion; a secondary reduction in renal perfusion secondary to dye-induced LV dysfunction; direct tubular injury; and a hypersensitivity reaction leading to immune-mediated intraluminal obstruction.[2,3] Patients with pre-existing renal insufficiency are most susceptible to dye-induced nephrotoxicity; those with diabetic nephropathy are highest risk. Other risk factors for renal dysfunction in high-risk patients include contrast load, baseline hypovolemia, and impaired left ventricular function. Once renal dysfunction develops, creatinine levels generally peak at 3-5 days and remain elevated for 1-2 weeks.[3,4] Oliguria occurs in 30% of patients. Although recovery is most common, some patients develop irreversible renal failure requiring temporary or permanent dialysis.

B. **PREVENTION.** Patients with pre-existing renal insufficiency, diabetic nephropathy, or a history of prior renal dysfunction following contrast exposure are at increased risk of dye-induced renal failure. Maintaining optimal intravascular volume status in the most important patient is goal of therapy, and may be challenging if the NPO, dye induced diuresis or blood loss. The administration of intravenous fluids (100-150cc/hr) for 8-10 hours prior to PTCA is common practice in the high risk group. Patients with left ventricular dysfunction at risk for renal failure may also require less pre-procedural

Table 25.1 Causes of Acute Renal Insufficiency in the PTCA Patient

ETIOLOGY	COMMENTS
A. PRERENAL	
Volume depletion	Oliguria usually responds quickly to fluids or blood as needed
• NPO status	
• Dye-induced diuresis	
• Blood loss (procedural, GI, retro-peritoneal)	
Diminished cardiac output	
• Dye-induced	May need nitrates and/or diuretics instead of volume expansion; use
• Ischemia	Swan-Ganz catheter to guide therapy. ECG to exclude threatened or acute closure
B. RENAL	
Acute tubular necrosis	Peak creatinine in 3-5 days, followed by slow recovery (days) and
• Dye-induced	post-azotemia diuresis. Oliguria in 30%. Fluid hydration, diuretics,
• Renal ischemia	mannitol, dopamine, stopping dipyridamole and starting theophylline
• Atheroembolism	may be of benefit
• Thromboembolism	Look for signs of embolic phenomenon (e.g., livedo reticular is).
• Aortic dissection	Check position of IABP. Discontinue recently prescribed ACE
• Malposition of IABP	inhibitors
• Drugs	
C. POST-RENAL	
Obstruction	Keep well hydrated. Avoid atropine. Foley catheter for diagnosis and
• Tubular (clots, dye-induced)	treatment
• Bladder outlet (prostatism, anticholinergic drugs)	

intravenous hydration and diuretics to maintain urine output. For patients with severe left ventricular dysfunction, pulmonary capillary wedge pressure measurements before, during and after the procedure may help guide fluid management. Noniomic contrast agents are associated with less volume overload than ionic agents, but do not decrease the risk of contrast nephropathy.[5,6]

In addition to optimizing hydration status, loop diuretics, mannitol, and dopamine are sometimes employed. Several small studies have reported equivocal results, but are limited by small sample size, lack of control group, and uncertain baseline volume status. Loop diuretics theoretically protect against contrast-induced nephropathy, but Weinstein[7] found that prophylactic furosemide had deleterious effects on renal function due to volume depletion. Therefore, loop diuretics as prophylaxis for renal failure should be accompanied by intravenous fluids or hemodynamic monitoring to avoid hypovolemia.

Mannitol (12.5-25gm IV) may provide prophylaxis against renal failure by increasing solute excretion and decreasing tubular obstruction, and may be of greater benefit in nondiabetic patients.[8] Mannitol may have an additional renal protective effects in intravascular hemolysis, hemoglobinuria, and extreme hyperuricemia. Since mannitol is a volume expander, it should be used with caution in patients with left ventricular dysfunction and congestive heart failure. Finally, the potential for mannitol associated dehydration may have similar deleterious effects as demonstrated with loop diuretics

Dopamine increases renal blood flow, sodium excretion and glomerular filtration rate, but the benefits in preventing contrast nephropathy are unclear. Weisberg[8] reported a benefit in non-diabetics, but there was a greater incidence of contrast nephropathy in diabetic patients. Given the role of endogenous intrarenal adenosine in the pathogenesis of contrast induced nephrotoxicity, a recent study demonstrated that contrast-induced renal dysfunction was exacerbated by dipyridamole,[11] and attenuated by theophylline (2.9 mg/kg PO Q 12 hrs x 4, starting one hour before contrast).[12] In summary, these pharmacologic agents may be useful as prophylaxis against renal failure, but they may need to be tailored to the individual patient with careful attention to fluid status and other medical conditions. Prospective randomized studies of hydration, diuretics, mannitol and dopamine are underway.

C. **MANAGEMENT.** Serum creatinine should be routinely obtained 12-24 hrs following PTCA. If the creatinine is elevated, follow-up measurements should be obtained and medical measures instituted until renal function has stabilized. For a decreasing urine output and/or a rising serum creatinine in the post-PTCA patient:

1. **Exclude Bleeding and Bladder Outlet Obstruction.** On occasion, retroperitoneal or GI bleeding, or bladder obstruction (particularly in males with prostatic enlargement) may first manifest as diminished urine output. These conditions must be excluded early, since they are readily reversible and their treatment is different from that of contrast nephropathy.

2. **Maintain Adequate Hydration and Urine Output.** Vigorous post-procedure hydration (100-150cc of crystalloid x 6-12 hrs; 1-2 L of water orally) help to maintain a stable blood pressure and urine output, thus facilitating excretion of the contrast agent. A helpful "rule of thumb" is to match urine output with IV fluids during the first 8-10 hrs post-procedure. If the urine output falls below 40-60cc/hr, intravenous fluids are increased (may give 200cc boluses of normal saline in those without evidence of congestive heart failure). If the patient is felt to have adequate intravascular volume, especially in the presence of baseline LV dysfunction or renal insufficiency, diuretics (furosemide 20-80mg IV over 1-2 minutes) will frequently relieve the prerenal state. Loop diuretics have an advantage over other diuretics because they are effective in patients with reduced glomerular filtration rate (GFR). Metolazone, a thiazide-like diuretic, is also effective in patients with reduced GFR. For severe oliguria, the combination of these agents has the theoretical advantage over either agent alone because they result in sequential nephron blockade.[9] Dopamine may add some additional benefit and is commonly added in low doses (5ug/min IV) for patients with severe oliguria. Right heart catheterization and hemodynamic monitoring should be considered in all cases of oliguria or anuria when the volume status is in question.

3. **Consult a Nephrologist.** Renal deterioration which is progressive or persistent should prompt consultation with a nephrologist. Additional noninvasive or invasive tests (e.g., renal scan, ultrasound, angiogram) as well as the institution of dialysis (primarily in cases of severe acute tubular necrosis or atheroembolism) should be performed as necessary.

CONTRAST REACTIONS

A. **TYPES OF CONTRAST AGENTS**
    1. **High-Osmolar Contrast Media.** These ionic agents are salts and consist of three iodine atoms bound to a fully substituted benzene ring (anion) and either a methylglucamine and/or sodium ion. In the aqueous phase, this results in the generation of two osmotically active particles. Given a minimum iodine content required for adequate coronary opacification of 320 mg/ml, this means that most ionic agents have an osmolarity (1400-2400 mOsm/L) which is 5-8 times higher than blood (275 mOsm/L) and a sodium content 1-7 times that of plasma. In addition, all ionic agents contain additives which bind ionized calcium.

    2. **Low Osmolar Contrast Media**
        a. **Ionic, Low-Osmolar Contrast Media.** The agent ioxaglate is an ionic dimer consisting of two, linked, benzene rings, each with 3 iodine atoms (anion) and a single cation. This results in two osmotically active particles for every 6 iodine atoms and a 50% reduction in osmolality compared to high-osmolar ionic agents.

        b. **Nonionic Media.** Nonionic agents consist of 3 iodine atoms attached to a fully substituted, uncharged benzene ring. These agents are not salts and enter the aqueous phase as an electrically-neutral, single, osmotically-active compound (i.e., one osmotically active particle for every 3 iodine atoms rather than two osmotic particles with first generation agents). The net result is that equivalent radiodensity can be delivered at half the osmotic load. The agents do not bind ionized calcium.

B. **ADVERSE DYE REACTIONS.** Despite excellent overall tolerance, contrast media can result in undesirable reactions, ranging from mild nausea to life-threatening anaphylaxis; overall mortality attributable to contrast agents in coronary angiography is 4-23 deaths per million patients.[10,11] Patients with a previous history of an adverse dye reaction are at highest risk of a subsequent a severe reaction; previous anaphylaxis carries a recurrence rate of 40% without premedication.[12] Asthmatics, especially those with nasal polyps, represent another high-risk group (6-9 fold risk compared to non-asthmatics).[13] Other predisposing conditions include dehydration, systemic illness, preexisting cardiac disease, and certain ethnic groups.[10,11]
    1. **Hemodynamic Effects.** Transient ventricular dysfunction and hypotension has been ascribed to

their hyperosmolar content and caclium-binding properties, and are more common following administration of first generation agents.

2. **Electrophysiologic Effects.** Bradycardia, AV block, ST segment and T wave changes, prolonged QT interval, and ventricular tachycardia/fibrillation have been attributed to the calcium chelating properties of the preservatives and buffers. Ionic agents differ in their ability to bind calcium and effect these electrophysiologic parameters. Additives in Renografin-76 (sodium EDTA, sodium citrate) chelate more calcium than Hypaque and Angiovist (calcium EDTA); this explains the greater incidence of hemodynamic and electrophysiologic alterations with Renografin-76.[14] Nonionic agents exhibit little if any calcium binding activity. In a randomized prospective study among patients undergoing PTCA, a trend was observed toward a lower incidence of contrast-induced ventricular tachycardia or fibrillation with the nonionic agent iopamidol (Isovue-370) compared to the high osmolar, ionic agent meglumine sodium diatrizoate (Renografin-76).[15]

3. **Minor Reactions.** In a large study of 337,647 patients, the five most frequent symptoms following intravenous contrast administration (nausea, urticaria, itching, heat sensation, vomiting) were reduced by low osmolar contrast agents.[16] Low osmolar contrast media also result in less patient discomfort during internal mammary artery and peripheral angiography.

4. **Allergic Reactions.** In this same report[16], severe reactions (i.e., dyspnea or hypotension requiring active therapy, loss of consciousness, cardiac arrest) were less frequent after administration of low osmolar agents.[16] In another report of patients with a previous reaction to high osmolar ionic agents, no reaction was observed in 95% of patients given a low osmolar agent.[17]

5. **Thrombosis (Table 25.2).** Routine use of non-ionic contrast media should be avoided in patients with acute ischemic syndromes undergoing percutaneous intervention. In-vitro and in-vivo studies have demonstrated that ionic contrast has anticoagulant and antiplatelet activities (prolongation of PTT and clotting time; inhibition of platelet aggregation and degranulation; and reduced time to thrombolysis) compared to non-ionic contrast. In prospective trials, to ionic contrast was associated with fewer complications than nonionic contrast after PTCA.[18,19] In one trial, ionic contrast reduced the risk of in-lab abrupt closure,[18] and in another, ionic contrast was associated with a decreased incidence of no-reflow, and recurrent ischemia.[19] The EPIC trial demonstrated a decreased incidence of abrupt closure, Q-wave MI and death with ionic contrast compared to non-ionic contrast in patients with recent MI, unstable angina, or high-risk lesion morphology.[20] However, in elective procedures on stable lesions, no differences were observed between ionic and nonionic contrast, suggesting that the presence of preexisting thrombus or hypercoagulable state contributes to the deleterious effects of non-ionic contrast.[21,22,23] In summary, nonionic contrast should be avoided if possible in patients with myocardial infarction and unstable angina. The low osmolar, ionic agent ioxaglate should be considered if hemodynamic instability or arrhythmias are present.

Table 25.2 Risk of Thrombosis with Ionic and Non-ionic Contrast

Study	N	Design	Results
Piessens[18]	500	Randomized Trial	Ionic contrast ↓ risk of acute thrombosis (8 vs. 18%; p<.05) compared to non-ionics
Aguirre[20]	1930	Retrospective review of EPIC	Ionic agents reduced incidence of abrupt closure (7 vs 10%; p=.003), Q-Wave MI (1.9 vs 7%; p=.018), and death (0.4 vs 1.5%; p=.016) compared to non-ionics
Grines[19]	211	Randomized trial in unstable angina and MI patients	Ionic contrast reduced post PTCA ischemia requiring urgent cath (3 vs 11.4%; p=.02), rePTCA in hospital (1 vs 5.8%; p=.06), and rest angina by 1 month (0 vs 5.9%; p=.04)

6. **Nephrotoxicity.** Among patients with baseline renal insufficiency, no difference was observed in the incidence of acute renal failure for high-osmolar and nonionic agents.[24,25] However, low osmolar agents may be preferred for patients with renal insufficiency requiring large contrast volumes, to minimize the osmolar volume load.

7. **Cost.** Low osmolar agents cost 15-20 times more than high osmolar agents (e.g., $100 vs $5 per 100cc.). It has been estimated that routine use of low osmolar agents for cardiac angiography would increase the annual budget for contrast agents by $100 million in the U.S. alone.

C. **RECOMMENDATIONS.** Low osmolar agents should be reserved for patients most likely to derive significant clinical benefit. Although limited data are available and opinions vary, our bias is to use a low-osmolar agent for PTCA patients with hemodynamic or electrophysiologic instability, decompensated heart failure, moderate-severe renal dysfunction who require large contrast volumes, and individuals with a prior history of a severe adverse contrast reactions. In addition, patients undergoing internal mammary artery PTCA may experience less discomfort when low osmolar agent is used. Due to the tendency toward thrombotic complications, the low osmolar nonionic agents should be avoided in patients with acute myocardial infarction, post-infarction angina, and unstable angina.

D. **PREVENTION**
The best approach is to plan ahead:
- Obtain history of previous contrast reaction and define other risk factors.
- Premedicate individuals with a known contrast allergy (see below).
- Minimize the contrast volume and have equipment, medications, and personnel ready to treat life-threatening reactions.

1. **Identify Patients at Risk.** The recommendations for prophylaxis against contrast reactions during cardiac catheterization are extrapolated from the radiologic experience with contrast reactions during radiologic procedures of all types. Shehadi[26] reported adverse reactions in 5.65%, severe reactions in 0.02% and death in 0.007% of 112,000 patients. Another study[27] of 302,083 patients

reported any reaction, severe reactions, and death in 4.7%, 0.07%, and 0.006% respectively. Patients at greatest risk for contrast reaction are those with a prior reaction, severe asthma, or multiple allergies. A history of hayfever and allergies doubled the chance of a contrast reaction; a prior contrast reaction tripled the chance of subsequent adverse reactions.[27] Low osmolar agents result in a decreased incidence of severe adverse reactions compared to high osmolar agents.[28,29]

2. **Pharmacologic Prophylaxis (Table 25.3).** Pretreatment with corticosteroids decreases the risk of contrast reactions:[30] had no difference in adverse reactions compared to untreated patients.[30] Thus, the timing of steroid administration is important for achieving prophylaxis against adverse events. In another study,[31] pretreatment with diphenhydramine and cimetidine resulted in fewer adverse reactions with ionic contrast.

E. TREATMENT

1. **Minor Contrast Reactions** - Infrequently require intervention
   a. **Symptoms.** Nausea, burning sensation, flushing, mild urticaria without hives, mild bradycardia or vasovagal episodes.

   b. **Comment.** Usually occur within minutes of exposure.

   c. **Treatment.** Supportive, including observation, cool compresses, oral diphenhydramine, atropine (0.5-1.0mg IV).

2. **Moderate Contrast Reactions** - Usually require intervention
   a. **Symptoms.** Persistent nausea and vomiting, anaphylactoid reaction (urticaria with hives and tongue swelling), persistent bradycardia or vasovagal episodes with hypotension.

   b. **Comment.** Usually occur within minutes to hrs of exposure.

   c. **Treatment.** Intravenous fluids, diphenhydramine, steroids (e.g. hydrocortisone 100mg IV), centrally-acting antiemetics (e.g. compazine 2mg IV., followed by a 25mg rectal suppository) and atropine (for bradycardia or vasovagal reactions). Anaphylactoid reactions are treated additionally with epinephrine (0.1-0.5cc of a 1:1,000 dilution subcutaneously, repeated every 5-15 minutes as necessary).

3. **Severe Contrast Reactions** - Life-threatening and require aggressive attention.
   a. **Symptoms.** Anaphylaxis, (bronchospasm laryngeal edema and/or profound hypotension) may occur immediately with a single contrast injection.

   b. **Comment.** Rare but requires prompt recognition and treatment.

Table 25.3 Premedication Protocol for Prevention of Contrast Allergy

DRUG	COMMENT
Prednisone	40 mg PO Q 6 hrs, starting 12-18 hours prior to contrast (Solumedrol 40 mg IV for emergency procedures)
Stop B-Blocker	Withhold β-blockers if possible (may blunt responsiveness to epinephrine)
Diphenhydramine	50 mg PO or IV before procedure
H$_2$ receptor antagonist	H$_2$ receptor antagonist is optional - no clear data to support its use. (ranitidine 150mg or cimetidine 300mg PO before procedure)
Low osmolar contrast	Use low osmolar contrast to reduce risk of reactions

   c.   **Treatment.** Epinephrine (1-5 cc of 1:10,000 dilution IV repeated every 2-5 minutes) steroids (e.g. hydrocortisone 100mg IV or solumedrol 125mg IV), diphenhydramine (50mg IV) and possible intubation. Bronchodilators (e.g. Albuterol aerosol 2.5mg nebulized mist treatments every 1-2 hrs) might be of additional benefit. Prolonged (2-10 hours) infusions of epinephrine (1-2 μg/min) or neosynephrine may be necessary for intermittent hypotension.

PERIPHERAL VASCULAR COMPLICATIONS

The explosive evolution of coronary interventional technology over the last few years has carried with it an increased incidence of peripheral vascular complications. The diagnosis, prevention, and management of these complications are discussed below:

A. AV FISTULA
   1.   **Definition.** During attempted vascular access, the needle may puncture both the femoral artery and vein creating an abnormal arterial venous communication (AV fistula) which may persist following sheath withdrawal. This results in a "continuous murmur" at the site of communication, distal arterial insufficiency, and a swollen, tender extremity due to venous dilatation. An increased number of femoral punctures, inappropriate low femoral puncture site, punctures which extends through both the anterior and posterior arterial wall and impaired clotting function all increase the risk for AV fistula formation. Additionally, when puncture of the superior aspect of the superficial femoral artery occurs, an increased propensity for an abnormal communication with the lateral circumflex femoral vein occurs. Therefore, meticulous attention to the details of arterial and

venous access is imperative to minimize local complications.

2. **Incidence.** Published reports indicate the incidence of AV fistula formation following diagnostic and therapeutic cardiac catheterization is between 0.1 and 1%. Wyman, et al.[32] has demonstrated the overall local vascular complication rate requiring repair to be 1.5% following PTCA. A more recent report of 2400 consecutive patients undergoing either diagnostic or interventional procedures demonstrated an incidence of 0.1 to 0.2% AV fistulas requiring surgical repair following the procedure.[33]

3. **Diagnosis.** A tender swollen extremity and/or the development of a continuous bruit in the vicinity of a recent arterial puncture should raise suspicion of AV fistula formation. Color flow Doppler imaging and ultrasonography are used to confirm the diagnosis.

4. **Management.** It is the practice of most vascular surgeons to repair all AV fistulas shortly after the diagnosis is made. Complications of delaying surgical repair include accelerated atherosclerosis, increased cardiac output and worsening of distal extremity swelling and tenderness. Surgical repair involves division or excision of the fistula, and occasionally synthetic grafting of the involved vessels. Ultrasound guided compression repair is being used with increasing frequency, but current experience with it is limited. One small series reported a success rate of 67% (6/9).[34]

B. PSEUDOANEURYSM AND HEMATOMA

1. **Definition.** A pseudoaneurysm is an encapsulated hematoma in communication with an artery. Often the diagnosis of pseudoaneurysm is difficult to distinguish from an expanding hematoma at the site of arterial puncture. Although hematomas generally resolve spontaneously, pseudoaneurysms usually require compression or surgical repair. The principle cause of pseudoaneurysm formation is inadequate compression following catheter removal or impaired clotting. Low femoral arterial puncture sites (superficial femoral artery or profundus artery) may also increase the likelihood for pseudoaneurysm development due to their deep anatomic location which is less accessible to compression following sheath removal.[36]

2. **Incidence.** The reported incidence of pseudoaneurysm formation after arterial cannulation varies widely. One report indicated that this complication may occur in 0.03%-0.05% of patients following routine coronary angiography.[35] Muller et al. demonstrated the incidence of pseudoaneurysm formation requiring surgery to be 0.3% in 2400 consecutive patients undergoing diagnostic or interventional procedures.[33] The incidence is increased with larger sheaths and prolonged anticoagulation.

3. **Diagnosis.** Any patient with a large hematoma should be evaluated for a pseudoaneurysm. The classic findings are a tender, pulsatile mass with a systolic bruit in the involved area. Confirmation may be made by local ultrasonography or repeat angiography.

4. **Management.** The need for repair of a pseudoaneurysm is dependent on size, expansion and

whether the patient requires long-term anticoagulation. Pseudoaneurysms of less than 3cm in size can often be followed clinically. A follow-up ultrasound 1-2 weeks after initial diagnosis often demonstrates spontaneous thrombosis and obviates the need for surgical repair. However, spontaneous thrombosis is less likely to occur when the pseudoaneurysm is ≥3cm in size on initial ultrasound evaluation. When the defect persists beyond two weeks or expands, the risk of femoral artery rupture necessitates correction. Ultrasound guided compression repair is commonly used with success related to the anticoagulation status and a pseudoaneurysm structure that can be readily visualized and compressed. Among patients not receiving anticoagulation, high success rates have been reported (92%-98%), with lower success rates (54%-86%) in those receiving anticoagulation.[34,37,38] There have been no randomized trials comparing ultrasound compression to surgical repair, but it seems reasonable to first attempt this noninvasive approach in patients with favorable anatomy prior to surgical repair.

C. THROMBOTIC OCCLUSION

1. **Incidence.** Although both arterial and venous thrombosis may occur following PTCA, the estimated incidence is <1%. Patients at increased risk include those of advanced age, and those with cardiomyopathy, peripheral vascular disease or hypercoagulation states. Major complications of post catheterization arterial thrombosis include severe symptomatic ischemia (21%), amputation (11%), and death (2%).[39]

2. **Diagnosis.** The fact that the majority of reported cases of arterial thrombosis occurred in the lower extremities (98% of 85 reported cases)[40] probably represents operator preference for the femoral approach. In a review of 222,553 patients who underwent cardiac catheterization, vascular complications occurred four times more frequently with brachial compared with femoral approaches (0.96% vs 0.22% p<.001).[41] Primary symptoms following arterial occlusion include the sudden onset of severe pain or numbness. Cyanosis, pallor, absence of a distal pulse with a cool extremity are common findings.

3. **Management.** Due to the potential complications of arterial thrombosis, heparinization and urgent thrombectomy are usually indicated. In addition to Fogarty catheter thrombectomy, surgical thrombectomy, bypass grafting or thromboendarectomy are common therapies for arterial thrombosis. The exact role for thrombolysis has yet to be defined in this setting.

D. ARTERIAL PERFORATION.
When advancing guidewires, catheters or other devices, the spectrum of vessel damage can range from minor trauma disrupting the endothelium to more serious complications including transmural vessel perforation.[42]

1. **Incidence and Diagnosis.** The incidence of arterial perforation remote from the puncture site has been estimated at 0.1%.[43] This complication should be suspected when the patient complains of acute pain simultaneous with guidewire and/or catheter manipulation. Contrast injections confirm with the diagnosis by demonstrating extravasation of blood, however, this may not be evident with small perforation.

2. **Management.** Most guidewire induced peripheral arterial perforations are benign and result in insignificant blood loss. Most will undergo spontaneous tamponade and rarely, pseudoaneurysm formation may occur.

E. DISSECTION

1. **Incidence.** The incidence of subintimal dissection or trauma resulting in subsequent hematoma formation ranges from 0.01% to 0.4%.[44-48] The most commonly recognized predisposing factor to peripheral arterial dissection is tortuosity and atherosclerosis of the distal aorta and iliac systems. Following subintimal disruption the development and entry into a "false lumen" may occur readily. High pressure injection into a false lumen will result in extensive dissection. However, iatrogenic dissection occurs infrequently and serious complications are few unless major branches of the aorta are involved.

2. **Management.** In the majority of cases, subintimal dissection occurs during retrograde catheter or wire advancement; thus, antegrade blood flow will usually "tack down" the flap and it requires no specific therapy. However, the need for immediate surgical treatment depends on the severity of the dissection (ie., involvement of the major aortic branches, distal flow characteristics, evidence of ischemia). If renal or visceral arteries are involved, emergency surgical intervention may be required. In this situation, stenting prosthetic insertion and/or bypass grafting may be required.

F. RETROPERITONEAL HEMORRHAGE

1. **Incidence.** Retroperitoneal hemorrhage is a complication that may occur when arterial access of the femoral artery is above the inguinal ligament. In this situation, effective compression may not be possible since the arterial structures are retroperitoneal and hemorrhage from the puncture site may accumulate posteriorly rather than the inguinal region. The reported incidence of retroperitoneal hematoma varies but is probably less than 1% of all interventional cases.

2. **Diagnosis.** Abdominal pain occurs in approximately 60% of patients with retroperitoneal hematomas, with back and flank pain in approximately 25%.[49,50] Although abdominal pain is generally vague and generalized in two-thirds of cases, occasionally pain may be localized over the site of hematoma formation. Physical exam may reveal a palpable mass with discoloration (Grey Turner sign) over the flank region or the abdomen. Digital rectal examination may also reveal a compressive mass. A sufficiently large hematoma may displace the ipsilateral ureter and kidney. Often the diagnosis is suspected from an asymptomatic drop in hemoglobin.

There is general agreement that CT scanning is the most precise tool in determining the diagnosis and extent of retroperitoneal hemorrhage. However, the diagnosis may also be established by ultrasound or abdominal x-rays which demonstrate a psoas shadow in 30% of patients, abdominal mass in 5% and a paralytic ileus in 8%.

3. **Treatment.** After confirmation of retroperitoneal hematoma, cessation of heparin and removal of arterial catheters with prolonged compression of the involved vessel is mandatory. The majority

of retroperitoneal bleeds will spontaneously tamponade. Although many patients may require a blood transfusion, most are hemodynamically stable. However, continued decline in hematocrit, signs of volume depletion, or hemodynamic instability despite reversal of anticoagulants indicate that hematoma expansion is likely and surgical exploration may be warranted.

G. ATHEROEMBOLIZATION

1. **Etiology.** Because of its often insidious clinical presentation, cholesterol emboli following coronary interventional procedures may be overlooked. In most cases, the etiology is catheter or guidewire induced mechanical trauma to a friable atherosclerotic lesion of the aorta. It is well recognized that distal embolization may occur to the lower extremities[51] as well as components of the abdominal viscera including the spleen, liver, kidney and pancreas. Most acute occlusions of a major arterial system are the result of macroemboli consisting of cholesterol crystals and thrombotic debris which arise from major atheromatous plaque.

   "Microemboli" generally result from the release of cholesterol crystals or other microscopic debris from an atheromatous plaque which may have undergone ulceration. Microemboli generally do not manifest clinical symptoms, however, severe showers of microemboli may result in glomerular obstruction, renal failure and/or livedo reticularis.

2. **Incidence.** Clinically recognized atheroembolic phenomena occur infrequently following invasive cardiac catheterization. However, autopsy series, have suggested that "spontaneous atheromatous embolism should be regarded as common "with an incidence of up to 10%."[52,53] In our experience, larger lumen catheters used for interventional devices (particularly left Judkins curves) can scrape atheroma into the guiding catheter.

3. **Diagnosis.** The clinician makes a diagnosis of atheroembolic disease primarily from the history and physical exam. Blue-toe syndrome or livedo reticularis involving the extremities and trunk may be the cardinal manifestation of peripheral microemboli. The chief manifestation of macroembolic disease may be acute arterial ischemia. In its most extreme and complicated form, gangerous transformation or ulceration of the distal extremity may rarely occur. Renal failure has been reported as a secondary manifestation of embolic disease. Generally, it is of insidious onset with manifestations taking days to months to become evident. Peripheral eosinophilia and episodic hypertension in addition to non-oliguric renal insufficiency may occur.[54,55]

4. **Management.** Prevention via the utilization of long guidewire (300cm) exchanges in patients with known or suspected atherosclerotic aortic involvement is recommended, as is allowing back bleeding from guiding catheters once the wire is removed, to allow atheroma to exit onto the cath table. The vast majority of microembolic cases can be managed by observation alone. Peripheral manifestations resolve over a period of days to weeks in the majority of patients. Some reports have advocated the use of anticoagulants, aspirin or dipyridamole; however, no randomized, controlled data are available to support or refute this approach.

The surgical management of atheroembolic disease has grown in popularity over the past decade. Especially when macroembolic involvement of the major arteries occurs, embolectomy is the favored approach. Adjunctive surgical elimination of the source of the atheroembolic material is advocated by some.[53]

H. BLEEDING COMPLICATIONS.   To determine the frequency and predictors of bleeding complications following interventional procedures we prospectively evaluated 2107 consecutive patients over a 12 month period.[56] Serious bleeding requiring transfusion occurred in 154/2107 (7.3%) patients and was related to bleeding at one or more of the following sites (access 5.8%, retroperitoneal 0.9%, gastrointestinal 1.8%, drop in hemoglobin of unknown etiology 3.7%). Regression analysis was used to find variables predictive of the need for transfusions. Clinical variables of female sex, low body weight, advanced age, urgent procedure, and low baseline hemoglobin were highly predictive of need for transfusion after PTCA.   Furthermore, long duration of case, larger sheath sizes, heparin dose/weight, thrombolytic use and multivessel disease contributed to bleeding complications. These data suggest that the majority of factors associated with bleeding relate to the underlying severity of patient illness.   Subsequent studies have reported similar findings.[57-62] Intracoronary stenting is associated with increased bleeding complications, undoubtedly due to the aggressive anticoagulation.[63] Bleeding risk was increased with the early use of new glycoprotein IIb/IIIa receptor antagonists, although when administered with low-dose heparin regimens combined with early sheath removal (EPILOG trial protocol), these antiplatelet agents were not associated with increased major bleeding events (Chapter 34). With recognition of the association between post-angioplasty bleeding risk and prolonged heparin use, there has been a trend toward less post-procedure heparin and early sheath removal. In a prospective trial involving 284 patients, Friedman[63] randomized angioplasty patients with good angiographic results to receive either 24 hours of continuous heparin or immediate discontinuation of heparin post procedure. In this study, there was no increased cardiac risk associated with early discontinuation of heparin. However, there was a greater risk of bleeding in the group receiving 24 hours of heparin infusion compared with immediate discontinuation of heparin post procedure (7% vs. 0%). Abbreviated heparin also translated into hospital savings in excess of $1300 per patient. In determining the appropriate use of post procedure heparin, the potential risks of cardiac events must be carefully weighed against the risk of bleeding, but it seems reasonable to discontinue heparin as early as possible in patients who receive favorable angioplasty results. Additional prospective studies investigating different heparin regimens are currently underway.

I.   Vascular Closure Devices. Recently, there has been an increased interest in vascular closure devices after percutaneous procedures. Many devices have been developed but most fall into 3 categories: collagen plugs, percutaneous suture, and compression girdles. Although the data on these devices are limited, the increase in coronary stent use and subsequent anticoagulation issues that accompany stent implantation have catalyzed interest in this area.

Biodegradable collagen insertion plugs (Vasoseal, Datascope, Inc.) for arterial sheath site sealing have shown equivocal results. One study reported a bleeding complication rate (all bleeds and hematomas) as high as 33% despite an initial success rate of 97% (154/159).[65] In this study, there was an association between sheath size and bleeding after collagen plug insertion and the conclusions were that the use of Vasoseal with sheath size greater than 8 FR is contraindicated. Another study reported a hematoma (size > 5cm) rate of 20% (7/35) in patients undergoing collagen plug arterial closure after stenting while maintained on full anticoagulation.[66] Silber[67] randomized 150 post angioplasty patients to conventional sheath removal or collagen plug closure and found no difference in bleeding complication rates (conventional: 34% vs. collagen plug: 25%) between these 2 sheath removal strategies. However, the patients who received the collagen plug perceived less discomfort associated with their hospitalization. In a small prospective study,[68] 32 patients undergoing coronary stent implantation were randomized to delayed sheath removal and pneumatic compression or immediate sheath removal and collagen plug closure. There was no difference in bleeding complication rates between these 2 sheath removal strategies. In summary, collagen plugs may improve patient comfort and allow for sheath removal while on anticoagulation, but they have not been shown to significantly reduce the rate of bleeding complications.

The second new device is the Prostar (Perclose Inc.) which allows percutaneous suture mediated closure of femoral artery access sites immediately following coronary interventions. This device utilizes a catheter that deploys four needles with 2 pairs of sutures around the hole of femoral artery access sites. The sutures are then tied to close the arteriotomy site mechanically to achieve immediate hemostasis. In a pilot study involving 91 patients, the device produced a 90% success rate in achieving immediate hemostasis despite full anticoagulation (ACT > 300 seconds).[69] Prospective, randomized trial data with this device are not yet available.

Finally, there are the pelvic girdle devices which apply direct pressure to the skin over the femoral artery access site. The prototype is the Femostop device which utilizes a pneumatic pressure device to achieve homeostasis. In one study of 200 angioplasty patients randomized to manual compression or Femostop after sheath removal, there was no significant difference in vascular complications.[70] In comparison to patients having angioplasty, patients undergoing coronary stenting may benefit more from Femostop. In a prospective trial of 82 stent patients randomized to receive either manual compression or Femostop compression, there was a significant decrease in vascular complications (pseudoaneurysm, AV fistula, hematoma requiring transfusion) associated with the Femostop device after stenting.[71] Other common pressure devices include C-clamps and sandbags. Clamps are generally regarded as a safe alternative to digital pressure.[72] Sandbags and/or pressure dressings are often used after hemostasis is achieved but a recent study suggested that they are ineffective in reducing vascular complications after angioplasty[73] and may simply mask an expanding hematoma. Our approach is to simply place a bandaid after sheath removal. This allows the nurse to easily inspect the site and quickly identify bleeding complications.

J. **Minor Vascular Problems.** We frequently encounter minor vascular problems during PTCA procedures. The majority of these problems can be easily managed as outlined in Table 25.4.

Table 25.4 Management of Common Vascular Problems in the PTCA Patient

Problem	Solution
• Difficult access	• Choose alternate site (see Chapter 27) • Use Doppler guided arterial puncture (Smart Needle®) ACS peripheral systems group
• Fibrotic groin or femoral bypass graft	• Successively dilate with 5,6,7,8,9F dilators, then insert 8F firm body sheath (Daig or Terumo)
• Difficulty negotiating tortuous atherosclerotic iliac vessels	• Obtain guiding shot by injection through sheath • Advance right Judkins or multipurpose catheter, torque into bend • Advance Glide®, (Terumo Corp) Wholey® or TAD (ACS peripheral systems group) wires into aorta • Insert long sheath
• Sheath or catheters kink due to sharp bends	• Insert firm bodied sheath (Terumo or Daig) over stiff wire (Amplatz) • Torque catheter with Amplatz or 0.063 inch wire inside (see Chapter 13)
• Bleeding around sheath	• Insert dilator to straighten kinks (distal 1/3 cut off) • Exchange for sheath 1-2F larger • Prolonged pressure over groin • Continued bleeding - remove sheaths

• Limb ischemia
   Acute: Probable thromboembolism
   Gradual: Probable sheath induced ischemia
	
	• Fogarty thrombectomy
	
	• Intraarterial nitroglycerin, remove sheath

• Expanding hematoma	• Prolonged direct pressure • Consider sheath removal and reversal of anticoagulation • Groin ultrasound, doppler • Vascular surgical consultation

INFECTION

During the course of vascular intervention, the introduction of antigenically active substances into the peripheral blood stream (proteins, endotoxin, etc.) may evoke a pyrogenic reaction. Local infection at the site of arterial puncture, phlebitis and fever occur in less than 1% of patients following interventional procedures. There are, however, case reports of epidemics due to infected water supplies with acinetobacteria or pseudomonas species.[74]

A. **CLINICAL MANIFESTATIONS.** Pyrogenic reactions following cardiac catheterizations generally commence within 60 minutes of the procedure and may be manifest as fevers, chills, rigors, and in some cases lethargy. Local reactions such as phlebitis occurring at the site of vascular access consists primarily of erythema, painful induration and rarely exudative drainage from the site.

B. **ETIOLOGY AND TREATMENT.** The therapy for infections following invasive procedures can be divided into systemic and local treatments. Critically important are the results of adjunctive tests (blood cultures, complete blood count, etc.).

1. **Local.** Phlebitis which is generally minor responds in most cases to hot soaks as well as elevation of the effected limb. Exudative drainage or clinical evidence of cellulitis may require institution of antibiotics.

2. **Systemic.** Fevers and/or rigors following invasive catheterization generally suggest a systemic transient bacteremia. It is imperative that indwelling catheters and sheaths be removed and blood cultures be obtained from several sites as well as urine and sputum cultures. The results of these cultures will be critically important in determining the intensity and time course of antibiotic therapy. Usually fevers and bacteremia resolve with discontinuation of indwelling lines. Empiric antibiotics should be considered in debilitated patients or those at high risk of developing endocarditis.

   The most common arterial etiologies for post-procedure fevers include the staphylococcus species (aureus, epidermitis).[75-77] Approximately 50% of all staphylococcus epidermitis and 20-30% of staphylococcus aureus species are methicillin resistant. Therefore, first line antibiotic therapy for bacteremia consists primarily of intravenous vancomycin. In the absence of documented endocarditis, an antibiotic course of 7 days is generally sufficient and it is not routinely recommended that patients be discharged on oral antibiotic therapy. Bacteremia due to gram negative enterics or Candida is sufficiently rare and therefore, antimicrobial treatment directed against these organisms is not routinely recommended in the absence of culture confirmation.

   Continued fevers and leukocytosis warrant continued antibiotics and a meticulous investigation as to the causative organism. Repeat blood cultures, infectious disease consultation and initiation of alternative antibiotic regimens should be considered depending on the clinical circumstances.

NEUROLOGIC COMPLICATIONS

A. ETIOLOGY. In patients undergoing cardiac catheterization and coronary arteriography, the incidence of peri-procedural neurologic events is 0.07%.[32,78-80] Common etiologies include: cardiac emboli (thrombus, calcium, vegetation), air embolus, and trauma to the aorta or carotid arteries from guidewire or catheter manipulation. Intracranial bleeding occurs infrequently. In patients undergoing PTCA, the risk of sustaining a focal neurological deficit is increased (0.1-0.5%); this is primarily due to the additional risk imposed by prolonged procedures, athero and air emboli from guiding catheters, the use of high-dose heparin and/or fibrinolytic agents, as well as cerebral hypoperfusion consequent to hypotension.[78,80,81]

B. MANAGEMENT. When confronted with a patient who has sustained an intra- procedural neurological event, a careful neurologic exam is performed, a neurology consult obtained, and the patient is sent for an emergent CT scan. Easily reversible causes of alteration in mental status including drug effects, hypoventilation, hypoperfusion, and metabolic abnormalities should be evaluated. In stable patients without critical coronary disease, heparin is reversed with protamine (10 mg/1,000 units of heparin i.v. over 5-15 minutes) prior to obtaining the CT scan. In patients with unstable angina, critical coronary disease with ulcerated, thrombus- containing lesion(s), or immediately following PTCA, the decision to reverse the patients anticoagulation and replete fibrinogen prior to obtaining the CT scan must be individualized. The risk of stroke extension must be balanced against the risk of acute vessel closure; this decision is usually based on the presumed etiology, extent and progression of the neurological deficit as well as the patient's clinical presentation, coronary anatomy and associated lesion morphology. In the absence of a cerebral bleed on CT scan, anticoagulation is continued. If the CT scan demonstrates the presence of an intracerebral hemorrhage, heparin and thrombolytic infusions should be immediately discontinued. Circulating heparin is neutralized by administering protamine, and the effects of thrombolytics by cryoprecipitate (10 units i.v.) and fresh frozen plasma (2 units).[81] If only low-dose intracoronary thrombolytics have been administered (e.g. i.c. urokinase <250,000u), a systemic lytic state is not achieved and fibrinogen repletion is usually not required.

* * * * *

REFERENCES

1. Porter GA. Experimental contrast-associated nephropathy and its clinical implications. Am J Cardiol 1990;66:18F-22F.
2. Cronin RE. Renal failure following radiologic procedures. Am J Med Sci 1989;298:342-356.
3. Porter GA. Contrast-associated nephropathy. Am J Cardiol 1989;64:22E-26E.
4. Manske CL, Sprafka JM, Strong JT, et al. Contrast nephropathy in azotemic diabetic patients undergoing coronary angiography. Am J Med 1990;89(5):615-620.
5. Davidson CJ, Hiatky M, Morris KG, et al. Cardiovascular and renal toxicity of a nonionic radiographic contrast agent after cardiac catheterization. A prospective trial. Ann Intern Med 1989;110:119-124.
6. Jeunikar AM, Finnie KJ, Dennis B, et al. Nephrotoxicity of high-and-low-osmolality contrast media. Nephron 1988;48:300-305.
7. Weinstein JM, Heyman S, Brezis M. Potential deleterious effect of furosemide in radiocontrast nephropathy. Nephron 1992;62:413-5.
8. Weisberg LS, Kurnid PB, Kurnid BRC. Risk of radiocontrast nephropathy in patients with and without diabetes mellitus. Kidney Int 1994;45:259-65.
9. Opie LH. Drugs for the heart.
10. Ansell G, Tweedie MCK, West CR, et al. The current status of reactions to intravenous contrast media. Invest Radiol 1980;15:532-539.
11. Bilazarian SD, Mittal S, Mills RM. Recognizing the extrarenal hazards of intravascular contrast agents. J Crit Illness 1991;6:859-869.
12. Lasser EC, et al. Pre-Treatment with corticosteroids to alleviate reactions to intravenous contrast material. N Engl J Med 1987;317:845-849.
13. Lang DM, Alpern MB, Visintainer PF, et al. Increased risk for Anaphylactoid reaction from contrast media in Patients on β-adrenergic blockers or with asthma. Ann Intern Med 1991;115:270-276.
14. Zuckerman LS, Friehling TD, Wolf NM, et al. Effect of calcium-binding additives on ventricular fibrillation and repolarization changes during coronary angiography. J Am Coll Cardiol 1987;10:1249-1253.
15. Lembo NJ, King SB III, Roubin GS, et al. Effects of nonionic versus ionic contrast media on complications of percutaneous transluminal coronary angioplasty. Am J Cardiol 1991;67:1046-1050.
16. Katayama H, Yamaguchi K, Kozuka T, et al. Adverse reactions to ionic and nonionic contrast media. Radiology 1990;175:621-628.
17. Fischer HW, Spataro RF. Use of low-osmolality contrast media in patients with previous reactions. Radiol 1988;23(Suppl I):S186-S188.
18. Piessens, et al. Cathet Cardiovasc Diagn 1993;28:99.
19. Grines CL, Zidar F, Jones D, et al. A randomized trial of ionic vs. nonionic contrast in myocardial infarction or unstable angina patients undergoing coronary angioplasty. Circulation 1993;88:1886.
20. Aguirre FV, Topol EJ, Donohue TJ, et al. Impact on ionic and non-ionic contrast media on post-PTCA ischemic complications: results from the EPIC trial. J Am Coll Cardiol 1995;March, Special Issue:8A.
21. Bonan R, Lesperance J, Gosselin G, et al. Recoil 15 minutes post-coronary angioplasty and contrast media: A randomized double-blind comparative study. Circulation 1994;90:I488.
22. Lembo NJ, King SB III, Roubin GS, et al. Effects of nonionic versus ionic contrast media on complications of percutaneous transluminal coronary angioplasty Am J Cardiol 1991;67:1046-50.
23. Schwab SJ, Hlatky MA, Pieper KS, et al. Contrast nephrotoxicity: A randomized controlled trial of a nonionic and an ionic radiographic contrast agent. N Engl J Med 1989;320:149-153.
24. Taliercio CP, Vlietstra RE, Ilstrup DM, et al. A randomized comparison of the nephrotoxicity of Iopamidol and diatrizoate in high risk patients undergoing cardiac angiography. J Am Coll Cardiol 1991;17:384-390.
25. Shehadi WH. Adverse reactions to intravascularly administered contrast media: a comprehensive study based on prospective survey. Am J Radiol 1975;124:145-52.
26. Shehadi WH, Toniolo G. Adverse reactions to contrast media. Radiology 1980;137:299-302.
27. Palmer FJ, The RACR survey of intravenous contrast media reactions: a preliminary report. Australas Radiol 1988;32:8-11.
28. Katayama H. Report of the Japanese committee on the safety of contrast media. Presented at the Radiological Society of North America Meeting, November, 1988.
29. Lasser EC, Berry CC, Talner LB, et al. Pretreatment with corticosteroids to alleviate reactions to intravenous contrast

material. N Engl J Med 1987;317:845-9.

30. Greenberg MA, Levine B, Menegus MA, et al. Single dose pre-treatment prevents adverse events associated with the use of ionic contrast agents. J Am Coll Cardiol 1995;March, Speical Issue:319A

31. Wyman RM, et al. Current complications of diagnostic and therapeutic cardiac catheterization. J Am Coll Cardiol 1988;12:1400.

32. Muller DWM, Shamir KJ, Ellis SG, et al. Peripheral vascular complications after conventional and complex percutaneous coronary interventional procedures. Am J Cardiol 1992;69:63-68.

33. Schaub F, Theiss W. Heinz M, et al. New Aspects in ultrasound-guided compression repair of post catheterization femoral artery injuries. Circulation 1994;90:1861-5.

34. Hessel SJ, Adams DF, Abrams HL. Complications of angiography. Radiology 1981;138:273-281.

35. Rappaport S, Sniderman KW, Morse SS. Pseudoaneurysm: A complication of faulty technique in femoral artery puncture. Radiology 1985;529-530.

36. Moote JJ, Hilborn MD, Harris KA, et al. Postarteriographic femoral pseudoaneurysms: treatment with ultrasound-guided compression. Annals of Vascular Surgery 1994;8:325-31.

37. Cox GS, Young JR, Gray BR, et al. Ultrasound-guided compression repair of postcatheterization pseudoaneurysms: results of treatment in one hundred cases. J Vascular Surg 1994;19:683-6.

38. Humphries AW, et al. Evaluation of the natural history and result of treatment involving the lower extremities: Fundamentals of vascular grafting. McGraw-Hill, New York 1973.

39. Raithel D. Surgical Treatment of acute embolization and acute arterial thrombosis. J Cardiovas Surgery. Barcelona, 1973.

40. Johnson LW, Lozner EC, Johnson S, et al. Coronary arteriography 1984-1987: A report of the registry of the society for cardiac angiography and interventions. Cathet Cardiovasc Diagn 1989;17:5-10.

41. Rooke TW. Vascular complications of interventional procedures. Radiology 1981;138;273-281.

42. Lauk EK. A survey of complications of percutaneous retrograde arteriography. Radiology 1963;81:257-263.

43. Bourassa MA, Noble J. Complication rate of coronary arteriography. Circulation. 1976;53:106-114.

44. Guss SB, Zin LM, Garrison HB, et al. Coronary occlusion during coronary angiography. Circulation 1975;52:1063-1068.

45. Feit A, Kahn R, Chowdry I, et al. Coronary artery dissection secondary to coronary arteriography: Case report and review. Cathet Cardiovas Diagn 1984;10:177-181.

46. Morise AP, Hardin NJ, Bovili EG, et al. Coronary artery dissection secondary to coronary arteriography: Presentation of three cases. Cathet Cardiovasc Diagn 1981;7:283-296.

47. Connors JP, Thanavaro S, Shaw RC, et al. Urgent myocardial revascularization for dissection of the left main coronary artery. J Thorac Cardiovasc Surgery 1982;84:349-352.

48. Shires TG. Principles of surgery. Fourth Edition. McGraw-Hill, New York, 1984:240-241.

49. Boylis SM, Lausing EH, Gilas NW. Traumatic retroperitoneal hematoma. Am J Surgery 1962;103:477.

50. Caravajial JA. A thrombolism. Arch Intern Med 1967;119:539.

51. Gore J, Collins WDP. Review of the literature and a report of 16 additional cases. Am J Clin Pathol 1960;33:416.

52. Haimovici H. Vascular emergencies. Appleton Century Crafts. 1982.

53. Colt HG, Begg RJ, Saporito JJ, et al. Cholesterol emboli after cardiac catheterization. Medicine 1988;57:389-400.

54. Gaines DA. Cholesterol embolization: A lethal complication of vascular catheterization. Lancet 1988;1(8578):168.

55. Grines CL, Glazier S, Bakalyar D, et al. Predictors of bleeding complications following coronary angioplasty. Circulation 1991;(Suppl II);84:II-591.

56. Brown KJ, Morcher JH, Whitman GR, et al. The incidence and analysis of bleeding and vascular complications following percutaneous coronary interventional procedures. Circulation 1994;88:I-196.

57. Hillgrass WB, Brott BC, Narins CR, et al. Predictors of blood loss and bleeding complications after angioplasty. J Am Coll Cardiol 1994;March, Special Issue:69A.

58. Mansour KA, Moscucce M, Kent C, et al. Vascular complications following directional coronary atherectomy or Palmaz-Schatz stenting. J Am Coll Cardiol;XX:136A.

59. Oweida SW, Roubin GS, Smith RB, et al. Postcatheterization vascular complication associated with percutaneous transluminal coronary angioplasty. J Vasc Surgery 1990;12:310-315.

60. Muller D, Shamir KJ, Ellis SG, et al. Peripheral vascular complications after conventional and complex percutaneous coronary interventional procedures. Am J Caridol 1992;69:63-68.

61. Popma JJ, Satler LF, Pichard AD, et al. Vascular complications after balloon and new device angioplasty. Circulation

1993;88:1569-1578.

62. Schweiger MJ, Wiseman A, Wolfe MW, et al. Bleeding complications of coronary angioplasty: A prospective multicenter study. Circulation 1994;90:I-621.

63. Friedman HZ, Cragg DR, Glazier SM, et al. Randomized prospective evaluation of prolonged versus abbreviated intravenous heparin therapy after coronary angioplasty. J Am Coll Cardiol 1994;24:1214-1219.

64. Carere RG, Webb JG, Dodek A. Collagen plug closure of femoral arterial punctures. Are complications excessive? Circulation 1994;90:I-621.

65. Webb JG, Carere RA, Dodek AA. Collagen plug hemostatic closure of femoral arterial puncture sites following implantation of intracoronary stents. Cathet Cardiovasc Diag 1993;30:314-6.

66. Silber S, Bjorvik A, Rosch A. Advantages of sealing arterial puncture sites after PTCA with a single collagen plug: a randomized prospective trial. J Am Coll Cardiol 1995;March, Special Issue:262A.

67. Camenzind E, Grossholz M, Urban P, et al. Mechanical compression (Femostop) alone versus combined collagen application (Vasoseal) and Femostop for arterial puncture site closure after coronary stent implantation: A randomized trial. J Am Coll Cardiol 1994;XX:355A.

68. Vetter JW, Hinohara T, Ribeiro EE, et al. Percutaneous vascular surgery: suture mediated percutaneous closure of femoral artery access site following coronary intervention. J Am Coll Cardio 1995;March, Special Issue:901-21.

69. Clark C, Popma JJ, Bucher TA, et al, A randomized study of the Femostop compression device to prevent vascular complications after coronary angioplasty. J Am Coll Cardiol 1994;March, Special Issue:106A.

70. Sridhar K, Porter K, Gupta B, et al. Reduction in peripheral vascular complications after coronary stenting by the use of a pneumatic vascular compression device. Circulation 1994;90:I-621.

71. Simon AW. Use of mechanical pressure device for hemostasis following cardiac catheterization. Am J Crit Care 1994;3:62-4.

72. Christensen BV, Iacarella CL. Manion RV, et al. Sandbags do not prevent complications after catheterization. Circulation 1994;90:I-205.

73. Reyes MP. Pyrogenic reactions after inadvertent infusion of endotoxin during cardiac catheterization. Ann Inter Med 1980;93:32.

74. McCready RA, Siderys H, Pittman JN, et al. Septic complications after cardiac catheterization and percutaneous transluminal coronary angioplasty. J Vasc Surg 1991;14:170-4.

75. Brummitt CF, Kravitz GR, Granrud GA, Herzog CA. Femoral endarteritis due to *staphylococcus aureus* complicating percutaneous transluminal coronary angioplasty. Am J Med 1988;86:822.

76. Frazee BW, Flaherty JP. Septic endarteritis of the femoral artery following angioplasty. Review of Infectious Diseases 1991;13:620-3.

77. Braunwald E, Swan HJC (eds). Cooperative study on cardiac catheterization. Circulation 1988;37(Suppl III):1.

78. Adams DF, Fraser DB, Abrams HL. The complications of coronary arteriography. Circulation 1973;48:609.

79. Kennedy JW, et al. Complications associated with cardiac catheterization and angiography. Cathet Cardiovasc Diagn 1982;8-5.

80. Califf RM. Risks and complications of thrombolytic therapy. Clinical Challenges in Acute Myocardial Infarction. 1989;1:3-6.

81. Hart RG. Cardiogenic embolism to the brain. Lancet 1992;339:589-594.

82. Katholi RE, Taylor GJ, McCann WP, Woods WT, Womack KA, McCoy CD, Katholi CR, Moses HW, Mishkel GJ, Lucore CL, Holloway RM, Miller BD, Woodruff RC, Dove JT, Mikell FL, Schneider JA. Nephrotoxicity from contrast media: Attenuation with theophylline. Radiology 1995;195:17-22.

26 CORONARY STENTS

Robert D. Safian, M.D.

In 1964, Dotter and Judkins proposed the concept of implanting intravascular stents to support the arterial wall following coronary angioplasty.[1] Since that time, stents have become the most important advance in mechanical techniques for percutaneous coronary revascularization. Although all stents share the common goals of enlarging the vascular lumen and decreasing the incidence of complications and restenosis, they differ in their fundamental designs.

A. STENT DESIGNS (Table 26.1, Figures 26.1, 26.2, 26.3, 26.4).

1. Self-Expanding Stents.

a. Wallstent. The prototype of the self-expanding stent is the Wallstent (Schneider, Minneapolis, MN), which has undergone extensive investigation in Europe but is not yet available in the United States.[2] This stent overcomes many of the problems of geometric instability and stent migration associated with earlier stent designs. The Wallstent consists of an interwoven mesh of 16 stainless steel wire filaments; a specially designed stent delivery system permits release of the stent within the target lesion, followed by continued expansion of the stent until an equilibrium is achieved between the elastic constraint of the vessel wall and the dilating force of the stent. Stents are selected to achieve diameters 0.5 mm larger than the size of the adjacent reference segment. European trials of the original prototype were interrupted over concerns about the high incidence of acute and subacute stent thrombosis.[3] A second generation Wallstent ("less-shortening" Wallstent) shortens by only 25% after deployment; this design may be less thrombogenic than the original prototype due to lower metal surface area, a decrease in the braiding angle of the mesh, and coating with a thromboresistant Biogold polymer. Several clinical trials are underway in the United States to evaluate the Wallstent in native coronary arteries and saphenous vein bypass grafts.

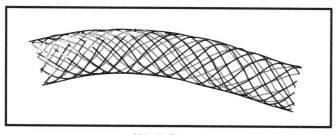

Wall Stent

Figure 26.1 The Self-Expanding Wallstent

b. **SciMed Stent.** A new self-expanding stent is currently under development (SciMed, Inc. Minneapolis, MN), and consists of a flexible slotted stainless steel tube. Advantages of the stent include its ease of deployment and shortening <5% after deployment. Clinical trials are expected to begin in 1996.

2. **Balloon-Expandable Stents.** Two balloon-expandable stents are currently approved for use in the United States: the Gianturco-Roubin stent and Palmaz-Schatz stents.

a. **Gianturco-Roubin Stent** (Flex-Stent, Cook, Inc., Bloomington, Indiana), the first coronary stent approved by the FDA, is a balloon-expandable stent formed by wrapping a single strand of stainless steel filament around a balloon dilatation catheter.[4] The final diameter of the stent is determined by the size of the inflated balloon. Potential advantages of this stent design are its flexibility, ease of insertion, radial expansion without stent shortening, and preserved access to sidebranches. A newer design (Flex-stent II) may have may added radial strength, enhanced trackability, and decreased thrombogenicity; new flatwire stent construction, lower profile, expanded diameters up to 5 mm, and stent length of 40 mm will be added features.

b. **Palmaz-Schatz Stent** (Johnson and Johnson, Inc., Somerville, New Jersey) consists of a slotted tube of stainless steel with two segments each measuring 7 mm in length, connected by a 1 mm bridge segment ("articulated" design).[5] This design enhances flexibility and eases insertion compared to the original nonarticulated design. Since 1990, a special supraselective guiding catheter ("delivery sheath") has been used to deliver the articulated stent to virtually any vessel with high degrees of success and reliability. The stent is crimped on a delivery balloon, and the final diameter of the stent is determined by the size of the largest balloon used to dilate the stent. This stent is highly resistant to elastic recoil, and provides an excellent scaffold to support the arterial wall. A newer heparin-coated Palmaz-Schatz stent with a spiral articulation is currently under investigation in Europe, and may further decrease the incidence of stent thrombosis. Disarticulated coronary stents may also be used.[6-12] Biliary stents (Johnson & Johnson Inc.), approved for use in the biliary system, have also been used in vein grafts and native coronary arteries ≥ 4 mm in diameter. These stents are available in 10-mm and 20-mm lengths, and the 20-mm stent is available in both articulated and nonarticulated designs; unlike the coronary stent, biliary stents have no delivery sheath.

c. **Other Stainless Steel Stents** include the MultiLink stent (Advanced Cardiovascular Systems, Inc., Santa Clara, CA), which consists of a stainless-steel cylinder with laser-etched overlapping loops and bridges. Some patients in Europe have received this stent, and human clinical trials have begun in the United States. The MicroStent (Applied Vascular Engineering, Santa Rosa, CA) has been widely used in Europe and may have unique characteristics which permit its application to small vessels and complex, tortuous anatomy. One or more stents can be crimped on a balloon to treat a wide range of lesion lengths. The Nir stent (SciMed, Inc., Minneapolis, MN) will be entering clinical trials within the next few months.

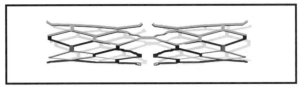

Palmaz-Schatz Stent

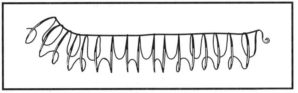

Gianturco-Roubin Stent

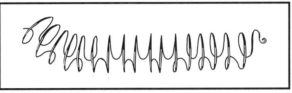

Gianturco-Roubin-II Stent

Figure 26.2 Balloon-Expandable Stents (FDA-Approved)

   d. **Tantalum Stents.** The Wiktor stent (Medtronic, Inc., Minneapolis, MN) consists of a single strand of tantalum wire wrapped around an angioplasty balloon in a U-shaped configuration; advantages of this stent include its flexibility and radiopacity.[13] The Cordis stent (Cordis Corp, Miami, FL), which has a low profile and good radiopacity, is currently under investigation, while the Strecker stent (Boston Scientific, Boston, MA) was recently withdrawn by the manufacturer.

3. **Thermal Memory Stents.** Unique metals such as the nickel and titanium alloy known as Nitinol have been used as stent materials in the peripheral circulation. Although Nitinol can expand from small to large diameters at certain temperatures, use of these stents in the coronary circulation is complex because of the need for refrigeration before insertion, and the risk of premature expansion in the guiding catheter before delivery.[14]

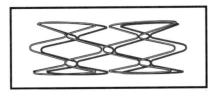

AVE Micro Stent

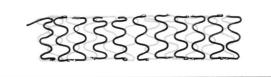

ACS Multilink Stent

Figure 26.3 Balloon-Expandable Stainless Steel Stents (Investigational)

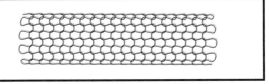

Strecker Stent

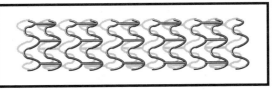

Cordis Stent

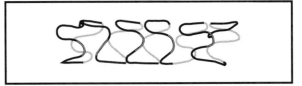

Wiktor Stent

Figure 26.4 Balloon-Expandable Nitinol Stents (Investigational)

B. STENT CHARACTERISTICS

1. **Biocompatibility.** Biocompatibility refers to the ability of the stent material to resist thrombosis and corrosion. Of all the stent materials currently under investigation, those made of stainless steel seem to be the most susceptible to thrombosis. The tendency for thrombosis can be minimized by using highly polished, ultra-pure grades of stainless steel, by minimizing the metal surface area of the stent, and possibly by thromboresistant coatings. Although experimental studies in animals suggest that tantalum and Nitinol may be less thrombogenic than stainless steel, further studies in humans are necessary. At present, all stent patients require medications to prevent stent thrombosis (see Adjunctive Therapy, Section F, below).

2. **Flexibility.** For practical reasons, stent flexibility is an extremely important consideration because of the tortuosity of the coronary arterial circulation and the angulated shape of many guiding catheters (particularly those for the left coronary artery). Of the balloon-expandable stents, the least flexible is the nonarticulated design of the Palmaz-Schatz stent, which has been replaced by the more flexible articulated design. Furthermore, the delivery sheath for the Palmaz-Schatz and MultiLink stent has improved the reliability of insertion into tortuous vessels. Although the flexibility of the Gianturco-Rubin and Wiktor stents appears to be excellent without a delivery sheath, these stents can be deformed by passage through severely angulated lesions or by roughened luminal surfaces; adequate predilation, extra-support guidewires, and ideal guiding catheter alignment are important for proper stent deployment. The MicroStent appears to be the most flexible stent; its short length and low profile permit its use in difficult anatomy. Early experience with the Nir stent suggests excellent flexibility, as well. Biliary stents are relatively inflexible compared to all coronary stents.

3. **Visibility.** The ability to visualize the stent by fluoroscopy is dependent on the stent material and design, as well as the X-ray equipment (Table 26.1). Optimal stent placement is highly dependent on the ability to visualize the stent; it is not sufficient to rely on balloon markers since the stent-balloon relationship may change slightly during advancement. Furthermore, most stents vary in length from 15-20 mm, mandating precise placement in long tubular lesions or in severe occlusive dissections. The radiopacity of tantalum stents (e.g., Wiktor, Cordis stents) is superior to stainless steel stents (Palmaz-Schatz, Gianturco-Roubin, AVE stents). Finally, biliary stents are easier to visualize than Palmaz-Schatz coronary stents because of their enhanced metal density.

4. **Reliable Expansion.** In general, balloon-expandable stents provide more reliable delivery and expansion than self-expanding or thermal-memory stents. Balloon-expandable stents permit expansion from 3.0-5.0 mm in diameter depending on the final size of the balloon used to dilate the stent (Table 26.1). Biliary stents permit expansion from 4.0-9.0 mm; they should not be used in smaller vessels because of the increased metal density (and risk of thrombosis) at diameters < 4 mm.

5. **Stent Surface Area.** In addition to the length of the lesion and the visibility of the stent, the ability to completely cover the lesion is dependent on the stent surface area, which varies from 7-20% for most stents (Table 26.1). However, there may be a relationship between the amount of metal surface

Table 26.1. Intracoronary Stents: Technical Features

	Wallstent* (Schneider)	Palmaz-Schatz ** (Johnson & Johnson)	Gianturco-Roubin (Cook)	MultiLink (ACS)
Design	Self expanding	Balloon expandable	Balloon expandable	Balloon expandable
Configuration	Woven wire mesh	Slotted tube	Flexible wire	Slotted tube with loops and bridges
Material	Stainless steel	Stainless steel	Stainless steel	Stainless steel
Strut diameter (mm/inch)	0.08/0.003	0.08/0.003	0.15/0.006	0.05/0.002
Delivery sheath	Yes	Yes	No	Yes
Length (mm)	15-43	15	12,20	15
Metal surface area (%)	10-15	12	10	10-15
Maximum guidewire (in)	0.018	0.014	0.018	0.014
Minimum guide ID (in)	0.077	0.084	0.086	0.075
Expanded diameter (mm)	3.5-6.0	3.0-5.0	2.0-4.5	3.0-3.85
Radio-opacity (Fluoroscopy)	Poor	Poor	Poor	Fair
Deployment pressure (ATM)	---	6-8	4-7	9

*   Less-shortening Wallstent-=second generation prototype; Less metal surface, shortens by 25%.

**   Biliary stents and peripheral stents have been used in large coronary arteries and saphenous vein grafts

***   Monorail design will accept a 0.014-inch guidewire

****   The Strecker stent (Boston Scientific) was withdrawn from the market.

area and the tendency toward thrombus formation, which may account for the higher rates of acute and subacute thrombosis with the original Wallstent compared to balloon-expandable stents.[3] On the other hand, stents with inadequate surface area may have insufficient radial strength; consequences include the inability to withstand elastic recoil of the arterial wall, and inadequate scaffolding of severe dissection flaps (or tufts of damaged plaque and endothelium protruding through the stent struts into the lumen), facilitating thrombus formation and/or restenosis. [15]   In some cases, multiple overlapping stents are needed to prevent recoil, which increases the metal surface area and may increase the risk of thrombosis and/or restenosis. Clearly, the ideal stent has not yet been developed; the relative merits of each stent design await further investigation.

C. TECHNIQUE OF STENT PLACEMENT
1. Self-Expanding Stents. To facilitate stent placement, target lesions must be predilated using a

Table 26.1. Intracoronary Stents: Technical Features (con't)

Self-Expanding Stent (SciMed)	MicroStent-II (AVE)	Wiktor (Medtronic)	Nir**** (SciMed)	Cordis
Self expanding	Balloon expandable	Balloon expandable	Balloon expandable	Balloon expandable
Slotted tube	Coil wire	Flexible wire	Wire mesh	Coil wire
Stainless steel	Stainless steel	Tantalum	Stainless steel	Tantalum
0.13/0.005	0.20/0.008	0.13/0.005	0.08/0.003	0.13/0.005
Yes	No	No	No	No
14, 20, 30	6-36	16	9, 16, 32	18
20	8.5	7-9	14-19	15
NA	0.014	0.018***	0.014	0.018
0.072	0.072	0.082	0.065	0.072
2.75-4.25	2.5-4.5	2.5-4.0	2.0-5.0	3.0-4.0
NA	Good	Good	Fair	Good
---	9-12	6	8	8

*   Less-shortening Wallstent-=second generation prototype; Less metal surface, shortens by 25%.
**   Biliary stents and peripheral stents have been used in large coronary arteries and saphenous vein grafts
***   Monorail design will accept a 0.014-inch guidewire
****   The Strecker stent (Boston Scientific) was withdrawn from the market.

conventional angioplasty balloon through a standard 8F or 9F guiding catheter. After predilation, the angioplasty balloon is exchanged for the stent/delivery system (Figure 26.5), which is positioned to completely cover the lesion. The stent is delivered by retracting the constraining sheath around the stent, resulting in expansion and shortening of the stent inside the vessel lumen (Figure 26.6). The selected stent should be 0.5 mm larger than the diameter of the adjacent normal reference segment; the inner surface of the stent may be smoothed by further balloon inflations. Greater degrees of stent oversizing may be necessary to resist elastic recoil and attenuate the impact of late intimal hyperplasia.[16]

2. **Balloon-Expandable Stents.** Two balloon expandable stents are approved by the FDA: the Gianturco-Roubin stent and the Palmaz-Schatz stent (Table 26.2). Predilation with a conventional angioplasty balloon is required prior to insertion of all balloon-expandable stents; to minimize the risk of unwanted dissection during planned stenting, the vessel should be slightly underdilated with a balloon measuring 0.5 mm less than the reference diameter. Besides facilitating stent insertion, predilation can confirm that the balloon (and therefore the stent) can be fully inflated, and will also allow the operator to visualize the "shoulders" of the original lesion, thereby facilitating complete

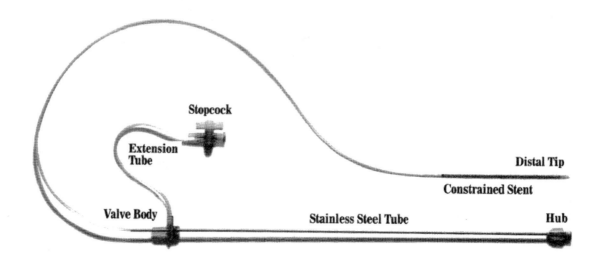

Figure 26.5 The Wallstent Delivery System

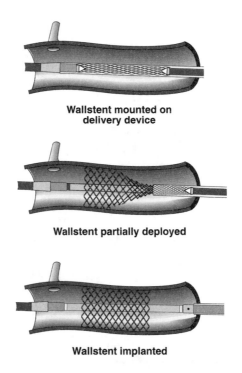

Wallstent mounted on
delivery device

Wallstent partially deployed

Wallstent implanted

Figure 26.6 Deployment of the Wallstent

Table 26.2. Comparison of the Palmaz-Schatz Stent and the Gianturco-Roubin Stent.

	Gianturco-Roubin Stent	Palmaz-Schatz Stent
FDA Approved	Yes	Yes
Indication	Bail-out	Elective
Vessel	Native, SVG	Native
Delivery sheath	No	Yes
Predilation	Proximal lesion, target	Target
Balloon markers	1-2 mm beyond stent	1-2 mm beyond stent
Balloon inflation	30-60 sec	5-15 sec
Balloon deflation	15-30 sec	5-15 sec
Adjunctive PTCA	Yes	Yes
Balloon/artery ratio	1.0-1.1	1.0-1.1
Inflation pressure	> 12 ATM	> 12 ATM
Typical appearance	Mildly scallopped	Smooth

coverage by the stent (Figure 26.7). The inability to fully dilate a rigid stenosis with a high-pressure balloon is a contraindication to stenting. In situations where a stent cannot be delivered because of proximal vessel tortuosity, techniques to enhance success include the use of guiding catheters that enhance coaxial alignment and optimize backup support; heavy duty or extra support guidewires to facilitate stent advancement; and the "buddy wire" approach to straighten tortuous segments (Table 26.3). The 0.014- or 0.018-inch Platinum-Plus guidewire (Meditech, Watertown, MA) provides the most straightening force and support, and is particularly useful for difficult procedures; pseudolesions, however, are commonly observed. Ideal placement of the stent should be confirmed by contrast injections prior to stent delivery. For the Palmaz-Schatz stent, the stent/balloon/delivery sheath should be advanced across the lesion (Figure 26.8). Once in position, the delivery sheath should be withdrawn into the guiding catheter, and the stent delivered by balloon inflation (Figure 26.9). For the Gianturco-Roubin stent, it is important to adequately predilate moderate lesions proximal to the target lesion, to facilitate passage of the stent without deforming it (Figures 26.10). In some cases, multiple stents may be required to cover long lesions or dissections. In general, it is desirable to place the most distal stent first; however, it may not always be possible to place a stent in the distal segment without first stenting the proximal segment (particularly for aorto-ostial lesions). In the earlier experience with balloon-expandable stents, adjunctive angioplasty was recommended using slightly oversized balloons at nominal inflation pressure. More recent experience suggests that post-stent angioplasty should be performed using high-pressure balloons matched to the normal reference diameter (balloon/artery ratio = 1.0-1.1) and inflated to 14-20 ATM;[17] intravascular ultrasound may be valuable for determining the actual reference vessel diameter and for confirming ideal stent apposition to the vessel wall (Figure

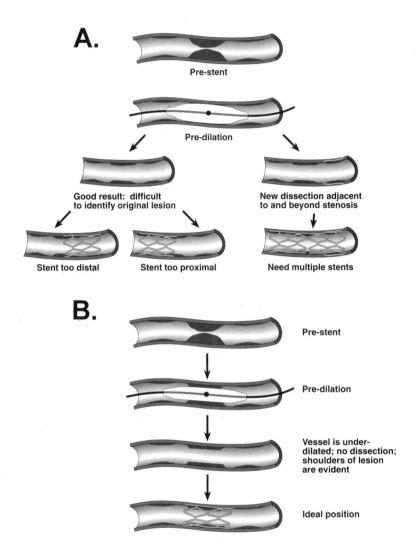

Figure 26.7 Adjunctive PTCA Before Stent Implantation: Importance of Balloon Size

A. PTCA with a full-size balloon (balloon/artery ratio ~ 1.0) may result in a "perfect" result (making it difficult to identify the original lesion), or in dissection beyond the original stenosis. Multiple stents may be needed to ensure complete coverage.

B. PTCA with an undersize balloon (0.5 mm smaller than the vessel diameter) results in underdilation; the shoulders of the original lesion are evident and there is no dissection. Ideal stent position can be achieved. Note: This technique should not be employed for aorto-ostial lesions or rigid lesions; initial PTCA should be performed with full-size balloons.

Table 26.3. Troubleshooting with Stents

Solution: Palmaz-Schatz Stent	Solution: Gianturco-Roubin Stent

Problem

1. Lesion < 5 mm

• Avoid placing articulation on lesion • Consider disarticulated stent(s)	• Use 12 mm stent

2. Moderate disease proximal to target lesion

• Place stent in target lesion; then reassess proximal disease	• Dilate proximal disease; if dissection occurs, stent that, too

3. Cannot predilate target lesion (rigid)

• Use high-pressure balloon alone, Rotablator, or DCA	• Use high-pressure balloon alone, Rotablator, or DCA

4. Proximal vessel tortuosity

• "Strong" guide support with excellent coaxial alignment ("push test")* • Heavy-duty or platinum-plus guide wire • "Buddy" wire approach** • Use disarticulated stent(s) • "Stentless" delivery sheath technique***	• "Strong" guide support with excellent coaxial alignment ("push" test)* • Heavy-duty or platinum-plus guide wire

5. Delivery system will not cross lesion

• Verify that the sheath is not leading the balloon • Advance delivery balloon to ensure tapered transition • Predilate with larger ballon • Improve guide support, alignment • Heavy duty or platinum-plus guidewire • "Buddy" wire approach* • Disarticulated stents(s) • "Stentless" delivery sheath technique*** • Bare-stent on lower profie balloon	• Predilate with larger balloon • Improve guide support, alignment • Heavy duty or platinum-plus guidewire

6. Inadvertent unstented proximal disease

• Insert another tandem stent (1 mm overlap)	• Insert another tandem stent (1 mm overlap)

Solution: **Palmaz-Schatz Stent**	Solution: **Gianturco-Roubin Stent**

7. Inadvertent unstented distal disease

• Post-dilate stent with high-pressure balloon • Optimize guide and guidewire • Insert another tandem stent (1 mm overlap)	• Post-dilate stent with high-pressure balloon • Optimize guide and guidewire • Insert another tandem stent (1 mm overlap)

8. Sidebranch occlusion

• Post-dilate stent with high-pressure balloon • Retrieve sidebranch with PTCA if indicated. Note: This is feasible with certain balloons (see reference #129)	• Post-dilate stent with high-pressure balloon • Retrieve sidebranch with PTCA if indicated

9. In-stent result is suboptimal

• Consider IVUS or angioscopy • Repeat PTCA with larger balloon or higher pressure • Overlapping stent	• Consider IVUS or angioscopy • Repeat PTCA with larger balloon or higher pressure • Prolonged balloon inflations • Overlapping stent

10. Loss of guidewire after stent deployment

• Must recross stent with large J-tip on floppy wire • Prolapse J-wire across stented segment • "Steering" a wire to avoid struts is unreliable	• Must recross stent with large J-tip on floppy wire • Prolapse J-wire across stented segment • "Steering" a wire to avoid coils is unreliable

11. Angulated lesion

• Avoid articulation on angle vertex • "Strong" guide support with excellent coaxial alignment • Heavy duty or platinum-plus guidewire • "Buddy" wire approach** • Use disarticulated stent(s) • "Stentless" delivery sheath technique • May need overlapping stents	• "Strong" guide support with excellent coaxial alignment • Heavy duty or platinum-plus guidewire • May need overlapping stents

Solution: Palmaz-Schatz Stent	Solution: Gianturco-Roubin Stent

12. Ostial lesions

• Predilate with noncompliant full size balloon	• Predilate with noncompliant full size balloon
• Consider debulking before stenting	• Consider debulking before stenting
• Avoid "aggressive" guiding catheters	• Avoid "aggressive" guiding catheters
• Heavy-duty or platinum-plus guidewire	• May need overlapping stents
• "Buddy" wire approach**	
• Use disarticulated stent(s)	
• "Stentless" delivery sheath technique***	
• May need overlapping stents	

13. Balloon rupture during stent deployment

• Gently advance and then slowly retract delivery balloon	• Gently advance and then slowly retract delivery balloon
• If unable to retract balloon, rapid inflation with full strength contrast may allow nearly-full balloon expansion	• If unable to retract balloon, rapid inflation with full strength contrast may allow nearly-full balloon expansion
• Use incremental increases in balloon size with low-profile balloon to further expand stent	• Use incremental increases in balloon size with low-profile balloon to further expand stent

14. Balloon rupture during post-stent PTCA

• Use noncompliant balloons	• Use noncompliant balloons
• Consider smaller noncompliant "kissing" balloons	• Consider smaller noncompliant "kissing" balloons

15. Tapering vessel

• Tapered balloon	• Tapered balloon

16. Removing an undeployed stent

• If stent is inside delivery sheath, remove entire delivery system	• Retract stent up to guide (not inside guide); remove guide, stent, and sheath en bloc over guidewire
• If stent is beyond delivery sheath, retract stent up to guide (not inside guide); remove guide, stent, and sheath en bloc over guidewire	

17. Accordioned stent

• Not applicable	• Inflate delivery balloon to 1 ATM
	• Retract delivery balloon up to (not inside) guide; remove guide, stent and sheath en bloc over guidewire

---

* Push test: Advance guiding catheter into proximal vessel; if it disengages, change to a different guide
** Buddy wire approach: Use double extra-support or heavy duty wires to straighten the vessel; once the stent delivery system is in position across the target lesion, remove the buddy wire; do not deploy the stent until the buddy wire has been removed.
*** Stentless delivery sheath technique: Remove the stent delivery balloon (and stent) from the delivery sheath and replace it with a low-profie 0.014-inch-compatible balloon catheter; advance the low-profile balloon/delivery sheath across the lesion. Once the delivery sheath is positioned distal to the target lesion, exchange the low-profile balloon for the stent delivery balloon (and stent). Retract the delivery sheath and deploy the stent.

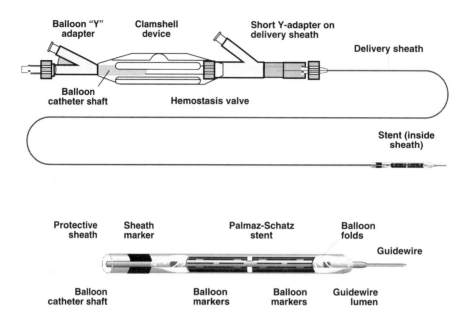

Figure 26.8 Palmaz-Schatz Stent: Delivery System

26.11).[17,18]   Preliminary data from the MUSCAT trial suggest that predilation, stent deployment, and adjunctive PTCA can be achieved with a special single balloon (Focus balloon; Cardiovascular Dynamics, Santa Clara, CA).[19]

3. **Radial Artery Technique.** Most operators use the percutaneous femoral artery approach for stent implantation. Recently, several centers in Europe have started using the percutaneous radial artery approach, even in patients who are fully anticoagulated on warfarin at the time of intervention. Advantages of this technique are primarily related to patient comfort, reduction in bleeding and vascular complications, and a potential reduction in hospital stay; in addition, radial artery stent implants may be performed on an outpatient basis.[20-23] The need for alternative sites to femoral access may diminish as the need for vigorous anticoagulation decreases (see Adjunctive Therapy, Section F, below).

D. **INDICATIONS FOR STENTING (Table 26.4)**. In 1996, indications for stenting may be broadly classified as "definite" indications (FDA approved; based on compelling observational data and randomized clinical trials); "probable" indications (FDA approval is likely; based on compelling observational data, but pending completion of randomized clinical trials); "possible" indications (stents

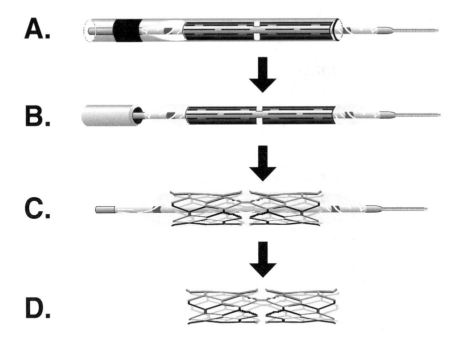

Figure 26.9 Palmaz-Schatz Stent: Deployment

A. After predilating, position the delivery system across the lesion.
B. Retract the delivery sheath and confirm ideal stent position.
C. Inflate the delivery balloon and deploy the stent. Further adjunctive PTCA is recommended with high-pressure balloons.
D. Final result.

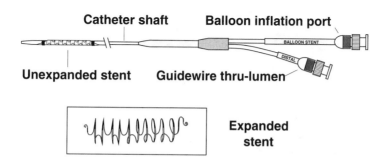

Figure 26.10   Gianturco-Roubin Stent Delivery System

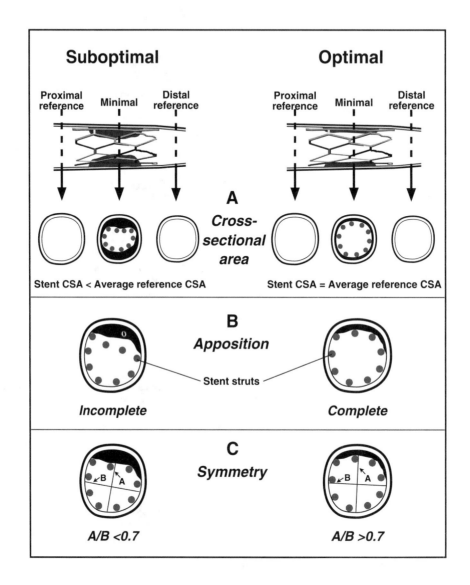

Figure 26.11   Optimal Stent Deployment: IVUS Criteria

A.   Cross-sectional area index > 0.8: The ratio of stent minimal CSA to normal reference vessel CSA (average CSA proximal and distal to stent).

B.   Apposition: Maximum gap < 0.1 mm between stent strut (or coil) and underlying wall.

C.   Symmetry index > 0.7: The ratio of the stent minor axis (A) to stent major axis (B).

Table 26.4. Indications for Stenting

Definite

    Abrupt closure (GRS)

    Threatened closure (GRS)

    Focal, de novo lesions in native vessel ≥ 3mm (PSS)

Probable

    SVG (focal or tubular lesions)

Possible

    SVG (degenerated)

    Bifurcation lesions

    Aorto-ostial lesions

    Restenotic lesions

    Vessels < 3mm

    Chronic total occlusion

    Lesions > 20mm

Contraindications

    Gross thrombus

Abbreviations: GRS = Gianturco-Roubin stent; PSS = Palmaz-Schatz stent; SVG = saphenous vein graft

are commonly employed, but data are lacking); and contraindications (stent implantation is not recommended). Non-FDA-approved (or "off-label") uses for stents may represent up to 40% of stent procedures in busy interventional practices.[24]

1. **Definite Indications for Stenting** (FDA approved; based on compelling observational data and randomized clinical trials)

    a. **Reversal of Abrupt Closure.** The overall incidence of abrupt closure after PTCA is 4-12%; standard methods to reverse abrupt closure (repeat balloon inflations, vasodilators, thrombolytic agents) may reduce the need for emergency surgery to ≤ 2%. In the randomized Trial of Angioplasty and Stents in Canada (TASC-II) and in several observational series (Table 26.5) (Chapter 20), primary stenting was more effective than prolonged balloon inflations for failed PTCA.[25-28] In the Hirulog Angioplasty Trial, abrupt closure occurred in 378 patients, representing 9.2% of patients enrolled; 40% were treated with bailout stenting and 60% were treated with repeat PTCA. Compared to patients treated with repeat PTCA,

Table 26.5. In-hospital Outcome After "Bail-Out" Stenting

Series	Stent	No. (pts)	In-hospital Complications (%)	
			Stent Thrombosis	**D / MI / CABG**
Goy[30] (1995)	PSS	32	13	8 / 6.3 / 0
Urban[31] (1995)	PSS	52	4	0 / 10 / 4
Metz[32] (1994)	PSS	88	9	3 / 26 / 8
Schomig[33] (1994)	PSS	339	6.9	1.3 / 4.0 / 9
Kiemeneij[34] (1993)	PSS	52	23	3 / - / 15
Reifart[35] (1992)	PSS	64	32	6 / 3 / 5
Hermann[36] (1992)	PSS	56	16	0 / 5.3 / 3.6
Chan[37] (1995)	GRS	42	4.8	0 / 4.8 / 7.1
Sutton[38] (1994)	GRS	415	-	3 / 5 / 12
Agrawal[39] (1994)	GRS	240	7	-
George[40] (1993)	GRS	518	8.7	2.2 / 5.5 / 4.3
Roubin[41] (1992)	GRS	115	7.6	1.7 / 16 / 4.2
Goy[30] (1995)	Wiktor	33	18	9 / 8 / 3
Vrolix[42] (1994)	Wiktor	180	13.3	3.3 / 12 / 16.5
Garratt[43] (1994)	Wiktor	308	3	3.7 / 2.7 / 8.7
Reifart[35] (1992)	Strecker	48	21	10 / 2 / 6
Ozake[44] (1995)	MicroStent	20	0	0 / 10 / 5

Abreviations: D = death; MI = myocardial infarction; CABG = emergency coronary artery bypass surgery; PSS = Palmaz-Schatz stent; GRS - Gianturco-Roubin stent; - = not reported stent patients had a lower incidence of emergency CABG (10% vs. 19%, p < 0.05) but more hemorrhagic complications (34% vs. 20%, p < 0.01); importantly, there was a lower incidence of recurrent ischemic events at 6 months in stented patients (54% vs. 71%, p < 0.001).[50] Intravascular stents have essentially replaced other approved or investigational devices for reversing abrupt closure, including DCA and thermal welding devices; in fact, some centers without cardiac surgery rely on stents alone for failed PTCA.[29] For emergency indications, numerous studies have demonstrated the favorable impact of stenting for threatened and established abrupt closure (Table 26.5);[17-31] successful stent delivery is accomplished in 90% of these cases. Almost all stents (Wallstent, Gianturco-Roubin stent, Wiktor stent, Palmaz-Schatz stent, Microstent) have been used successfully in patients with abrupt closure; in the United States, the only FDA-approved stent for reversal of abrupt closure is the Gianturco-Roubin stent. Despite the success of stents for reversing abrupt closure, there is still significant patient morbidity, including stent thrombosis (0-32%), myocardial infarction (2-16%), emergency bypass surgery (0-16.5%), and death (0-10%). Although unplanned use of stents is associated with a higher incidence of adverse in-hospital events and lower procedural success compared to planned elective stenting, most adverse events relate to abrupt closure *prior* to stenting, rather than stent failure per se.[46] Many dissections leading to abrupt closure exceed 20 mm in length but can be managed by multiple tandem stents;[47-49] focal dissections (10-15 mm) are ideally suited for placement of a single stent.

Stents are the most important advance for treating abrupt closure; nevertheless, several issues await resolution:

- **Thrombotic Closure.** Although a minority of abrupt closures are due to thrombosis, these might be managed better by other methods, such as thrombolytic therapy, extraction atherectomy, PTCA, perfusion balloon angioplasty, or local drug delivery. Stenting in the setting of a large untreated thrombus is relatively contraindicated due to the risk of further thrombus formation, but could be considered if thrombus can be removed or dissolved.

- **Timing of Stenting.** The timing of stent implantation for abrupt closure appears to be important; the risk of MI is nearly 3-fold higher when stents are used for established abrupt closure than for threatened abrupt closure.[51] Since delayed stenting appears to be associated with an increased risk of ischemic complications, early (pre-emptive) stenting for threatened closure may be indicated. However, other studies suggest that stenting for threatened abrupt closure was not better than conventional therapy without stenting.[52,53]

- **Threatened Closure.** There appears to be no difference in major ischemic complications, vascular injury, or late outcome when Gianturco-Roubin stents are implanted for failed PTCA with moderate dissection compared to failed PTCA with severe dissection;[54] preliminary data suggest that emergency stenting after failed PTCA is less costly than emergency CABG, resulting in a cost-savings of 17%.[55]

- **Temporary Stents.** Other strategies using temporary stents are also under investigation. Although temporary stenting with the Flow Support Catheter has been shown to stabilize dissection and avoid the need for a permanent implant,[56] this device was withdrawn from the market. A heat-activated recoverable temporary stent (HARTS) is also under investigation for treatment of failed PTCA.[57]

b. **Prevention of Restenosis.** Current data indicate that stenting can be performed with high (>95%) success and low complication rates (< 5%) despite the presence of high-risk clinical and anatomical factors (Tables 26.6, 26.7).[58-71] In addition, randomized and observational studies demonstrate that stenting results in a large, smooth lumen and a lower incidence of restenosis compared to PTCA.

1. **Incidence of Stent Restenosis.** Quantitative angiographic assessment of lumen dimensions after stenting frequently reveals a residual stenoses < 5% (without dissection or luminal abnormalities)[3,58-73] and restenosis rates < 20% (Tables 26.6, 26.7).[33,36,38,40,58,63,64,67,74] Recently, two multicenter randomized trials compared immediate and longterm results of elective Palmaz-Schatz stenting vs. PTCA in de novo lesions in native coronary arteries (Table 26.8);[75,76] both studies confirmed that stenting resulted in better lumen enlargement, higher procedural success, lower restenosis rates, fewer repeat procedures, and better event-free survival. Elective stenting of de novo lesions resulted in less restenosis compared to restenotic lesions (14% vs. 39%).[63]

2. **Mechanism of Beneficial Effect.** The favorable impact of stenting on restenosis relates to its ability to achieve superior lumen enlargement (final diameter stenosis from minus 5% to 10%), to minimize elastic recoil (usually < 8%; possibly less recoil after Palmaz-Schatz vs. Gianturco-Roubin stent[83]), and to virtually eliminate arterial remodeling.[79-82,290] PTCA vs. stent trials suggest *more* intimal thickening after stenting, but this was more than offset by its other beneficial effects.

3. **Time Course for Restenosis.** The time course of restenosis is similar to PTCA,[84,85] but several angiographic studies suggest that in-stent minimal lumen diameter improves between 6 months and 3 years after implantation; 6 month angiography may actually *underestimate* the longterm benefit of stenting.[86,87] As discussed in Chapter 24, restenosis is inversely proportional to acute gain, and is due to elastic recoil, intimal thickening, and arterial remodeling. Recurrent ischemia beyond 6-12 months after Gianturco-Roubin or Palmaz-Schatz stenting is virtually always due to progressive disease in a nonstented vessel.

4. **Predictors of Stent Restenosis and Event-Free Survival (Table 26.9).** Comparison of studies of late outcome after stenting are hampered by different

Table 26.6. Results of Stents in Native Coronary Arteries.

Series	Stent	N	Thrombosis (%)	Comments
Hall[58] (1995)	PSS	411	0.8	Optimal stenting with IVUS; no Coumadin
Morice[59] (1995)	All	1250	1.7	No Coumadin; French Registry
Colombo[60] (1995)	MicroStent	16	0	Small vessels (reference diameter 2.8mm)
Hamasaki[61] (1995)	Cordis	63	0	Major complication (0%)
Karouny[62] (1995)	Wiktor	225	4	Death (2.2%); CABG (4.4%); RS (27%)
Dawkins[69] (1995)	MultiLink	56	0	CABG (1.9%); Coumadin
Chevalier[70] (1995)	MicroStent	100	3	Death (0); CABG (1%); perforation (1%)
Goy[71] (1995)	PSS	60	-	6-month EFS (88%); RS (23%)
Goy[71] (1995)	Wiktor	42	-	6-month EFS (76%); RS (47%)
Savage[63] (1994)	PSS	300	4.7	
Popma[64] (1994)	PSS	108	-	IVUS guidance; CABG (3.7%), RS (9.3%)
Webb[65] (1994)	MicroStent	27	0	Success (100%); no complications
deJaeger[66] (1993)	Wiktor	109	12	
Carrozza[67] (1992)	PSS	220	0.4	CABG (0.4%); RS (25%)
Strauss[68] (1992)	Wallstent	265	15	
Serruys[3] (1991)	Wallstent	105	24	

Abbreviations: PSS = Palmaz-Schatz stent; CABG = emergency coronary artery bypass surgery; RS = restenosis; IVUS = intravascular ultrasound; EFS = event-free survial; - = not reported

Table 26.7. Late Outcome After Stenting

Series	Stent	IND	F/U (m)	rePTCA/CABG/MI/D	Comments
Ortiz[286] (1996)	PSS	FPTCA	8	-	RS (15%), EFS (85%)
Ortiz[286] (1996)	GRS	FPTCA	8	-	RS (44%), EFS (70%)
Wong[74] (1995)	PSS	Elect	8	7.9 / 5.4 / 3.5 / 4.9	EFS 83% at 6 mos, 76% at 12 mos
Hall[58] (1995)	PSS	All	6	11.4 / 6.2 / 4.9 / 2.1	Optimal stenting
Savage[63] (1994)	PSS	Elect	12	13 / 8 / 3.7 / 0.7	RS 14% (de novo), 39% (restenotic); 1 year EFS 80%
Sutton[38] (1994)	GRS	Elect	3	- / 6 / 0.5 / 3	Recurrent ischemia 9%
Sutton[38] (1994)	GRS	FPTCA	3	- / 12 / 5 / 2	Recurrent ischemia 20%
Schomig[33] (1994)	PSS	FPTCA	1	6.3 / 1.0 / 4.0 / 1.3	2 yr EFS 71%
George[40] (1993)	GRS	FPTCA	6	- / 11.2 / 7.1 / 3.6	
Hermann[36] (1992)	PSS	FPTCA	1	- / 13 / 19 / 3.6	SAT 16%
Carrozza[67] (1992)	PSS	Elect	36	9 / 3.7 / 1.3 / 2.3	AR 25% (19% for de novo); 3 yr EFS 70%
Debbas[92] (1995)	Wall	All	6	9 / 8 / 11 / 6	9 yr EFS 55%
Laham[91] (1995)	PSS	All	54	- / - / 13 / 14	Late TLR 5%; Any revascularization 39%
Kern[93] (1995)	PSS	All	61	14 / 10 / 5 / 6	

Abbreviations: PSS = Palmaz-Schatz stent; GRS = Gianturco-Roubin stent; Wall = Wallstent; FPTCA = failed PTCA; F/U = Follow-up interval after stent (months); - = not repored; ARS = angiographic restenosis; EFS = event-free survival; SAT = subacute thrombosis; RS = restenosis; TLR = target lesion revascularization; IND = indication; Elect = elective stent

Table 26.8. Results of Multicenter Randomized Trials of PTCA and Palmaz-Schatz Stent.

	STRESS[75] (n=407)		BENESTENT[76] (n=516)	
	PTCA	**Stent**	**PTCA**	**Stent**
In-hospital results				
Procedural Sucess (%)	89.6	96.1**	91	92.7
Final DS (%)	35	19*	33	22*
All ischemic events (%)	7.9	5.9	6.2	6.9
Death	1.5	0	0	0
Q-MI	3.0	2.9	0.8	1.9
nQMI	2.0	1.5	2.3	1.5
CABG	4.0	2.0	3.9	3.1
PTCA	1.0	2.0	1.2	0.4
Bleeding/Vascular (%)	4.0	7.3	3.1	13.5*
Vessel occlusion (%)+	10.2	3.4	6.2	3.5
LOS (day)	2.8	5.8*	3.1	8.5*
6 Month Follow-up (%)				
Angiographic restenosis	42	31**	32	22*
Ischemic events	23	17	24	14
TLR	22	14**	27	18**
EFS	72	78**	60	70**

Abbreviations: STRESS = Stent Restenosis Study; BENESTENT = Belgium-Netherlands Stent Trial; DS = diameter stenosis; nQMI = non-Q-wave myocardial infarction; CABG = emergency coronary artery bypass surgery; LOS = length of stay; TLR = target lesion revascularization; EFS = event-free survival.
* $p < 0.001$
** $p < 0.005$
+   vessel occlusion due to abrupt closure (PTCA group) or stent thrombosis (stent group)

Table 26.9. Predictors of Adverse Outcome After Stents

In-hospital Ischemic Complications After Bailout Stenting[38,45]
    Delayed stent implantation
    Sidebranch occlusion
    Multiple stents
    Residual dissection
    Stent diameter

Stent Thrombosis[39,106,107]
    Post-stent residual dissection/distal disease
    Stent diameter < 3mm
    Residual filling defect in stent
    Multiple stents
    Bailout stent

Late Cardiac Events After Bailout Stenting[38]
    Stent for Abrupt Closure
    Multivessel disease
    Small stent size

Stent Retenosis[94-96]
    Multiple stents
    Restenosis lesion
    Post-stent residual stenosis > 10%

indications for stents (abrupt closure, elective stents), different stent designs (Palmaz-Schatz stent, Gianturco-Roubin stent), and different target lesions (native vessels, vein grafts). Nevertheless, there appears to be a higher incidence of stent restenosis under the following conditions: Multiple stents, vessel diameter < 3.0 mm, restenotic lesions, and lesion length > 10 mm.[94-96] While these angiographic variables have been associated with stent restenosis, several clinical variables have been associated with less favorable event-free survival, including diabetes, post-procedural non-Q-wave MI, and multivessel disease.[38,91]

5. **Patterns of Stent Restenosis.** In one report, angiographic patterns of stent restenosis included diffuse in-stent restenosis (33%), focal restenosis at the edges of the stent (26%), and focal in-stent restenosis involving the articulation (33%) or the body of the stent (8%);[101] focal in-stent restenosis of the body of the stent was identified in 17% of stent restenosis in another study.[102]

6. **Treatment of Stent Restenosis.** Treatment of in-stent restenosis is relatively straightforward. Conventional PTCA has been applied most commonly;[47,96,103] success rates generally exceed 90%, although recurrent restenosis occurs in 50%.[96] (PTCA

generally results in compression and extrusion of intimal tissue rather than stent-expansion.[47]) Rotablator atherectomy should not be used due to the risk of burr entrapment. ELCA and DCA have been used rarely, but offer no clear advantage over PTCA. In the multicenter Palmaz-Schatz stent registry, stent restenosis was managed by medical therapy (3%), CABG (13.6%), and re-PTCA (40%). There is probably no need for oral anticoagulation after PTCA for stent restenosis.

2. **Probable Indications For Stenting** (FDA approval is likely; based on compelling observational data but pending completion of randomized clinical trials)

   a. **Saphenous Vein Bypass Grafts.** In general, intravascular stents offer the best opportunity for immediate enlargement of the vascular lumen, particularly in large vessels. Acute and longterm results suggest that stents may be the treatment of choice for focal or tubular lesions in nondegenerated vein grafts.

      1. **Nondegenerated Grafts (Table 26.10).** Although virtually all stents have been implanted in saphenous vein grafts, the largest experience is with the Palmaz-Schatz coronary stent and the Palmaz-Schatz biliary stent:[68,74,108-119] Numerous studies suggest that successful stent delivery can be accomplished in 95-100% of lesions, with a low incidence of stent thrombosis (0-3.4%), emergency CABG (0-2.8%), myocardial infarction (0-4.3%), and death (0-2%). Restenosis rates after Palmaz-Schatz stenting range between 17-35%. In the multicenter prospective randomized trial of PTCA vs. Palmaz-Schatz coronary stents in vein grafts (SAVED), preliminary data suggest that stenting achieves superior immediate lumen enlargement (final diameter stenosis 12% vs. 33%, $p < 0.001$), higher procedural success (96% vs. 85%, $p < 0.05$), and a lower incidence of emergency CABG (0% vs. 6.7%, $p < 0.05$);[121] preliminary follow-up data suggest similar total- and event-free survival at 3 months, but complete 6-month angiographic and clinical outcomes are pending.[282] In contrast to PTCA, stenting of vein grafts does not appear to be influenced by graft age; acute and longterm results were similar for vein grafts less than or greater than 4 years of age.[122] However, similar to PTCA, 2-year event-free survival after vein graft stenting is only 55%; this attrition in late outcome is due to increasing mortality, recurrent ischemia, and unfavorable clinical characteristics of many patients treated with previous CABG.[123,124] Stenting of the internal mammary bypass graft is also feasible,[125] but data are limited.

      2. **Degenerated Grafts.** The ideal intervention for degenerated vein grafts is unknown. Some operators recommend TEC atherectomy followed by immediate stent implantation to achieve definitive lumen enlargement and reduce restenosis.[126] Others recommend a strategy of initial TEC followed by 1-2 months of oral warfarin and staged stent implantation; compared to immediate stenting, this deferred stent strategy resulted in less distal embolization (10.7% vs. 22.7%) and fewer in-hospital ischemic complications (0% vs. 11.4%), but silent total occlusion occurred in 15%.[127] In some cases, intragraft urokinase may facilitate

Table 26.10. Results of Stents in Saphenous Vein Bypass Grafts

Series	Stent	No. Lesion	Success (%)	SAT (%)	D/MI/CABG (%)	VSR /XF*	RS (%)
Wong[74] (1995)	PSS	624	98.8	1.4	1.7 / 0.3 / 0.9	8.0 / 6.3	30
Rechavia[108] (1995)	PSS, Biliary	29	100	0	0 / 0 / 0	3.4 / 6.8	-
Wong[109] (1995)	PSS, Biliary	205	95.3	1.7	1.3 / 0.9 / 0.4	15.9 / 25	-
Piana[110] (1994)	PSS, Biliary	200	98.5	0.6	0.6 / 0 / 0	8.5 / 14.0	17
Eeckhout[111] (1994)	Wallstent, Wiktor	58	100		2 / 0 / 2	14	25
Keane[112] (1994)	New Wallstent	29	97	3.4	0 / 0 / 0	3.4 / 6.8	32
Fenton[113] (1994)	PSS	209	98.5	0.5	0.4 / 0 / 0	17.2 / 12	34
Leon[114] (1993)	PSS	589	97	1.4	1.7 / 0.3 / 0.9	7.5 / 15.5	30
Fortuna[115] (1993)	Wiktor	101	90	2	1 / 3 / 1	-	-
Pomerantz[116] (1992)	PSS	84	99	0	0 / 0 / 0	5	25
Bilodeau[117] (1992)	GRS	37	-	-	0 / 2.5 / 0	-	35
Strauss[68] (1992)	Wallstent	145	-	8	-	-	39
deScheerder[118] (1992)	New Wallstent	69	100	10	1.4 / 4.3 / 2.8	33	47
Urban[119] (1989)	Wallstent	14	100	0	0 / 0 / 0	7.7 / 7.7	20

Abbreviations: VSR = vascular surgical repair; XF = blood transfusion; SAT = subacute thrombosis, D = death; MI = myocardial infarction; CABG = emergency coronary artery bypass surgery; RS = restenosis
* single numbers indicate combined incidence of vascular repair and/or blood transfusion.

stenting; in one report, procedural success was achieved in 93.3%, with stent thrombosis in 6.7%, Q-wave MI in 3.3%, and serious vascular injury in 16.7%.[128]

3. **Possible Indications for Stenting** (Not FDA approved; stents are sometimes employed, but data are lacking).

   a. **Bifurcation Lesions (Chapter 10).** Experimental data have shown that flow into nondiseased sidebranches is well-preserved after stent placement, and several angiographic studies suggest a low incidence of sidebranch occlusion (see below). Nevertheless, stents should be used cautiously in patients with stenoses involving significant sidebranches. While sidebranches may still be accessible by PTCA after Gianturco-Roubin and other coil stent implantation, there may be a greater chance of balloon entrapment in the struts of slotted tubular stents (e.g., Palmaz-Schatz).[129] However, occluded sidebranches can be successfully retrieved by PTCA through 86% of Palmaz-Schatz stents and 75% of Gianturco-Roubin stents.[287] Important considerations include the likelihood of immediate and future revascularization of the sidebranch, the size of the sidebranch, and the amount of myocardium served by that branch. In general, jeopardy of acute marginal branches of the right coronary artery, small diagonal branches of the LAD, and small obtuse marginal branches of the left circumflex do not represent significant contraindications to stent placement. In some anatomically suitable vessels, these are now several reports of "kissing" articulated and disarticulated stents (Figure 26.12); these techniques are technically demanding and should be reserved for experienced stent operators (Figure 26.13).[130-131,288]

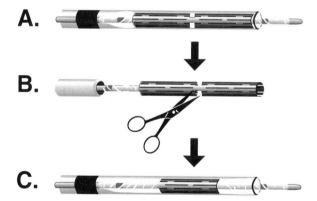

Figure 26.12   Technique for Disarticulating the Palmaz-Schatz Stent

A. Remove the Palmaz-Schatz stent delivery system from its package.
B. Retract the stent delivery sheath, and slide the stent forward on the delivery balloon until the articulation is freely exposed. Cut the stent at the articulation using sterile scissors. Save the half-stent.
C. Reposition the other half-stent in the middle of the stent delivery balloon, and gently crimp it with your fingers. Gently advance the delivery sheath back over the stent.

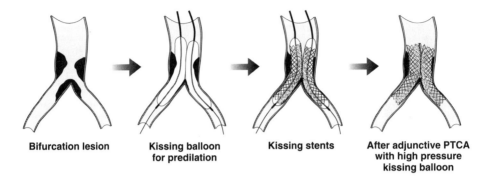

Bifurcation lesion   Kissing balloon   Kissing stents   After adjunctive PTCA
for predilation   with high pressure
                                          kissing balloon

Figure 26.13   Bifurcation Lesions: Stent Technique

b. **Ostial Lesions (Table 26.11).** PTCA of aorto-ostial lesions is frequently suboptimal because of the elasticity and rigidity of the aorta; final diameter stenoses > 50% are common. Stent implantation in the aorto-ostial location is technically challenging because of difficulties seating the guiding catheter, obtaining adequate images to optimize stent placement, ensuring proper stent position to adequately cover the entire lesion (i.e., the proximal end of the stent must be flared in the aorta), and stent migration or embolization (Figure 26.14). For calcified aorta-ostial lesions, stents should probably be avoided because of the risk of incomplete stent expansion, unless pretreatment with Rotablator and/or high-pressure balloons allows full balloon inflation before stenting. Intravascular ultrasound may be valuable in aorto-ostial lesions to assess the degree and depth of calcification, to ensure adequate stent sizing, and to confirm complete stent apposition and lesion coverage. In several small observational studies, stents have been successfully implanted in > 95% of ostial lesions; restenosis rates range from 15% (for native vessels) to 62% (for vein grafts).[108,132-137] In a small randomized study of PTCA and Wiktor stents in ostial RCA lesions, stents resulted in better lumen enlargement, but there was no difference in early or late outcome.[138] For aorto-ostial vein graft lesions, the results of stenting have been shown to be superior to those of DCA.[137] Unprotected origin lesions of the LAD or left circumflex may be unsuitable for stenting since proper lesion coverage requires stenting of the distal left main.

c. **Restenotic Lesions.** Although not an approved FDA indication, Palmaz-Schatz coronary stents are commonly used to treat restenotic lesions. In a study of 97 restenotic lesions, procedural success was achieved in 95%; adverse events included major complications in 3%, subacute thrombosis in 2%, and restenosis in 19%.[139] In the Trial of Angioplasty and Stents in Canada (TASC-I), stenting

Table 26.11. Results of Stenting for Special Lesion Subsets

Series	Stent	Morphology	N	Success (%)	SAT (%)	Comments
Colombo[291] (1996)	PSS, GRS, Wiktor	ostial	35	100	-	ARS (23%)
Rechavia[108] (1995)	PSS	ostial	29	100	-	CRS (15%)
Rocha-Singh[133] (1995)	PSS	ostial	41	100	10	Death (7.3%)
Wong[135] (1994)	PSS	ostial SVG	104	97	-	Coronary & biliary stents; death (1%), CABG (1%), ARS (62%)
Fenton[136] (1994)	PSS	ostial SVG	20	-	-	ARS (60%)
Sato[279] (1996)	-	CTO	30	-	0	ARS (36%); TLR (32%)[+]
Medina[146] (1995)	PSS	CTO	30	100	9	RS (22%)
Hsu[147] (1994)	PSS, Wiktor	CTO	36	-	5	RS (20%)*
Ooka[148] (1994)	PSS, GRS	CTO	33	-	5	RS (24%)**
Ooka[174] (1995)	PSS, GRS	CTO	47	-	10	RS (44%)***
Goldberg[175] (1995)	PSS	CTO	60	98	5	ARS (20%); 14-month EFS (77%)
Maiello[149] (1995)	PSS, GRS, Wiktor	diffuse	89	93	1.2	RS (35%)
Reimers[150] (1995)	PSS, GRS, Wall	diffuse	48	94	4	ARS (25%)
Shaknovich[151] (1995)	PSS	diffuse	54	98.2	3.7	
Mintz[176] (1995)	PSS	calcified	88	100	-	Adjunctive Rotablator in all lesions
Teirstein[141] (1995)	PSS	vessel < 3mm	145	96.5	0	IVUS; final DS (19%)
Hall[142] (1995)	GRS	vessel < 3mm	68	-	3	RS (31%); IVUS; final DS (1%)
Colombo[60] (1995)	MicroStent	vessel < 3mm	16	93.7	0	

Abbreviations: ARS = angiographic restenosis; CRS = clinical restenosis; SAT - subacute thrombosis; DS = diameter stenosis; PSS = Palmaz-Schatz stent; GRS = Gianturco-Roubin stent; Wall; Wallstent; - = not reported
*   Reocclusion 22% and restenosis 61% for PTCA   **   Reocclusion 35% and restenosis 68% for PTCA
***   Reocclusion 35% and restenosis 68% for PTCA   +   Randomized study of stents vs. PTCA; for PTCA: ARS (33%), TLR (29%)

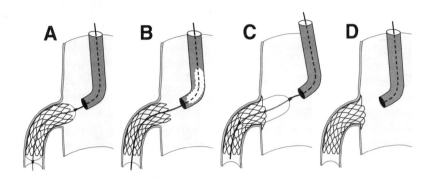

Figure 26.14   Aorto-Ostial Lesions: Stent Technique

A. Position the stent-delivery balloon so 1-2 mm of stent extends into the aorta. The guide must be retracted 1-2 cm before deploying the stent.
B. Remove the delivery balloon while maintaining backward tension on the guide, to prevent it from advancing into the ostium and damaging the stent.
C. Perform adjunctive PTCA with a high pressure balloon to ensure full stent expansion and apposition. Flaring the proximal end of the stent with a slightly larger balloon is useful.
D. Final result.

of restenotic lesions was associated with fewer late cardiac events (4.8% vs. 20%) compared to PTCA, but a higher incidence of in-hospital major complications (6.5% vs. 1.7%) due to stent thrombosis.[140] Preliminary data from the prospective randomized trial of Palmaz-Schatz stents versus PTCA for restenotic lesions (REstenosis Stent study, REST) suggest less need for target vessel revascularization after stenting (11.7% vs. 37%).[283]

d. **Small Vessels (Table 26.11).** FDA guidelines do not recommend elective stenting in vessels < 3 mm. Nevertheless, several stents (some without chronic anticoagulation[141,142]) have been successfully implanted in small vessels with excellent results,[60] although elastic recoil may be as high as 15%.[145] Preliminary subgroup analysis in the STRESS trial suggested that compared to PTCA, the relative impact of stents on restenosis was actually better in vessels < 3 mm than in vessels > 3 mm.[143] A meta-analysis of 1109 patients in the STRESS and Benestent trials found that the greatest benefit of stenting was observed in vessels 2.6-3.4 mm in diameter.[144]

e. **Chronic Total Occlusion / Diffuse Disease (Table 26.11).** There are several small observational studies of stents for chronic total occlusion and diffuse disease;[146-152,174,175] subacute thrombosis and restenosis occurred in 1.2-5% and 20-35%, respectively. A randomized study of stents versus PTCA for chronic total occlusions is in progress;

preliminary data in 53 lesions suggest significantly better immediate angiographic results after stenting,[153] but angiographic restenosis (36% vs. 33%) and target lesion revacsularization (32% vs. 29%) were similar at 3-6 months.[285]

4. **Contraindications to Stenting: Lesions with Gross Thrombus.** Although it is best to avoid placing stents in lesions with significant thrombus, stenting may be reasonable if thrombus can be removed.[154] Potentially useful adjuncts include TEC atherectomy;[126,155,156] systemic or intracoronary infusion of thrombolytics;[128] or local delivery of heparin or lytics.[157] For patients who are clinically stable, a 3-7 day infusion of heparin or a 2-3 week course of warfarin may "clean-up" the vessel and permit stent implantation. Coronary angioscopy may be especially useful in saphenous vein grafts to help guide interventional strategy in clinical situations in which thrombus is likely to be present.[126,155]

E. SPECIAL CLINICAL SITUATIONS

1. **Acute MI**. The primary concern about stenting patients in the setting of acute MI is stent thrombosis. Nevertheless, small observational studies have reported successful bailout stenting for failed PTCA in 80-94%; subacute thrombosis rates have varied between 1.8-30%.[158-164,280] In one report, major in-hospital complications were similar to those obtained after successful PTCA for acute MI.[161] Because of these findings, we have initiated a pilot study to determine the feasibility of planned STenting in Acute MI (STAMI). Although the proper regimen for prophylaxis against stent thrombosis is unknown in this setting, we routinely employ aspirin (325 mg BID), ticlopidine (250 mg BID) and warfarin (INR 2-3) for 1 month after stenting.[165] (The need for warfarin has been called into question.) Other studies using the heparin-bonded stent are now in progress in Europe. In reviewing 565 lesions treated by PTCA for acute MI, 63% were anatomically suitable for stent implantation based on vessel diameter ≥ 3 mm and other angiographic characteristics.[161] Taken together, these data suggest that stents should not be withheld from appropriate patients with acute MI.

2. **Unstable Angina.** The immediate and longterm results for stent implantation in patients with stable and unstable angina are similar.[166] In a study of 62 patients with unstable angina and post-MI angina, procedural success for Palmaz-Schatz stenting was 94%, with in-hospital death in 3%, Q-wave MI in 3%, and serious vascular complications in 5%. Stent thrombosis did not occur. Adjunctive lytic therapy was used in 38% and warfarin in 37% of patients.[167] Available data suggest that stenting is reasonable and safe in patients with unstable angina.

3. **Single Patent Vessel**. Stenting of a single patent coronary artery or bypass graft may be considered for patients who are not candidates for CABG, when the target lesion is anatomically suitable for ≤ 3 stents and there is good distal runoff. Technical considerations include predilatation of the lesion (to ensure full balloon inflation and maximize the chance of rapid stent deployment); use of large lumen 9F guides with sideholes (to permit passive perfusion during interventions); use of prophylactic IABP or CPS; possible use of IVUS (to ensure optimal stenting); and possible surgical removal of vascular sheaths (to allow uninterrupted heparin therapy). Warfarin (INR 2-3), soluble

aspirin (325 mg QD-BID), and ticlopidine (250 mg BID) are routinely prescribed for 1 month.

4. **Unprotected Left Main.** The approach to stenting patients with unprotected left main disease is similar to that of patients with a single patent vessel. In general, the operator must decide whether to use a kissing stent technique (to ensure patency of the LAD and left circumflex for left main bifurcation lesions; Chapter 10) or to stent the body of the left main alone. Palmaz-Schatz and Gianturco-Roubin stents have been used successfully in small numbers of patients with unprotected left main lesions (Chapter 4).[168]

5. **Sealing Perforations and Pseudoaneurysms.** There have been a few experimental[169] and clinical [170-172] reports of stents with vein allografts, which have been used to seal perforations and/or coronary pseudoaneurysms (Figure 26.15). This technique is technically challenging, and is not appropriate for inexperienced stent operators or for patients with profound hemodynamic collapse.

6. **Women.** In the STRESS trial of elective stenting, women were older, had smaller vessels, and more vascular complications than men; nevertheless, restenosis and longterm outcomes were similar.[173]

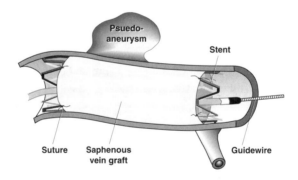

Figure 26.15   Stent-Vein Allograft for Coronary Pseudoaneurysm

F. ADJUNCTIVE THERAPY. For all stent patients, adjunctive medical therapy is required to prevent stent thrombosis. Despite a multitude of studies testing a variety of different drug combinations, the medical regimen is largely empiric (Table 26.12).

1. **Conventional Anticoagulation Regimen.** The FDA-approved regimen for prophylaxis against stent thrombosis includes aspirin (325 mg QD, started at least 24 hours before intervention), dipyridamole (50-75 mg TID or QID), dextran 40 (started immediately prior to intervention), and continuous heparin infusion (aPTT = 60-80 sec.) until the patient is therapeutically anticoagulated with oral warfarin (continued for 4-8 weeks, INR 2.5-3.5). This regimen has been recommended in the United States for all patients receiving either the Gianturco-Roubin or Palmaz-Schatz coronary stent. This regimen has been associated a low incidence of stent thrombosis (< 5% for elective procedures), but a high incidence of bleeding and vascular complications (up to 25% require transfusion or surgical repair); a long hospital stay (average 5-7 days), and high costs (patient charges are 80-100% higher than PTCA). Meticulous attention to clotting parameters, prolonged groin compression, and bedrest are necessary to minimize stent thrombosis (from inadequate anticoagulation) or hemorrhage (from excessive anticoagulation) (Table 26.13). One experimental stent study reported a 2-fold increase in platelet deposition after aspirin/Coumadin compared to aspirin/ticlopidine,[177] suggesting that Coumadin-based regimens may not be superior to other antiplatelet regimens for preventing stent thrombosis.

2. **Low-Intensity Anticoagulation Regimens.** Several alternative anticoagulation regimens have been proposed in the hope of decreasing bleeding/vascular complications, length of stay, and cost (Tables 26.14, 26.15, 26.16).[58,59,142,165,182-210] The majority of these regimens use "optimal stenting" (post-stent angioplasty with high-pressure balloons inflated to 14-20 ATM), and consist of intraprocedural heparin (ACT > 300 sec.) followed by post-procedural antiplatelet drugs (soluble aspirin [325 mg BID] and ticlopidine [250 mg QD] for 4-8 weeks) with or without subcutaneous heparin.[17,211,212] Dipyridamole, Dextran, prolonged heparin, and warfarin are generally omitted from these low-intensity regimens, which may be particularly useful in the elderly in reducing the risk of bleeding (1%), vascular (2%), and ischemic complications (<5%).[294] In highly selected cases, heparin effect may be reversed with protamine without complication;[215] however, the utility of this approach is uncertain, and it is not routinely recommended. Even in centers that commonly use a low-intensity regimen after optimal stenting, conventional anticoagulation is often prescribed in the following situations (Table 26.17) (Figure 26.16):

   · Vessel diameter < 3 mm.
   · Final post-stent inflation pressure < 14 atm.
   · The presence of significant disease or dissection distal to the stent.
   · Incomplete stent expansion by angiography or IVUS (see below).
   · Filling defects inside or adjacent to the stent.
   · Other clinical indications for prolonged heparin therapy or warfarin.
   · Final TIMI flow < 3
   · Stent placement in a single patent vessel
   · Persistent stenosis

Table 26.12. Anticoagulation Regimens for Stent Patients

A.	Conventional (FDA-approved) Regimen:		
	PRE	**DURING**	**POST**
Aspirin (325 mg QD)	✓	--	✓
Dipyridamole (75 mg TID)	✓	--	✓
Dextran-40[+]	✓	✓	✓
Heparin*	--	✓	✓
Warfarin**	--	--	✓

*	Heparin: ACT 300-350 sec during procedure; PTT 60-80 sec after procedure, until therapeutic INR
**	Warfarin: adjust INR 2.5-3.5; continue for 4-8 weeks
+	Dextran 40: 200cc bolus before procedure; 50 cc/hr for next 24 hours

B.	Low-Intensity Medical Regimen for Stent Patients		
	PRE	**DURING**	**POST**
Soluble aspirin (325 mg QD or BID)	✓	--	✓
Heparin*	--	✓	--
Ticlopidine** (250 mg QD)	✓	--	✓
SQ Heparin[+]	--	--	✓

*	Heparin: ACT - 300 sec during procedure
**	Ticlopidine: May be started 4 days prior or 500 mg BID for 48 hrs, then 250 mg QD for 4-6 weeks (Check LFTs and WBC count).
+	SQ Heparin: Some regimens include Lovenox or SQ heparin for 4-6 weeks; maintain PTT 50-60 sec

Two or more of the following: Stent in LAD, bailout stent for abrupt closure, major sidebranch within the stented segment, adjacent stenosis >50%, unstented dissection, TIMI flow < 3, recent MI within 2 weeks, thrombus, chronic total occlusion, or minimal cross-sectional area < 8 mm^2 by IVUS.[217]

Using these guidelines, 10-20% of patients may require use of the conventional anticoagulation regimen. A prospective randomized trial of aspirin, aspirin plus warfarin, and aspirin plus ticlopidine is now in progress (STent Anti-Thrombotic Regimen Study, STARS).[218]

Table 26.13. General Patient Management After Stent Implantation

	Conventional Regimen*	Low-Intensity Regimen**
Sheath removal	ACT < 140 sec	ACT < 140 sec
Groin compression	≥ 1 hour	Standard
Pressure dressing	Yes	No
Heparin bolus	No	No
Heparin infusion	10-13 ug/kg/hr	No
Bedrest	48 hrs	Standard
Ambulation	Gradual	Standard
PTT	60-80 sec	Not Applicable
Warfarin	INR 2.5-3.5	Not Applicable

*   Conventional regimen: restart heparin after sheaths removed; oral anticoagulation with Warfarin
**   Low-intensity regimen: no additional heparin; no Warfarin

3.   **Intravascular Ultrasound (IVUS)**

   a.   **Use of IVUS (Table 26.17, Figure 26.11).**   Potential uses of IVUS include accurate measurement of reference vessel dimensions, assessment of the degree and distribution of calcium (to guide the need for other adjunctive devices), identification of the adequacy of lesion coverage by the stent; and assessment of the parameters for optimal stent implantation. Such parameters include stent *expansion* (minimum stent cross-sectional area/average reference cross-sectional area ≥ 0.8-0.9), *symmetry* (ratio of minimum/maximum stent diameter > 0.7), and *apposition* (flush axial and radial contact between the stent and vessel wall). Similar IVUS criteria have also been used to identify suitable patients for low-intensity anticoagulation with aspirin and ticlopidine.[58,190,211] Using IVUS after biliary stent implantation in vein grafts, adequate stent expansion was identified in 9%, symmetry in 85%, and apposition in 63%.[211]   Dynamic 3-D reconstruction using an EKG-gated pullback device may further enhance image analysis.[219]

   b.   **Impact of IVUS on Stent Results.**   Although IVUS may add cost and time (21 minutes on average),[221] routine use of high-pressure PTCA does not ensure optimal stent implantation by IVUS criteria;[222,223,285,289] in a study of 96 stents implanted with "optimal technique," IVUS revealed improper stent expansion in 60%.[224]   In another study, 80% of stents underwent further PTCA after IVUS because of inadequate results.[220]   In addition, IVUS can improve stent apposition not discernible by angiography;[204,222,227-230] however, the discrepancy between IVUS and quantitative angiography decreases with progressively

Table 26.14. Summary of Two French Registries with Low Intensity Medical Regimens[59,178]

Phase	Period	Medical Regimen	No.	SAT (%)[59]
1	3/92-12/92	ASA 250 mg* IV Heparin 2d LMH 2 mos	145	10.4
2	12/92-12/93	ASA 100 mg* Ticlopidine 250 mg* IV Heparin 2d LMH 1 mo	237	1.3
3	12/93-4/94	ASA 100 mg* Ticlopidine 250 mg* IV Heparin 2d LMH 2 wks	523	1.7
4	5/94-10/94	ASA 100 mg* Ticlopidine 250 mg* LMH 1 wk	491	1.8

Phase	Period	Medical Regimen	No.	SAT (%)	Bleeding (%)
1	3/89-6/93	ASA Heparin IV Warfarin IP > 11 Atm	752	6.5	6.9
2	7/93-12/94	ASA Ticlopidine LMH IP ≥ 17 Atm	553	0.7	2
3	1/95-3/95	ASA 100 mg Ticlopidine 250 mg IP ≥ 17 Atm	263	1.1	1.1

Abreviations: ASA = aspirin; LMH = low molecular weight heparin; SAT = subacute thrombosis; IP = inflation pressure
* Treatment for 1 month

higher inflation pressures.[231] Despite data to suggest that IVUS can be used to optimize lumen enlargement and stent expansion, other data indicate that excellent results can be achieved using post-stent high-pressure (14-16 atm.) inflations without IVUS.[232] At the present time, the interventional community is divided over the routine use of IVUS-guided stenting. The prospective multicenter Angiography Versus Intravascular ultrasound-Directed stent placement (AVID) will help resolve this important issue; preliminary data in 163 patients indicated that even after high-pressure balloons, 33% of patients with angiographic optimal stenting failed

Table 26.15. Results of BENESTENT-II Pilot Study[179-181,295]

	Phase 1	Phase 2	Phase 3	Phase 4
No. of pts.	51	51	51	88
Heparin IV (hrs)*	6	12	36	None
In-hospital events (%)	0	2	0	0
Stent Thrombosis (%)	0	0	0	0
Bleeding requiring treatment (%)	7.9	5.9	4.0	0
Length-of-stay (d)	7.4	6.1	7.2	3.1
ASA (mg QD)	100	100	100	100
Ticlopidine (mg QD)	0	0	0	250
Restenosis (%)	15	20	11	6
7-mo. EFS (%)	84	74	94	92
IVUS (%)	12	8	20	8
PTCA (%)	82	86	84	92
IP > 12 ATM (%)	43	71	67	72
Final B/A	1.01	1.06	1.06	1.08

Abbreviations: EFS = event-free survival (freedom from death, MI, CABG, or repeat PTCA); IVUS = intravascular ultrasound; PTCA = post-stent adjunctive PTCA; IP = inflation pressure; B/A = balloon/artery ratio; - = not reported
* Time interval between sheath removal and restarting heparin infusion

to satisfy IVUS criteria, but IVUS had no impact on 30-day clinical event rates.[285] A new IVUS imaging guidewire and on-line 3-dimensional reconstruction may have useful applications for stent implantation in the future.[236,237]

c. **Impact of IVUS on Stent Complications.** IVUS may also have an impact on complications: In one preliminary study, use of IVUS-guided stent deployment was associated with a lower incidence of subacute stent thrombosis (0% vs. 4.2%, p. < 0.01), but a higher incidence of emergency CABG (6.6% vs. 1.4%, p < 0.05) compared to angiography-guided stent deployment; there were no differences in overall success (98%) or major complications (8%).[234] Final balloon/artery ratio > 1.2 may be an independent predictor of ischemic complications; careful attention to balloon sizing (perhaps using IVUS guidance) may limit these complications.[235] Currently, the precise role of IVUS is uncertain and further study is needed.

Table 26.16. Studies of Reduced Anticoagulation Regimens After Stent

Series	Regimen	N	Stent	In-hospital Complications (%) SAT	D/MI/CABG	Comments
Lefevre[294]	A,T,LMH	245	All	2.0	3 / 1.6 / 0	Age >75; French Registry
Morice[276] (1996)	A,T	260	PSS	1.2	- / 1.9 / 0.4	MUST Trial; preliminary results
Goods[277] (1996)	A,T	296	GRS	0.7	0.3 / - / 0.7	Optimal stenting; no IVUS
Goods[277] (1996)	A	46	GRS	6.6	4.4 / - / 0	Optimal stenting; no IVUS
Marco[278] (1996)	A,T	18	GRS-II	0	0 / 0 / 0	Second generation GRS
Elias[279] (1996)	A,T,LMH	240	Wiktor	3.6	1.2 / - / 1.2	Phase II, III, IV study
Elias[279] (1996)	A,T	182	Wiktor	1.0	1 / - / 0	Phase V study
Morice[59] (1995)	A,T,LMH	1250	All	1.7	0.7 / 0.6 / 0.4	French Registry; Vascular (3.5%)
Morice[182] (1995)	A,T,LMH	397	PSS, GRS, Wiktor	1.5	1.0 / 0.3 / 1.0	Vascular (3.8%)
Morice[183] (1995)	A,T,LMH	246	Strecker, PSS, GRS, Wiktor	1.2	0.4 / 0 / 0.8	Vascular (3.7%)
LaBlanche[184]	A,T,D	98	PSS, GRS, Wiktor	0	2.0 / 4.0 / 3.0	Vascular (4%)
Hall[58] (1995)	A or T	411	PSS	1.0	0.3 / 1.0 / 0.5	Optimal stenting; IVUS; vascular (0.5%)
Barragan[185] (1995)	A,T	208	GRS, PSS	0.5	1.0 / 1.0 / 0.5	Optimal stenting; no IVUS; vascular (0.5%)
Colombo[186] (1995)	A,T	60	GRS	0	1 / - / 4.0	Restenosis (32%); optimal stenting; IVUS

Series	Regimen	N	Stent	In-hospital Complications (%)		Comments
				SAT	D/MI/CABG	
Wong[187] (1995)	A,T	33	PSS	0	0 / 0 / 0	Vein grafts; optimal stenting with IVUS (RAVES)
Buszman[188] (1995)	A,LMH,C	100	PSS	1.0	1.0 / - / -	Vascular (1%); optimal stenting, no IVUS
Fajadet[189] (1995)	A,T,LMH	119	PSS	0	0.8 / - / -	Transradial approach
Blasini[190] (1995)	A,T	60	PSS	0	0	
Colombo[191] (1995)	-	59	Wiktor	1.7	1.7 / - / 3.4	Optimal stenting with IVUS; restenosis (23%)
Colombo[192] (1995)	A or T	359	PSS	0.9	1.1 / 3.9 / 3.9	Optimal stenting with IVUS; vascular (0.3%)
Mehan[193] (1995)	A	8	PSS	0	0 / 0 / 0	Half-articulated stents
Reifart[194] (1995)	A,T,O	98	GRS	-	1 / 0 / 1	Pilot phase GRACE trial
Lablanche[195] (1995)	A,T,O	334	-			TASTE Registry
Russo[196] (1995)	A,T	105	PSS	0	- / - / -	Optimal stenting; IVUS; 6-mos TLR (13%)
Hall[142] (1995)	A,T	68	GRS	3.0	1.5 / - / -	RS (31%); vessels < 3mm
Haase[197] (1995)	A,T	46	PSS	0	0 / 0 / 0	Bailout stenting
Goods[198] (1995)	A,T	152	GRS	0.7	0 / 0 / 0.7	Vascular (2%); transfusion (1.3%); no IVUS
Belli[199] (1995)	A,T	88	-	0	0 / 0 / 0	Vascular (4.5%); IVUS

Series	Regimen	N	Stent	In-hospital Complications (%)		Comments
				SAT	D/MI/CABG	
Morice[200] (1995)	A,T	1156	PSS, GRS, Wiktor, Micro	1.6	0.3 / 2.7 / 0.3	Vascular (0.6%); no IVUS
Saito[165] (1995)	A,T	32	PSS	0	- / - / -	Restenosis (18%); acute MI patients
Carvalho[201] (1994)	A,T,LMH	87	GRS	1.1	0 / 0 / 0	Vascular injury (2.3%)
Barragan[202] (1994)	T,SQH	238	Strecker, PSS	3.8	1.6 / 1.2 / 0	Vascular (4.6%)
Jordan[203] (1994)	A,T,LMH	132	PSS	0	- / - / -	
Wong[204] (1994)	A,T	28	PSS	0	0 / 0 / 0	Optimal stenting; IVUS (RAVES)
Colombo[205] (1994)	A,T	50	Wiktor	2.2	- / - / -	Optimal stenting; IVUS
Elias[206] (1994)	A,T,LMH	79	Wiktor	1.3	0 / 0 / 0	
Hall[207] (1994)	A,T	44	GRS	0	- / - / -	Optimal stenting; IVUS
Aubry[208] (1994)	A,T,LMH	643	PSS, GRS, Wiktor	2.5	3.7 / 3.7 / 1.3	
Blengino[209] (1994)	A; A,T	74	PSS, GRS, Wiktor	0	- / - / -	Randomized study of A vs. A,T

Abbreviations: PSS = Palmaz-Schatz stent; GRS = Gianturco-Roubin stent; SAT = subacute thrombosis; MI = myocardial infarction; CABG = emergency coronary artery bypass surgery; A = aspirin; T = Ticlopidine; LMH = low-molecular weight heparin; SQH = subcutaneous heparin; IVUS = intravascular ultrasound; - = not reported; O = other antiplatelet agents

4. **Thrombolytic Therapy.** Although intracoronary urokinase was originally recommended for patients receiving the Wallstent, thrombolytic therapy is not necessary for the vast majority of patients receiving stents. Intracoronary urokinase (250,000-500,000 U bolus over 5-15 min. or continuous infusion of 50,000-200,000 U/hr for 8-24 hr) has been used as an adjunct to recanalize vessels with stent thrombosis [160] or in degenerated vein grafts.[128] Urokinase is not recommended for intraluminal haziness unless thrombus in confirmed by angioscopy.

Table 26.17. Guidelines for Conventional Anticoagulation Regimen in Stent Patients[17,211-217]

Angiographic Criteria

Unstented disease distal to stent (DS > 50%)

Unstented dissection distal to stent

Vessel < 3mm

Filling defect in stent

Final diameter stenosis > 10%

Post-stent inflation pressure < 14 ATM

TIMI flow < 3

Ultrasound Criteria

Symmetry index (minor/major stent diameter) < 0.7

Minimal stent CSA < 8 mm^2

Stent CSA/reference CSA < 0.8

Incomplete stent apposition to vessel wall

Unstented dissection distal to stent

Intrastent CSA < distal reference CSA

Residual plaque adjacent to stent > 60% of adjacent reference CSA

Clinical Criteria

Stent in single patent vessel

Stent in acute MI setting

Abbreviations: DS = diameter stenosis; ATM = atmospheres; CSA = cross-sectional area; MI = myocardial infarction.

5. **Vasodilators.** Most interventional cardiologists empirically treat stent patients with long-acting nitrates and calcium channel blockers, beginning 24 hrs prior to stent placement and continuing for 6 weeks after discharge. This regimen seems reasonable to prevent vasospasm in arterial segments adjacent to the stent, but its value has not been rigorously tested.

6. **Antibiotics.** There are no data to suggest the benefit of routine antibiotics in patients receiving intravascular stents. Although endovascular infections have not yet been reported in stent patients, it is reasonable to prescribe prophylactic antibiotics for patients who require dental procedures, endoscopy, or other invasive procedures within 3 months of stent placement (until intimalization is complete).

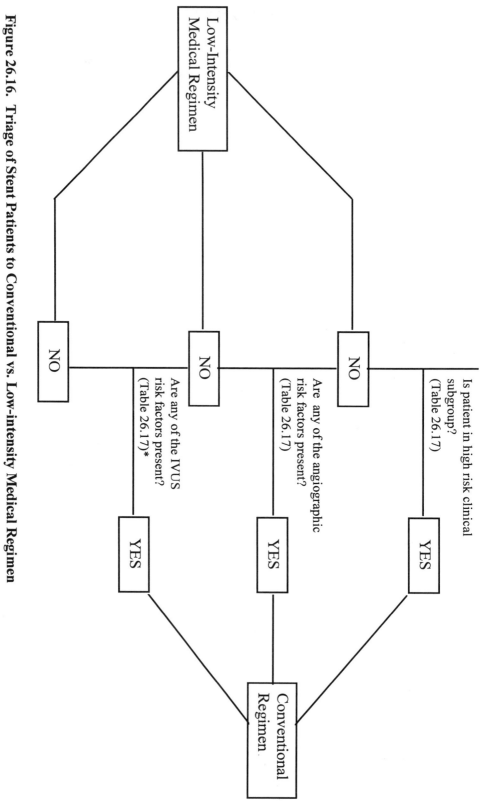

Successful Stent Deployment

Is patient in high risk clinical subgroup? (Table 26.17)

Are any of the angiographic risk factors present? (Table 26.17)

Are any of the IVUS risk factors present? (Table 26.17)*

Low-Intensity Medical Regimen

Conventional Regimen

NO / YES

Figure 26.16. Triage of Stent Patients to Conventional vs. Low-intensity Medical Regimen

* If IVUS is not used, triage is based on clinical and angiographic factors

7. **Other Medications.** The use of potent platelet antagonists (ReoPro, Trilofiban, Xemlofiban, Integrelin) is theoretically attractive but of unproven benefit in stent patients. Several studies of platelet IIb/IIIa inhibitors are planned; preliminary findings from IMPACT-II suggest improved 3-month outcome with Integrelin compared to placebo in patients who received stents for abrupt closure.[284] Subcutaneous and low molecular weight heparin have been prescribed, but their value is unknown. There are no data to support the use of corticosteroids, colchicine, or antiproliferative drugs.

8. **Angioscopy.** Angioscopy may have a limited role in the evaluation of thrombus after TEC atherectomy or intracoronary thrombolysis (and prior to stent implantation).[126] While angioscopy has been used to identify incomplete stent apposition or residual dissection,[238] IVUS is far superior to angioscopy in assessing stent size, geometry, and optimal implantation.[239]

9. **Doppler Flow.** Data from our own institution suggest that stenting may normalize coronary flow reserve after otherwise "successful" PTCA. These data and others [240-242] suggest that Doppler techniques may be used to identify angiographically inapparent residual disease or dissection after "successful" PTCA.

10. **Debulking with Atherectomy or ELCA.** DCA[243] and Rotablator[176] have been used as adjuncts to stenting. In one report, the combination of DCA followed by stenting achieved better immediate lumen enlargement than DCA followed by PTCA;[243] further follow-up is needed to determine the impact on restenosis. In calcified lesions in vessels ≥ 3mm, combined Rotablator and Palmaz-Schatz stenting was performed in 88 lesions; quantitative angiography and IVUS suggested better results compared to Rotablator and adjunctive PTCA.[176] Both TEC[126,155,156,281] and ELCA[281] have been used in high-risk vein grafts as adjuncts to stenting.

G. COMPLICATIONS

1. Stent Thrombosis

a. **Incidence (Tables 26.5, 26.6, 26.8, 26.10, 26.11).** Stent thrombosis is the most feared complication of stenting, due to the high incidence of ischemic complications (death in 7-19%, MI in 57-85%, emergency CABG in 30-44%). Acute stent thrombosis (i.e., before the patient leaves the cath lab) is rare (< 1%) and is virtually always associated with readily identifiable causes such as incomplete stent expansion and uncovered dissection. In general, the risk of stent thrombosis is highest at 3-5 days and is rare after 2 weeks, although the risk of Wiktor stent thrombosis is highest within the first 24 hours.[244] (The incidence and timing may depend on operator experience and technique, stent design and material, and adjunctive medical therapy). For planned elective stenting, the risk of stent thrombosis appears to be lower for the Palmaz-Schatz stent (0.4-4.7%) than either the Wallstent (15-24%) or Wiktor stent (12%). Subacute stent thrombosis has been reported in 0-32% of bailout procedures with the Gianturco-Roubin stent: The strongest predictors of stent thrombosis include unstented distal disease or dissection (odds ratio 10.6), stent diameter < 3mm (odds ratio 14.7), residual filling defect inside the stent (odds ratio 14.7); and multiple stents (odds ratio 3.7);[39] the rate of stent thrombosis increased from 5.6% to 9.4% to 16.7%, when none, 1 or 2 of these factors were present, respectively (Table 26.9).[106, 107]

b. **Prevention.** The proper medical regimen for preventing stent thrombosis is a subject of intense investigation. Because of the tendency of intravascular metals to form blood clots, original guidelines for medical management focused on the use of aggressive anticoagulation regimens to prevent stent thrombosis (Section F1, above). In the early Wallstent experience in Europe, stent thrombosis occurred in 20-25% of lesions, despite the use of aspirin, persantine, heparin, urokinase, dextran, and warfarin. In contrast, when the medical regimen was changed from aspirin alone to aspirin, persantine and warfarin, the incidence of stent thrombosis after Palmaz-Schatz stenting of chronic total occlusions decreased from 16% to 2%. Nevertheless, these aggressive anticoagulation regimens were associated with a high incidence of bleeding and vascular complications, prolonged hospital stay, and increased cost.

Largely due to the pioneering work of Colombo and colleagues, stent thrombosis is now viewed as a mechanical problem that can be prevented by optimal stent implantation technique without the need for aggressive anticoagulation. "Optimal stenting" requires meticulous technique to ensure complete coverage of the lesion, complete apposition of the stent to the vessel wall, full stent expansion, and stent symmetry. Adjunctive angioplasty after stent implantation using high-pressure balloons inflated to at least 15 ATM is a key component of "optimal stenting," and IVUS may be valuable to confirm "optimal" technique. Using this approach, the incidence of stent thrombosis is < 2% despite elimination of prolonged heparin infusions, dextran, persantine, and warfarin. Alternative medical regimens under evaluation include aspirin alone; aspirin and ticlopidine; and aspirin, ticlopidine, and subcutaneous heparin (Table 26.16).

c. **Treatment and Outcome.** Clinical manifestations of stent thrombosis are similar to abrupt closure after other devices and usually include chest pain and ST segment elevation. Thrombosis of a previously occluded vessel, however, may be clinically silent. In most cases, emergency catheterization and revascularization are recommended; potential remedial causes should be sought and corrected if possible, including inadequate stent apposition (IVUS may be useful), improper stent sizing, and failure to adequately cover distal disease or dissection. Rarely, stent occlusion may be secondary to intimal flaps protruding through stent struts or coils; this can be managed by overlapping stents.

Most cases of stent thrombosis can be successfully managed by repeat PTCA. When crossing the stented segment with a guidewire, it is important to put a large J-curve on the wire tip; otherwise, the wire may pass between the stent and the vessel wall. If this occurs and goes unrecognized — excessive resistance to balloon advancement is an important clue — subsequent balloon inflations can separate the stent from the vessel wall and lead to stent compression, stent embolization, and further thrombus formation. Potentially useful adjuncts for treating stent thrombosis include an intracoronary bolus of thrombolytics (urokinase

250,000-500,000 over 2-5 min.); a prolonged (8-24 hr) intracoronary infusion of thrombolytics (100,000-200,000 U/hr through an infusion wire); or local delivery of thrombolytic drugs directly into the stented segment.[245] Patients who are successfully revascularized should be treated with a prolonged heparin infusion (aPTT 60-80 sec. until a "therapeutic" warfarin level is achieved), and oral warfarin (INR 2.5-3.5) for 4-6 weeks; soluble aspirin (325 mg QD-BID) and ticlopidine (250 mg QD) are also prescribed. The use of new platelet glycoprotein receptor IIb/IIIa antagonists is theoretically attractive, but of unproven value. For refractory stent thrombosis, CABG is usually advised. Stent thrombosis is associated with significant patient morbidity and mortality, including death in 7-19%, nonfatal myocardial infarction in 57-88%, and emergency CABG in 30-44%.

2. **Ischemic Complications.** Ischemic complications arise as a consequence of failed PTCA or stent thrombosis. When stents are used to reverse abrupt closure, significant patient morbidity should be anticipated, including nonfatal myocardial infarction (2-26%), emergency CABG (0-16%), and death (0-10%). In one study the overall incidence of ischemic complications was 28%. Independent predictors of ischemic complication included delayed use of stents for abrupt closure, sidebranch occlusion, need for multiple stents, and incomplete coverage of dissection.[45,246] In contrast, the overall incidence of ischemic complications when stents are used for non-emergent indications is 0-6.9%.

3. **Bleeding and Vascular Injury.** In the recent multicenter randomized trials of PTCA vs. stents, significant bleeding or vascular repair occurred in 7.3-13.5% of stent patients due to the intensive anticoagulation regimen. In contrast, major bleeding occurred in 1% and major vascular complications in 2.5% of 1232 patients treated without warfarin after optimal stent technique.[59] Risk factors for vascular complications include age > 70 years, female gender, multiple procedures during the same hospitalization,[249] and the use of warfarin.[249,250] If prolonged intravenous heparin therapy is needed after stent implantation, sheaths should be removed immediately after the procedure; compared to overnight heparin and sheath removal the following morning, this strategy resulted in a 2-3 fold reduction in bleeding and vascular complications.[247] Finally, gradual ambulation over 48 hours, and the use of collagen hemostatic devices may reduce groin complications (Chapter 25).[248]

4. **Stent Embolization** occurs in < 1% of patients receiving coronary stents, may occur more often in those receiving biliary stents, and can be managed by stent deployment at the site of embolization.[251,252] Stent retrieval with a wire snare is feasible, but difficult.

5. **Sidebranch Occlusion.** Experimental and clinical studies have shown that flow into sidebranches is usually preserved after stenting the parent vessel.[253] In fact, stenting often results in reappearance of sidebranches that are initially occluded after PTCA.[254] The management of sidebranch occlusion is more straightforward after the Gianturco-Roubin stent, since guidewires and balloons can readily be passed through the stent coils and into sidebranches. In contrast, while sidebranches have been retrieved by PTCA through slotted stents (Palmaz-Schatz), there is a greater risk of balloon

entrapment or damage to the stent struts. Experimental studies have identified a number of balloons which will, or will not, pass through a fully deployed Palmaz-Schatz stent and return intact without damaging the stent;[129] in general, low-profile balloons work best (Chapter 1).

6. **Perforation.** Coronary perforation occurs more often after percutaneous laser and atherectomy than after PTCA. In contrast, two contemporary studies of coronary perforation did not report perforation after coronary stenting, although coronary artery rupture was mentioned as a serious complication after high-pressure adjunctive PTCA.[192,235] In our own stent experience, we have observed several cases of coronary artery perforation, which were usually related to one of the following: use of an oversized balloon (balloon-to-artery ratio > 1.2) during stent deployment or adjunctive PTCA; high-pressure balloon inflations outside the stent; stenting of vessels with significant tapering; stenting of contained perforations after other devices; recrossing lesions with antecedent severe dissections or abrupt closure; and stenting total occlusions when there has been unrecognized subintimal passage of the guidewire.

H. OTHER ISSUES

1. **Cost.** Compared to PTCA, the elective use of Palmaz-Schatz stenting in the STRESS trial was associated with a 90% increase in length of hospital stay, a 37% increase in cath lab costs, and a 27% increase in initial hospital costs. However, stenting was associated with a 25% reduction in repeat revascularization at 1 year, and a 58% reduction in follow-up hospital costs — overall costs at 1 year were virtually identical.[255,256] It is anticipated that stent costs will be reduced by less intensive anticoagulation regimens, which will result in fewer bleeding and vascular complications, shorter hospital stay, and fewer repeat revascularizations.[256-260] In fact, preliminary data from the Reduced Anticoagulation VEin graft Stent trial (RAVES) suggest that IVUS-guided optimal stent implantation and reduced anticoagulation may reduce overall costs by 38% compared to conventional Coumadin-based regimens due to reductions in length of stay and complications.[261] In another study, IVUS-guided stent implantation and reduced anticoagulation resulted in a 13% increase in procedural cost, but an 18% reduction in total hospital cost compared to conventional treatment.[262]

2. **Future Directions.** Stents are clearly the most important advance in mechanical techniques for percutaneous coronary revascularization. Over the next few years, we can expect vast improvements in stent technology and design, including biodegradable stents, drug-delivery stents,[263] coated stents to inhibit thrombosis,[179,264-266] radioactive stents to inhibit intimal proliferation,[267-270] endoluminal paving,[271] catheter-based radiation therapy,[272,273,293] and genetically engineered endothelial cell seeding.[274] Stent-grafts using PTFE (Teflon), PET (Dacron), and other materials are also under investigations for treatment of vein grafts, aneurysms, and other problems.[275] Finally, optimal use of adjunctive pharmacotherapy, IVUS, Doppler, percutaneous arteriotomy closure devices, radial/brachial technique, and other devices (e.g., Rotablator followed by stenting for calcified lesions) will allow for even safer and more effective stenting. It is quite likely that this revolutionary technology may ultimately account for > 50% of all percutaneous interventions.

REFERENCES

1. Dotter CT, Judkins MR. Transluminal treatment of arteriosclerotic obstructions. Circulation 1964;30:654.

2. Sigwart U, Puel J, Mirkovitch V, et al. Intravascualr stents to prevent occlusion and restenosis after transluminal angioplasty. N Engl J Med 1987;316:701.

3. Serruys PW, Strauss BH, Beatt KJ, et al. Angiographic follow-up after placement of a self-expanding coronary-artery stent. N Engl J Med 1991 324:13.

4. Macander PJ, Agrawal SK, Roubin GS. The Gianturco-Roubin balloon-expandable intracoronary flexible coil stent. J Interven Cardiol 1991;3:85.

5. Schatz RA. A view of vascular stents. Circulation 1989;79:445.

6. Medina A, Hernandez E, de Lezo J, Pan M. Divided Palmaz-Schatz stent for discrete coronary stenosis. J Inv Cardiol 1992;4:389-392.

7. Nordrehaug JE, Priestly K, Chronos N, Buller N, Sigwart U. Implantation of half Palmaz-Schatz stents in short aorto-ostial lesions of saphenous vein grafts. Cathet Cardiovasc Diagn 1993;30:141-143.

8. Mehan V, Kaufmann U, Salzmann C, Meier B. Use of half (disarticulated) Palmaz-Schatz stents for thrombus-containing coronary lesions. Cathet Cardiovasc Diagn. 1994;33:370-372.

9. Mehan V, Kaufmann U, Urban P, Chatelain P, Meier B. Stenting with the half (disarticulated) Palmaz-Schatz Stent. Cathet Cardiovas Diagn. 1995;34:122-127.

10. Wong P, Wong CM, Ko P. Clinical application of a new Palmaz-Schatz coronary stent delivery system with a short (8mm) nonarticulated stent. Cathet Cardiovasc Diagn. 1995;34:82-87.

11. Koh, Tai-Hai. Method of preparing, mounting, and implanting a Palmaz-Schatz coronary half-stent from the stent delivery system. Cathet Cardiovasc Diagn 1995;36:164-170.

12. Satler, Lowell F. Editorial Comment. Cathet Cardiovasc Diagn 1995;35:171-172.

13. Buchwald A, Unterberg C, Werner G, et al. Initial clinical results with the Wiktor stent: A new balloon-expandable coronary stent. Clin Cardiol 1991;14:374.

14. Cragg A, Lund G, Rysavy J, et al. Nonsurgical placement of arterial endoprostheses: A new technique using nitinol wire. Radiol 1983;147:261.

15. den Heijer P, van Dijk R, Twisk SP, Lie K. Early stent occlusion is not always caused by thrombosis. Cathet Cardiovasc Diagn. 1993;29:136-140.

16. Ozaki Y, Keane D, Ruygrok P, vd Giessen W, de Feyter P. Six-month clinical and angiographic follow-up of the new less shortening Wallstent in native coronary arteries. Circulation 1995;92:I-79.

17. Colombo A, Hall P, Martini G. Ultrasound-guided coronary stenting without anticoagulation. In: Current Review of Interventional Cardiology, Second Edition. Topol EJ, Serruys PW (eds). Current Medicine, Philadelphia, PA. 1995, pg. 115.

18. Kiemeneij F, Laarman G, Slagboom T. Mode of deployment of coronary Palmaz-Schatz stents after implantation with the stent delivery system: An intravascular ultrasound study. Am Heart J 1995;129:638-644.

19. Mudra H, Regar E, Wener F, Rothman MftMI. A focal high pressure dilatation of Palmaz-Schatz stents can safely achieve maximal stent expansion using a single balloon catheter approach. First results from the MUSCAT Trial. Circulation 1995;92:I-280.

20. Kiemeneij F, Laarman GJ, Slagboom T, Stella P. Transradial Palmaz-Schatz coronary stenting on an outpatient basis: Results of a prospective pilot study. J Inv Cardiol 1995;7:5A-11A.

21. Kiemeneij F, Laarman GJ. Transradial artery Palmaz-Schatz coronary stent implantation: Results of a single center feasibility study. Am Heart J 1995;130:14-21.

22. Kiemeneij F, Laarman GJ, Slagboom T. Percutaneous tranradial coronary Palmaz-Schatz stent implantation, guided by intravascular ultrasound. Cathet Cardiovasc Diagn. 1995;34:133-136.

23. Kiemeneij F, Laarman G, Slagboom T, van der Wieken R. Transradial coronary stenting in outpatients. Circulation 1995;92:I-535.

24. Holmes D, Berger P, Garratt K, Bell M, Bresnahan J. Stenting in cardiac interventional practice, off label versus

approved indication. Circulation 1995;92:I-85.

25. Penn I, Ricci D, Brown R, et al. Randomized study of stenting versus prolonged balloon dilatation in failed angioplasty (PTCA): Preliminary data from the trial of Angioplasty and Stents in Canada (T.A.S.C. II). Circulation 1993;88:I-601.

26. Ricci D, Buller C, O'Neill B, et al. Coronary stent vs. prolonged perfusion balloon for failed coronary angioplasty. A randomized trial. Circulation 1994;90:I-651.

27. Ray S, Penn I, Ricci D, et al. Mechanism of benefit of stenting in failed PTCA. Final results from the trial of Angioplasty and Stents in Canada (TASC II). J Am Coll Cardiol 1995;25:156A.

28. Ricci D, Ray S, Buller C, et al. Six month followup of patients randomized to prolonged inflation or stent for abrupt occlusion during PTCA-clinical and angiographic data: TASC II. Circulation 1995;92:I-475.

29. Hui N, Brass N, Klinke P. Effect of coronary stents on PTCA practice in a hospital without cardiac surgery. Circulation 1995;92:I-409.

30. Goy JJ, Eeckhout E, Stauffer J-C, Vogt P, Kappenberger L. Emergency endoluminal stenting for abrupt vessel closure following coronary angioplasty: A randomized comparison of the Wiktor and Palmaz-Schatz stents. Cathet Cardiovasc Diagn. 1995;34:128-132.

31. Urban P, Chatelain P, Brzostek T, Jaup T, Verine V, Rutishauser W. Bailout coronary stenting with 6F guiding catheters for failed balloon angioplasty. Am Heart J 1995;129:1078-83.

32. Metz D, Urban P, Camenzind E, Chatelain P, Hoang V, Meier B. Improving results of bailout coronary stenting after failed balloon angioplasty. Cathet Cardiovasc Diagn. 1994;32:117-124.

33. Schomig A, Kastrati A, Mudra H, et al. Four-year experience with Palmaz-Schatz stenting in coronary angioplasty complicated by dissection with threatened or present vessel closure. Circulation 1994;90:2716-2724.

34. Kiemeneij F, Laarman G, van der Wieken R, Suwarganda J. Emergency coronary stenting with the Palmaz-Schatz stent for failed transluminal coronary angioplasty: results of a learning phase. Am Heart J 1993;126:23-31.

35. Reifart N, Haase J, Preusler W, Schwartz F, Storger H. Randomized trial comparing two devices: The Palmaz-Schatz stent and the Strecker stent in bail-out situations. J Interven Cardiol 1994;7:539-547.

36. Herrmann H, Buchbinder M, Cleman M, et al. Emergent use of balloon-expandable coronary artery stenting for failed percutaneous coronary angioplasty. Circulation 1992;86:812-819.

37. Chan C, Tan A, Koh T, Koh P. Intracoronary stenting in the treatment of acute or threatened closure in angiographically small coronary arteries (<3.0 mm) complicating percutaneous transluminal coronary angioplasty. Am J Cardiol 1995;75:23-25.

38. Sutton J, Ellis S, Roubin G, et al. Major Clinical events after coronary stenting. The multicenter registry of acute and elective Gianturco-Roubin stent placement. Circulation 1994;89:1126-1137.

39. Agrawal S, Ho D, Liu M, et al. Predictors of thrombotic complications after placement of the flexible coil stent. Am J Cardiol 1994;73:1216-1219.

40. George B, Voorhees W, Roubin G, et al. Multicenter investigation of coronary stenting to treat acute or treated closure after percutaneous transluminal coronary angioplasty: Clinical and angiographic outcomes. J Am Coll Cardiol 1993;22:135-143.

41. Roubin G, Cannon A, Agrawal S, et al. Intracoronary stenting for acute and threatened closure complicating percutaneous transluminal coronary angioplasty. Circulation 1992;85:916-927.

42. Vrolix MC, Rutsch W, Piessens J, Kober G, Wiegand V. Bail-out stenting with Medtronic Wiktor: Results from the European stent study group. J Interven Cardiol 1994;7:549-555.

43. Garratt K, White C, Buchbinder M, Whitlow P, Heuser R. Wiktor stent placement for unsuccessful coronary angioplasty. Circulation 1994;90:I-279.

44. Ozaki Y, Keane D, Ruygrok P, de Feyter P, Stertzer S, Serruys P. Acute clinical and angiographic results with the new AVE micro coronary stent in bailout management. Am J Cardiol 1995;76:112-116.

45. Metz D, Urban P, Hoang V, Camenzind E, Chatelain P, Meier B. Predicting ischemic complications after bailout stenting following failed coronary angioplasty. Am J Cardiol 1994;74:271-274.

46. Carrozza J, George C, Curry C. Palmaz-Schatz stenting for non-elective indications: Report from the new approaches to coronary intervention (NACI) Registry. Circulation 1995;92:I-86.

47. Gordon P, Gibson M, Cohen D, Carrozza J, Kuntz R, Baim D. Mechanisms of restenosis and redilation within coronary

stents-quantitative angiographic assessment. J Am Coll Cardiol 1993;21:1166-1174.

48. Hermiller J, Fry E, Peters T, Orr C, Van Tassel J, Pinkerton C. Multiple Gianturco-Roubin stent for long dissections causing acute and threatened coronary artery closure. J Am Coll Cardiol 1994;23:73A.

49. Sankardas M, Garrahy J, McEniery PT. Sequential implantation of dissimilar tandem stents for long dissections complicating percutaneous transluminal coronary angioplasty. Cathet Cardiovasc Diagn. 1995;34:155-158.

50. Meckel C, Kjelsberg M, Ahmed W, et al. Bailout stenting for abrupt closure during coronary angioplasty. Circulation 1995;92:I-688.

51. Agrawal S, Liu M, Hearn J, et al. Can preemptive stenting improve the outcome of acute closure? J Am Coll Cardiol 1993;21:291A.

52. Lincoff M, Topol E, Chapekis A, et al. Intracoronary stenting compared with conventional therapy for abrupt vessel closure complicating coronary angioplasty: A matched case-control study. J Am Coll Cardiol 1993;21:866-875.

53. Stauffer JC, Eeckhout E, Goy JJ, et al. Major dissection during coronary angioplasty: Outcome using prolonged balloon inflation versus coronary stenting. J Invas Cardiol 1995;7:221-227.

54. Garratt K, Voorhees W, Bell M, et al. Complications related to intracoronary stents placed for moderate and severe dissections: Cook FlexStent Registry report. J Am Coll Cardiol 1994;23:102A.

55. Pilon C, Foley JB, Penn I, Brown R. A costing study of coronary stenting in failed angioplasty. J Am Coll Cardiol 1994;23:73A.

56. Gaspard P, Didier B, Lienhart Y, et al. Emergency temporary stenting should be preferred to permanent stenting for abrupt closure during coronary angioplasty. J Am Coll Cardiol 1994;23:103A.

57. Mahrer J, Eigler N, Khorsandi M, et al. Development of the Heat Activated Recoverable Temporary Stent (HARTS) with a slotted-tube design for coronary application. J Am Coll Cardiol 1994;23:103A.

58. Hall P, Nakamura S, Maiello L, et al. Clinical and angiographic outcome after Palmaz-Schatz stent implantation guided by intravascular ultrasound. J Inv Cardiol 1995;7:12A-22A.

59. Morice M-C. Advances in post stenting medication protocol. J Inv Cardiol 1995;7:32A-35A.

60. Colombo A, Maiello L, Nakamura S, et al. Preliminary experience of coronary stenting with the MicroStent. J Am Coll Cardiol 1995;25:239A.

61. Hamasak N, Nosaka H, Nobuyoshi M. Initial experience of Cordis stent implantation. J Am Coll Cardiol 1995;25:239A.

62. Karouny E, Khalife K, Monassier J-P, et al. Clinical experience with Medtronic Wiktor stent implantation: A report from the French Multicenter Registry. J Am Coll Cardiol 1995;25:239A.

63. Savage M, Fischman D, Schatz R, et al. Long-term angiographic and clinical outcome after implantation of a balloon-expandable stent in the native coronary circulation. J Am Coll Cardiol 1994;24:1207-1212.

64. Popma J, Colombo A, Chuang YC, et al. Late angiographic outcome after ultrasound-guided stent deployment in native coronary arteries using adjunct high pressure balloon dilatation. Circulation 1994;90:I-612.

65. Webb J, Abel J, Allard M, Carere R, Evans E, Dodek A. AVE Microstent: Initial human experience. Circulation 1994;90:I-612.

66. de Jaegere P, Serruys P, Bertrand M, et al. Angiographic predictors of recurrence of restenosis after Wiktor stent implantation in native coronary arteries. Am J Cardiol 1993;72:165-.

67. Carrozza J, Kuntz R, Levine M, et al. Angiographic and clinical outcome of intracoronary stenting: Immediate and long-term results from a large single-center experience. J Am Coll Cardiol1992;20:328-337.

68. Strauss B, Serruys P, Bertrand M, et al. Quantitative angiographic follow-up of the coronary Wallstent in native vessels and bypass grafts (European experience--March 1986 to March 1990). Am J Cardiol 1992;69:475-481.

70. Chevalier B, Royer T, Glatt B, Diab N, Rosenblatt E. Preliminary experience of coronary stenting with the MicroStent. Circulation 1995;92:I-409.

71. Goy J, Eeckhout G, Stauffer J-C, Vogt P. Stenting of the right coronary artery for de novo stenoses. A comparison of the Wiktor and the Palmaz-Schatz stents. Circulation 1995;92:I-536.

72. Levine M, Leonard B, Burke J, et al. Clinical and angiographic results of balloon-expandable intracoronary stents in right coronary artery stenoses. J Am Coll Cardiol 1990;16:332-339.

73. Fischman D, Savage M, Zalewski A. Overview of the Palmaz-Schatz stent. J Interven Cardiol 1991;3:75.

74.   Wong SC, Baim D, Schatz R, et al. Immediate results and late outcomes after stent implantation in saphenous vein graft lesions: The multicenter U.S. Palmaz-Schatz Stent Experience. J Am Coll Cardiol 1995;26:704-712.

75.   Fischman DL, Leon MB, Baim DS, Schatz RA, et al. A randomized comparison of coronary stent placement and balloon angioplasty in the treatment of coronary artery disease. N Engl J Med 1994;331:496-501.

76.   Serruys P, de Jaegere P, Kiemeneij F, et al. A comparison of balloon expandable stent implantation with balloon angioplasty in patients with coronary artery disease. N Engl J Med 1994;331:489-495.

77.   Mashman W, Gatlin S, King S, Klein L. Medtronic Wiktor TM stent implantation and follow-up: results from the core laboratory. J Am Coll Cardiol 1994;23:117A.

78.   Kuntz RE, Safian RD, Levine MJ, Reis GJ, Diver D, Baim D. Novel approach to the analysis of restenosis after the use of three new coronary devices. J Am Coll Cardiol 1992;19:1493-1499.

79.   de Jaegere P, Serruys P, van Es G, et al. Recoil following Wiktor stent implantation for restenotic lesions of coronary arteries. Cathet Cardiovasc Diagn 1994;32:147-156.

80.   Rodriguez A, Santaera O, Larribau M, et al. Coronary stenting decreases restenosis in lesions with early loss in luminal diameter 24 hours after successful PTCA. Circulation 1995;91:1397-1402.

81.   Penn I, Ricci D, Almond D, et al. Coronary artery stenting reduces restenosis: Final results from the Trial of Angioplasty and Stents in Canada (TASC) I. Circulation 1995;92:I-279.

82.   Mintz G, Pichard A, Kent K, et al. Endovascular stents reduce restenosis by eliminating geometric arterial remodeling: A serial intravascular ultrasound study. J Am Coll Cardiol 1995;25:36A.

83.   Fernandez-Ortiz A, Goicolea J, Perez-Vizcaynio M, et al. Is coronary stent recoil different for Gianturco-Roubin and Palmaz-Schatz stent? Circulation 1995;92:I-94.

84.   Kastrati A, Schomig A, Dietz R, Neumann F-J. Time course of restenosis during the first year after emergency coronary stenting. Circulation 1993;87:1498-1505.

85.   Kimura T, Nosaka H, Yokoi H, Iwabuchi M, Nobuyoshi M. Serial angiographic follow-up after Palmaz-Schatz stent implantation: Comparison with conventional balloon angioplasty. J Am Coll Cardiol 1993;21:1557-1163.

86.   Kimura T, Yokoi H, Tamura T, Nakagawa Y, Nosaka H, Nobuyoshi M. Three years clinical and quantitative angiographic follow-up after the Palmaz-Schatz coronary stent implantation. J Am Coll Cardiol 1995;25:375A.

87.   Hermiller J, Fry E, Peters T, et al. Late lesion regression within the Gianturco-Roubin Flex stent. J Am Coll Cardiol 1995;25:375A.

88.   Macaya C, Serruys P, Suryapranata H, et al. One year clinical follow-up of the Benestent trial. J Am Coll Cardiol 1995;25:374A.

89.   Hermiller J, Fry E, Berkompas D, et al. Five-year clinical follow-up of the Gianturco-Roubin stent: No late stent restenosis. Circulation 1995;92:I-280.

90.   Painter J, Mintz G, Wong C, Popma J. Serial intravascular ultrasound studies fail to show evidence of chronic palmaz-schatz stent recoil. Am J Cardiol 1995;75:398-400.

91.   Laham R, Carrozza J, Berger C, Cohen D, Baim D. Long-term (4-6 year) outcome of Palmaz-Schatz coronary stenting. Circulation 1995;92:I-281.

92.   Debbas N, Sigwart U, Eeckhout E, Stauffer J-C, Vogt P, Goy J-J. Late clinical follow-up 9 years after intracoronary stenting with the Wallstent. Circulation 1995;92`:I-280.

93.   Kern M, Rupprecht H, Wolf T, Meyer J. Five year follow-up after Palmaz-Schatz coronary stent implantation. Circulation 1995;92:I-686.

94.   Ali N, Lowry R, Tawa C, et al. Predictors of restenosis after Gianturco-Roubin coronary stent deployment. Analysis of 135 consecutive patients from a single center. J Am Coll Cardiol 1994;23:71A.

95.   Ellis S, Savage M, Dischman D, Baim D, Leon M, Goldberg S. Restenosis after placement of palmaz-schatz stents in native coronary arteries. Initial results of a multicenter experience. Circulation 1992;86:1836-1844.

96.   Baim D, Levine M, Leon M, Levine S, Ellis S, Schatz R. Management of restenosis within the palmaz-schatz coronary stent (the U.S. multicenter experience). Am J Cardiol 1993;71:364-366.

97.   Wong SC, Zidar J, Chuang YC, et al. Stents improve late clinical outcomes: Results from the combined (I + II) STent REStenosis Study. Circulation 1995;92:I-281.

98.   Hall P, Nakamura S, Maiello L, et al. Factors associated with late angiographic outcome after intravascular ultrasound

guided Palmaz-Schatz coronary stent implantation: A multivariate analysis. J Am Coll Cardiol 1995;25:36A.

99. Wong SC, Chuang Y, Schatz R, et al. Predictors for adverse clinical events are different in stents and PTCA: Results from the Stent Restenosis Study. J Am Coll Cardiol 1995;25:125A.

100. Segal J, Reiner J, Thompson M, et al. Residual stenosis and MLD following coronary stenting do not predict restenosis in the Strecker stent. J Am Coll Cardiol 1994;23:134A.

101. Yokol H, Kimura T, Nobuyoshi M. Palmaz-Schatz coronary stent restenosis: Pattern and management. J Am Coll Cardiol 1994;23:117A.

102. Ikari Y, Hara K, Tamura T, Saeki F, Tamaguchi T. Luminal lost and site of restenosis after palmaz-schatz coronary stent implantation. Am J Cardiol 1995;76:117-120.

103. Macander P, Roubin G, Agrawal S, Cannon A, Dean L, Baxley W. Balloon angioplasty for treatment of in-stent restenosis: Feasibility, safety, and efficacy. Cathet Cardiovasc Diagn. 1994;32:125-131.

104. Ribichini F, Steffenino G, Dellavalle A, et al. Restenosis after coronary stenting is associated with high plasma angiotensin-converting enzyme levels. Circulation 1995;92:I-86.

105. Markovitz J, Roubin G, Parks JM. Platelet activation and restenosis following intracoronary stenting. Circulation 1995;92:I-87.

106. Haude M, Erbel R, Issa H, et al. Subacute thrombotic complication after intracoronary implantation of palmaz-schatz stents. Am Heart J 1993;126:15-22.

107. Liu MW, Voohees W, Agrawal S, Dean L, Roubin G. Stratification of the risk of thrombosis after intracoronary stenting for threatened or acute closure complicating coronary balloon angioplasty: A Cook registry study. Am Heart J 1995;130:8-13.

108. Rechavia E, Litvack F, Macko G, Eigler N. Stent implantation of saphenous vein graft aorto-ostial lesions in patients with unstable ischemic syndromes: Immediate angiographic results and long-term clinical outcome. J Am Coll Cardiol 1995;25:866-870.

109. Wong SC, Popma J, Pichard A, Kent K. Comparison of clinical and angiographic outcomes after saphenous vein grafts angioplasty using coronary versus "biliary" tubular slotted stents. Circulation 1995;91:339-350.

110. Piana R, Moscucci M, Cohen D, et al. Palmaz-Schatz stenting for treatment of focal vein graft stenosis: Immediate results and long-term outcome. J Am Coll Cardiol 1994;23:1296-304.

111. Eeckhout E, Goy J, Stauffer J, Vogt P, Kappenberger L. Endoluminal stenting of narrowed saphenous vein grafts: Long-term clinical and angiographic follow-up. Cathet Cardiovasc Diagn 1994;32:139-146.

112. Keane D, Buis B, Reifart N, Plokker TH. Clinical and angiographic outcome following implantation of the new less shortening Wallstent in aortocoronary vein grafts: Introduction of a second generation stent in the clinical arena. J Interven Cardiol 1994;7:557-564.

113. Fenton S, Fischman D, Savage M, et al. Long-term angiographic and clinical outcome after implantation of balloon-expandable stents in aortocoronary saphenous vein grafts. Am J Cardiol 1994;74:1187-1191.

114. Leon MB, Wong SC, Pichard A. Balloon expandable stent implantation in saphenous vein grafts. In Hermann HC, Hisrschfeld JW (Eds). Clinical use of the Palmaz-Schatz Intracoronary Stent. Futura Publishing Company Inc. 1993; 111-121.

115. Fortuna R, Heuser R, Garratt K, Schwartz R, M B. Intracoronary stent: experience in the first 101 vein graft patients. J Am Coll Cardiol 1993;26:I-308.

116. Pomerantz R, Kuntz R, Carrozza J, et al. Acute and long-term outcome of narrowed saphenous venous grafts treated by endoluminal stenting and directional atherectomy. Am J Cardiol 1992;70:161-167.

117. Bilodeau L, Iyer S, Cannon A, et al. Flexible coil stent (Cook, Inc) in saphenous vein grafts: Clinical and angiographic follow-up. J Am Coll Cardiol 1992;19:264A.

118. de Scheerder I, Strauss B, de Feyter P, et al. Stenting of venous bypass grafts: A new treatment modality for patients who are poor candidates for reintervention. Am Heart J 1992;123:1046-1054.

119. Urban P, Sigwart U, Golf S, Kaufmann U. Intravascular stenting for stenosis of aortocoronary venous bypass grafts. J Am Coll Cardiol 1989;13:1085-1091.

120. Wong SC, Kent K, Chuang YC, et al. Is bigger really better for stent placement in large saphenous vein grafts? Circulation 1994;90:I-279.

121. Savage M, Douglas J, Fischman D, et al. Coronary stents versus balloon angioplasty for aorto-coronary saphenous vein bypass graft disease: Interim results of a randomized trial. J Am Coll Cardiol 1995;25:79A.

122. Wong SC, Chuang Y, Hong M, et al. Stent placement is safe and effective in the treatment of older (>4 years) saphenous vein graft lesions. J Am Coll Cardiol 1995;25:79A.

123. Sketch M, Wong C, Chuang Y, et al. Progressive deterioration in late (2-year) clinical outcomes after stent implantation in saphenous vein grafts: The Multicenter JJIS experience. J Am Coll Cardiol 1995;25:79A.

124. Wong SC, Chuang Y, Popma J, et al. Comparative analysis of long term clinical outcomes after native coronary versus saphaneous vein graft stent implantation. J Am Coll Cardiol 1995;25:198A.

125. Hadjimiltiades S, Gourassas J, Louridas G, Tsifodimos D. Stenting the distal anastomotic site of the left internal mammary artery graft: A case report. Cathet Cardiovasc Diagn. 1994;32:157-161.

126. Kaplan BM, Safian RD, Grines CL, Goldstein JA, et al. Usefulness of adjunctive angioscopy and extraction atherectomy before stent implantation in high-risk aortocoronary saphenous vein grafts. Am J Cardiol 1995;76:822-824.

127. Hong M, Pichard A, Kent K, et al. Assessing a strategy of stand-alone extraction atherectomy followed by staged stent placement in degenerated saphenous vein graft lesions. J Am Coll Cardiol 1995;25:394A.

128. Denardo SJ, Morris NB, Rocha-Singh KJ, Curtis GP, et al. Safety and efficacy of extended urokinase infusion plus stent deployment for treatment of obstructed, older saphenous vein grafts. Am J Cardiol 1995;76:776-780.

129. Guarneri E, Sklar M, Russo R, Claire D, Schatz R, Teirstein P. Escape from Stent Jail: An in vitro model. Circulation 1995;92:I-688.

130. Nakamura S, Hall P, Maiello L, Colombo A. Techniques of Palmaz-Schatz stent deployment in lesions with a large side branch. Cathet Cardiovas Diagnos 1995;34:353-361.

131. Colombo A, Gaglione A, Nakamura S. "Kissing" stents for bifurcational coronary lesion. Cathet Cardiovas Diag. 1993;30:327-330.

132. Zampieri P, Colombo A, Almagor Y, Mairello L, Finci L. Results of coronary stenting of ostial lesions. Am J Cardiol 1994;73:901-903.

133. Rocha-Singh K, Morris N, Wong C, Schatz R, Teirstein P. Coronary stenting for treatment of ostial stenoses of native coronary arteries or aortocoronary saphenous venous grafts. Am J Cardiol 1995;75:26-29.

134. Maiello L, Hall P, Nakamura S, et al. Results of stent implantation for diffuse coronary disease assisted by intravascular ultrasound. J Am Coll Cardiol 1995;25:156A.

135. Wong SC, Hong M, Popma J, et al. Stent placement for the treatment of aorto-ostial saphenous vein graft lesions. J Am Coll Cardiol 1994;23:118A.

136. Fenton S, Fischman D, Savage M, et al. Does stent implantation in ostial saphenous vein graft lesions reduce restenosis? J Am Coll Cardiol 1994;23:118A.

137. Wong SC, Popma J, Hong M, et al. Procedural results and long term clinical outcomes in aorto-ostial saphenous vein graft lesions after new device angioplasty. J Am Coll Cardiol 1995;25:394A.

138. Eeckhout E, Stauffer J-C, Vogt P, Debbas N, Kappenberger L, Goy J-J. A comparison of intracoronary stenting with conventional balloon angioplasty for the treatment of new onset stenoses of the right coronary artery. J Am Coll Cardiol 1995;25:196A.

139. Colombo A, Almagor Y, Maiello L, et al. Results of coronary stenting for restenosis. J Am Coll Cardiol 1994;23:118A.

140. Penn I, Ricci D, Almond DG, et al. Stenting results in increased early complications and fewer late reinterventions: Final clinical data from the trial of Angioplasty and Stents in Canada (TASC) I. Circulation 1995;92:I-475.

141. Teirstein P, Schatz R, Russo R, Guarneri E, Stevens M. Coronary stenting of small diameter vessels: Is it safe? Circulation 1995;92:I-281.

142. Hall P, Colombo A, Itoh A, et al. Gianturco-Roubin stent implantation in small vessels without anticoagulation. Circulation 1995;92:I-795.

143. Wong SC, Hirshfeld J, Teirstein P, Schatz R, Shaknovich A, Nobuyoshi M. Differential impact of stent versus PTCA on restenosis in large (> or less 3 mm) vessels in the Stent Restenosis Trial. J Am Coll Cardiol 1995;25:375A.

144. Azar AJ, Detre K, Goldberg S, Kiemeneij F, et al. A meta-analysis on the clinical and angiographic outcomes of stents vs PTCA in the different coronary vessel sizes in the Benestent-I and Stress ½ trials. Circulation 1995;92:I-475.

145. Rechavia E, Litvack F, Macko G, Eigler NL. Influence of expanded balloon diameter on Palmaz-Schatz stent recoil. Cathet Cardiovasc Diagn 1995;36:11-16.

146. Medina A, Melian F, deLezo J, et al. Effectiveness of coronary stenting for the treatment of chronic total occlusion in angina pectoris. Am J Cardiol 1994;73:1222-1224.

147. Hsu Y-S, Tamai H, Ueda K, et al. Clinical efficacy of coronary stenting in chronic total occlusions. Circulation 1994;90:I-613.

148. Ooka M, Suzuki T, Kosokawa H, Kukkutomi T, Yamashita K, Hayase M. Stenting vs. non-stenting after revascularization of chronic total occlusion. Circulation 1994;90:I-613.

149. Maiello, Luigi, Hall, Patrick, Nakamura, Shigeru Blengino, Simonetta, et al. Results of stent implantation for diffuse coronary disease assisted by ultravascular ultrasound. J Am Coll Cardiol 1995;25:156A.

150. Reimers B, Di Mario C, Nierop P, Pasquetto G, Camenzind E, Ruygrok P. Long-term restenosis after multiple stent implantation. A quantitative angiographic study. Circulation 1995;92:I-327.

151. Shaknovich A, Moses J, Undemir C, et al. Procedural and short-term clinical outcomes of multiple Palmaz-Schatz stents (PSS) in very long lesions/dissections. Circulation 1995;92:I-535.

152. Akira I, Hall P, Maielli L, et al. Coronary stenting of long lesions (greater than 20 mm)-A matched comparison of different stents. Circulation 1995;92:I-688.

153. Sato Y, Kimura T, Nosaka H, Nobuyoshi M. Randomized comparison of balloon angioplasty (BA) versus coronary stent implantation (CS) for total occlusion (TO): Preliminary result. Circulation 1995;92:I-475.

154. Kaul U, Agarwal R, Mathur A, Wasir HS. Intracoronary stent placement in thrombus containing vein graft lesions. J Inv Cardiol 1995;7:248-250.

155. Annex BH, Ajluni SC, Larkin TJ, et al. Angioscopic guided interventions in a saphenous vein bypass graft. Cathet Cardiovasc Diagn 1994;31:330-333.

156. Hong MK, Pichard A, Kent KM, et al. Assessing a strategy of stand-alone extraction atherectomy followed by staged stent placement in degenerated saphenous vein graft lesions. J Am Coll Cardiol 1995;25:394A.

157. Glazier J, Kiernan F, Bauer H, et al. Treatment of thrombotic saphenous vein graft stenoses/occlusions with local urokinase delivery with the dispatch catheter-initial results. Circulation 1995;92:I-671.

158. Walton AS, Oesterle SN, Yeung AC. Coronary artery stenting for acute closure complicating primary angioplasty for acute myocardial infarction. Cathet Cardiovasc Diagn. 1995;34:142-146.

159. Ahmad T, Webb JG, Carere RR, Dodek A. Coronary stenting for acute myocardial infarction. Am J Cardiol 1995;76:77-80.

160. Wong PH, Wong CM. Intracoronary stenting in acute myocardial infarction. Cathet Cardiovasc Diagn. 1994;33:39-45.

161. Benzuly KH, Goldstein JA, Almany SL, et al. Feasibility of stenting in acute myocardial infarction. Circulation 1995;92:I-616.

162. Iyer S, Bilodeau L, Cannon A, et al. Stenting the infarct related artery within 15 days of the acute event: Immediate and long term outcome using the Flexible Metallic Coil stent. J Am Coll Cardiol 1993;21:291A.

163. Capers Q, Thomas C, Weintraub W, King S, Douglas J, Scott N. Emergent stent placement: Worse out come in the patients with a recent myocardial infarction. J Am Coll Cardiol 1994;23:71A.

164. Levy G, De Boisgelin X, Volpiliere R, Gallay P, Bouvagnet P. Intracoronary stenting in direct angioplasty: Is it dangerous? Circulation 1995;92:I-139.

165. Saito S, Kim K, Hosokawa G, Hatano K, Tanaka S. Primary Palmaz-Schatz implantation without coumadine in acute myocardial infarction. Circulation 1995;92:I-796.

166. Malosky S, Hirshfeld J, Herrmann H. Comparison of results of intracoronary stenting in patients with unstable vs. stable angina. Cathet Cardiovasc Diagn 1994;31:95-101.

167. Guarneri EM, Schatz RA, Sklar MA, Norman SL, et al. Acute coronary syndromes: Is it safe to stent? Circulation 1995;92:I-616.

168. Fajadet J, Brunel P, Jordan C, Cassagneau B, Marco J. Is stenting of left main coronary artery a reasonable procedure? Circulation 1995;92:I-74.

169. Stefanadis C, Vlachopoulos C, Kallikazaros I, et al. Autologous vein graft coating applied to vascular stents: the ideal

coated stent? J Am Coll Cardiol 1994;23:135A.

170. Dorros G, Jain A, Kumar K. Management of coronary artery rupture: Covered stent or microcoil embolization. Cathet Cardiovasc Diagn. 1995;36:148-154.

171. Kaplan BM, Stewart RE, Sakwa MP, et al. Repair of a coronary pseudoaneurysm with percutaneous placement of a saphenous vein allograft attached to a biliary stent. Cathet Cardiovasc Diagn 1996 (in-press).

172. Stefanadis C, Tsiamis E, Toutouzas K, et al. Autologous vein graft-coated stent in coronary artery disease: The first implantation in de novo lesions in humans. Circulation 1995;92`:I-544.

173. Fenton S, Fischman D, Savage M, Rake R, Goldberg S. Influence of gender on outcome after elective coronary stent implantation. Circulation 1995;92:I-86.

174. Ooka M, Suzuki T, Yokoya K, et al. Stenting after revascularization of chronic total occlusion. Circulation 1995;92:I-94.

175. Goldberg SL, Colombo A, Maiello L, Borrione M, et al. Intracoronary stent insertion after balloon angioplasty of chronic total occlusion. J Am Coll Cardiol 1995;26:713-719.

176. Mintz G, Dussaillant G, Wong SC, et al. Rotational atherectomy followed by adjunct stents: The preferred therapy for calcified lesions in large vessels? Circulation 1995;92:I-329.

177. Kruse, Tanguay J-F, Armstrong B, Phillips h. Coumadin versus Ticlopidine in an animal model of stent thrombosis: A comparative study. Circulation 1995;92:I-485.

178. Brunel P, Jordon C, Fajadet J, Cassagneau B, Marco J. Successive steps in the management of coronary stenting. Circulation 1995;92:I-87.

179. Heyndrickx G. Benestent-II Pilot Study: In-hospital results of phase I,2,3, and 4. Circulation 1995;92:I-279.

180. Serruys P. Benestent-II Pilot Study: 6 months follow-up of phase I,II. Circulation 1995;92:I-542.

181. Suryapranata H, Group ObotBS. Evolving changes in technique of stent deployment during the course of the BENESTENT-II Pilot Study. Circulation 1995;92:I-687.

182. Morice M-C, Bourdonnec C, Lefevre T, et al. Coronary stenting without coumadin. Phase III. Circulation 1994;90:I-125.

183. Morice M, Zemour G, Benveniste E, et al. Intracoronary stenting without coumadin: One month results of a french multicenter study. Cathet Cardiovasc Diagn. 1995;35:1-7.

184. Lablanche J-M, Grollier G, Danchin N, et al. Full antiplatelet therapy without anticoagulation after coronary stenting. J Am Coll Cardiol 1995;25:181A.

185. Barragan P, Silverstri M, Sainsous J, et al. Prevention of subacute occlusion after coronary stenting with ticlopidine regimen without intravascular ultrasound guided stenting. J Am Coll Cardiol 1995;25:182A.

186. Colombo A, Nakamura S, Hall P, Maiello L, Ferraro M, Martini G. A prospective study of Gianturco-Roubin coronary stent implantation without anticoagulation. J Am Coll Cardiol 1995;25:50A.

187. Wong C, Popma J, Chuang Y, et al. Economic impact of reduced anticoagulation after saphenous vein graft stent placement. J Am Coll Cardiol 1995;25:80A.

188. Buszman P, Clague J, Gibbs S, et al. Improved post stent management: High gain at low risk. J Am Coll Cardiol 1995;25:182A.

189. Fajadet J, Jordon C, Carvalho H, et al. Percutaneous transradial coronary stenting without coumadin can reduce vascular access complications and hospital stay. J Am Coll Cardiol 1995;25:182A.

190. Blasini R, Mudra H, Schuhlen H, et al. Intravascular ultrasound guided optimized emergency coronary Palmaz-Schatz stent placement without post procedural systemic anticoagulation. J Am Coll Cardiol 1995;25:197A.

191. Colombo A, Nakamura S, Hall P, Maiello L, Finci L, Martini G. A prospective study of Wiktor coronary stent implantation without anticoagulation. J Am Coll Cardiol 1995;25:239A.

192. Colombo A, Hall P, Nakamura S, et al. Intracoronary stenting without anticoagulation accomplished with intravascular ultrasound guidance. Circulation 1995;91:1676-1688.

193. Mehan V, Saizmann C, Kaufmann U, Meier B. Coronary stenting without anticoagulation. Cathet Cardiovasc Diagn. 1995;34:137-140

194. Reifart N, Haase J, Vandormael M, et al. Gianturco-Roubin Stent Acute Closure Evaluation (GRACE): Thirty-day outcomes compared to drug regimen. Circulation 1995;92:I-409.

195. Lablanche J-M, Grollier G, Bonnet J-L, et al. Ticlopidine Aspirin Stent Evaluation (TASTE); A French multicenter study. Circulation 1995;92:I-476.

196. Russo R, Schatz R, Morris N, Stevens M, Teirstein P. Ultrasound-guided coronary stent placement without warfarin anticoagulation: Six-month clinical follow-up. Circulation 1995;92:I-543.

197. Haase H, Reifart N, Baier T, et al. Bail-out stenting (Palmaz-Schatz) without anticoagulation. Circulation 1995;92:I-795.

198. Goods C, Al-Shaibi K, Iyer S, et al. Flexible coil coronary stenting without anticoagulation or intravascular ultrasound: A prospective observational study. Circulation 1995;92:I-795.

199. Belli G, Whitlow P, Gross L, et al. Intracoronary stenting without oral anticoagulation: The Cleveland Clinic Registry. Circulation 1995;92:I-796.

200. Morice M, Breton C, Bunouf P, et al. Coronary stenting without anticoagulant, without intravascular ultrasound. Results of the French Registry. Circulation 1995;92:I-796.

201. Carvalho H, Fajadet J, Jordan C, Cassagneau B, Robert C, Marco J. A lower rate of complications after Gianturco-Roubin coronary stenting using a new antiplatelet and anticoagulant protocol . Circulation 1994;90:I-125.

202. Barragan P, Sainsous J, Silestri M, et al. Ticlopidine and subcutaneous heparin as an alternative regimen following coronary stenting. Cathet Cardiovasc Diagn. 1994;32:133-138.

203. Jordan C, Carvalho H, Fajadet J, Cassagneau B, Robert G, Marco J. Reduction of acute thrombosis rate after coronary stenting using a new anticoagulant protocol. Circulation 1994;90:I-125.

204. Wong SC, Popma J, Mintz G, et al. Preliminary results from the Reduced Anticoagulation in Saphenous Vein Graft Stent (RAVES) Trial. Circulation 1994;90:I-125.

205. Colombo A, Nakamura S, Hall P, Maiello L, Blengino S, Martini G. A prospective study of Wiktor Coronary stent implantation treated only with antiplatelet therapy. Circulation 1994;90:I-124.

206. Elias J, Monassier JP, Puel J, et al. Medtronic Wiktor stent implantation without coumadin: Hospital outcome. Circulation 1994;90:I-124.

207. Hall P, Colombo A, Nakamura S, Maiello L, Blengino S. A prospective study of Gianturco-Roubin coronary stent implantation without subsequent anticoagulation. Circulation 1994;90:I-124.

208. Aubry P, Royer T, Spaulding C, et al. Coronary stenting without coumadin: Phase II and III, the bail-out group. Circulation 1994;90:I-124.

209. Blengino S, Maiello L, Hall P, Nakamura S, Martini G, Colombo A. Randomized trial of coronary stent implantation without anticoagulation: aspirin vs. ticlopidine. Circulation 1994;90:I-124.

210. Gaglion A, Tiecco F, Hall P, et al. High pressure assisted intracoronary stent implantation without subsequent anticoagulation. Circulation 1994;90:I-622.

211. Painter J, Mintz G, Wong C, et al. Intravascular ultrasound assessment of biliary stent implantation in saphenous vein graft. Am J Cardiol 1995;75:731-734.

212. Fajadet J. New coronary stenting management. J Inv Cardiol 1995;7:30A-31A.

213. May A, Neumann F-J, Gawaz M, Ott I. Monocyte function after coronary stent implantation. Effect of two different antithrombotic regimens. Circulation 1995;92:I-86.

214. Ho Jeong M, Owen W, Staab M, et al. Does ticlopidine affect platelet deposition and acute stent thrombosis? Circulation 1995;92:I-489.

215. Colombo A, Hall P, Nakamura S, et al. Preliminary experience using protamine to reverse heparin immediately following a successful coronary stent implantation. J Am Coll Cardiol 1995;25:182A.

216. Russo R, Schatz R, Sklar M, Johnson A, Tobis J, Teirstein P. Ultrasound-guided coronary stent placement without prolonged systemic anticoagulation. J Am Coll Cardiol 1995;25:50A.

217. Schuhlen H, Blasini R, Mudra H, Klauss V, Kastrati A, Zitzmann E. Stenting for progressive dissection during PTCA: Clinical, angiographic and intravascular ultrasound criteria to define a low-risk group not requiring subsequent anticoagulation. J Am Coll Cardiol 1995;25:125A.

218. Schomig A, Schuhlen H, Blasini R, et al. Anticoagulation versus antiplatetet therapy after intracoronary Palmaz-Schatz placement-A prospective randomized trial. Circulation 1995;92:I-280.

219. Bruining N, di Mario C, Prati F, et al. Dynamic three-dimensional reconstruction of implanted intracoronary stent

structures using IVUS images based on an ECG gated pull-back device. Circulation 1995;92:I-17.

220. Nakamura S, Colombo A, Gaglione A, et al. Intracoronary ultrasound observations during stent implantation. Circulation 1994;89:2026-2034.

221. Mudra H, Klauss V, Blasini R, Kroetz M. Ultrasound guidance of Palmaz-Schatz intracoronary stenting with a combined intravascular ultrasound balloon catheter. Circulation 1994;90:1252-1261.

222. Caputo R, Lopez J, Ho K, et al. Intravascular ultrasound analysis of routine high pressure balloon post-dilatation after Palmaz-Schatz stent deployment. J Am Coll Cardiol 1995;25:49A.

223. Gorge G, Haude M, Ge J, et al. Intravascular ultrasound after low and high inflation pressure coronary artery stent implantation. J Am Coll Cardiol 1995;26:725-730.

224. Gil R, Prati F, Ligthart J, von Birgelen C, van Camp G, Serruys P. Is quantitative angiography a substitute for intracoronary ultrasound in guidance of stent deployment? Circulation 1995;92:I-327.

225. Fitzgerald P. Lesion composition impacts size and symmetry of stent expansion: Initial report from the STRUT registry. J Am Coll Cardiol 1995;25:49A.

226. Metz J, Mooney M, Walter P, et al. Significance of edge tears in coronary stenting: Initial observations from the STRUT Registry. Circulation 1995;92:I-546.

227. Popma J, Colombo A, Mintz G, Wong SC, Pichard A. The impact of intravascular (IVUS) on post-stent deployment balloon dilatation. J Am Coll Cardiol 1995;25:49A.

228. Jain S, Liu M, Iyer S, Parks M, Babu R, Yadav S. Do high-pressure balloon inflations improve acute gain within flexible metallic coil stents? An intravascular ultrasound assessment. J Am Coll Cardiol 1995;25:49A.

229. Mudra H, Klauss V, Blasini R, et al. Intracoronary ultrasound guidance of stent deployment leads to an increase of luminal gain not discernible by angiography. J Am Coll Cardiol 1994;23:71A.

230. Nunez B, Foster-Smith K, Berger P, Melby S, Garratt K, Higano S. Benefit of intravascular ultrasound guided high pressure inflations in patients with a "perfect" angiographic result: The Mayo Clinic Experience. Circulation 1995;92:I-545.

231. Blasini R, Schuhlen H, Mudra H, et al. Angiographic overestimation of lumen size after coronary stent placement impact of high pressure dilatation. Circulation 1995;92:I-223.

232. Caputo R, Ho K, Lopez J, Stoler R, Cohen D, Carrozza J. Quantitative angiographic comparison of Palmaz-Schatz stent implantation with and without intravascular ultrasound. Circulation 1995;92:I-545.

233. Russo R, Teirstein P. Angiography versus intravascular ultrasound-directed stent placement. Circulation 1995;92:I-546.

234. Goldberg S, Colombo A, Almagor Y, et al. Has the introduction of intravascular ultrasound guidance led to different clinical results in the deployment of intracoronary stents? Circulation 1994;90:I-612.

235. Hall P, Nakamura S, Maiello L, Blengino S, Martini G, Colombo A. Factors associated with procedural complications during high pressure optimized Palmaz-Schatz intracoronary stent implantation. Circulation 1994;90:I-612.

236 Hall P, Maiello L, Colombo A, et al. In vivo evidence that Palmaz-Schatz stents do not recoil immediately following deployment. Circulation 1995;92:I-327.

237. Prati F, Di Mario C, Gil R, et al. Usefulness of on-line three-dimensional reconstruction of intracoronary ultrasound for guidance of stent deployment. Circulation 1995;92:I-546.

238. Teirstein P, Schatz R, Wong C, Rocha-Singh K. Coronary stenting with angioscopic guidance. Am J Cardiol 1995;75:344-347.

239. Shaknovich A, Lieberman S, Kreps E, et al. Qualitative comparison of intravascular ultrasound and angioscopy with angiographic assessment of Palmaz-Schatz (PS) coronary stents. J Am Coll Cardiol 1994;23:72A.

240. Kern M, Aguirre F, Thomas D, Bach R, Caracciolo E. Impact of lumen narrowing of coronary flow after angioplasty and stent: Intravascular ultrasound Doppler and imaging data in support of physiological-guided coronary angioplasty. Circulation 1995;92:I-263.

241. Verna E, Gil R, Di Mario C, Sunamura M, Gurne O, Porenta GobotDSG. Does coronary stenting following balloon angioplasty improve distal coronary flow reserve? Circulation 1995;92:I-536.

242. Haude M, Baumgart D, Caspari G, Erbel R. Does adjunct coronary stenting in comparison to balloon angioplasty has an impact of Doppler flow velocity parameters? Circulation 1995;92:I-547.

243. Mintz G, Pichard A, Dussalilant G, et al. Acute results of adjunct stents following directional coronary atherectomy. Circulation 1995;92:I-328.

244. Holmes D, Garratt K, Schwartz R. Timing of stent occlusion/thrombosis after stent placement. J Am Coll Cardiol 1994;23:70A.

245. Mitchel J, McKay R. Treatment of acute stent thrombosis with local urokinase therapy using catheter-based, drug delivery systems: A case report. Cathet Cardiovasc Diagn. 1995;34:149-154.

246. Metz D, Urban P, Hoang V, Camenzin E, Chatelain P. Predicting the risk of ischemic complications after bail-out stenting for failed angioplasty. J Am Coll Cardiol 1994;23:72A.

247. Moscucci M, Mansour K, Kuntz R, et al. Vascular complications of Palmaz-Schatz stenting: Predictors, management and outcome. J Am Coll Cardiol 1994;23:134A.

248. Bartorelli A, Sganzerla P, Fabbiocchi F, et al. Prompt and safe femoral hemostasis with a collagen device after intracoronary implantation of Palmaz-Schatz stents. Am Heart J 1995;130(1):26-32.

249. Mansour K, Moscucci M, Kent C, et al. Vascular complications following directional coronary atherectomy or Palmaz-Schatz stenting. J Am Coll Cardiol 1994;23:136A.

250. Dean L, Voorhees W, Sutor C, Roubin G. Female gender: A risk factor for complications following intracoronary stenting? A Cook multicenter registry report. Circulation 1994;90:I-620.

251. Cishek MB, Laslett L, Gershony G. Balloon catheter retrieval of dislodged coronary artery stents: A novel technique. Cathet Cardiovasc Diagn 1995;34:350-352.

252. Rozenman Y, Burstein M, Hasin Y, Gotsman M. Retrieval of occluding unexpanded palamaz-Schatz stent from a saphenous aorto-coronary vein graft. Cathet Cardiovasc Diagn. 1995;34:159-161.

253. Iniguez A, Macaya C, Alfonso F, Goicolea J. Early angiographic changes of side branches arising from a Palmaz-Schatz stented coronary segment: Results and clinical implications. J Am Coll Cardiol 1994;23:911-915.

254. Mazur W, Grinstead C, Hakim A, et al. Fate of side branches after intracoronary implantation of the Gianturco-Roubin flex-stent for acute or threatened closure after percutaneous transluminal coronary angioplasty. Am J Cardiol 1994;74:1207-1210.

255. Cohen D, Krumhotz H, Sukin C, et al. Economic outcomes in the randomized stent restenosis study (STRESS): In-hospital and one-year follow-up costs. Circulation 1994;90:I-620.

256. Cohen D, Breall J, Ho K, et al. Evaluating the potential cost-effectiveness of stenting as a treatment for symptomatic single-vessel coronary disease. Use of a decision-analytic model. Circulation 1994;89:1859-1874.

257. Cohen D, Baim D. Coronary stenting: Costly or cost-effective? J Inv Cardiol 1995;7:36A-42A.

258. Weintraub W, Bernard J, Hicks F, Canup D, Mauldin P, Becker E. How coronary stents impact costs in interventional cardiology. Circulation 1995;92:I-436.

259. Eccleston D, Eisenberg M. Ticlopidine without intravascular ultrasound or coumadin reduces high marginal costs of elective coronary stent deployment. Circulation 1995;92:I-796.

260. Goods C, Liu M, Iyer S. A cost analysis of coronary stenting without anticoagulation versus stenting with anticoagulation using warfarin. Circulation 1995;92:I-796.

261. Wong SC, Popma JJ, Chuang YC, et al. Economic impact of reduced anticoagulation after saphenous vein graft stent placement. J Am Coll Cardiol 1995;25:80A.

262. Blengino S, Nakamura S, Hall P, et al. A cost analysis of intravascular ultrasound guided coronary stenting without anticoagulation vs. the traditional method of stenting with anticoagulation. J Am Coll Cardiol 1995;25:197A.

263. Aggarwal R, Ireland D, Azrin M, Ezekowitz M, de Bono D, Gershlick A. Antithrombotic properties of stents eluting platelet glycoprotein IIb/IIIa antibody. Circulation 1995;92:I-488.

264. Chronos N, Robinson K, Kelly A, et al. Thrombogenicity of tantalum stenosis decreased by surface heparin bonding: Scintigraphy of 111 in-plaletet deposition in baboon carotid arteries. Circulation 1995;92:I-490.

265. De Scheerder I, Wang K, Wilczek K, Meuleman D, Piessens J. Heparin coating of metallic coronary stents decrease their thrombogenicity but does not decreases neointimal hyperplasia. Circulation 1995;92:I-537.

266. Chronos N, Robinson K, Kelly A, et al. Thromboresistant phosphorylcholine coating for coronary stents. Circulation 1995;92:I-685.

267. Laird J, Carter A, Kufs W, et al. Inhibition of neointimal proliferation with a beta particle emitting stent. J Am Coll

Cardiol 1995;25:287A.

268. Wiedermann J, Marboe C, Amois H, Schwartz A, Weinberger J. Intracoronary irradiation fails to reduce neointimal proliferation after oversized stenting in a porcine model. Circulation 1995;92:I-146.

269. Hehrlein C, Kaiser S, Kollum M, Kinscherf R, Fehsenfeld P. Effects of very low dose endovascular irradiation via an activated guidewire on neointima formation after stent implantation. Circulation 1995;92:I-146.

270. Hehrlein C, Gollan C, Donges K, Metz J, et al. Low-dose radioactive endovascular stents prevent smooth muscle cell proliferation and neointimal hyperplasia in rabbits. Circulation 1995;92:1570-1575.

271. Slepian M, Massia S, Weselcouch E, Khosravi F, Roth L. Photopolymerization of hydrogel barriers on endoluminal surfaces of porcine stented arteries reduces stent and adjacent arterial wall thrombogenicity. Circulation 1995;92:I-687.

272. Waksman R, Robinson KA, Crocker IR, Gravanis MB, et al. Intracoronary radiation before stent implantation inhibits neointima formation in stented porcine coronary arteries. Circulation 1995;92:1383-1386.

273. Teirstein P, Massullo V, Jani S, et al. Catheter-based radiation therapy to inhibit restenosis following coronary stenting. Circulation 1995;92:I-543.

274. Sawa H, Vinogradsky B, Guala A, Fujii S. Genetically engineered endothelial cells: Increased surface fibrinolysis and potential adaptation to endovascular stenting. Circulation 1995;92:I-537.

275. Murphy JG, Schwartz R, Edwards W, Camrud A. Percutaneous polymeric stents in porcine coronary arteries. Initial experience with polethylene terephthalate stents. Circulation 1992;86:1596-1604.

276. Morice MC, Valelx B, Marco J, et al. Preliminary results of the MUST trial, major clinical events during the first month. J Am Coll Cardiology 1996;March Special Issue.

277. Godds CM, Al-Shaibi KF, Dean LS, et al. Is ticlopidine a necessary component of antiplatelet regimens following coronary artery stenting. J Am Coll Cardiology 1996;March Special Issue.

278. Marco J, Fajadt J, Brunel P, et al. First use of the second-generation Gianturco-Roubin stent without coumadin. Am J Cardiol 1996 (in-press).

279. Ekuas Hm Nibassuer JP, Carrie D, et al. Final results of phases II, III, IV and V of Medtronic Wiktor stent implantation without coumadin. J Am Coll Cardiology 1996;March Special Issue.

280. Monassier JP, Ellias J, Meyer P, et al. STENTIM I: The French Registry of stenting of acute myocardial infarction. J Am Coll Cardiology 1996;March Special Issue.

281. Hong MK, Wong SC, Popma JJ, et al. Favorable results of debulking followed by immediate adjunct stent therapy for high risk saphenous vein graft lesions. J Am Coll Cardiology 1996;March Special Issue.

282. Douglas JS, Savage MP, Bailey S, Bailey R, et al. Randomized trial of coronary stent and balloon angioplasty in the treatment of saphaneous vein graft stenosis. J Am Coll Cardiology 1996;March Special Issue.

283. Erbel R, Hande M, Hopp HW, et al. REstenosis STent (REST) study: Randomized trial comparing stenting and balloon angioplasty for treatment of restenosis after balloon angioplasty. J Am Coll Cardiology 1996;March Special Issue.

284. Zidar JP, Kruse KR, Thel MC, et al. Integrelin for emergency coronary artery stenting. J Am Coll Cardiology 1996;March Special Issue.

285. Sato Y, Nosaka H, Kimura AT, et al. Randomized comparison of balloon angioplasty versus coronary stent implantation for total occlusion. J Am Coll Cardiology 1996;March Special Issue.

286. Fernandez-Ortiz A, Goicoles J, Perez-Vizcayno MJ, et al. Late clinical and angiographic outcome of bailout coronary stenting. A comparison between Gianturco-Roubin and Palmaz-Schatz stents. J Am Coll Cardiology 1996;March Special Issue.

287. Caputo RP, Chafizedeh ER, Stoler RC, et al. "Stent Jail"— A minimum security prison. Am J Cardiol 1996 (in-press).

288. Colombo A, Maiello L, Itoh A, Hall P, et al. Coronary stenting of bifurcation lesions immediate and follow-up results. J Am Coll Cardiology 1996;March Special Issue.

289. Golderberg SL, Hall P, Nakamura S, et al. Is there a benefit from intravascular ultrasound when high-pressure stent expansion is routinely performed prior to ultrasound imaging? J Am Coll Cardiology 1996;March Special Issue.

290. Serruys PQW, Azar AJ, Sigwart U, et al. Long-term follow-up of "stent-like" ($\leq$ 30% diameter stenosis post) angioplasty: A case for provisional stenting. J Am Coll Cardiology 1996;March Special Issue.

291. Colombo A, Itoh A, Maiello L, et al. Coronary stent implantation in aorto-ostial lesions: Immediate and follow-up results. J Am Coll Cardiology 1996;March Special Issue.

292. Russo RJ, Teirstein PS, et al. Angiography versus intravascular ultrasound-directed stent placement. J Am Coll Cardiology 1996;March Special Issue.

293. Teirstein P, Massullo V, Shirish J, et al. A Randomized, Clinical Trial of Radiation Therapy to Reduce Restenosis Following Coronary Stenting-Early Results. J Am Coll Cardiology 1996;March Special Issue.

294. Lefevre T, Morice M, Labrunie B, et al. Coronary stenting in elderly patients. Results from the Stent Without Coumadin French Registry. J Am Coll Cardiology 1996;March Special Issue.

295. Serruys P, Emanuelsson H, van der Giessen W, et al. Heparin-coated Palmaz-Schatz Stents in human coronary arteries. Early outcome of the Benestent-II pilot study. Circulation 1996;93:412-422.

27 ROTABLATOR ATHERECTOMY

Mark Reisman, M.D.

A. DESCRIPTION. The Rotablator system (Heart Technology, Inc. Redmond, WA) (Figures 27.1, 27.2) consists of a reusable console that controls the rotational speed of a disposable advancer. The advancer consist of an olive-shaped, nickel-plated, brass burr, which is coated on its leading edge with 20-30 micron diamond chips and is bonded to a flexible drive shaft. The drive shaft is enclosed in a 4.3 F flexible Teflon sheath, which protects the arterial wall from the rotating drive shaft and serves as a conduit for saline flush solution, which cools and irrigates the system. The speed of burr rotation is regulated by a compressed-air or nitrogen-driven turbine, which is controlled by the console and activated by a foot pedal; rotational speed is monitored by a fiberoptic tachometer (Figure 27.3). The specialized 0.009-inch stainless steel Rotablator guidewire is 310 cm long, and has a floppy 3.7cm (type C wire) or a stiff 2.6 cm (type A wire) distal platinum spring with 00.017-inch radiopaque tip. To perform atherectomy, the guidewire is steered into the target vessel so that the platinum tip is distal to the lesion (the burr will not advance over the large diameter tip). The burr/drive shaft is then advanced over the guidewire until it lies just proximal to the stenosis. Thereafter, the saline flush is infused, rotation is initiated, and using a control knob on the top of the advancer, the rotating burr (160,000-180,000 rpm depending on burr size) is slowly advanced through the lesion.

B. PHYSICAL PRINCIPLES AND DESIGN CHARACTERISTICS. The two physical principles that enable the Rotablator system to preferentially ablate atherosclerotic plaque are differential cutting and orthogonal displacement of friction:

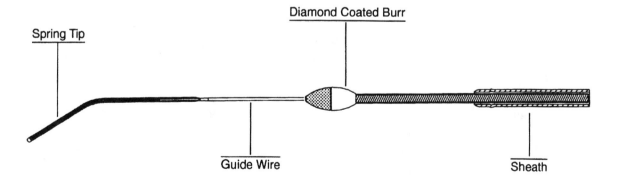

Figure 27.1 The Rotablator Burr

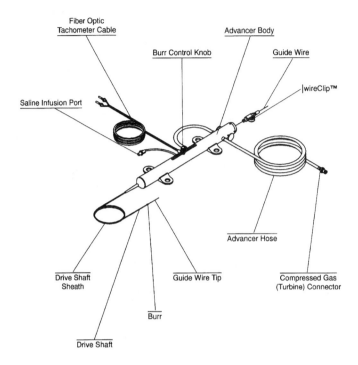

Figure 27.2 The Rotablator Setup

1. **Differential Cutting** is defined as the ability of a device to selectively cut one material while maintaining the integrity of another, based on differences in substrate composition. In the case of high-speed rotational atherectomy, this results in pulverization of inelastic material such as fibrotic atheromatous plaque and lipid-rich tissue; in contrast, nondiseased vessel segments, which retain their viscoelastic properties, are deflected away from around the advancing burr and spared from ablation.

2. **Orthogonal Displacement of Friction** explains the easy passage of the burr through tortuous and diseased segments of the coronary vasculature. At a rotational speed of 60,000 rpm, the longitudinal friction vector is virtually eliminated, resulting in reduced surface drag and unimpeded advancement and withdrawal of the burr.

C. IMPACT OF HIGH-SPEED ROTATIONAL ABLATION
1. **Effect On The Vessel Wall.** Histological[1] and IVUS[2,3] studies have demonstrated

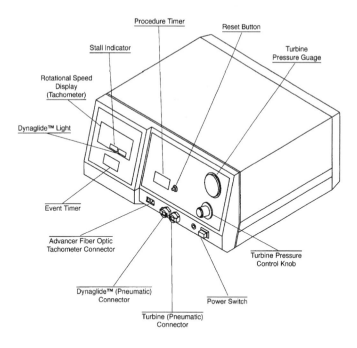

Figure 27.3 The Rotablator Control Panel

that fibrotic, calcified, and soft plaque are removed after Rotablator, leaving a smooth internal surface devoid of endothelium without medial injury. The segments proximal and distal to the treatment site show no change in diameter at follow-up angiography 3 and 6 months after atherectomy, suggesting that Rotablator does not accelerate atherosclerosis.[4]

2. **Microparticulate Debris.** The size of microparticulate debris generated during atherectomy is determined by the size of the diamond chips and by the speed and pressure of the advancing burr. Larger particles and heat are generated at slow (< 75,000 rpm)[5] burr speeds and during forceful advancement of the burr characterized by a fall in rpm > 5000.[54] Conversely, smaller particles and a lower particulate burden are generated at speeds > 140,000 rpm and during gentle advancement of the burr. Experimental studies have found that 77% of the particles generated by the Rotablator were < 5 microns and 88% were < 12 microns,[5] and that particulate concentrations 10-30 times greater than those observed in human Rotablator studies were needed to reduce coronary blood flow.[6] Most particles pass harmlessly through the circulation and are cleared by the liver, lungs, and spleen;[7] studies using positron emission tomography (PET) [8]and simultaneous transesophageal echocardiography[9] found no effect on hemodynamic performance, global LV function, or regional wall motion. In contrast, another study[10] demonstrated a transient (30-40 minutes) decrease in regional wall motion of 28% due primarily to myocardial stunning.[11] Studies with the Doppler

wire demonstrated an increase in average peak velocity after the Rotablator, but coronary flow reserve remained abnormal.[12]

3. **Efficiency of Ablation.** Quantitative angiographic analyses suggest that Rotablator atherectomy achieves a lumen that is 90% of the selected burr size;[13] lumen dimensions may increase even further over the following 24 hours,[14] possibly due to release of elastic recoil and/or vasospasm. Intravascular ultrasound (IVUS) studies show that the primary mechanism of lumen enlargement after the Rotablator is plaque ablation; Kovach et al[15] demonstrated a decrease in plaque plus media area (plaque removal), an increase in lumen diameter, no change in external elastic membrane area (no arterial expansion), and a significant decrease in the arc of target lesion calcium. In contrast, adjunctive PTCA was shown to enlarge the lumen primarily through arterial expansion (an increase in external elastic membrane in 80% of lesions) and not by plaque removal (no change in plaque pulse media). Typical IVUS findings after Rotablator atherectomy included an intimal-luminal interface that was distinct and circular, and lumen dimensions that were frequently in excess of final burr diameter. Deviations from cylindrical geometry were noted only in areas of calcified plaque manifesting superficial tissue disruption, and in areas of soft plaque.[16]

4. **Costs.** In an environment of cost containment, any incremental cost of a procedure must be weighed against its ability to improve acute and long-term outcome. In the case of the Rotablator, limited data are available concerning cost-effectiveness.[17,18] In a randomized trial of PTCA, Rotablator atherectomy and excimer laser angioplasty, the incremental cost of Rotablator over PTCA was 23%; however, this was accompanied by an increase in procedural success (93% vs. 83% for PTCA) and a decrease in length of stay (2.5 days vs. 4.2 days for PTCA).

D. ROTABLATOR PROCEDURE

1. **Pre-procedural Assessment.** The approach to Rotablator is similar to PTCA; however, several factors are worth special emphasis. For target lesions in a dominant RCA, dominant circumflex or ostial LAD, or when using a 2.5 mm burr, the high incidence of bradyarrhythmias and heart block warrants prophylactic insertion of a temporary pacemaker. Bradycardia usually occurs immediately upon burr activation and typically reverses within 5-60 seconds after ablation is terminated or after cough. The mechanism of bradycardia is unknown, but may be due to microcavitation, microparticulate embolization, vasospasm, guidewire vibration or an unknown reflex. Continuous monitoring of pulmonary artery pressure and prophylactic placement of an intra-aortic balloon pump are strongly recommended when Rotablator atherectomy is used in patients with significant LV dysfunction,[53] or when the target vessel supplies a large myocardial territory to prevent hemodynamic instability should transient myocardial dysfunction occur.

2. **Adjunctive Medication.** As for all interventions, aspirin (325 mg/d beginning at least 1 day prior to atherectomy) is mandatory. Adequate hydration and calcium channel blockers are also recommended prior to the case and may reduce the frequency of vasospasm, which may occur in up to 15% of patients. During the procedure, heparin (10,000 units IV bolus with supplements as

needed) is used to maintain the ACT > 350 seconds throughout the case. Although severe vasospasm is uncommon, generous doses of intracoronary nitroglycerin are recommended; a common technique is to administer a 100-150 mcg bolus after each ablation run. Intracoronary verapamil or diltiazem (injected through a balloon or transport catheter into the distal vessel) may be helpful in reversing cases of slow-flow or no-reflow (Chapter 21). Finally, some operators prepare a "cocktail" of nitroglycerin, verapamil and heparin in the flush solution, to provide continuous delivery of coronary vasodilators during Rotablation, which may reduce the incidence of no-reflow.[19,55,56]

3. **Rotablator Technique**

   a. **Guide Catheter Selection and Guidewire Placement.** A critical step in the procedure is selection of the guide catheter: Coaxial alignment will ensure that the guidewire is oriented in the center of the lumen. Since ablation occurs along the path of the guidewire, tangential orientation of the guidewire (guidewire bias) may result in directing the burr into the arterial wall, thereby increasing the risk of dissection or perforation.[20] The internal diameter of the guiding catheter must be 0.004-inch larger than the burr; the 1.25 mm, 1.50 mm, 1.75 mm and 2.0 mm burrs can be advanced through a giant-lumen 8F guide (ID $\geq$ 0.086-inch); 2.25 mm burrs with a 9F (ID > 0.092-inch); 2.38 mm burrs with a giant-lumen 9F guide (ID $\geq$ 0.098-inch); and 2.50 mm burrs with a 10F guiding catheter.

   b. **Burr Selection and Placement.** A two-burr approach, beginning with a burr-to-artery ratio of 0.5-0.6 and ending with a burr-to-artery ratio of 0.75-0.8, is often recommended to minimize the microparticulate burden and allow the operator to assess the progress of the procedure. After the burr is tested outside the body, it is advanced to a position just proximal to the target lesion (i.e., the "platform segment"). The burr must have free unimpeded rotation in the platform segment; if the burr is activated while in contact with the arterial wall, the risk of vessel injury is greatly increased. Free flow of contrast dye around the burr will confirm adequate positioning. Prior to activating the burr, all forward tension accumulated by advancing the device should be neutralized by gentle pulling back on the drive shaft itself; no resistance should be felt when the advancer known is loosened and "jiggled." If tension remains in the drive shaft, activation of the device will cause the burr to lurch forward, possibly resulting in dissection. Once tension is released, the burr is activated in the platform segment and platform speed (RPM proximal to lesion) is adjusted according to the burr size; larger burrs (> 2 mm) should have a platform speed of 160,000 RPM while smaller burrs ($\leq$ 2 mm) should have a platform speed of 180,000 RPM.

   c. **Ablation Technique.** The most recent modification of Rotablator technique is the use of RPM surveillance to guide slow and careful advancement of the burr through the lesion. Aggressive burr advancement, indicated by excessive deceleration (rotational speed falls below 5,000 RPM of the platform speed), increases the risk of vessel trauma and ischemic complications caused by frictional heat and the formation of large particles. Contrast injections are intermittently performed to provide visual assessment of burr advancement; these injections identify the borders of the lesion, the orientation of the device in tortuous segments, the burr-to-artery relationship, and may also provide secondary benefit by inducing reactive hyperemia. If egress of contrast is not observed, the burr is withdrawn slightly to re-establish antegrade flow and allow the clearance of particles. The optimal duration of ablation is based on lesion morphology, distal runoff, and hemodynamic and clinical parameters. In general, each run lasts 15-30 seconds, with time between runs (30 sec. to 2 min. depending on patient's response) sufficient to allow particle clearance and the administration of vasodilators. When ECG changes, significant chest discomfort or hemodynamic compromise occurs, the interval between ablations should be increased until the patient is clinically stable. Several average 2-4 ablation runs are usually required to completely treat the lesion (i.e., minimal tactile resistance and no drop in RPM during burr advancement).

d. **Adjunctive Treatment.** Since most burrs are small in relation to the target vessel, adjunctive PTCA is required to achieve definitive lumen enlargement in about 90% of lesions; the technique of adjunctive PTCA (low-pressure inflations with slightly oversized balloons vs. standard inflation pressures using balloons matched to the reference vessel (diameter) is under evaluation. Rotablator atherectomy followed by directional atherectomy has been applied synergistically to calcified lesions in large diameter vessels. In one report,[21] diameter stenosis decreased from 79% pretreatment to 50% after the Rotablator to 17% after directional atherectomy; the arc of calcium decreased with each procedure and the Rotablator appeared to render calcified plaque more susceptible to directional atherectomy. There is growing interest in the use of Rotablator followed by stenting (RotaStent) for calcified stenoses. Compared to adjunctive PTCA, adjunctive stenting resulted in a larger lumen and smaller final stenosis.[22] An IVUS study of Rotablator followed by PTCA, DCA, or stent for calcified lesions in vessels > 3 mm found that Rotablator/stent resulted in the largest lumen and lowest residual stenosis.[52] Several centers are planning a trial to investigate this promising interventional strategy. Finally, IVUS has been used to assess the extent and distribution of lesion calcium and guide interventional strategy: The preferred treatment of superficial calcium is the Rotablator, whereas lesions with deep calcium (without superficial calcium) can be treated by PTCA, DCA, or stenting (Chapter 12).

e. **Postprocedure Management**. In uncomplicated cases, the pacemaker may be removed at the end of the procedure. Nitrates (IV nitroglycerin 10-50 mcg/min or oral agents) are usually administered overnight to minimize vasospasm.

E. **RESULTS.** Available Rotablator data are based on earlier techniques; important modifications in technique (as described above) may have significant beneficial impact or immediate and longterm results.

1. **Success.** In a multicenter registry of 2976 patients (3717 lesions), procedural success was achieved in 94.5%.[24] In the majority of cases (~ 90%), adjunctive angioplasty was needed to obtain a

residual stenosis of < 30%. Procedural success was greater in restenotic lesions than de novo lesions, but was not predicted by patient age, gender, multivessel disease or unstable angina. Results from other studies are similar (Table 27.1). An angiographic study revealed further lumen enlargement 24 hours post-Rotablator, suggesting release of elastic recoil and/or vasospasm.[14]

Table 27.1. Rotablator Atherectomy: Procedural Success and Restenosis

Series	N	Results (%)			
		Success[†]	PTCA	Final Stenosis	Restenosis
MacIsaac[35] (1995)	2161	94.5	74	22	-
Safian[26] (1994)	116	95.2	77	30	51
Vandormael[27] (1994)	215	91	-	31	62
Ellis[34]* (1994)	400	89.9	-	27	-
Warth[32]* (1994)	874	94.7	42	-	38
Barrione[29] (1993)	166	95	100	24	-
Guerin[30] (1993)	67	93.4	100	-	-
Gilmore[31] (1993)	143	91.7	-	-	-
Stertzer[33]* (1993)	346	94	77	-	37
Dietz[28] (1991)	106	73	67	32	42

Abbreviation: - = not reported
†   Residual stenosis < 50% without death, Q-wave MI, or emergency bypass surgery
††   PTCA = adjunctive PTCA
*   Subsets of the multicenter Registry

2. **Complications.** In the multicenter registry, clinical complications rates were similar to those reported for PTCA, including death in 1.0%, Q-wave MI in 1.2%, and emergency CABG in 2.5%.[24] Clinical complications for the different studies are shown in Table 27.2. Elevated CK-MB more than 2 times normal — the most conservative definition of non-Q-wave MI — occurred in 6-8% of patients; there is growing concern that patients experiencing these "minor" elevations in CK-MB may have a poorer long-term prognosis.[25] As shown in Table 27.3, angiographic complications include dissection (10-13%), abrupt closure (1.8-11.2%), slow-flow (1.2-7.6%), perforation (0-1.5%), and severe spasm (1.6-6.6%); differences in complication rates

Table 27.2. Rotablator Atherectomy: In-Hospital Complications

Series	N	Complications (%)				
		Death	**CABG**	**Q-MI**	**non-Q-MI**	**Other**
MacIsaac[35] (1995)	2161	0.8	2.0	0.7	8.8	
Ellis[34]* (1994)	316	0.3	0.9	2.2	5.7	
Vandormael[27] (1994)	215	-	-	-	-	Major complications (2.3%)
Warth[32]* (1994)	743	0.8	1.7	0.9	3.8	Vascular (2.2%); Arrhythmia (1.9%)
Safian[26] (1993)	104	1	1.9	4.8	2.9	Bleeding (7.7%); Vascular (2.9%); Arrhythmia (1.8%)
Barrione[29] (1993)	166	1.8	0	0.6	8.4	
Guerin[30] (1993)	61	0	1.6	1.6	6.6	Arrhythmia (6.6%)
Gilmore[31] (1993)	108	0.9	2.8	0.9	2.8	
Stertzer[33]* (1993)	302	0	1.0	2.6	-	
Dietz[28] (1991)	106	0	1.9	0	4.7	

Abbreviations: CABG = emergency coronary bypass grafting; Q-MI = Q-wave myocardial infarction; non-Q-MI = non-Q-wave myocardial infarction; - = not reported

† Need for transfusion, drop in hemoglobin ≥ 3 gm/dL, or hematoma > 4 cm

* Subsets of multicenter Registry

Table 27.3. Rotablator Atherectomy: Angiographic Complications

| Series | N | Complications (%) | | | | | |
		Acute Closure	Slow Flow	Perf	Diss	SBO	Severe Spasm
MacIsaac[35]* (1995)	2161	3.6	-	0.7	13	-	-
Ellis[34] (1994)	400	5.5	7.6	1.5	-	-	-
Warth[32]* (1994)	874	3.1	1.2	0.5	10.5	0.1	1.6
Safian[26] (1993)	116	11.2	6.1	0	-	1.8	-
Barrione[29] (1993)	166	1.8	-	-	-	-	-
Guerin[30] (1993)	67	0.9	-	-	-	-	4.5
Dietz[28] (1991)	106	-	-	-	-	1.9	6.6

Abbreviation: Perf = perforation; Diss = dissection; SBO = sidebranch occlusion; - = not reported
* Data from subsets of the multicenter registry

between series are likely the result of different definitions, the growth in operator experience, and evolving technique. Due to the slightly larger sheath size ($\geq$ 8F), significant bleeding (need for transfusion, decrease in hemoglobin > 3 gm/dL, or hematoma > 4 cm) occurred in 1.0 - 7.7%, while groin complications requiring surgery occurred in 2-3% of patients. In high-risk patients undergoing Rotablator, prophylactic insertion of an IABP may reduce the incidence of hypotension and non-Q-wave MI.[53]

3. **Restenosis.** Restenosis rates appear comparable to balloon angioplasty and have ranged from 39% in the multicenter registry to 62% in the randomized Excimer Laser Rotablator Balloon Angioplasty Comparison (ERBAC) trial.[27] A study of restenosis by lesion length and calcium showed that restenosis was 1.86 times more likely in long lesions and 2.54 times more likely in noncalcified lesions;[36] restenosis rates were lowest (6.3%) for short calcified lesions and highest (37.2%) for noncalcified lesions greater than 20 mm in length.[36]

4. **Impact of Plaque Composition on Results (Table 27.4)**

a. **Calcification.** Procedural success and major complications are similar among calcified and noncalcified lesions treated with the Rotablator.[35,37] Reports differ with respect to restenosis; the multicenter Registry reported no difference,[35] while another report found a lower restenosis rate among calcified lesions.

b. **Soft Plaque.** Intravascular ultrasound has shown that Rotablator is capable of ablating soft plaque; in a study of 10 noncalcified lesions, Rotablator led to a significant increase in lumen volume, although diffuse vasospasm occurred in 60%.[38]

5. **Impact of Lesion Morphology on Results (Table 27.4)**

a. **Complex Lesions.** The ERBAC trial compared Rotablator atherectomy, PTCA and excimer laser angioplasty in type B and C lesions.[27] Despite its use in more B2 and C lesions compared to PTCA (85% vs. 72%), Rotablator had higher success (91% vs. 80%), lower residual stenosis (27% vs. 35%), and fewer ischemic complications (1.5% vs. 7.0%); restenosis rates at 6-months were similar (PTCA 51.4%, Rotablator 62%; p = NS).

b. **Long Lesions.** In the multicenter Registry, there was no difference in procedural success or restenosis for lesions 1 - 10 mm, 11 - 15 mm, and 15 - 25 mm in length.[39] In a retrospective study[40] of lesions 10 - 20 mm in length, procedural success and major complications were higher after Rotablator than after PTCA (success: 95% vs. 91%; complications: 1.4% vs. 0.5%); success was also higher after the Rotablator in lesions > 20 mm (84% vs 76% for PTCA), but there was a high (10%) incidence of major complications in both groups.

c. **Ostial Lesions.** Treatment of ostial lesions by the Rotablator has been analyzed in four reports.[41-44] The largest of these studies[42] (105 patients) reported success in 97%, dissections in 17%, spasm in 2.8%, and CABG in 1.9%; angiographic restenosis was evident in 32%.

d. **Chronic Total Occlusions.** Among 145 chronic total occlusions in the multicenter Registry crossed with a guidewire, Rotablator success was achieved in 91% and correlated with vessel diameter.[45] In-hospital death and non-Q-wave MI occurred in 1.4% and 4.3%, respectively. Restenosis was present in 62.5%, although angiographic follow-up occurred in only 49% of patients. Multivariate predictor of success and restenosis were vessel diameter and diabetes, respectively.

e. **Undilatable Lesions.** The Rotablator has proven to be particularly useful for the management of fibrocalcific lesions resistant to PTCA.[46-49] Brogan et al[47] achieved procedural success in 37/41 (90%) of such lesions. In this report, the Rotablator was shown to improve lesion compliance, rendering the lesion more responsive to subsequent PTCA. Recurrent symptoms and restenosis developed in 24% and 35% of patients respectively, while 3 patients died suddenly during follow-up without recurrent symptoms.

Table 27.4. Procedural Success by Lesion Morphology

Series	Lesion Type	N	Success (%)
MacIsaac[35] (1995)	Calcified	1078	94
	Non calcified	1083	95
Altmann[37] (1993)	No/mild Calcified	-*	96
	Moderate Calcified	-	96
	Heavy Calcified	-	92
Vandormael[27] (1994)	Complex**	215	91
Reisman[39] (1993)	< 10 mm	953	95
	11-15 mm	180	97
	15-25 mm	143	92
Favereau[40]	10-20 mm	215	95
	20 mm	73	84
Koller[41] (1994)	Ostial	29	93
Zimarino[43] (1994)	Ostial	69	92
Popma[42] (1993)	Ostial	105	97
Omoigui[45] (1995)	Chronic TO	145	91
Reisman[46] (1993)	Undilatable	34	97
Brogan[47] (1993)	Undilatable	41	90
Sievert[49] (1993)	Undilatable	32	97
Rosenblum[48] (1992)	Undilatable	40	97
Bass[50] (1992)	Restenotic	428	97
Chevalier[51] (1994)	Angulated	123	86

Abbreviation: TO = total occlusion
* Total number of lesion = 675; subgroup data not available
** Type B_2 (72%), Type C (13%)

f. **Restenotic Lesions.** Comparison of de novo and restenotic lesions from the multicenter Registry revealed a higher initial success rate in restenotic lesions with no difference in restenosis (38%) at follow-up.[50]

g. **Angulated Lesions.** Compared to Rotablator atherectomy of nonangulated lesions, lesion angulation > 45 degrees resulted in lower procedural success (86% vs. 94%), more death (2.7% vs. 0.3%), and a higher incidence in total ischemic events (5.4% vs 1.3%).[51] When performing Rotablator in angulated lesions, it is important to adjust the guidewire to minimize vessel distortion, begin with smaller burrs, use a maximum burr-to-artery ratio of 0.6-0.7, and plan to use adjunctive PTCA or stenting. Lesions on the outer curve may be better suited for the Rotablator than inner curve lesions (Chapter 11) (Figure 27.4).

h. **Other Lesions.** The Rotablator is not recommended in thrombus-containing lesions or saphenous vein grafts due to the risk of distal embolization and no-reflow. Fibrous plaque at vein graft anastomoses, however, has been successfully treated.

F. **CLINICAL TRIALS.** At present, 3 large multicenter trails are enrolling patients to further explore the effectiveness of the Rotablator system.

1. **STRATAS (Study to Determine Rotablator System and Transluminal Angioplasty Strategy)** is a technique trial to evaluate whether maximal debulking (burr-to-artery ratio of 0.8 - 0.9)

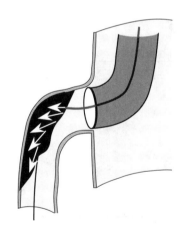 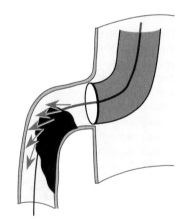

Lesion on Outer Curve:
Device directed into lesion

Lesion on Inner Curve:
Device deflected into disease-free wall

Figure 27.4 Angulated Lesions: Impact of Lesion Location

Angulated lesions with plaque situated along the outer curve may sometimes be considered for ELCA, TEC, or Rotablator. In contrast, when plaque is situated along the inner curve, these devices may deflect away from the plaque and into the disease-free wall, increasing the risk of dissection or perforation.

followed by no or low-pressure PTCA is better than moderate debulking (burr-to-artery ratio < 0.75) followed by systematic adjunctive PTCA using conventional balloon pressure (3 atm). The trial will randomize 500 patients with lesions indicated for the Rotablator. The primary endpoint is angiographic restenosis.

2. **DART (Dilation vs. Ablation Revascularization Trial)** is a two-arm randomized trial of Rotablator atherectomy versus balloon angioplasty in noncomplex (Type A and B1) lesions < 3 mm diameter; 1,000 patients at 25 centers will be enrolled. The primary endpoint is clinical and angiographic restenosis, with a subset of 500 patients undergoing 6-8 month angiographic follow-up. DART will include substudies comparing angiography with intravascular ultrasound, examining cost effectiveness, and measuring quality of life.

3. **CARAT (Coronary Angioplasty and Rotablator Atherectomy Trial)** is a prospective multicenter randomized trial which compares the results of Rotablator using small burrs (final burr-to-artery ratio < 0.7) versus large burrs (final burr-to-artery ratio > 0.7). The primary endpoint is final diameter stenosis; secondary endpoints include target lesion revascularization and cost. The study will enroll approximately 600 patients.

4. **RotaStent.** Several centers are planning a trial of Rotablator prior to stenting to determine if Rotablator pretreatment will increase lesion compliance and improve stent deployment. In a study of 88 calcified lesions subjected to RotaStenting, a final diameter stenosis of 12% was achieved without major in-hospital complications.[22]

G. **SUMMARY.** Rotational atherectomy has emerged as one of the second generation devices to expand the therapeutic opportunities of percutaneous revascularization. The device is more closely related to a surgical scalpel and therefore is best suited for well-trained interventional cardiologists. Lesions that benefit most from plaque ablation are typically calcified or have a fibrocalcific component. Lesion modification (debulking) as a method of improving vessel compliance has been an important indication for the Rotablator, particularly in diffusely diseased vessels, as well as aorto-ostial and branch-ostial stenoses. The role of rotational atherectomy used syngeristically with other second generation devices such as stents are presently been defined.

* * * * *

REFERENCES

1. Fourrier JL, Stankowiak C, Lablanche JM, et al. Histopathology after rotational angioplasty of peripheral arteries in human beings. J Am Coll Cardiol 1988;11:109A.

2. Kovach J, Mintz G, Pichard A, Kent K, et al. Sequential intravascular ultrasound characterization of the mechanisms of rotational atherectomy and adjunct balloon angioplasty. J Am Coll Cardiol 1993;22:1024-32.

3. Mintz G, Potkin B, Keren G, Satler L, et al. Intravascular ultrasound evaluation of the effect of rotational atherectomy in obstructive atherosclerotic coronary artery disease. Circulation 1992; 86:1383-1393.

4. Cowley M, Buchbinder M, Warth D, Dorros G, et al. Effect of coronary rotational atherectomy abrasion on vessel segments adjacent to treated lesions . J Am Coll Cardiol 1992;19:333A.

5. Prevosti LG, Cook JA, Unger EF, Sheffield CD, et al. Particulate debris from rotational atherectomy: size distribution and physiologic effect. Circulation 1988;78:II-83.

6. Friedman HZ, Elliott MA, Gottlieb GJ, O'Neill WW. Mechanical rotary atherectomy: The effects of microparticle embolization on myocardial blood flow and function. J Interv Cardiol 1989;2:77-83.

7. Hansen DD, Auth DC, Hall M, Ritchie JL. Rotational endarterectomy in normal canine coronary arteries: preliminary report. J Am Coll Cardiol 1988; 11:1073-77.

8. Sherman C, Brunken R, Chan A, et al. Myocardial perfusion and segmental wall motion after coronary rotational atherectomy. Circulation 1992;86:I-652.

9. Pavlides G, Hauser A, Grines C, et al. Clinical, hemodynamic, electrocardiographic, and mechanical events during nonocclusive coronary atherectomy and comparison to balloon angioplasty. Am J Cardiol 1992;70:841-845.

10. Williams MJA, Dow CJ, Weyman AE, et al. Myocardial dysfunction after rotational coronary atherectomy: Serial evaluation by echocardiography. Circulation 1994;90:I-395.

11. Huggins GS, Williams MJA, Yang J, et al. Transient wall motion abnormalities following rotational atherectomy are reflective of myocardial stunning more than myocardial infarction. J Am Coll Cardiol 1995;25:96A.

12. Nunez BD, Keelan ET, Lerman A, et al. Coronary hemodynamics after rotational atherectomy. J Am Coll Cardiol 1995;25:95A.

13. Safian R, Freed M, Lichtenberg A, et al. Are residual stenoses after excimer laser angioplasty and coronary atherectomy due to inefficient or small devices? Comparison with balloon angioplasty. J Am Coll Cardiol 1993;22:628-1634.

14. Reisman M, Buchbinder M, Bass T, et al. Improvement in coronary dimensions at early 24-hour follow-up after coronary rotational ablation: Implications for restenosis. Circulation 1992;86:I-332.

15. Kovach JA, Mintz GS, et al. Sequential intravascular ultrasound characterization of the mechanisms of rotational atherectomy and adjunct balloon angioplasty. J Am Coll Cardiol 1993;22:1024-32.

16. Mintz GS, Douek P, et al. Target lesion calcification in coronary artery disease: An intravascular ultrasound study. J Am Coll Cardiol 1992;20:1149-55.

17. Nino C, Free M, Blankenship L, et al. Procedural cost and benefits of new interventional devices. Am J Cardiol 1994;74:1165-1166.

18. Vandormael M, Reifart N, Preusler W, et al. In-hospital costs comparison of excimer laser angioplasty, rotational atherectomy (rotablator) and balloon angioplasty for complex coronary lesions: A randomized trial (ERBAC). J Am Coll Cardiol 1994;89:223A.

19. Cohen B, et al. Intracoronary cocktail infusion during rotational ablation: Safety and Efficacy. Cathet Cardiovasc Diagn (in press).

20. Reisman M, Harms V. Guidewire bias: A potential source of complications with rotational atherectomy. Cathet Cardiovasc Diagn (in press).

21. Mintz GS, Pichard AD, et al. Transcatheter device synergy: preliminary experience with adjunct directional coronary atherectomy following high-speed rotational atherectomy or excimer laser angioplasty in the treatment of coronary artery disease. Cathet Cardiovasc Diagn 1993;28 Suppl(1):37-44.

22. Mintz GS, Dussaillsnt GR, Wong SC, et al. Rotational atherectomy followed by adjunct stents: The preferred therapy for calcified large vessels? Circulation 1995;92:I-329.

23. Mintz GS, Pichard AD, et al. Impact of preintervention intravascular ultrasound imaging on transcatheter treatment strategies in coronary artery disease. Am J Cardiol 1994;73:423-430.

24. MacIsaac A, Whitlow P, Cowley M, Buchbinder M. Angiographic predictors of outcome of coronary rotational atherectomy from the completed multicenter registry. J Am Coll Cardiol 1994;23:353A.

25. Redwood SR, Popma JJ, Kent KM, Pichard AD, et al. "Minor" CPK-MB elevations are associated with increased mortality following new-device angioplasty in native coronary arteries. Circulation 1995;92:I-544.

26. Safian RD, Niazi KA, et al. Detailed angiographic analysis of high-speed mechanical rotational atherectomy in human coronary arteries. Circulation 1993;88:961-8.

27. Vandormael M, Reifart N, Preusler W, et al. Comparison of excimer laser, rotablator and balloon angioplasty for the treatment of complex lesions: ERBAC study final results. J Am Coll Cardiol, 1994;23:57A.

28. Dietz UR, Erbel R, et al. Angiographic and histologic findings in high frequency rotational ablation in coronary arteries in vitro. Zeitschrift fur Kardiologie 1991;80:222-9.

29. Borrions M, Hall P, et al. Treatment of simple and complex coronary stenosis using rotational ablation followed by low pressure balloon angioplasty. Cath Cardiovasc Diagn 1993;30:131-7.

30. Guerin Y, Rahal S, et al. Coronary angioplasty combining rotational atherectomy and balloon dilatation. Results in 67 complex stenoses. Arch Mal du Coeur 1993;86:1535-41.

31. Gilmore PS, Bass TA, et al. Single site experience with high-speed coronary rotational atherectomy. Clin Cardiol 1993;16:311-6.

32. Warth DC, Leon MB, et al. Rotational atherectomy multicenter registry: Acute results, complications and 6-month angiographic follow-up in 709 patients. J Am Coll Cardiol 1994;24:641-8.

33. Stertzer SH, Rosenblum J, et al. Coronary rotational ablation: initial experience in 302 procedures. J Am Coll Cardiol 1993;21:287-95.

34. Ellis SG, Popma JJ, et al. Relation of clinical presentation, stenosis morphology, and operator technique to the procedural results of rotational atherectomy and rotational atherectomy facilitated angioplasty. Circulation 1994;89:882-92.

35. MacIsaac AI, Bass TA, Buchbinder M, et al. High speed rotational atherectomy: Outcome in calcified and noncalcified coronary artery lesions. J Am Coll Cardiol 1995;26:531-6.

36. Leguizamon JH, Chambre DF, Torresani EM, et al. High speed coronary rotational atherectomy: Are angiographic factors predictive of failure, major complications or restenosis? J Am Coll Cardiol 1995;25:95A.

37. Altmann D, Popma J, Kent K, et al. Rotational atherectomy effectively treats calcified lesions. J Am Coll Cardiol 1993;21:443A.

38. Dussaillant GR, Mintz GS, Walsh CL, et al. Volumetric intravascular ultrasound analysis shows that rotational atherectomy effectively ablates soft atherosclerotic plaque. Circulation 1995;92:I-17.

39. Reisman M, Cohen B, Warth D, Fenner J, et al. Outcome of long lesions treated with high speed rotational ablation. J Am Coll Cardiol 1993;21:443A.

40. Favereaux X, Chevalier B, Commeau P, et al. Is rotational atherectomy more effective than balloon angioplasty for the treatment of long coronary lesions? SCA & I Meeting Abstracts, 92.

41. Koller PT, Freed M, Grines CL, O'Neill WW. Success, complications, and restenosis following rotational and transluminal extraction atherectomy of ostial stenoses. Cathet and Cardiovas Diagn 1994;31:255-260.

42. Popma J, Brogan W, Pichard A, et al. Rotational coronary atherectomy of ostial stenoses. Am J Cardiol 1993;71:436-438.

43. Zimarino M, Corcos T, Favereau X, et al. Rotational coronary atherectomy with adjunctive balloon angioplasty for the treatment of ostial lesions. Cathet Cardiovas Diagn 1994;33:22-27.

44. Sabri MN, Cowley MJ, DiSciascio G, DeBottis D, et al. Immediate results of interventional devices for coronary ostial narrowing with angina pectoris. Am J Cardiol 1994;73:122-125.

45. Omoigui N, Booth J, Reisman M, et al. Rotational atherectomy in chronic total occlusions. J Am Coll Cardiol 1995;25:97A.

46. Reisman M, Devlin P, Melikian J, et al. Undilatable noncompliant lesions treated with the Rotablator: outcome and angiographic follow-up. Circulation 1993;88: I-547.

47. Brogan W, Popma J, Pichard A, Satler L, et al. Rotational coronary atherectomy after unsuccessful coronary balloon angioplasty. Am J Cardiol 1993;71:794-798.

48. Rosenblum J, Stertzer S, Shaw R, et al. Rotational ablation of balloon angioplasty failures. J Inva Cardiol 1992;4:312-317.

49. Sievert H, Tonndorf S, Utech A, Schulze R. [High frequency rotational angioplasty (rotablation) after unsuccessful balloon dilatation] Z Cardiol 1993;82:411-414.

50. Bass T, Gilmore P, Buchbinder M, et al. Coronary rotational atherectomy (PTCA) in patients with prior coronary

revascularization: a registry report. Circulation 1992;86:I-653.

51. Chevalier B, Commeau P, Favereau X, et al. Limitations of rotational atherectomy in angulated coronary lesions. J Am Coll Cardiol 1994;23:285A.

52. Dussaillant GR, Mintz GS, Pichard AD, et al. The optimal strategy for treating calcified lesions in large vessels: Comparison of intravascular ultrasound results of rotational atherectomy + adjunctive PTCA, DCA, or stents. J Am Coll Cardiol 1996;March Special Issue.

53. O'Murchu B, Foreman RD, Shaw RE, et al. Role of intraaortic balloon pump counterpulsation in high risk coronary rotational atherectomy. J Am Coll Cardiol 1995;26:1270-5.

54. Reisman M, DeVore LJ, ferguson M, et al. Analysis of heat generation during high-speed rotational ablation: Technical implications. J Am Coll Cardiol 1996;March, Special Issue

55. Coletti RH, Haik BJ, Wiedermann JG, et al. Marked reduction in slow-reflow after rotational atherectomy through the use of a novel flushing solution. TCT Meeting 1996;Washington DC

56. Stertzer SH, Pomerantsev EV, Fitzgerald PJ, et al. Effects of technique modification on immediate results of high speed rotational atherectomy in 710 procedures on 656 patients.

28 DIRECTIONAL CORONARY ATHERECTOMY

Robert D. Safian, M.D.

A. **DESCRIPTION.** Directional coronary atherectomy (DCA) (Devices for Vascular Intervention, Inc. Redwood City, CA) is a percutaneous, over-the-wire cutting and retrieval system (Figure 28.1). The prototype of the directional atherectomy catheter is the Simpson Coronary AtheroCath™ which consists of a metal housing with an affixed balloon, a nosecone collection chamber, and a hollow torque tube which accommodates a 0.014" guidewire. A cup-shaped cutter inside the housing is attached to a flexible drive shaft, and is activated by a hand-held battery-operated motor drive unit (Figure 28.2). The AtheroCath is advanced into the lesion over a 0.014" wire with the cutting window oriented toward the atheroma. The balloon is inflated, pushing the plaque into the cutting window and holding the housing in place. A lever on the motor drive unit allows the operator to activate and slowly advance the cutter through the lesion as it rotates at 2,000 rpm. Excised atheroma is stored in the distal nosecone collection chamber. The balloon is deflated, the AtheroCath rotated and reoriented, and the process repeated until the desired angiographic result is achieved.

B. **DCA EQUIPMENT.** Since FDA approval of the Simpson Coronary AtheroCath in 1990, there have been several important improvements in the design of the AtheroCath and ancillary hardware. These improvements have addressed many of the limitations of the early atherectomy devices.

1. **Guiding Catheters** (Figure 28.3, Table 28.1). Over the last few years, almost the entire line of 11F guiding catheters has been replaced by 9.5F and 10F guiding catheters with enhanced torque response. Rather than the typical primary and secondary curves of conventional left Judkins

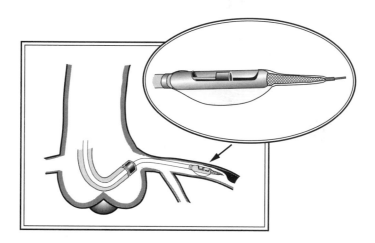

Figure 28.1 Directional Coronary Atherectomy (DCA)

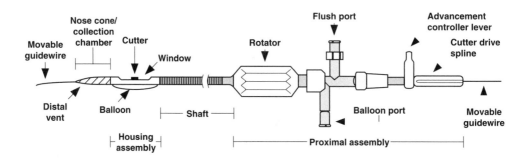

Figure 28.2 Directional Coronary Atherectomy: AtheroCath Components

catheters, DCA guiding catheters for the left coronary artery have gentle C-curves (originally called JCL guides), which permit easy cornering of the AtheroCath through the guiding catheter. Standard sizes for the left coronary artery include JL3.5, JL4.0, JL4.5, and JL5.0, depending on the diameter of the aortic root. For the right coronary artery, the JR4.0 is available in standard-length and short-tip designs. Additional guides for the RCA include the JR4 IF (for inferior takeoff), the Hockey Stick (for horizontal, anterior, or superior takeoff) and the JRG (for superior takeoff or Shepherd Crook origin). For bypass grafts, available guiding catheters include the JRG (for anterior grafts with gentle upward takeoff), the JLG (for anterior grafts with marked superior takeoff), and the multipurpose guide (for grafts with vertical takeoff). The manufacturer is currently developing giant lumen 9F guides for all vessels.

2.   **AtheroCath Designs (Table 28.2).** There are 3 generations of AtheroCaths:
   - **First Generation: SCA-1.** This was the original design, and is only available as a 7F Graft cutter.

   - **Second Generation: SCA-EX.** Enhanced torque and an improved nosecone design were the key modifications of this second generation AtheroCath. In addition, the Surlyn balloon on the SCA-1 device was replaced by a less compliant PET balloon. The EX has a 9 mm cutting window and is available in all sizes, including a 7F Graft. The EX is also available with a short (5 mm) window, which may be better suited for very focal lesions and tortuous vessels, and is available in all sizes except the 7F Graft.

   - **Third Generation: SCA-GTO.** This third generation AtheroCath is available in all sizes except the 7F Graft. The GTO has a redesigned shaft with better support and torque control than the EX (Figure 28.4). Within the next year, further additions to the line of available AtheroCaths will include a GTO-short housing device; better cutters for treating large vessels

Table 28.1. Guiding Catheter Selection for DCA.

Vessel	Configuration	Guiding Catheter
LCA	Normal	JL 4.0
	Narrow aortic root or superior origin	JL 3.5
	Wide aortic root or posterior origin	JL 4.5, JL 5.0
RCA	Normal	JR 4.0 ST, JR 4.0
	Anterior origin	Hockey stick
	Horizontal origin	Hockey stick
	Superior origin or Shepherd Crook	Hockey stick, JRG
	Inferior origin	JR 4.0 IF, JR 4.0 ST
Vein Grafts to LCA	Normal	JR 4.0, JR 4.0 ST, Hockey stick
	Superior origin	Hockey stick, JRG, JLG
Vein Grafts to RCA	Normal	Multipurpose, JR 4.0 IF
	Horizontal origin	JR 4.0, Hockey stick

Abbreviations: LCA = left coronary artery; RCA = right coronary artery; JL = Judkins left; JR = Judkins right; ST = short tip; JRG = modified right graft; IF = inferior; JLG = modified left graft

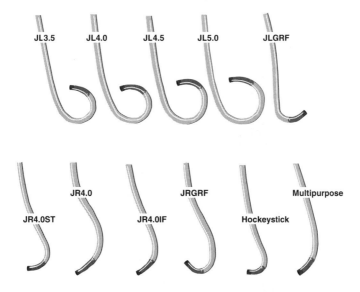

Figure 28.3 Directional Coronary Atherectomy: Guiding Catheters

Table 28.2. AtheroCaths for Directional Coronary Atherectomy

Type	Balloon Material	Housing Length (mm) Rigid/Window	Sizes
SCA-1	Suryln	17 / 10	7FG
SCA-EX	PET	17 / 9	5F, 6F, 7F, 7FG
SCA-EX short	PET	12 / 5	5F, 6F, 7F
AtheroCath GTO	PET	16 / 9	5F, 6F, 7F

Abbreviations: SCA = Simpson Coronary AtheroCath; GTO = greater torque output; PET = polyethylene terephthalate (Dacron); F = French size; G = graft cutter

(3.75-5.0 mm); a Power Blade device with a tungsten carbide-coated cutter for enhanced excision of heavily calcified lesions; and an ultrasound-guided atherectomy device (GDCA).

3. **Ancillary Equipment.** Other ancillary equipment for DCA includes a large-bore rotating hemostatic valve (internal diameter > 0.094-inch), the motor drive unit (MDU), and 0.014-inch guidewires. Guiding catheters may be advanced into the central circulation using either a 7F tapered introducer and a 0.035" guidewire, or a 0.063" guidewire without the introducer. The new MDU has a locking mechanism to prevent cutter movement while the device is advanced through the target vessel.

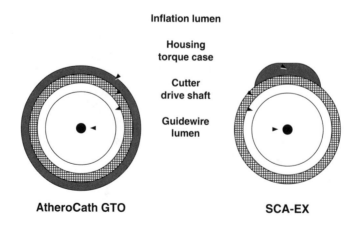

Figure 28.4 Directional Coronary Atherectomy: Construction

Comparison of the GTO and SCA-EX devices.

C. DCA TECHNIQUE. Many interventional cardiologists have achieved considerable experience with directional atherectomy; general guidelines for lesion selection are based on operator experience (Table 28.3). Several aspects of this procedure facilitate the technique and improve results:

1. **Preparation of the AtheroCath.** Unlike the SCA-EX, which required a single negative aspiration prep, preparation of the GTO requires a *triple* negative aspiration prep, each for 30-45 seconds. The balloon should then be inflated to 2-3 ATM for a few seconds, and then deflated completely. This technique ensures elimination of air and permits adequate visualization of the balloon during inflation.

2. **Guiding Catheter Manipulation.** Because of the caliber and rigidity of the AtheroCath, proper guiding catheter position is crucial. The most important feature is coaxial alignment of the tip of the guide with the vessel ostium (Table 28.1); guiding catheter maneuvers such as over rotation and deep-seating increase the risk of vessel injury and should be avoided.

Table 28.3. Recommendations for DCA Based on Operator Experience and Lesion Morphology

Morphology	Level 1: Requires 0 to 5 cases	Level 2: Requires > 5 cases	Level 3: Requires > 20 cases	Level 4: Not recommended
Vessel	Proximal & mid LAD	Ostial LAD	Distal LAD, RCA, non-degenerated SVG, LCX, protected LM	Degenerated SVG unprotected LM
Angulation of takeoff	Shallow	Shallow	Moderate	Severe
Tortuosity (proximal or distal to lesion)	None	Mild	Moderate	Severe
Lesion length	≤ 10mm	≤ 10mm	11-20 mm	> 20mm
Vessel diameter	≥ 3.0 mm	≥ 3.0 mm	≥ 2.5 mm	< 2.5 mm
Vessel dissection	Absent	Absent	Focal flap, not angulated	Severe flap, angulated, long or spiral dissection
Lesion morphology	Eccentric, concentric	Ulcerated	Thrombus	Heavily calcified
Lesion type	Restenosis	De novo	All	Friable, grumous
Calcification	None	Mild	Moderate	Heavy, especially in tortuous vessels

Abbreviations: LAD = left anterior descending coronary artery; RCA = right coronary artery; SVG = saphenous vein graft; LCx = left circumflex coronary artery; LM = left main coronary artery

3. **AtheroCath Deployment.** To properly position the AtheroCath, it is important to gently rotate and advance the device into the lesion; forward advancement without rotation will increase resistance and can result in proximal vessel dissection or failure to cross the lesion. In contrast to PTCA, the AtheroCath should never be "jack-hammered" across a lesion; if the device does not cross, ensure coaxial alignment of the guiding catheter, exchange for a heavier-duty guidewire, and use more device rotation (to "screw" it across the lesion); changing to a smaller or short-cutter device or predilating the lesion with a 2.0 mm balloon will also improve crossing rates. To avoid perforation, the window should be oriented towards angiographically-apparent plaque before initiating the cutting sequence. Periodic contrast injections should be performed every 6-8 cuts to assess progress. Free mobility of the distal guidewire should be maintained at all times. Loss of wire mobility after several cuts suggests that the nosecone collection chamber is full; forceful removal of the device at this point greatly increases the risk of guidewire fracture. If free mobility cannot be achieved, the guidewire and AtheroCath should be removed together as a single unit.

4. **Adjunctive Medical Therapy.** Adjunctive medical therapy for DCA is similar to PTCA, including preprocedural aspirin (325 mg/d starting at least 1 day prior to DCA) and intraprocedural heparin (to maintain the ACT >300 seconds). Long acting nitrates and/or calcium antagonists are administered at the discretion of the operator to minimize vasospasm. If a satisfactory angiographic result is obtained, heparin is discontinued at the end of the case and the vascular sheaths are removed 4-6 hours later. Other platelet antagonists such as dipyridamole, Dextran, and sulfinpyrazone are not routinely prescribed. In high-risk patients (e.g, unstable ischemic syndromes, high-risk lesion morphology), bolus and infusion of c7E3 has been shown to decrease the incidence of major complications and possibly restenosis (Chapter 34).[1]

5. **Adjunctive Devices.** PTCA, Rotablator, and ELCA have been used to facilitate subsequent passage of the AtheroCath when it fails to cross the lesion;[2,3] this is more common in aorto-ostial, angulated and calcified lesions, and in tortuous vessels. Intravascular ultrasound may be particularly useful to assess the depth and extent of calcification; for superficial calcification, Rotablator may be preferable to PTCA, but for deep calcification, DCA alone or DCA followed by PTCA may be considered.

6. **Optimal Atherectomy.** The goal of optimal atherectomy is to create the largest lumen diameter possible without complications. Optimal atherectomy can be achieved as follows:
   - For initial DCA passes, begin with an AtheroCath according to the practical guidelines in Table 28.4. Initial cuts should be directed toward angiographically-apparent plaque (as guided by multiple orthogonal views). Initial balloon inflation pressures of 10-20 psi are used, and the AtheroCath is usually removed and emptied after 6-8 cuts. If repeat angiography demonstrates a residual stenosis > 15%, additional atherectomy is performed using higher inflation pressures (20-40 psi).

   - If a residual stenosis > 15% is still evident, the decision to perform DCA with a larger cutter (vs. PTCA or stenting) depends on the cutter-to-artery ratio; if upsizing complies with the

Table 28.4. Recommendations for DCA Sizing and Normal Vessel Diameter

Size (F)	Vessel diameter (mm)*	Vessel diameter (mm) Practical **
5F	2.5-2.9	≤ 2.5
6F	3.0-3.4	2.5-3.0
7F	3.5-3.9	3.0-3.5
7FG	≥ 4.0	3.5-4.0

Abbreviations: F = French size; G = graft cutter
*   These guidelines are based on the product label; recommended by the FDA
**   These guidelines are not approved by the FDA, but may allow for more "optimal atherectomy"

sizing guidelines in Table 28.4, DCA is performed; if the next size cutter is too large for the target vessel, PTCA or stenting is performed. PTCA should be performed using a balloon-to-artery ratio of 1.0-1.2 and inflation pressures of 4-6 atm. In one report, adjunctive stenting resulted in superior immediate lumen enlargement compared to PTCA.[10]

Although preliminary data suggest that intravascular ultrasound can be used to achieve larger lumen diameters,[4-7] other data suggest that comparable lumen enlargement can be achieved using angiography alone.[8,9] The "ideal" residual stenosis is unknown; one study suggested a reduction in late cardiac events when the final diameter stenosis was 10-20%, with no incremental benefit for residual stenoses < 10%.[11] Most operators attempt to achieve a residual stenosis < 15-20%.

D.   MECHANISM OF LUMEN ENLARGEMENT. Although DCA can excise tissue and plaque, the amount of tissue removal (usually 6-45 mg) may not fully account for the magnitude of luminal enlargement. IVUS studies suggest that tissue removal accounts for about 75% of the luminal improvement after DCA, [15-18] the rest being due to a combination of Dotter and balloon dilating effects.

E.   PROCEDURAL RESULTS. The results of DCA have been reported in numerous single and multicenter observational studies (Tables 28.5, 28.6, 28.7, 28.8), and in three large multicenter prospective randomized trials (Table 28.9). Further studies of optimal atherectomy (with and without ultrasound guidance) are also in progress (Tables 28.10, 28.11).

1.   **Immediate Angiographic Results.** As shown in Tables 28.5 and 28.6, observational studies report DCA success in 83-99%, final diameter stenoses of 5-29%, and major complications in 1.5-10% of patients. In the three largest randomized studies comparing DCA and PTCA in native vessels (CAVEAT-I, CCAT) and vein grafts (CAVEAT-II), DCA resulted in better immediate lumen enlargement, higher procedural success, and similar major complications rates (Table 28.9).

Table 28.5. Immediate Results and Clinical Complications after DCA

Series	N (pts)	Final DS (%)	Success (%)	MC (%)	Comments
Fortuna[11] (1995)	310	16	95%	5	VSR (1.3%), TLR (28%)
Safian[4] (1990)	67	5	88	1.5	VSR (3%); nQMI (4.5%)
Umans[12] (1994)	150	29	90	10	Worse 2 year EFS with unstable angina
Popma[13] (1993)	306	14	95	2.6	nQMI (5.6%); CRS (28% at 1 year)
Cowley[14] (1993)	300	-	95%	4.6	
Baim[15] (1993)	873	-	92%	4.9	US DCA Registry: ARS (42%); nQMI (5%); VSR (1.1%)
Feld[16] (1993)	116	8	99	4%	Matched comparison with PTCA;* nQMI (6%)
Fishmann[17] (1992)	190	7	97	3	nQMI (7.4%); ARS (32%); 1 yr. EFS (74%); nQMI (7.4%)
Popma[18] (1992)	1020	-	83	-	Death (0.2%), MI (1.7%); CABG (2.5%)
Garratt[19] (1992)	158	-	91	7	ARS (58%)
Ellis[20] (1991)	378	-	88	6.3	
Hinohara[21] (1991)	339	15	94	3.4	Success: 78% (noncalcified), 52% (calcified)
Rowe[22] (1990)	83	14	95	2.2	
Kaufmann[23] (1989)	50	15	89	4%	nQMI (4.2%), VSR (1.4%)

Abbreviations: MC = major in-hospital complication (death, Q-wave myocardial infarction, emergency coronary artery bypass surgery); nQMI = non-Q-wave myocardial infarction; VSR = vascular surgical repair; TLR = target lesion revascularization; EFS = event-free survival; - = not reported; ARS = angiographic restenosis, CRS = clinical restenosis
* After PTCA: Success 98%; fewer dissections with DCA (13% vs. 22%); major complications 1.6%

Table 28.6. Immediate Results and Clinical Complications After DCA in Vein Grafts

Series	N (Lesions)	Success (%)	Major Complications** (%)
Cowley[24] (1993)	363	86	2.5*
Garratt[19] (1992)	26	96	4.2
Pomerantz[25] (1992)	35	94	0
DiScasio[26] (1992)	96	97	1.4
Ghazzal[27] (1992)	286	87	2.1
Selmon[28] (1991)	87	91	2.6
Kaufmann[29] (1990)	14	93	7

* US DCA Registry: vascular repair 3.5%; non-Q-wave myocardial infarction 3%; restenosis rate 57% (38% de novo lesions, 75% restenotic lesions)
** In-hospital death, MI, emergency bypass surgery

Although adjunctive PTCA after DCA was initially discouraged, PTCA may actually improve DCA outcome and can often result in residual stenoses <10%.[4,5,8,9] In lesions with ≥ 3 complex characteristics, the success rate of atherectomy decreased from 97% to 84%, but increased to nearly 90% after adjunctive PTCA.[28] In another study, adjunctive PTCA was performed if the immediate post-DCA result was considered suboptimal (residual stenosis 10-50%, residual luminal irregularity); final diameter stenosis was 9%, which was similar to the 6% residual stenosis after DCA alone. Interestingly, although the incidence of major complications was similar, 6-month event-free survival was better in patients treated with adjunctive PTCA (81% vs. 52%, p<0.05).[56] Two prospective trials of optimal atherectomy are in progress or have just been completed (Table 28.10): In the Optimal Atherectomy Restenosis Study (OARS), 199 patients were prospectively treated with DCA, using ultrasound guidance and adjunctive PTCA if necessary. Findings include a final diameter stenosis of 7% (adjunctive PTCA was used in 89%), major complications in 2.5%,[4] and perforation in 0.9%;[100] similar results were reported in the pilot phase of the Balloon vs. Optimal Atherectomy Trial (BOAT),[8,9] which did not use ultrasound guidance (Table 28.11).

2. **Angiographic Complications (Table 28.7).** In general, the overall incidence of angiographic complications after DCA is probably similar to that after PTCA.[12,19-58]

    a. **Dissection and Abrupt Closure.** Nonocclusive dissection and severe dissection leading to abrupt closure occur in 20%[29] and 0-7% of cases, respectively (Tables 28.7 and 28.9). In CAVEAT-II and CCAT, the incidence of abrupt closure after DCA and PTCA were similar (Table 9). In CAVEAT-I, abrupt closure was more common after DCA (8% vs. 3.8%, p = 0.005) and occurred at a site *other* than the target lesion in 42% (from guide catheter or nosecone trauma).[98] Finally, reports from the NACI Registry[99] and OARS[100] indicated abrupt closure rates of only 1.3% and 1%, respectively. Whereas the principal mechanism of abrupt closure after PTCA is dissection, vessel thrombosis is more often the cause after DCA. In the U.S. Directional Atherectomy Registry of 1020 procedures, abrupt closure was caused by thrombosis in 51%, dissection in 30%, guide catheter-induced in 9% (all in RCA), and was indeterminate in 9%. Treatment of abrupt closure included immediate CABG without PTCA (21%), attempted PTCA (74%), and medical therapy without further revascularization (5%). Salvage PTCA for abrupt closure was successful in 50%.[25] Dissection may be caused by the guiding catheter (particularly for the RCA), the guidewire, and the atherectomy device itself (from the cutting mechanism, integrated balloon, or nosecone). Guiding catheter-induced injury can be reduced by avoiding over rotation and "deep-seating."

    b. **Thrombosis.** Although angiography is often insensitive for detecting thrombus, local thrombosis is felt to complicate approximately 2% of DCA procedures, and may account for ≥50% of acute vessel closures after DCA.[25,57] Treatment includes PTCA and thrombolytic agents (local drug delivery, intracoronary, or intravenous), or CABG for refractory cases (Chapter 9).

    c. **Distal Embolization and No-Reflow.** Distal embolization causing abrupt cutoff of the target vessel beyond the original target lesion has been reported in 0-13.4% of DCA procedures (Tables 28.7, 28.9). This type of macroembolization is usually due to dislodgement of thrombus or friable plaque from the target vessel, or less often, from release or incomplete capture of tissue stored in the nosecone collection chamber. Distal embolization occurs more often after DCA in vein grafts than in native vessels, probably due to the frequent presence of loose friable atherothrombotic debris in vein grafts. Treatment includes disruption or dissolution of the embolus with a guidewire, balloon, or thrombolytic therapy; emergency CABG is usually reserved for refractory cases if clinically indicated. In contrast to distal embolization of the epicardial vessels, no-reflow may be secondary to embolization and/or spasm of the coronary microvasculature. Like distal embolization, no-reflow is more frequent after DCA (and other percutaneous interventions) in vein grafts or in lesions with thrombus. Intracoronary calcium antagonists are the most effective form of therapy, whereas nitrates, thrombolytic agents, and CABG are usually ineffective in restoring flow (Chapter 21).

Table 28.7. Angiographic Complications after DCA

Series	N (lesions)	Vessel	Complications (%)			
			AC	DE No-reflow	Branch Occlusion	Perforation
Stephan[30] (1995)	160	N, SVG	4.0	4.0	-	-
Fortuna[11] (1995)	396	N, SVG	3.6	-	-	-
Umans[12] (1994)	150	N	1.3	0	0.7	0
Popma[13] (1993)	306	N, SVG	2.3	1.3	0.7	0.3
Cowley[14] (1993)	318	SVG	1.9	7.2	0.3	0.6
Baim[15] (1993)	1032	N, SVG	3.9	1.8	3.8	0.6
Pomerantz[25] (1992)	35	SVG	0	2.9	0	0
Fishman[31] (1992)	225	N, SVG	3.2	0	3.7	0.5
Popma[18] (1992)	1140	N, SVG	4.2	-	-	0.6
Garratt[19] (1992)	165	N, SVG	-	2.0	1.0	-
Hinohara[21] (1991)	382	N, SVG	3.7	2.1	2.6	0.8
Rowe[22] (1990)	91	N	2.2	-	7.7	-
Safian[4] (1990)	76	N, SVG	1.5	1.5	1.5	0
Kaufmann[23] (1989)	50	N, SVG	4.0	4.0	2	0

Abbreviations: N = native vessel; SVG = saphenous vein graft; AC= abrupt closure; DE = distal embolization;
- not reported

d. **Vasospasm.** Severe epicardial vasospasm is an infrequent (< 2%) complication of DCA,[55,99] probably because most patients are routinely pretreated with parental nitrates at the time of intervention. Spasm may occur at the site of the original lesion, but more commonly occurs distal to the lesion, probably from nosecone vibration. Spasm generally responds readily to intracoronary nitroglycerin or gentle, low-pressure balloon inflations (Chapter 19).

e. **Perforation.** Coronary artery perforation is an important complication because of its associated morbidity and mortality (Chapter 22). The incidence of perforation after DCA is < 1% (Tables 28.7, 28.11), which is probably lower than other devices that ablate or remove plaque (TEC, ROTA, ELCA), but higher than the 0.2% incidence after PTCA. Some perforations occur when DCA is used to reverse abrupt closure by excising flow-limiting dissection; vessel perforation can be minimized in this situation by use of an undersized device and low-pressure (10 psi) atherectomy (Chapter 20).[59] Treatment is identical to perforation of any cause including prolonged balloon inflations, and pericardiocentesis (Chapter 22). Contained perforations treated without surgery may lead to focal ectasia, pseudoaneursym, and restenosis.[60]

f. **Sidebranch Occlusion.** The overall incidence of significant sidebranch occlusion after DCA is 0.7-7.7% (Table 28.7). However, among true bifurcation lesions, sidebranch narrowing or occlusion may occur in up to 37%. Fortunately, most cases can be managed by PTCA; for suitable vessels (diameter ≥ 3mm without severe lesion angulation), DCA can be used to salvage the sidebranch.[61] Risk factors for sidebranch occlusion are similar to PTCA and include origin of the sidebranch from the target lesion and baseline narrowing of the sidebranch origin.[62]

3. **Clinical Complications (Tables 28.5, 28.6, 28.8, 28.9, 28.11).** Abrupt closure is the most common cause of clinical complications after DCA (and other devices). In one report, abrupt closure was associated with a 16-fold increase in mortality and a 23-fold increase in MI.[25]

   a. **Major Clinical Complications.** The incidence of death, MI, or emergency CABG after DCA is 0-10% and similar to other devices. In one report, indications for emergency CABG included obstructive complications at the target lesion (57%), perforation (9%), guiding catheter injury (13%), device-related complications (8%), and complications related to adjunctive PTCA (11%).[57]

   b. **Non-Q-Wave MI.** In most observational studies of DCA, the reported incidence of non-Q-wave MI is 3-12.5% (Tables 28.5, 28.8, 28.9). In CAVEAT-I, but not in CCAT or CAVEAT-II, there was a higher incidence of non-Q-wave MI after DCA compared to PTCA. Risk factors for CK-MB elevation include high-risk patients, de novo lesions, and complex lesion morphology.[63] The clinical significance of non-Q-wave MI in the absence of other signs of ischemia is uncertain; while some studies suggest an adverse prognosis,[64] others do not.[65] Patients with high CK-MB levels (i.e., > 50 IU/L) appear to be at risk for adverse clinical outcome at 2 years.[65] Results from the EPIC trial suggest that the risk of non-Q-MI can be reduced by c7E3, invoking a platelet-dependent mechanism.[66] The CK-MB ratio may be useful for identifying clinically significant enzyme elevations.[67]

Table 28.8. DCA for Special Situations

Series	Situation	N	Success (%)	D / QMI / CABG (%)	Comments
Bergelson[32] (1994)	Failed PTCA	16	100	0 / 0 / 0	Final DS (17%); Restenosis (17%) at 9 months
Harris[33] (1994)	Suboptimal PTCA	16	63	0 / 6.3 / 6.3	Final DS (41%), 21% if DCA success
McCluskey[34] (1993)	Suboptimal PTCA	103	91	2.0 / 6.0 / 6.0	Perforation (1%)
Movsowitz[35] (1993)	Failed PTCA	40	80	0 / 10 / 7.5	Procedural success (38%) for severe dissection; (88-100%) for focal dissection, elastic recoil, or thrombus.
Hofling[36] (1992)	Failed, Suboptimal PTCA	40	92	0 / 5 / 12.5	All MI due to SBO; All CABG had AC before DCA
Stephen[30] (1995)	Ostial	160	87	0 / 0 / 0.6	nQMI (9%); restenosis: (48%) de novo; (61%) restenotic; (93%) restenotic SVG
Popma[37] (1991)	Ostial (RCA)	7	86	0 / 0 / 0	Final DS (14%), ARS (14%)
Lewis[38] (1994)	Bifurcation lesions (2 wires)	30	97	0 / 0 / 3	nQMI (67%); SBO (37%)
Mooney[30] (1993)	Lesions > 10mm	88	97	0 / 1.0 / 1.0	AC (4.6%), Final DS (18%)
Laster[40] (1994)	Left main (protected)	25	88%	0 / 0 / 4.5	nQMI (4.5%); CRS (16%), EFS (89%) at 2 yrs
Dick[41] (1991)	Total occlusion	7	86	0 / 0 / 0	Final DS (32%); duration of occlusion 5-10 days
Baldwin[42] (1993)	MI	11	91	0 / - / 9	Adjunctive PTCA 73% (pre), UK (45%); AC (18%)
Emmi[43] (1993)	Thrombus	58	76	1.7 / 3.4 / 10.3	More CABG compared to lesions without clot (3.9%, p = 0.03); no difference in success or final outcome.

Abbreviations: D = death; N = # of lesions; QMI = Q-wave myocardial infarction; CABG = emergency coronary artery bypass surgery; SBO = sidebranch occlusion; AC = abrupt closure; DS = diameter stenosis; ARS = angiographic restenosis; CRS = clinical restenosis; EFS = event-free survival; UK = urokinase; AC = acute closure; - = not reported

c. **Vascular Injury (Tables 28.5, 28.6, 28.8).** The incidence of vascular injury requiring blood transfusion or vascular repair is approximately 1-5%. The incidence of any peripheral vascular complication in CAVEAT-I was 6.6% and was similar between PTCA and DCA groups.[68] Steps to minimize vascular complications are described in Chapter 25.

4. **Restenosis and Late Outcome.** Several observational studies have reported restenosis rates of 25-58% after DCA (Tables 28.5 and 28.6), but comparisons between studies are hindered by incomplete follow-up, different definitions, and different patient populations and target lesions. Three large multicenter randomized trials failed to demonstrate differences in restenosis between DCA and PTCA in native vessels (CAVEAT-I, CCAT) or in saphenous vein grafts (CAVEAT-II) (Table 28.9).[53-55] A comparative study of PTCA and DCA using matched lesions with similar baseline and immediate post-intervention results reported greater late loss of lumen diameter after DCA than PTCA (2.0 vs. 1.8mm, p = 0.001); these data support the use of optimal atherectomy to overcompensate for the greater late loss.[70] Using "optimal" atherectomy technique, restenosis was only 30% in OARS[100] (compared to 50% in CAVEAT-I). The major mechanism of restenosis after DCA is controversial: Data from OARS suggest that vascular remodeling accounts for 84% of late loss of lumen diameter after DCA;[72,73] however, IVUS studies suggest that intimal proliferation (not vascular remodeling) is the major mechanism of restenosis.[74] Drugs that show promise in reducing restenosis include tranilast[75] and ReoPro: In the EPIC trial, high-risk DCA patients (unstable angina, acute MI, high-risk lesion morphology) treated with bolus + infusion of ReoPro had lower 30-day and 6-month ischemic complication rates compared to placebo (Chapter 34).

In CAVEAT and CCAT, the need for target vessel revascularization and event-free survival at 6 months were similar. However, at 1-year, CAVEAT patients initially treated by DCA experienced more death (2.2% vs. 0.6 for PTCA, p < 0.05) and MI (8.9% vs. 4.4% for PTCA, p < 0.01).[69] The major criticism of these randomized studies was that optimal atherectomy technique was not routinely employed; longterm follow-up in OARS and BOAT will determine whether optimal atherectomy can reduce the excess deaths and myocardial infarctions seen in earlier trials.

5. **Correlates of Outcome**
   a. **Angiographic Results.** Lesion morphologies associated with lower procedural success include lesion calcification, lesion length > 10 mm, restenotic lesions, lesion angulation, proximal tortuosity, and thrombus. As the number of unfavorable Type B or C characteristics increases, DCA success decrease (B_1 success = 88%, B_2 success = 75%; C = 75%).[27] Of all lesion morphologies, heavy calcification is the most powerful predictor of procedural failure; in one report, DCA was successful in only 52% of calcified lesions.[76]

   b. **Complications.** The development of angiographic complications was associated with operator experience (relative risk 6.6), treatment of a de novo lesion (relative risk 2.2), and lesion angulation (relative risk 2.7).[27]

Table 28.9. Results of Randomized Trials of PTCA vs. DCA

In-hospital (%)	CAVEAT-I [44]		CCAT [45]		CAVEAT-II [46]	
	PTCA (n=500)	DCA (n=512)	PTCA (n=136)	DCA (n=138)	PTCA (n=156)	DCA (n=149)
Final DS	36	29	33	25**	38	32**
Success	76	82*	88	94+	79	89*
Abrupt closure	3	7	5.1	4.3	2.6	4.7
Death, QMI, CABG	4.4	5	4.4	2.1	5.7	4.7
Any MI	8	19**	3.7	4.3	11.5	17.4
Distal embolization	-	-	-	-	5.1	13.4*
Follow-up (6 months) (%)						
Final DS $\geq$ 50%	57	50	4.3	46	46	51
TLR	37.2	36.5	26.4	28.3	26	19
EFS	63	60	71	71	56	60

Abbreviations: CAVEAT = Coronary Angioplasty Versus Excisional Atherectomy Trial (I = native vessels; II = saphenous vein grafts); CCAT = Canadian Coronary Atherectomy Trial (LAD only); DS = diameter stenosis; QMI = Q-wave myocardial infarction; CABG = emergency coronary artery bypass surgery; TLR = target lesion revascularization; EFS = event-free survival; N = number of patients; - = not reported
* $p < 0.05$
+ $p = 0.06$
** $p < 0.01$

c.   **Restenosis.**   Several observational studies reported different predictors of restenosis; these differences are secondary to differences in patient population, lesion morphology, and definitions of restenosis. In these studies, risk factors included target lesion in a vein graft or the LAD, or hypertension, lesion length $\geq$ 10 mm, vessel diameter < 3 mm, use of a 6F device, final lumen diameter < 3 mm, cholesterol > 200 mg%, and diabetes.[21,37,77,78] In CAVEAT, the most important determinant of 6-month lumen diameter was the final lumen diameter after intervention; less important determinants included reference vessel diameter, a history of diabetes, and target lesion in the proximal LAD.[53] In CCAT, the only predictor of 6-month restenosis was the presence of unstable angina before intervention.[54]

Table 28.10. Multicenter Trials of DCA in Native Coronary Arteries

	CAVEAT-I[44]	CCAT[45]	OARS[2]	BOAT[3]
N (pts)	1012	548	200	1000
Year[a]	1993	1993	1995	1995
# Cases/Operator[b]	50	-	> 200	> 200
Qualify[c]	No	No	Yes	Yes
AtheroCath[d]	Suryln, EX	Surlyn, EX	EX, GTO	EX, GTO
PTCA[e]	No	No	Yes	Yes
IVUS[f]	No	No	Yes	No
Goal (final DS %)[g]	< 50	< 50	< 15	< 15

Abbreviations: CAVEAT-I = Coronary Angioplasty Versus Excisional Atherectomy Trial (native vessels); CCAT = Canadian Coronary Atherectomy Trial (LAD); OARS = Optimal Atherectomy Restenosis Study;
BOAT = Balloon vs. Optimal Atherectomy Trial; - not reported
[a]　Year of primary publication
[b]　Co-investigators had to perform a minimum number of DCA cases
[c]　Co-investigators had to submit angiograms to Core Lab to document their ability to achieve good results
[d]　Type of AtheroCaths used during study period
[e]　Use of adjunctive PTCA: No = not permitted; Yes = permitted
[f]　Routine use of IVUS
[g]　Co-investigators attempted to achieve a predefined target diameter stenosis

F.　SPECIAL CONSIDERATIONS

1.　**Deep Tissue Resection.** Deep wall components (media and advential) can be identified in up to 2/3 of DCA cases.[12,79] Although immediate post-procedure lumen diameter is an important determinant of restenosis and is the central theme of the "bigger-is-better" hypothesis,[80] there is concern among some interventionalists that achieving large lumen diameters by partial excision of plaque and deep vessel wall components may increase the risk of perforation, restenosis, and aneurysm formation.[81] Although perforation is slightly more frequent after DCA than PTCA, there does not appear to be any relationship between retrieval of deep wall components and perforation. The issue of restenosis is more controversial: one study in 52 patients with prior restenosis or vein graft lesions suggested a higher incidence of restenosis if deep wall components were recovered,[81] while another study in 374 lesions found no such correlation.[82] Finally, no relationship was observed between deep tissue resection and the late development of coronary aneurysms.[83]

Table 28.11. Optimal Atherectomy Trials

	OARS[*4,5]	BOAT PILOT[**8,9]
No. Lesions	218	192
Procedure Success (%)	97	96
Adjunctive PTCA (%)	89	67
Final DS (%)	8	10
Complications (%)		
Death	0	0.5
nQMI/QMI	11 / 1.5	17 / 1.6
CABG	1.0	1.0
Perforation	0.5	0.5
Angiographic restenosis	30.3	-

Abbreviations: DS = diameter stenosis; nQMI = non-Q-wave myocardial infarction; CABG = emergency coronary artery bypass surgery, - = Not reported
* OARS = Optimal Atherectomy Restenosis Study
** BOAT = Balloon versus Optimal Atherectomy Trial

2. **Unstable Angina.** The use of DCA for patients with unstable ischemic syndromes is controversial. In many early observational studies, high procedural success and low complication rates were achieved, despite inclusion of many patients with unstable angina. However, other reports indicate that 2-year event-free survival may be lower in patients with unstable angina (54% vs. 69% for stable angina, $p < 0.02$).[20,84]

3. **Acute MI.** The results of DCA after recent MI are less favorable than those in patients without previous infarction, primarily due to a higher incidence of dissection (7.1% vs. 2.8%, $p < 0.05$) and abrupt closure (4.7% vs. 1.2%, $p < 0.05$).[85] Other studies reported more angiographic[85] and major ischemic complications after recent MI (9.7% vs. 2.6%, $p < 0.01$) despite overall procedural success rates of 92-97%.

4. **Elderly.** While there may be a higher incidence of major complications (4.2-10.9%), procedural failure (3.3-13.8%), and need for blood transfusion (3.3-17%) in the elderly,[8] final diameter stenosis (18-22%), abrupt closure (0.8-4.9%), perforation (0-0.8%), and stroke (0-2.4%) appear to be unrelated to age.[88]

G. LESION-SPECIFIC APPLICATIONS

1. **Ostial Lesions (Table 28.8).** Percutaneous intervention on ostial lesions is frequently limited by lesion rigidity and elastic recoil, leading to suboptimal results. For noncalcified ostial lesions in vessels ≥3mm, DCA is associated with procedural success in 86-87% and major complications in <1% of patients.[36,46] Although immediate angiographic results in highly selected lesions are excellent, DCA of ostial lesions is limited by a high incidence of restenosis (48% in de novo lesions, 61% in restenotic lesions, and 93% in restenotic vein graft lesions).[36]

2. **Bifurcation Lesions (Table 28.8).** Percutaneous intervention on bifurcation lesions is sometimes complicated by "shifting plaque," leading to "snow-plow" injury, sidebranch occlusion, or suboptimal results. As with PTCA, the risk of sidebranch occlusion with DCA is greatest when the sidebranch originates from the target lesion and when the origin of the branch is stenotic. The approach to atherectomy of bifurcations includes DCA of the main vessel followed by sequential PTCA or DCA of the branch, depending on vessel size, calcification, and angulation. In some cases, a double guidewire technique can be used; nitinol guidewires are resistant to injury after DCA an can be used to protect sidebranches during atherectomy of the main vessel.[45] In highly selected cases, procedural success has been reported in 97-100% with major complications in 0-3% (Figure 28.5).[43,44,47] In these studies, transient sidebranch occlusion occurred in 37% but was successfully retrieved in most patients by PTCA or DCA; final diameter stenosis was 6-12% in the main vessel and 0-17% in the branch. In CAVEAT-I, DCA of bifurcation lesions was associated with higher success (88% vs. 74%, $p < 0.001$), more ischemic complications (9.5% vs. 3.7%, $p < 0.01$), and less restenosis (50% vs. 61%, $p < 0.001$) compared to PTCA.[90]

3. **Thrombus-Containing Lesions.** DCA should not be used in vessels that contain a large clot burden (i.e., thrombus length ≥ vessel diameter) due to the risk of acute closure. When a lesser amount of clot is present, DCA (± adjunctive intracoronary lytic therapy) may be performed with high success and low complication rates.[27] In one study, the presence of thrombus was associated with a higher incidence of emergency CABG, but no difference in success or other complications compared to lesions without thrombus.[52] In another series, the presence of a "complex, probable thrombus-containing" lesion was actually predictive of *higher DCA success*,[27] although vessels with a large clot burden were generally not treated by DCA. Intracoronary thrombolytic therapy (Chapter 5) and prolonged (12-48 hours) post-procedural heparin infusions are frequently employed in this setting.

4. **Saphenous Vein Grafts.** For focal lesions in nondegenerated vein grafts, numerous observational studies report procedural success in 86-96% and major complications in 0-7% (Table 28.6). Although one study reported angiographic restenosis in 25%,[32] another reported restenosis in 57%, including 38% for de novo lesions and 75% for restenotic lesions.[31] In the CAVEAT-II study, DCA resulted in better lumen enlargement and higher procedural success, but no difference in angiographic restenosis, target lesion revascularization, or event-free survival compared to PTCA (Table 28.9).[55]

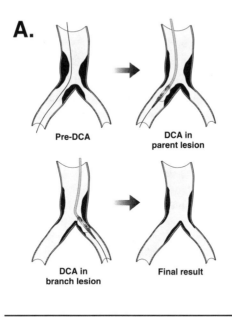

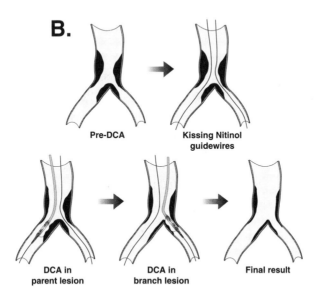

Figure 28.5 Bifurcation Lesions: DCA Techniques

A.   Sequential guidewires and sequential DCA.
B.   Kissing nitinol guidewires and sequential DCA.

5. **Left Main Disease.** Stenoses in the left main coronary artery are well-suited for DCA because of their proximal location and large vessel caliber. In one study of protected left main lesions, procedural success was 88% and emergency CABG was required in 4.5%.[49]

6. **Suboptimal PTCA (Table 28.8).** DCA may be applied to lesions after suboptimal PTCA due to dissection, thrombus, elastic recoil, or abrupt closure. In highly selected focal lesions in large vessels, DCA success has ranged from 63-92%, with death, Q-wave MI, and emergency CABG reported in 0-2%, 0-6.3%, and 0-12.5% of patients, respectively.[38-42,56] Because of the risk of perforation, DCA should not be used to excise spiral dissections, deep dissections extending beyond the lumen into the vessel wall, long dissections ($\geq$ 10 mm), or dissections in vessels < 3 mm. When used to excise focal dissections after PTCA, undersized devices and low inflation pressures are recommended. Although DCA can treat failed PTCA, stents have become the preferred salvage modality (Chapter 20).

7. **Restenotic Lesions.** In a recent study of 1087 patients with restenotic lesions, procedural success was 94-96% for conventional PTCA, DCA, and Palmaz-Schatz stenting. Although DCA and stents resulted in significantly better immediate lumen enlargement compared to PTCA, the incidence of major in-hospital complications, 6-month cardiac events (clinical restenosis), and 3-year event free survival were similar for all 3 devices.[91] For restenotic ostial lesions, recurrent restenosis after DCA was 61% in native vessels and 93% in vein grafts.[35]

8. **Stent Restenosis.** Although DCA has been used to treat in-stent restenosis,[89] there are no data to suggest superiority over conventional PTCA. In fact, there have been several instances of partial excision of stent struts and complete extraction of stent coils. Histologic studies of DCA for in-stent restenosis confirm a high incidence of intimal hyperplasia, virtually identical to that observed after restenosis following other interventions.

H. **TISSUE ANALYSIS.** The application of DCA to patients with peripheral vascular and coronary artery disease has provided the first opportunity for sampling of atherosclerotic vascular tissue from living patients. The availability of such tissue has led to several interesting observations, which may have important implications for further understanding and treatment of atherosclerosis:
- De novo lesions frequently consist of fibrosis, necrotic debris, foam cells, cholesterol, and calcium are typical findings of atherosclerosis.

- In 20% of de novo lesions, intimal proliferation is evident and is indistinguishable from similar cellular proliferation in restenotic lesions.[92] Thus, intimal proliferation is not specific for restenosis, but is a nonspecific response to injury. Such injury may be due to spontaneous events (plaque rupture), to interventional devices, or to other causes.

- Immunohistochemical studies confirm that proliferative tissue consists primarily of cells of smooth muscle cell origin.

- There is a higher prevalence of mural thrombus and plaque hemorrhage in unstable compared to stable angina (22% vs. 2% in one study; 44% vs. 17% in another); this is lower than the prevalence of thrombus in angiographic studies, but similar to that of necropsy studies.[92,93]

- Intimal hyperplasia is observed in 93% of restenotic lesions and in 44% of de novo lesions.[94] Intimal hyperplasia in de novo lesions was associated with younger age and lesions in the LAD, and was not associated with higher rates of restenosis than de novo lesions without intimal hyperplasia.

- There is a higher prevalence of thrombus and inflammatory cells as the severity of the acute ischemic syndrome increases from stable angina, to crescendo angina, to rest angina, to acute MI.[95,96]

- Human tissue factor, a crucial activator of blood coagulation and intimal proliferation, is detectable in 43% of patients with unstable coronary syndromes and only 12% of patients with stable coronary syndromes.[97]

* * * * *

REFERENCES

1. Topol E, Califf R, Weisman H, et al. Randomized trial of coronary intervention with antibody against platelet IIb/IIIa integrine for reduction of clinical restenosis: results at six months. Lancet 1994;343:881-886.

2. Mintz GS, Pichard AD, Kent KM, Kovach JA, Popma JJ, Satler LF, Leon MB. Transcatheter device synergy: Preliminary experience with adjunct directional coronary atherectomy following high-speed rotational atherectomy or excimer laser angioplasty in the treatment of coronary artery disease. Cathet Cardiovasc Diagn 1993;Suppl 1:37-44.

3. Dussaillant GR, Griffin J, Weaver TK, Deible RA, Pichard AD. Transcatheter device synergy: Intravascular ultrasound assessment of rotational atherectomy followed by adjunct directional coronary atherectomy in the treatment of calcified coronary artery disease. Circulation 1995;92:I-329.

4. Leon M, Kuntz R, Popma J, et al. Acute angiographic, intravascular ultrasound and clinical results of directional atherectomy in the optimal atherectomy restenosis study. J Am Coll Cardiol 1995;25:137A.

5. Simonton CA, Leon MB, Kuntz RE, et al. Acute and late clinical and angiographic results of directional atherectomy in the optimal atherectomy restenosis study (OARS). Circulation 1995;92:I-545.

6. Doi T, Tamai H, Ueda K, Hsu YS, Ono S, et al. Impact of intracoronary ultrasound-guided directional atherectomy on restenosis. Circulation 1995;92:I-545.

7. Bauman RP, Yock PG, Fitzgerald PJ, Annex BH, et al. "Reference Cut" method of intracoronary ultrasound guided directional coronary atherectomy: Initial and six month results. Circulation 1995;92:I-546.

8. Baim D, Kuntz R, Popma J, Leon M. Results of directional atherectomy in the "Pilot" phase of BOAT. Circulation 1994;90:I-214.

9. Baim DS, Kuntz RE, Sharma SK, Fortuna R, Feldman R, et al. Acute results of the randomized phase of the balloon versus optimal atherectomy trial (BOAT). Circulation 1995;92:I-544.

10. Mintz GS, Pichard AD, Dussaillant GR, Satler LF, Wong SC, Walsh CL, et al. Acute results of adjunct stents following directional coronary atherectomy. Circulation 1995;92:I-326.

11. Waksman R, Weintraub WS, Ghazzal ZMB, Douglas JS, et al. Directional coronary atherectomy (DCA): Is much bigger much better? Circulation 1995;92:I-329.

12. Safian R, Gelbfish J, Erny R, Schnitt S, Schmidt D, Baim D. Coronary atherectomy. Clinical, angiographic, and histological findings and observations regarding potential mechanisms. Circulation 1990;82:69-79.

13. Baim D, Kuntz R. Directional coronary atherectomy: How much lumen enlargement is optional? Am J Cardiol 1993;72:65E-70E.

14. Penny W, Schmidt D, Safian R, Erny R, Baim D. Insights into the Mechanism of Luminal Improvement After Directional Coronary Atherectomy. Am J Cardiol 1991;67:435-437.

15. Matar F, Mintz G, Farb A, Douek P. The contribution of tissue removal to lumen improvement after directional coronary atherectomy. Am J Cardiol 1994;74:647-650.

16. Tenaglia AN, Buller CE, Kisslo KB, Stack RS. Mechanisms of balloon angioplasty and directional coronary atherectomy as assessed by intracoronary ultrasound. J Am Coll Cardiol 1992;20:685-691.

17. Braden G, Herrington D, Downes T, et al. Qualitative and quantitative contrasts in the mechanisms of lumen enlargement by coronary balloon angioplasty and directional coronary atherectomy. J Am Coll Cardiol 1994;23:40-48.

18. Umans V, Baptisla J, di Mario C, et al. Angiographic, ultrasound, and angioscopic assessment of the coronary artery wall and lumen area configuration after directional atherectomy: The mechanism revisited. Am Heart J 1995;130:217-227.

19. Fortuna R, Walston D, Hansell H, Schulz G. Directional coronary atherectomy: Experience in 310 patients. J Invas Cardiol 1995;7:57-64.

20. Umans V, de Feyter P, Deckers J, et al. Acute and long-term outcome of directional coronary atherectomy for stable and unstable angina. Am J Cardiol 1993;74:641-646.

21. Popma J, Mintz G, Satler L, et al. Clinical and angiographic outcome after directional coronary atherectomy: A qualitative and quantitative analysis using coronary arteriography and intravascular ultrasound. Am J Cardiol

1993;72:55E-64E.

22. Cowley M, DiSciascio G. Experience with directional coronary atherectomy since pre-market approval. Am J Cardiol 1993;72:12E-20E.

23. Baim D, Tomoaki H, Holmes D, et al. Results of directional coronary atherectomy during multicenter preapproval testing. Am J Cardiol 1993;72:6E-11E.

24. Feld H, Schulhoff N, Lichstein E, et al. Coronary atherectomy versus angioplasty: The CAVA study. Am Heart J 1993;126:31-38.

25. Popma J, Topol E, Hinohara T, et al. Abrupt vessel closure after directional coronary atherectomy. J Am Coll Cardiol 1992;19:1372-1379.

26. Garratt K, Holmes D, Bell M, et al. Results of directional atherectomy of primary atheromatous and restenosis lesions in coronary arteries and saphenous vein grafts. Am J Cardiol 1992;70:449-454.

27. Ellis S, DeCesare N, Pinkerton C, Whitlow P. Relation of stenosis morphology and clinical presentation to the procedural results of directional coronary atherectomy. Circulation 1991;84:644-653.

28. Hinohara T, Rowe MH, Robertson GC, et al. Effect of lesion characteristics on outcome of directional coronary atherectomy. J Am Coll Cardiol 1991;17:1112-20.

29. Rowe MH, Hinohara T, White NW, Robertson GC. Comparison of dissection rates and angiographic results following directional coronary atherectomy and coronary angioplasty. Am J Cardiol 1990;66:49-53.

30. Kaufmann UP, Garratt KN, Vlietstra RE, Menke KK. Coronary atherectomy: First 50 patients at the Mayo Clinic. Mayo Clin Proc 1989;64:747-752.

31. Cowley M, Whitlow P, Baim D, Hinohara T, et al. Directional coronary atherectomy of saphenous vein graft narrowings: Multicenter investigational experience. Am J Cardiol 1993;72:30E-34E.

32. Pomerantz R, Kuntz R, Carrozza J, et al. Acute and long-term outcome of narrowed saphenous venous grafts treated by endoluminal stenting and directional atherectomy. Am J Cardiol 1992;70:161-167.

32a. DiScasio G, Cowley MJ, Vetrovec GW, Goudreau E, et al. Directional coronary atherectomy of saphenous vein graft lesions unfavorable for balloon angioplasty: Results of a single center experience. Cathet Cardiovasc Diagn 1992;26:75.

33. Ghazzal ZMB, Douglas JS, Holmes DR, et al. Directional atherectomy of saphenous vein grafts: Recent multicenter experience. J Am Coll Cardiol 1991;17:219A.

34. Selmon MR, Hinohara T, Robertson GC, Rowe MH, et al. Directional coronary atherectomy for saphenous vein graft stenoses. J Am Coll Cardiol 1991;17:23A.

35. Kaufmann U, Garratt K, Vlietstra R, Holmes D. Transluminal atherectomy of saphenous vein aortocoronary bypass grafts. Am J Cardiol 1990;65:1430-1433.

36. Stephan W, Bates E, Garratt K, Hinohara T, Muller D. Directional atherectomy of coronary and saphenous vein graft ostial stenoses. Am J Cardiol 1995;75:1015-1018.

37. Fishman R, Kuntz R, Carrozza J, et al. Long-term results of directional coronary atherectomy: Predictors of restenosis. J Am Coll Cardiol 1992;20:1101-1110.

38. Bergelson B, Fishman R, Tomaso C, et al. Acute and long-term outcome of failed percutaneous transluminal coronary angioplasty treated by directional coronary atherectomy. Am J Cardiol 1994;73:1224-1226.

39. Harris W, Berger P, Holmes D, Garratt K. "Rescue" directional coronary atherectomy after unsuccessful percutaneous transluminal coronary angioplasty. Mayo Clin Proc 1994;69:717-722.

40. McCluskey E, Cowley M, Whitlow P. Multicenter clinical experience with rescue atherectomy for failed angioplasty. Am J Cardiol 1993;72:42E-46E.

41. Movsowitz H, Emmi R, Manginas A, et al. Directional coronary atherectomy for failed balloon angioplasty: Outcome depends on the Underlying pathology. Circulation 1993;88:I-601.

42. Hofling B, Gonschior P, Simpson L, Bauriedel G. Efficacy of directional coronary atherectomy in cases unsuitable for percutaneous transluminal coronary angioplasty (PTCA) and after unsuccessful PTCA. Am Heart J 1992;124:341-348.

43. Mansour M, Fishman RF, Kuntz RE, Carrozza JP. Feasibility of directional atherectomy for the treatment of bifurcation

lesions. Cor Art Dis 1992;3:761-765.

44. Eisenhauer AC, Clugston RA, Ruiz CE. Sequential directional atherectomy of coronary bifurcation lesions. Cathet Cardiovasc Diagn 1993;Suppl 1:54-60.

45. Groassman ED, Leya FS, Lewis BE, Johnson SA, et al. Examination of common PTCA guide wires used for side branch protection during directional coronary atherectomy of bifurcation lesions performed in vivo and in vitro. Cathet Cardiovasc Diagn 1993;1:48-53.

46. Popma JJ, Dick RJL, Haudenschild CC, Topol EJ, Ellis S. Atherectomy of right coronary ostial stenoses: Initial and long-term results, technical features and histologic findings. Am J Cardiol 1991;67:431-433.

47. Lewis B, Leya F, Johnson S, et al. Acute procedural results in the treatment of 30 coronary artery bifurcation lesions with a double-wire atherectomy technique for side-branch protection. Am Heart J 1994;127:1600-1607.

48. Mooney M, Mooney-Fishman J, Madison J, Nahhan A, Van Tassel R. Directional atherectomy for long lesions: Improved results. Cathet Cardiovasc Diagn 1993;1:26-30.

49. Laster S, Rutherford B, McConahay D, Giorgi L, Johnson W. Directional atherectomy of left main stenoses. Cathet Cardiovasc Diagn 1994;33:317-322.

50. Dick RJL, Haudenschild CC, Popma JJ, Ellis SG. Directional atherectomy for total coronary occlusions. Cor Art Dis 1991;2:189-199.

51. Baldwin TF, Lash RE, Whitfeld SS, Toalson WB. Directional coronary atherectomy in acute myocardial infarction. J Inv Cardiol 1993;5:288-294.

52. Emmi R, Movsoqitz H, Manginas A, et al. Directional coronary atherectomy in lesions with coexisting thrombus. Circulation 1993;88:3204.

53. Topol E, Leya F, Pinkerton C, et al. A comparison of directional atherectomy with coronary angioplasty in patients with coronary artery disease. N Engl J Med 1993;329:221-227.

54. Adelman A, Cohen E, Kimball B, et al. A comparison of directional atherectomy with balloon angioplasty for lesions of the left anterior descending coronary artery. N Engl J Med 1993;329:228-233.

55. Holmes D, Topol E, Califf R, et al. A multicenter, randomized trial of coronary angioplasty versus directional atherectomy for patients with saphenous vein bypass graft lesions. Circulation 1995;91:1966-1974.

56. Gordon P, Kugelmass A, Cohen D, et al. Balloon postdilation can safety improve the results of successful (but suboptimal) directional coronary atherectomy. Am J Cardiol 1993;72:71E-79E.

57. Carrozza J, Baim J. Complications of directional coronary atherectomy: Incidence, causes, and management. Am J Cardiol 1993;72:47E-54E.

58. Carrozza JP, Baim DS, Safian RD, et al. Risks and complications of coronary atherectomy. In: Atherectomy, eds. Holmes DR, Garratt KN; Blackwell Scientific Publication, 1992, p.132-148.

59. Van Suylen RJ, Serruys PW, Simpson JB, et al. Delayed rupture of right coronary artery after directional coronary atherectomy for bail-out. Am Heart J 1991;121:914-917.

60. Selmon MR, Robertson GC, Simpson JB, et al. Retrieval of media and adventitia by directional coronary atherectomy and angiographic correlation. Circulation 1990;82:III-624.

61. Safian R, Schreiber T, Baim D. Specific indications for directional coronary atherectomy: Origin left anterior descending coronary artery and bifurcating lesions. Am J Cardiol 1993;72:35E-41E.

62. Campos-Esteve M, Laird J, Kufs W, Wortham CD. Side-branch occlusion with directional coronary atherectomy: Incidence and risk factors. Am Heart J 1994;128:686-690.

64. Tauke JT, Kong TW, Meyers SN, et al. Prognostic value of creatinine kinase elevation following elective coronary artery interventions. J Am Coll Cardiol 1995;25:269A.

63. Hinohara T, Vetter JW, Robertson GC, Selmon MR, et al. CK MB elevation following directional coronary atherectomy. Circulation 1995;92:I-544.

65. Kugelmass AD, Cohen DJ, Moscucci M, et al. Elevation of the creatine kinase myocardial isoform following otherwise successful directional coronary atherectomy and stenting. Am J Cardiol 1994;74:748-754.

66. Lefkovits J, Anderson K, Weisman H, Topol E. Increased risk of non-Q MI following DCA: Evidence for a platelet

dependant mechanism from the EPIC Trial. Circulation 1994;90:I-214.

67. Cutlip DE, Ho KKL, Senerchia C, Baim DS, et al. Classification of myocardial infarction after directional coronary atherectomy and relation to clinical outcome: Results of the OARS trial. Circulation 1995;92:I-616.

68. Omoigui N, Califf R, Pieper K, et al. Peripheral vascular complications in the coronary angioplasty versus excisional atherectomy trial (CAVEAT-I). J Am Coll Cardiol 1995;26:922-930.

69. Elliott J, Berdan L, Holmes D, et al. One-year follow-up in the coronary angioplasty versus excisional atherectomy trial (CAVEAT I). Circulation 1995;91:2158-2166.

70. Umans V, Keane D, Foley D, Boersma E, et al. Optimal use of directional coronary atherectomy is required to ensure long-term angiographic benefit: A study with matched procedural outcome after atherectomy and angioplasty. J Am Coll Cardiol 1994;24:1652-1659.

71. Morris D, Weintraub W, Liberman H, Douglas J, King S. A case matched comparison of directional atherectomy to balloon angioplasty. Circulation 1993;88:3232.

76. Popma JJ, DeCesare NB, Ellis SG, Holmes DR. Clinical, angiographic and procedural correlates of quantitative coronary dimensions after directional coronary atherectomy. J Am Coll Cardiol 1991;18:1183-1189.

77. Umans V, Robert A, Foley D, et al. Clinical, histological and quantitative angiographic predictors pf restenosis after directional coronary atherectomy: A multivariate analysis of the renarrowing process and late outcome. J Am Coll Cardiol 1994;23:49-58.

78. Hinohara T, Robertson G, Selmon M, et al. Restenosis after directional coronary atherectomy. J Am Coll Cardiol 1992;20:623-632.

72. Mintz GS, Fitzgerald PJ, Kuntz RE, Simonton CA, et al. Lesion site and reference segment remodeling after directional coronary atherectomy: An analysis from the optimal atherectomy restenosis study. Circulation 1995;92:I-93.

74. Mitsuo K, Degawa T, Nakamura S, Ui K, et al. Serial intravascular ultrasound evaluation of the mechanism of restenosis after directional coronary atherectomy. Circulation 1995;92:I-149.

75. Kosuga K, Tamai H, Ueda K, Hsu YS, et al. Efficacy of tranilast on restenosis after directional coronary atherectomy (DCA). Circulation 1995;92:I-346.

73. Mintz GS, Kent KM, Satler LF, Wong SC, Hong MK, Griffin J, Pichard AD. Dimorphic mechanisms of restenosis after DCA and stents: A serial intravascular ultrasound study. Circulation 1995;92:I-546.

79. Garratt KN, Kaufmann UP, Edwards WD, Vlietsra RE. Safety of percutaneous coronary atherectomy with deep arterial resection. Am J Cardiol 1989;64:538-542.

80. Kuntz RE, Gibson MC, Nobuyoshi M, Baim DS. Generalized Model of Restenosis After Conventional Balloon Angioplasty, Stenting and Directional Atherectomy. J Am Coll Cardiol 1993;21:15-25.

81. Garratt K, Holmes D, Bell M, et al. Restenosis after directional coronary atherectomy: Differences between primary atheromatous and restenosis lesions and the influence of subintimal resection. J Am Coll Cardiol 1990;16:1665-1671.

82. Kuntz R, Hinohara T, Safian R, Selmon M, Simpson J, Baim D. Restenosis after directional coronary atherectomy. Effects of luminal diameter and deep wall excision. Circulation 1992;86:1394-1399.

83. Bell M, Garratt K, Bresnahan J, Edwards W, Holmes D. Relation of deep arterial resection and coronary artery aneurysms after directional coronary atherectomy. J Am Coll Cardiol 1992;20:1474-1481.

84. Abdelmeguid A, Ellis S, Sapp S, Simpfendrofer C. Directional coronary atherectomy in unstable angina. J Am Coll Cardiol 1994;24:46-54.

85. Ghazzal Z, Hinohara T, Scott N, et al. Directional coronary atherectomy in patients with recent myocardial infarction. A NACI Registry Report. J Am Coll Cardiol 1993;21:32A.

86. Robertson G, Hinohara T, Vetter J, et al. Directional coronary atherectomy for patients with recent myocardial infarction. J Am Coll Cardiol 1994;23:219A.

87. Poelnitz AV, Backa D, Bauriedel G, Nerlich A. Coronary directional atherectomy: Rescue for failed balloon angioplasty and treatment of complicated lesions. J Interven Cardiol 1991;4:5-11.

88. Movsowitz H, Manginas A, Emmi R, et al. Directional coronary atherectomy can be successfully performed in the

elderly. Am J Cardiol 1994;31:261-263.

89.   Strauss B, Umans V, van Suylen R-J, et al. Directional atherectomy for treatment of restenosis within coronary stents: Clinical, angiographic and histologic results. J Am Coll Cardiol 1992;20:1465-1473.

90.   Lewis B, Leya F, Johnson S, et al. Outcome of angioplasty (PTCA) and atherectomy (DCA) for bifurcation and non-bifurcation lesions in CAVEAT. Circulation 1993;88:I-601.

91.   Waksman R, Weintraub WS, Ziyad MB, Douglas JS, Shen Y, King SB. Balloon angioplasty, Palmaz-Schatz stent, and directional coronary atherectomy for restenotic lesions: Retrospective comparison in a single center. J Am Coll Cardiol 1995;25;330A.

92.   Escaned J, van Suylen R, MacLeod D, et al. Histologic characteristics of tissue excised during directional coronary atherectomy in stable and unstable angina pectoris. Am J Cardiol 1993;71:1442-1447.

93.   Rosenschein U, Ellis S, Haudenschild C, et al. Comparison of histopathologic coronary lesions obtained from directional atherectomy in stable angina versus acute coronary syndromes. Am J Cardiol 1994;73:508-510.

94.   Miller M, Kuntz R, Friedrich S, et al. Frequency and consequences of intimal hyperplasia in specimens retrieved by directional atherectomy of native primary coronary artery stenoses and subsequent restenoses. Am J Cardiol 1993;71:652-657.

95.   DiSciascio G, Cowley M, Goudreau E, Vetrovec G, Johnson D. Histopathologic correlates of unstable ischemic syndromes in patients undergoing directional coronary atherectomy: In vivo evidence of thrombosis, ulceration, and inflammation. Am Heart J 1994;128:419-26.

96.   Arbustini E, De Servi S, Bramucci E, et al. Comparison of coronary lesions obtained by directional coronary atherectomy in unstable angina, stable angina, and restenosis after either atherectomy or angioplasty. Am J Cardiol 1995;75:675-682.

97.   Annex B, Denning S, Channon K, et al. Differential expression of tissue factor protein in directional atherectomy specimens from patients with stable and unstable coronary syndromes. Circulation 1995;91:619-622.

98.   Holmes DR, Simpson JB, Berdan LG, et al. Abrupt closure: The CAVEAT I Experience. J Am Coll Cardiol 1995;26:1494-500.

99.   Mehta S, Popma J, Margolis JR, et al. Complications with new angioplasty devices. Are these device specific? J Am Coll Cardiol 1996;March Special Issue.

100. Popma JJ, Baim DS, Kuntz RE, Mintz GS, et al. Early and late quantitative angiographic outcomes in the Optimal Atherectomy Restenosis Study (OARS). J Am Coll Cardiol 1996;March Special Issue.

TRANSLUMINAL EXTRACTION ATHERECTOMY

29

Barry M. Kaplan, M.D.
Cindy L. Grines, M.D.
Robert D. Safian, M.D.

A. DESCRIPTION. The Transluminal Extraction Catheter (TEC) (InterVentional Technologies, Inc., San Diego, CA) is a percutaneous over-the-wire cutting and aspiration system that consists of a conical cutting head with two stainless steel blades attached to the distal end of a flexible hollow torque-tube (Figure 29.1). The proximal end of the catheter attaches to a battery-powered hand-held motor drive unit and to a vacuum bottle for aspiration of excised atheroma, thrombus and debris (Figure 29.2). A trigger on the bottom of the motor drive unit activates cutting blade rotation and aspiration, and a lever on top of the unit allows advancement/retraction of the cutter. During atherectomy, warmed (37°C) Lactated Ringers solution is infused under pressure to create a slurry of blood and tissue which facilitates aspiration. A special 0.014-inch stainless steel guide wire allows coaxial passage of the catheter and has a radiopaque floppy tip with a terminal 0.021" ball to prevent wire tip entrapment or advancement of the cutting blades beyond the guidewire (Figure 29.3). A large-bore rotating hemostatic valve contains a side arm for contrast injections and infusion of pressurized flush solution.

B. EQUIPMENT

1. **Cutters (Table 29.1).** TEC cutters for coronary application are available in sizes from 5.5-7.5 F (1.8-2.5 mm). The conical cutter head — fabricated from a cylindrical base of proprietary stainless

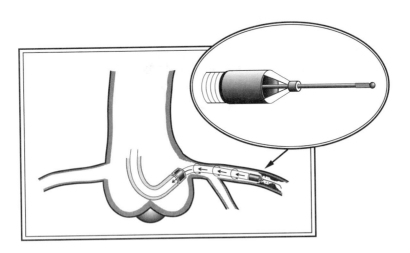

Figure 29.1 Transluminal Extraction Atherectomy (TEC)

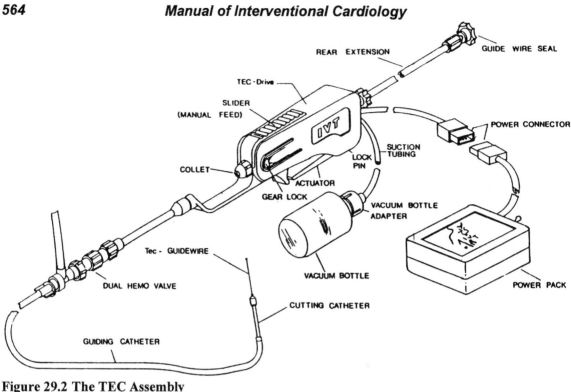

Figure 29.2 The TEC Assembly

steel — is bonded to the distal end of the catheter and contains microtome-sharp cutting edges that rotate at 750 rpm when the motor-drive is activated. The shaft of the cutter consists of a hollow inner-core through which excised material is aspirated and evacuated.

2. **Guiding Catheters (Table 29.2).** Special 10F tungsten-braided, soft-tip guiding catheters are available in the following sizes and tip configurations: JR 4.0; JL 3.5, 4.0, 5.0; modified Amplatz; hockey stick; multipurpose; and right bypass graft. 10F guides from other manufacturers can be used if necessary. For TEC cutters ≤ 6.5F (2.2mm), 9F guiding catheters may be used; the 8F giant lumen (ID = 0.086 inches) guide can only accommodate the 5.5F cutter. Pressure damping and poor contrast opacification are common when using guiding catheters < 10F.

C. **TECHNIQUE**
1. **Guiding Catheter Manipulation.** The TEC guiding catheters are stiffer than conventional angioplasty guides; overrotation and deep seating greatly increase the risk of vessel injury and should be avoided. During advancement of the TEC guide to the aortic root, blood loss can be minimized by tracking the guide over a 0.063-inch guidewire, or alternatively, over a 0.035-inch guidewire through a 6F multipurpose catheter.

2. **Hemostatic Valve.** A special rotating hemostatic valve (RHV), connects the TEC motor-drive

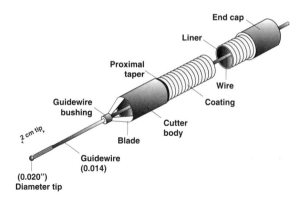

Figure 29.3 The TEC Cutter and Guidewire

handle to the guiding catheter. To minimize the risk of air embolism, it is extremely important to aspirate blood from the guiding catheter (once attached to the RHV), and to thoroughly flush all air from the RHV.

3. **Guidewires.** Because the stiff 300-cm stainless-steel TEC guidewire is less steerable than conventional PTCA guidewires, a conventional guidewire should be used to cross tortuous vessels or complex lesions. Once in position, the PTCA guidewire can be exchanged for the TEC guidewire using any suitable transport catheter that will accommodate the 0.021-inch ball. For simple anatomy, the TEC guidewire can be used as the primary wire, but a bare-wire technique must be employed (i.e., TEC wire advanced beyond the lesion without the TEC catheter). It is important to advance

Table 29.1. Cutters for TEC Atherectomy

Cutter Size (F)	Cutter Diameter (mm)	Vessel Diameter* (mm)	Guide ID** (inch)
5.5	1.8	2.5	0.086
6.0	2.0	2.75	0.092
6.5	2.17	3.0	0.092
7.0	2.33	3.25	0.104
7.5	2.5	3.5	0.104

*   Minimum vessel diameter to be used with TEC cutters
** Minimum guide catheter internal diameter

the floppy, radiopaque portion of the wire well beyond the lesion to ensure that atherectomy is performed along the stiff, radiolucent segment. Due to the stiffness of the TEC guidewire, pseudolesions are common but generally resolve after removal of the guidewire.

4. **Cutter Deployment.** Ideal cutter selection criteria have not been identified. We prefer to undersize the cutter by at least 1mm in relation to the distal reference segment (i.e., cutter-to-artery ratio of 0.5-0.7). In diffusely diseased vessels, subtotal stenoses, angulated lesions, or vessels < 3 mm, our bias is to use a 5.5F cutter followed by definitive lumen enlargement with adjunctive PTCA or stenting. While step-by-step instruction and lesion-specific techniques are detailed in the Device Guide, several important principles deserve emphasis here:

- The TEC cutter must be activated proximal to the lesion; activation within the lesion increases the risk of distal embolization and dissection and should be avoided.

- The cutter should be advanced slowly (10 mm/30 seconds) through the lesion to achieve a continuous stream of blood entering the vacuum bottle. Never advance a rotating cutter in the absence of flow into the vacuum bottle due to the risk of dissection and distal embolization. If blood does not flow into the vacuum bottle, determine if the vacuum has been lost, and change bottles. Adequate removal of thrombus and atheroma usually requires the filling of 5-10 vacuum bottles.

Table 29.2. Guiding Catheters for TEC Atherectomy

Target Vessel	Configuration	Guiding Catheter
RCA	Normal	JR 4
	Anterior origin	Mod.-Amplatz, Hockey Stick
	Horizontal origin	Hockey Stick
	Superior origin; Shepherd Cook	Hockey Stick, RBG
	Inferior origin	JR 4, Multipurpose
LCA	Normal	JL 4.0
	Narrow root or superior origin	JL 3.5
	Wide root or posterior origin	JL 3.0
SVG to LCA	Normal	JR 4
	Superior origin	Mod.-Amplatz, Hockey Stick
		Mod.-Amplatz, RBG
SVG to RCA	Normal	Mod.-Amplatz, Multipurpose, RBG
	Horizontal origin	JR 4, Hockey Stick, Mod.-Amplatz

Abbreviations: JR = right Judkins; JL = left Judkins; Mod.-Amplatz = modified Amplatz; RBG = right bypass graft; RCA = right coronary artery; LCA = left coronary artery; SVG = saphenous vein graft

- The cutter should not be activated in the guiding catheter or in nondiseased segments, particularly when traversing a bend.

- Be sure the pressurized flush is turned on while cutting, and turned off between cutter passes.

- After completing 2-5 slow passes through the lesion, the TEC cutter should be retracted and the lesion reassess. If a filling defect persists and there is no evidence for dissection, a larger TEC cutter may be used. If there is significant residual stenosis but no residual filling defect, adjunctive PTCA, DCA, or stenting should be performed.

5. **Adjunctive Medical Treatment.** Medications are the same as those prescribed for PTCA: All patients should receive aspirin ($\geq$ 325 mg/d at least 1 day prior to the procedure), heparin (to achieve and maintain an ACT $\geq$ 300 seconds during the case), and intracoronary nitroglycerin (100-200 mcg just prior to cutting to attenuate spasm). In addition, intracoronary verapamil (100 mcg/min up to 1-1.5 mg), intracoronary urokinase (250,000-500,000 units over 5-30 min), and IV ReoPro (Chapter 34) may be of value for no-reflow, intraluminal thrombus, and high-risk angioplasty, respectively.

6. **Adjunctive Intervention.** If a suboptimal result is obtained, the TEC cutter may be exchanged for a larger cutter, PTCA balloon, or stent; the rotating hemostatic valve, TEC guidewire, and guiding catheter are compatible with all coronary stents and articulated biliary stents, angioscopy, and intravascular ultrasound.

D. **MECHANISM OF ACTION.** Angioscopy studies demonstrate partial or complete thrombus removal in 75-100% of thrombotic lesions after TEC;[1,2] dissection, however, has been noted in virtually all cases by angioscopy[1,2] (including occlusive dissections in 75% in one report)[3] and in 36% of cases by IVUS.[4] Although gross examination of aspirated material sometimes demonstrates yellowish debris, histologic studies have failed to reveal evidence for tissue removal. It is likely that a "Dotter" effect contributes to angiographic improvement after TEC.[5]

E. **RESULTS**
1. **Native Coronary Arteries (Table 29.3)**
   a. **Immediate Results.** Procedural success in native coronary arteries has been achieved in 84-94%, [6,7] although adjunctive PTCA was required in 79-84% of lesions to enlarge lumen dimensions (72%), salvage technical failures (1%), or manage TEC-induced vessel occlusion (11%).[7] In one study, quantitative angiography revealed a residual diameter stenosis of 61% after TEC and 36% after adjunctive PTCA. The extent of elastic recoil after TEC was approximately 30%, similar to conventional PTCA.[8]

Table 29.3. In-hospital Results of TEC Atherectomy in Native Coronary Arteries

	IVT[6] (1995)	Safian[7] (1994)
No. lesions	783	181
Adjunctive PTCA (%)	79	84
Success (%)	94	84
Complications (%)		
MI	0.6	3.4
Death	1.4	2.3
Acute closure	8.0	11.0
Distal embolization	1.6	0.5
No-reflow	0	0

    b.   **Clinical Complications.** Major in-hospital complications after TEC include death (1.4-2.3%), emergency CABG (2.6-3.4%), and Q-wave MI (0.6-3.4%).[6,7] In one report, abrupt closure immediately after TEC — regardless of whether or not it was reversed by adjunctive PTCA — was the strongest independent correlate of major clinical complications.[7]

    c.   **Angiographic Complications.** Angiographic evidence for dissection was reported in 39% after TEC, but in only 6.6% lesions after adjunctive PTCA.[7] Abrupt closure was observed in 8-11%, coronary artery perforation in 0.7-2.2%, distal embolization in 0.5-1.6%, and sidebranch occlusion in 2.7%.[6,7]

    d.   **Follow-up.** Angiographic restenosis (> 50% stenosis) has been reported to occur in 56-61% of native vessels treated by TEC,[6,7] and was not affected by the use of adjunctive PTCA. Clinical restenosis (the need for target vessel revascularization, MI, or death) occurred in 29% of patients.[7] In a study on 26 patients who underwent angiography 1 day, 3 months and 6 months after TEC, elastic recoil at 1 day was shown to contribute to early restenosis.[9]

2.   **Saphenous Vein Grafts (Table 29.4)**
    a.   **Immediate Results.** For vein graft lesions treated with TEC, procedural success rates were 82-92%;[4,6,10-12] adjunctive PTCA was required in 74-95% of lesions. In the multicenter TEC registry, procedural success was 90% in thrombotic lesions, 97% in ulcerated lesions, and 97% in grafts > 3 years old.[6]

    b.   **Clinical Complications.** Major clinical complications after vein graft TEC include death in 0-10.3%, MI in 0.7-3.7%, and CABG in 0.2%.[4,6,10-12]

Table 29.4. In-hospital Results of TEC Atherectomy in Saphenous Vein Grafts

	Meany[11] (1995)	Twidale[12] (1994)	Safian[16] (1992)	Popma[4] (1992)
No. lesions	650	88	158	29
Adjunctive PTCA (%)	74	95	91	86
Success (%)	89	86	84	82
Complications (%)				
MI	0.7	3.4	2.0	3.7
Death	3.2	0	2.0	10.3
Acute closure	2.0	5.0	5.0	-
Distal embolization	2.0	4.5	11.9	17
No-reflow	-	-	8.8	-

Abbreviation: - = not reported

    c. **Angiographic Complications.** Serious angiographic complications after vein graft TEC are similar to conventional PTCA and include distal embolization in 2-17%, no-reflow in 8.8%, and abrupt closure in 2-5%. No-reflow occasionally responds to intragraft verapamil (100-300 mcg),[13-15] and the value of prophylactic intragraft verapamil prior to intervention is currently under investigation. In one report, distal embolization was more likely to occur in grafts with one or more intraluminal filling defects, and in older grafts.[16] In a recent NACI Registry report, distal embolization was associated with a higher incidence of in-hospital mortality and myocardial infarction; multivariate predictors of distal embolization included noncardiac disease, stand-alone TEC, thrombus, and large vessel size.[17] To minimize the risk of distal embolization and no-reflow, some operators recommend TEC followed by staged (1-2 months later) rather than immediate stent implantation; in one report, this approach resulted in less distal embolization,[18,19] although 15% of grafts occluded before stenting.[18] A multicenter randomized trial comparing TEC followed by stent vs. PTCA (TEC-BEST) will be initiated shortly.

    d. **Follow-up.** Angiographic restenosis has been reported in 64-69% of vein graft lesions treated with TEC,[6,10] with a 29% incidence of late total occlusion in one report.[10]

F. SPECIAL CONSIDERATIONS. TEC atherectomy may have special utility in several clinical situations:
    1. **Acute Ischemic Syndromes.** TEC may have a role in primary revascularization for acute MI, rescue after failed thrombolysis, post-infarct MI angina, and unstable angina associated with a thrombotic lesion. In a study of 110 patients with acute ischemic syndromes, overall procedural success was 94%; in-hospital complications included death in 4.3% (only 1.4% of patients not presenting in cardiogenic shock), CABG in 2.9%, repeat PTCA in 5.7%, and blood transfusion in 20%.[20] At 6 months, vessel patency was 90% and angiographic restenosis 68%. A multicenter randomized trial comparing TEC vs. PTCA (TOPIT) in acute ischemic syndromes is in progress.

2. **Thrombus.** Angiographic thrombus increases the risk of an adverse outcome in virtually all studies of percutaneous interventional devices. However, in the initial TEC registry, procedural success was equally high with and without thrombus, offering hope that TEC's ability to excise and aspirate thrombus would fill an important void in the interventional arena. Some of these hopes were dashed when studies of TEC in thrombotic vein grafts reported lower procedural success, and more angiographic and clinical complications.[4,21] Nevertheless, TEC is currently under investigation as a bailout technique after failed PTCA in the setting of acute MI,[22] and to pretreat thrombotic lesions prior to stenting.[2]

3. **Saphenous Vein Bypass Grafts.** Angioscopy reveals that TEC effectively removes thrombus and friable debris from degenerated vein grafts, albeit at an increased risk of no-reflow and distal embolization.[23] Patients in whom filling defects persist or transient no-reflow occurs after TEC are at increased risk for no-reflow and distal embolization after adjunctive PTCA or stenting. An angioscopic-guided study recently completed at our institution demonstrated the effectiveness of TEC followed by stenting for thrombotic and degenerated saphenous vein grafts:[2] partial and complete thrombus extraction was evident in 100% and 65%, respectively, and all 32 high-risk lesions were successfully treated without Q-wave MI, need for emergency CABG, or death. Debulking high risk vein grafts with TEC prior to stenting results in high procedural success and low complication rates.[24]

4. **Ostial Lesions.** Recent studies suggest that a combined strategy of TEC followed by PTCA results in an incremental increase in lumen diameter of 22% compared to PTCA alone.[8] In the TEC registry, high procedural success (94%) and low complications (similar to other lesions subtypes) were achieved.[6]

5. **Contraindications.** Certain lesions are unsuitable for TEC, including moderate-to-heavily calcified lesions, severely angled stenoses, highly eccentric lesions, bifurcation lesions, and lesions in vessels < 2.5 mm. TEC is absolutely contraindicated in the setting of dissection caused by another device due to the risk of extending the dissection and perforating the vessel. Since it is often difficult to distinguish dissection from thrombus by angiography alone, adjunctive imaging techniques such as angioscopy and intravascular ultrasound can be used to guide subsequent use of TEC (for thrombus) or stents (for dissection).

G. **FUTURE DIRECTIONS.** Current TEC cutters are hampered by their small size (≤ 2.5 mm) and limited ability to aspirate. Larger cutters with improved cutting and aspiration are under development. An expandable cutter may allow the use of larger cutters without the need for larger guiding catheters. Finally, adjustments in cutter angles and sharpness may create smoother cuts and decrease complications.

REFERENCES

1. Annex BH, Larkin TJ, O'Neill WW, Safian RS. Evaluation of Thrombus Removal by Transluminal Extraction Coronary Atherectomy by Percutaneous Coronary Angioscopy. Amer J Cardiol 1994;74:606-9.

2. Kaplan BM, Safian RS, Grines CL, Goldstein JA, et al. Usefulness of adjunctive angioscopy and extraction atherectomy before stent implantation in high risk narrowings in aorto-coronary artery saphenous vein grafts. Amer J Cardiol 1995;76:822-824.

3. Moses JW, Lieberman SM, Knopf WD, et al. Mechanism of transluminal extraction catheter (TEC) atherectomy in degenerative saphenous vein grafts (SVG): An Angioscopic Observational Study. J Am Coll Cardiol 1993;21:442A.

4. Popma JJ, Leon MB, Mintz GS, et al. Results of coronary angioplasty using the transluminal extraction catheter. Am J Cardiol 1992;70:1526-1532.

5. Pizzulli L, Kohler U, Manz M, Luderitz B. Mechanical dilatation rather than plaque removal as major mechanism of transluminal extraction atherectomy. J Intervent Cardiol 1993;6:31-39.

6. IVT Coronary TEC Atherectomy Clinical Database. 1995.

7. Safian RS, May MA, Lichtenberg A, et al. Detailed clinical and angiographic analysis of complex lesions in native coronary arteries. J Am Coll Cardiol 1995;25:848-854.

8. Safian RD, Freed M, Reddy V, et al. Do excimer laser and rotational atherectomy facilitate balloon angioplasty? Implications for lesion-specific coronary intervention. J Am Coll Cardiol (in-press)

9. Ishizaka N, Ikari Y, Hara K, Saeki F, et al. Angiographic follow-up of patients after transluminal extraction atherectomy. Am Heart J 1994; 128(4): 691-696.

10. Safian RS, Grines CL, May MA, et al. Clinical and angiographic results of transluminal extraction coronary atherectomy in saphenous vein bypass grafts. Circulation 1994; 89(1): 302-312.

11. Meany TB, Leon MB, Kramer BL, et al. Transluminal extraction catheter for the treatment of diseased saphenous vein grafts: A multicenter experience. Cathet Cardio Diagn 1995; 34: 112-120.

12. Twidale N, Barth III, CW, Kipperman RM, et al. Acute results and long-term outcome of transluminal catheter atherectomy for saphenous vein graft stenoses. Cath and Cardio Diagn 1994; 31: 187-91.

13. Kaplan BM, Benzuly KH, Bowers TR, et al. Prospective study of intracoronary verapamil and nitroglycerin for the treatment of no-reflow after interventions on degenerated saphenous vein grafts. Circ 1995; 92:I-330.

14. Piana RN, Paik GY, Moscucci M, Cohen DJ, et al. Incidence and treatment of "no-reflow" after percutaneous coronary intervention. Circulation 1994; 89(6): 2514-2518.

15. Pomerantz RM, Kuntz RE, Diver DJ, Safian RD, Baim DS. Intracoronary verapamil fir the treatment of distal microvascular coronary artery spasm following PTCA. Cathet Cardio Diagn 1991; 24: 283-285.

16. Hong MK, Popma JJ, Pichard AD, Kent KM, et al. Clinical significance of distal embolization after transluminal extraction atherectomy in diffusely diseased saphenous vein grafts. Am Heart J 1994; 127(6): 1496-1503.

17. Moses JW, Yeh W, Popma JJ, Sketch Jr. MH, NACI Investigators. Predictors of distal embolization with the TEC catheter: A NACI Registry Report. Circ 1995; 92:I-329.

18. Hong MH, Pichard AD, Kent KM, et al. Assessing a strategy of stand-alone extraction atherectomy followed by staged stent placement in degenerated saphenous vein graft lesions. J Amer Coll Cardiol 1995;27:394A.

19. Al-Shaibi KF, Goods CM, Jain SP, et al. Does transluminal extraction atherectomy reduce distal embolization in saphenous vein grafts? Circ 1995; 92:I-329.

20. Kaplan BM, Larkin TJ, Safian RS, O'Neill WW, et al. A Prospective pilot trial of direct and rescue extraction atherectomy for acute myocardial infarction. 1995 (to be submitted for publication).

21. Dooris M, Hoffman M, Glazier S, et al. Comparative results of transluminal extraction coronary atherectomy in saphenous vein graft lesions with and without thrombus. J Am Coll Cardiol 1995; 25: 1700-1705.

22. Kaplan BM, O'Neill WW, Grines CL, et al. Rescue extraction atherectomy after failed primary angioplasty in right coronary artery infarction. Am J cardiol (in-press)

23. Tilli FV, Kaplan BM, Safian RD, Grines CL, O'Neill WW. Angioscopic plaque friability: a new risk factor for procedural complications following saphenous vein graft interventions. J Am Coll Cardiol (in-press).

EXCIMER LASER CORONARY ANGIOPLASTY

30

Ashish Parikh, M.D.
Neal Eigler, M.D.
Frank Litvack, M.D.

A. **BACKGROUND.** The name "excimer" is an acronym for e̲x̲cited di̲me̲r. Laser energy is produced when the active medium (e.g. HCl gas) is excited by electrical energy and emits monochromatic, coherent light. Laser energy can be emitted as a continuous or pulsed wave. The excimer laser emits pulsed ultraviolet laser light at 308 nm. Excimer laser energy ablates inorganic material by photochemical mechanisms that involve the breaking of molecular bonds without generation of heat.[1] In vivo, the precise mechanism of tissue ablation is unknown, but it probably consists of photochemical, localized thermal, and mechanical effects. Some ultrasound studies in humans have demonstrated lumen enlargement due to atheroablation and vessel expansion,[2] while other demonstrate little or no plaque ablation.[3] In blood or radiographic contrast, ultraviolet laser energy is avidly absorbed, inducing significant acoustic effects, tissue disruption, and dissection.[4] Accordingly, ELCA should be performed only after blood and contrast are displaced from the coronary artery.

B. **EQUIPMENT**

1. **Laser Unit.** Advanced Interventional Systems, Inc. and Spectranetics, Inc. received FDA approval independently and are now merged, operating under the Spectranetics name. The latest version of the Spectranetics laser unit is the CVX-300 system, which utilizes XeC1 as the active medium (wavelength 308 nm, catheter output 30-60 mJ/mm², maximum repetition rate 40 Hz, pulse width 125-200 nsec). The laser has a warm-up time of only 5 minutes.

2. **Laser Catheters (Table 30.1).** Conventional excimer laser catheters are front-firing, concentric, and track over conventional coronary angioplasty guidewires (Figure 30.1). The current concentric designs use greater than 200 individual, small fibers concentrically arranged around the guidewire lumen. Limitations of concentric catheters include the inability to treat highly eccentric lesion on an inner curve of a severe bend; the catheter may deflect off the plaque and into the normal wall, resulting in dissection and/or perforation (Figure 11.2). Other limitations include the need for definitive lumen enlargement by PTCA or stenting.

    To overcome some of these limitations, a first generation directional excimer laser catheter has been developed (Figure 13.1). The catheter shaft has an eccentric fiberoptic bundle opposite the guidewire lumen, which runs through a tapered tip. During the procedure, the catheter is rotated so the fiberoptic bundle is in contact with the plaque; the guidewire and protective tip are positioned along the normal wall. Directional ELCA allows selective ablation of eccentric plaque, minimizing injury to the normal wall.

Table 30.1 Excimer Laser Catheters

Catheter Type	Diameter mm	F	Guidewire* (inch)	Guide ID * (inch)	Vessel Diameter* (mm)
Over-the-Wire					
Extreme	1.4	4.3	0.014	0.084	2.4
Extreme	1.7	4.7	0.018	0.084	2.7
Extreme	2.0	5.9	0.018	0.092	3.0
Monorail					
Vitesse	1.4	4.3	0.014	0.072	2.4
Vitesse	1.7	4.7	0.018	0.080	2.7
Vitesse	2.0	5.9	0.018	0.092	3.0

Abbreviations: F = French size; ID = internal diameter; * = maximum guidewire, minimum guide ID, maximum vessel diameter

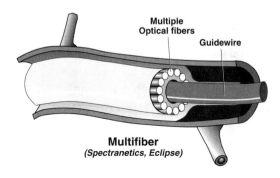

Figure 30.1 Excimer Laser

In 1994, Spectranetics introduced a rapid exchange version of the co-axial laser catheter (trade name "Vitesse") in diameters of 1.4 mm, 1.7 mm and 2.0 mm. In addition to the rapid exchange feature, these devices produce more axial force transmission and tip control than earlier over-the-wire systems. The 1.4 mm device is compatible with a 0.014-inch guidewire, but the 1.7 and 2.0 mm catheters will accept 0.018-inch guidewires.

Recently, a laser guidewire (Prima™) has been developed for crossing chronic total occlusions (Figure 8.9). This wire has a shapeable tip and 12 individual front firing, small diameter (45 micron) laser fibers running through it. The device is currently in clinical trial in the U.S. and Europe.[5]

C. CLINICAL RESULTS

1. **Observational Studies (Table 30.2).** In the original ELCA Registry, laser success was 83% and procedural success was 90%.[6-8] The mean baseline diameter stenosis decreased to $50 \pm 22\%$ after ELCA and to $24 \pm 17\%$ after adjunctive PTCA. In later series, ELCA success increased and complications decreased,[9] which may have been due to advances in catheter design and more operator experience.[26] The influence of lesions morphology on in-hospital outcome is described in Table 30.3. There was no difference in success or complications for long lesions, total occlusions, saphenous vein grafts, and aorto-ostial lesions, suggesting that selected complex lesions can be well treated with ELCA.[9-11]

2. **Non-Randomized Comparative Studies.** In a matched comparison of 696 patients undergoing ELCA or Rotablator at a single institution, ELCA was an independent predictor of lower procedural success, acute complications and a trend toward more frequent target lesion.[12] In a case-controlled series of 53 lesions treated with ELCA compared to 53 lesions treated with PTCA, restenosis rates were higher after ELCA (57% vs. 34%, p = 0.02).[13] Neither study employed the saline infusion technique.

Table 30.2. ELCA Success and Complications: Influence of Operator Experience[9]

Outcome (%)	Pt # 1-2000	Pt # 2001-3000	P Value
Laser Success	83	86	.04
Procedure Success	90	90	NS
Adjunctive PTCA	71	95	< .001
Perforation	1.6	0.4	< .005
CABG	4.0	3.4	NS
Q Wave MI	2.3	1.7	NS
Death	0.7	0.9	NS

Abbreviations: Pt = patient; PTCA = percutaneous transluminal coronary atherectomy; CABG = emergency coronary artery bypass grafting; Q-Wave-MI = in-hospital Q-wave myocardial infarction; NS = not significant

Table 30.3. ELCA Success and Complications: Influence of Lesion Morphology [9-11]

Lesion Type	Laser Success (%)	Procedure Success (%)	Major Complications (%)
Lesion Length (mm)			
< 10	86	91	6.0
10-19	83	92	4.6
20 - 29	79	89	6.6
≥ 30	85	87	7.3
Morphology			
Aorto Ostial	88	89	6.9
Vein Graft	88	92	3.9
Total Occlusion	84	89	2.4
All Others	82	90	6.4

3. **Randomized Trials.** Randomized clinical trials have shown similar angiographic results for conventional PTCA and ELCA, but restenosis rates are higher after ELCA. In the Dutch AMRO study,[14-16] there were no differences in angiographic success, dissection, or perforation; however, there was a 10-fold higher incidence of transient vessel occlusion and a trend toward higher restenosis after ELCA (Table 30.4). However, lesions >20 mm were excluded. The German ERBAC study[17] randomized complex lesions to conventional PTCA, ELCA and Rotablator. As outlined in Table 30.5, higher rates of acute complications and restenosis were observed after ELCA compared to PTCA. However, chronic total occlusions and long lesions were excluded.

4. **Laser Wire for Total Occlusions.** Table 30.6 summarizes recent results using the new Prima™ laser wire designed to treat total occlusions refractory to conventional PTCA guidewires (Table 30.2).[5]

5. **Complications.** In the ELCA Registry, in-hospital death occurred in 0.8%, Q-wave myocardial infarctioning 2.1%, non-Q-wave MI in 2.3%, and in-hospital bypass surgery in 3.8% of patients. Laser perforations occurred in 1% of lesions but decreased significantly from 1.4% in the first 2,592 lesions to 0.3% in last 1,000 lesions;[9] 62% of perforations were treated conservatively. Coronary dissection occurred in 13% of lesions, but sustained occlusions occurred in 3.1% of lesions. Risk factors for dissection include the use of larger ELCA catheters, high energy per pulse, lesion length >10 mm, and presence of a sidebranch.[18-20] The incidence of perforation was higher in women, total occlusions, bifurcation lesions, and when the target vessel size was < 0.1 mm larger than the laser catheter.[26] There appears to be a significant learning curve with ELCA,

Table 30.4. Dutch AMRO Study: Comparison of ELCA and Conventional PTCA[14-16]

	PTCA (n = 157)	ELCA (n = 151)
Angiographic Success (%)	79	80
Angiographic Complications (%)		
Dissection	55	47
Spasm	1	4
Perforation	1	3
Transient Occlusion	0.7	7*
Clinical Events at 6 months (%)		
Death	0	0
Myocardial Infarction	5.7	4.6
Coronary artery bypass surgery	10.8	10.6
Repeat PTCA	18.5	21.2
Overall clinical events	29.9	33
Restenosis stenosis > 50%	41.3	51.6

* p = 0.005

Table 30.5. ERBAC Study: PTCA vs. ELCA vs. Rotablator Atherectomy for Complex Lesions[17]

Lesion Type (%)	PTCA (n = 210)	ELCA (n = 195)	Rotablator (n = 215)
Immediate results (%) B2/C lesions	60/12	68/10	72/13
Final diameter stenosis	36	32	31
Major Complications	4.8	6.2*	2.3*
Follow-up results (%) Angiographic restenosis	54	60	62
Target lesion revascularization	35	46*	46*
Q-wave myocardial infarction	3.8	0.7	3.2
Death	3.1	0	2.6

* p < 0.05 compared to PTCA

Table 30.6. Excimer Laser Guidewire: Preliminary Results[5]

Patients: 306

Age: 60 ± 10 yrs

Lesion length: 18 ± 10 mm

Occlusion Duration: 27 weeks (range 2-1040 weeks)

Successful crossing with laser wire: 58%

Wire perforation: 21%

In hospital events: 2.4%

since the incidence of complications decreases after performing 50 laser procedures. Risk factors for restenosis after ELCA include small target vessels and more severe stenoses before and after intervention.[21,22]

6. **New Techniques to Improve Results.** As demonstrated in Table 30.7, the saline infusion technique eliminates blood and contrast from the laser field, resulting in a significant decrease in dissection.[23,24] In addition, many operators are now using smaller laser probes and slightly larger balloons to achieve better angiographic results, as well as the directional laser for lesions unfavorable for the conventional laser.[25]

D. **RECOMMENDATIONS AND CASE SELECTION.** Clinical data suggest that ELCA is most useful in complex lesions not well suited for PTCA. It is not a "stand-alone" procedure, and should be considered an adjunct to PTCA or stenting. To date, there are no data supporting reduction of

Table 30.7. ELCA Results: Influence of Saline Infusion Technique[23]

	Saline	No Saline
Baseline Stenosis (%)	79	71
ELCA Success (%)	97	96
Dissection (%)	7	24

Table 30.8. Potential Indications for ELCA

- Diffuse disease

- Long lesions (> 20 mm)

- Chronic total occlusions (crossable with guidewire)

- Aorto-ostial lesion

- Saphenous vein grafts

- In-stent restenosis

- Non-dilatable or non-crossable lesion by PTCA

- Total occlusions uncrossable by guidewire (laser wire)

restenosis.[13-17] The procedure should be considered to facilitate PTCA or stenting by debulking[27] and increasing plaque compliance. The cost of the ELCA system has limited its application. Possible indications and contradictions are described in Tables 30.8 and 30.9

E. TECHNICAL DETAILS. Excimer laser coronary angioplasty equipment is user friendly. Nonetheless, the procedure should be performed by operators with sufficient training and skill. Case selection, choice of equipment, technique and judgement are critical.

1.   **Patient Preparation and Catheter Selection.** Patients should be on aspirin and a calcium channel blocker. Select a laser catheter no more than two-thirds the reference vessel diameter (Table 30.1); further undersizing is recommended if the lesion is distal, very eccentric, severely calcified or if the proximal artery is tortuous. Larger catheter are used for aorto-ostial and saphenous vein graft lesions.

2.   **The ELCA Procedure.** After vascular access, intravenous heparin should be administered (10-15,000 units) to maintain the ACT $\geq$300 seconds. The selection of a guide catheter is crucial to provide coaxial alignment and support, and extra-support guidewires are recommended. Always keep the guidewire tip as distal as possible to allow tracking over the stiff portion of the wire.

For lasing, use energy densities between 40-60 mJ/mm^2 at frequencies of 10-30 Hz, beginning at lower energies and increasing only if the lesion cannot be crossed with the catheter. Do not attempt to cross a lesion without laser energy. Saline infusion is recommended to minimize dissection (using normal saline or lactated ringers solution): Advance the laser catheter in contact with the lesion, and eliminate all contrast from the manifold and guide. When the primary operator is ready to lase, the assistant should inject a 10 cc bolus of saline via the guide catheter and continue to inject slowly at a rate of 1 to 3 cc per second. The primary operator should start lasing immediately

Table 30.9. Contraindications to ELCA

- Bifurcation lesions*
- Highly eccentric lesions*
- Severe lesions angulation
- Prior dissection (laser or balloon induced)
- Extreme vessel tortuosity
- Inability to cross total occlusion with guidewire**

*   Consider directional excimer laser
** Consider excimer laser guidewire

after the 10 cc bolus of saline is given, and continue for 2 to 4 seconds. The laser catheter should be advanced 1 mm per second. Terminate the saline injection at the end of lasing, and repeat the procedure for each lasing burst.

To create a larger lumen one may exchange for a larger laser catheter, particularly when debulking an aorto-ostial or saphenous vein graft lesion. Adjunctive PTCA and/or stent placement should be performed in most cases with the goal of obtaining the largest lumen diameter. Post-procedural management is identical to that for routine PTCA.

3. **Trouble Shooting.** Exchange for a more flexible, smaller catheter if the device cannot negotiate a bend. Never apply additional laser energy once dissection has occurred. If the 1.4 mm catheter cannot cross a rigid lesion on a straight segment of the artery, the energy density may be increased to 60 mJ/mm^2, or the frequency increased to 30 Hz, to facilitate crossing. If the catheter will not cross, ELCA should be abandoned.

F. **SUMMARY.** In summary, excimer laser angioplasty is a useful technique for treating selected complex lesions which are not well suited for PTCA. Using concentric catheters, such lesions include diffuse, long, ostial, calcified, undilatable, vein grafts, and total occlusions. Using the newer directional catheter, highly eccentric or bifurcation lesions may be treated. As with all new interventional technologies, case selection is crucial. Significant coronary dissection, the most unpredictable of the excimer laser complications, has been nearly eliminated by the use of saline flush technique.

* * * * *

REFERENCES

1. Grundfest WS, Segalowitz J, Laudenslager J, et al. The physical and biological basis for laser angioplasty: In coronary laser angioplasty. Litvack F (ed), Blackwell Scientific Publications, 1992.

2. Mintz GS, Kovach JA, Javier SP, et al. Mechanisms of lumen enlargement after excimer laser coronary angioplasty: An intravascular ultrasound study. Circulation. 1995;92:3408-3414.

3. Honye J, Mahon DJ, Nakamura S, Wallis J, et al. Intravascular ultrasound imaging after excimer laser angioplasty. Cathet Cardiovasc Diagn 1994;32:213-222.

4. van Leeuwen TG, Meertens JH, Velema E, et al. Intraluminal vapor bubble induced by excimer laser pulse causes microsecond arterial dilation and invagination leading to extensive wall damage in the rabbit. Circulation 1993;87:1258-1263.

5. Serruys PW, Leon MB, Hamburger JN, et al. Recanalization of chronic total coronary occlusions using a laser guide wire: The European and US total experience. J Am Coll Cardiol 1996;March Special Issue.

6. Bittl JA, Sanborn TA. Excimer laser-facilitated coronary angioplasty. Circulation 1992;86:71-80.

7. Margolis JR, Mehta S. Excimer laser coronary angioplasty. Am J Cardiol 92;69:3F-11F.

8. Litvack F. Excimer Laser Coronary Angioplasty. In Textbook of Interventional Cardiology. Topol (ed) Second Edition, 1990, pp. 840-858.

9. Litvack F, Eigler N, Margolis J, et al. Percutaneous excimer laser coronary angioplasty: Results in the first consecutive 3,000 patients. J Am Coll Cardiol 1994;23:323-329.

10. Bittl JA, Sanborn RA, Tcheng JE, et al. Clinical success complications and restenosis rates with excimer laser coronary angioplasty. Am J Cardiol 1992;70:1553-1539.

11. Bittl JA, Sanborn TA, Siegel RM, et al. Which complex lesions are suitable for excimer laser coronary angioplasty: Multivariate analysis in 701 patients. J Am Coll Cardiol 1992;263A.

12. Dussaillant GR, Popma JJ, Picard AD, et al. Rotational atherectomy vs. excimer laser angioplasty: A multivariable analysis of early and late procedural outcome. Abstract presented at TCT, 1995.

13. Strikwerda S, vanSwijndregt EM, Foley DP, et al. Immediate and late outcome of excimer laser and balloon coronary angioplasty: A quantitative angiographic comparison based on matched lesions. J Am Coll Cardiol 1995;26:939-46.

14. Foley DP, Appelman YE, Piek JJ on behalf of the AMRO group. Comparison of angiographic restenosis propensity of excimer laser coronary angioplasty (ELCA) and balloon angioplasty (BA) in the Amsterdam Rotterdam (AMRO) Trial. Circulation 1995;92: I-477.

15. Koolen J, Appelman Y, Strikwerda S, et al. Initial and long-term results of excimer laser coronary angioplasty versus balloon angioplasty in functional and total coronary occlusions. Eur Heart Journal 1994:832.

16. Appelman YEA, Piek JJ, Strikwerda S, et al. Randomized trial of excimer laser angioplasty versus balloon angioplasty for treatment of obstructive coronary artery disease. Lancet 1996;347:79-84.

17. Vandormael M, Reifart N, Preusler W, et al. Six months follow-up results following excimer laser angioplasty, rotational atherectomy and balloon angioplasty for complex lesions: ERBAC Study. Circulation 1994;90:I-213.

18. Ghazzal ZM, Hearn JA, Litvack F, et al. Morphological predictors of acute complications after percutaneous excimer laser coronary angioplasty. Circulation 1992;86:820-827.

19. Baumbach A, Bittl JA, Fleck E, et al. Acute complications of coronary excimer laser angioplasty: Analysis of 2 multicenter registries. Circulation 1992;86:4 510.

20. Baumbach A, Bittl JA, Fleck E, et al. Coinvestigators of the U.S. and European percutaneous excimer laser coronary angioplasty (PELCA) registries. J Am Coll Cardiol 1994;23:1305-13.

21. Bittl JA, Kuntz RE, Estella P, et al. Analysis of late lumen narrowing after excimer laser-facilitated coronary angioplasty. J Am Coll Cardiol 1994;23:1314.

22. Ghazzal ZMB, Burton E, Wintraub, WS, et al. Predictors of restenosis after excimer laser coronary angioplasty. Am J Cardiol 1995;75:1012-1014.

23. Deckelbaum LI, Natarajan MK, Bittl JA, et al. For the percutaneous excimer laser coronary angioplasty (PELCA) investigators: Effect of intracoronary saline infusion on dissection during excimer laser coronary angioplasty: A randomized trial. J Am Coll Cardiol 1995;26:1264-9.

24. Tcheng JE, Wells LD, Phillips HR, et al. Development of a new technique for reducing pressure pulse generation during 308-nm excimer laser coronary angioplasty. Cathet Cardiovasc Diagn 1995;34:15-22.

25. Rechavia E, Federman J, Shefer A, et al. Usefulness of a prototype directional catheter for excimer laser coronary angioplasty in narrowings unfavorable for conventional excimer or balloon angioplasty. Am J Cardiol 1995;76:1144-1146.

26. Bittl JA, Brinker JA, Sanborn TA, et al. The changing profile of patient selection, procedural techniques, and outcomes in excimer laser coronary angioplasty. J Interven Cardiol 1995;8:653-660.

CORONARY INTRAVASCULAR ULTRASOUND

31

Steven E. Nissen MD
Anthony C. De Franco MD,
E. Murat Tuzcu MD

The traditional approach to percutaneous revascularization employs visual assessment by fluoroscopy and angiography; yet the angiographic assessment of lesion severity, vessel morphology, calcification, dissection, and thrombus is subjective and difficult to quantitate. In the 1990's, intravascular ultrasound (IVUS) was established as an important complementary imaging modality for diagnostic and interventional cardiac catheterization. IVUS represents a radically different approach to vascular anatomy: Unlike angiography, which displays the coronary artery as a silhouette of the contrast-filled lumen, IVUS generates a cross-sectional tomographic image of the lumen and vessel wall.

A. LIMITATIONS OF ANGIOGRAPHY

1. **Stenosis Severity.** In the 1960's, investigators first began to question the accuracy and reproducibility of coronary angiography.[1,2] Multiple studies demonstrated that visual interpretation of angiograms was associated with significant inter- and intra-observer variability, and that there were major discrepancies between angiographic lesion severity and post-mortem examination. Recent studies have demonstrated major differences between angiographic lesion severity and the physiologic significance of stenoses by Doppler flow techniques.[3] Quantitative angiography has improved the reproducibility of angiographic measurements, but requires that the angiographer identify and measure the diameter of the "normal" reference segment. Since post-mortem and IVUS studies have shows that coronary atherosclerosis is a diffuse process, a "normal" reference segment may not be identifiable. In such cases, angiography will underestimate lesion severity (Figure 31.1).

2. **Post-Intervention Assessment.** Many mechanical interventions enlarge the lumen by fracturing or dissecting the atheroma.[4] The physical disruption of plaque permits contrast extravasation into the atheroma, leaving the angiographic appearance of an enlarged, "hazy" lumen. Since angiography depicts complex coronary cross-sectional anatomy from a 2-dimensional silhouette of the contrast-filled lumen, the hazy angiographic result may overestimate vessel dimensions and the actual gain in lumen size (Figure 31.2).

B. **IVUS EQUIPMENT** consists of two principal components: A catheter with a miniaturized transducer, and a console to reconstruct the image. IVUS catheters range in size from 2.9 to 3.5 F (0.96-1.17 mm) (Table 31.1). Excellent image quality is a result of high operating frequency (20 to 30 MHZ) and close proximity of the transducer to the target; nominal axial and lateral resolution are approximately 0.08 mm and 0.20 mm, respectively. The two principal designs of IVUS catheters are mechanical devices and multi-element electronic devices:

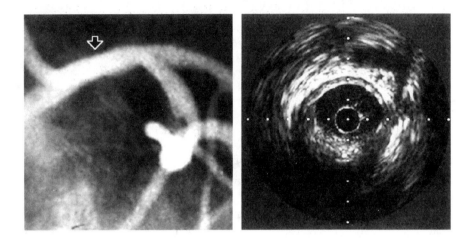

Figure 31.1 Underestimation of Atherosclerosis by Angiography

Although the angiogram is nearly normal, ultrasound shows a large crescent-shaped atheroma (3 to 9 o'clock).

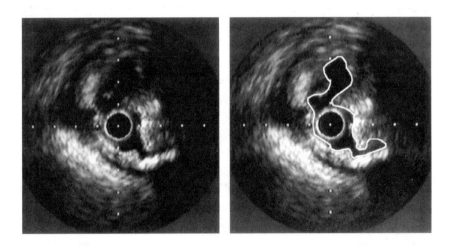

Figure 31.2 Lumen Irregularity Following Angioplasty

A complex luminal shape is frequently observed following PTCA (the intimal edge is outlined on the right).

Table 31.1. Intravascular Ultrasound Systems.

Manufacturer	Type	Diameter (F)	Frequency (MHZ)	Catheter Configuration	Ultrasound Scanner
Boston Scientific*	Mechanical	3.5 Fr	30	Short Monorail; No Sheath	HP Sonos 100™
Boston Scientific*	Mechanical	3.0 Fr	30	Shared Lumen; Moveable Imaging Core in Sheath	CVIS Insight™ or HP Sonos 100™
Cardiovascular Imaging Systems*	Mechanical	2.9 Fr	30	Shared Lumen; Moveable Imaging Core in Sheath	CVIS Insight™ or HP Sonos 100™
Cardiovascular Imaging Systems**	Mechanical	3.2 Fr	30	Short Monorail; Moveable Imaging Core in Sheath	CVIS Insight™ or HP Sonos 100™
Endosonics Corporation	Electronic	3.5 Fr	20	Monorail or over-the-wire	Endosonics Cathscanner™

* No Longer Marketed

** Marketed by Scimed Life Systems

1. **Mechanical Devices** employ an external motor and drive shaft to rotate a single piezoelectric transducer mounted near the distal end of the catheter. Mechanical transducers typically operate at 1800 rpm, which yields 30 frames per second. In the United States, Scimed Life Systems (Minneapolis, Minn.) currently markets several FDA-approved mechanical catheters; these IVUS systems were originally developed by Cardiovascular Imaging Systems (Mountain View, CA) and Boston Scientific Corporation (Table 31.1). In Europe, a mechanical system is manufactured by DuMED Corporation (Rotterdam, The Netherlands) and marketed by Endosonics Corp (Pleasanton, CA).

2. **Electronic Devices** employ an annular array of 32-64 elements mounted near the distal tip of the catheter. Advantages of this design include excellent flexibility, absence of rotational artifacts, and excellent guidewire tracking; however, many experts feel that the image quality of electronic devices is inferior to mechanical devices. A unique version of an electronic IVUS catheter employs an imaging transducer mounted proximal to a standard angioplasty balloon; this device was recently approved by the FDA (Oracle-Micro ™ Endosonics Corp) and allows examination of the vessel before and after PTCA, without a catheter exchange. Despite their current limitations, electronic ultrasound devices have tremendous potential; once perfected, the small size, lack of moving parts, and freedom from rotational artifacts may allow electronic transducers to be readily coupled to a variety of interventional devices.

C. IMAGE INTERPRETATION

1. **Normal Lumen Features.** The normal coronary artery has been characterized by IVUS.[5-7] At low frequency transducers (20 MHZ), the vessel lumen is sonolucent; at higher frequencies ($\geq$30 MHZ), blood appears as faint, finely textured specular echoes that move and swirl during active blood flow (Figure 31.3). Blood echogenicity assists image interpretation by identifying the communication between tissue planes and the lumen, thereby confirming the presence of a dissection channel; lumen echogenicity can identify the lumen-wall interface.

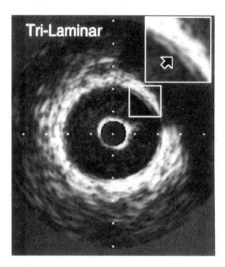 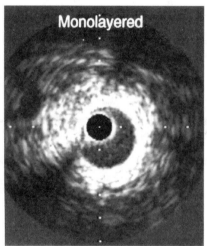

Figure 31.3 Normal Coronary Artery Morphology by IVUS

Distinct trilaminar appearance (left) and a single-layered appearance (right).

2. **Normal Wall Anatomy.** Normal coronary artery morphology consists of a circular lumen surrounded by distinct layers exhibiting variable echogenicity (Figure 31.3).[5-7] Some normal vessels demonstrate three discrete vessel wall layers: 1) an inner layer, which represents the internal elastic lamina; 2) a middle sonolucent layer, which represents the media; and 3) an outer layer, which has a characteristic "onionskin" appearance and represents the adventitia and peri-adventitial tissues. About 50% of normal coronary arteries have a monolayered appearance.

3. **Plaque Composition and Distribution (Table 31.2).** Patients with coronary disease have a wide spectrum of abnormal features reflecting the distribution, severity, and composition of the

Table 31.2. Advantages of IVUS

Precise quantitative measurements

- Lumen diameter

- Reference vessel diameter

- Cross-sectional area (CSA)

Characterization of plaque

- Distribution

    Eccentric
    Concentric

- Composition

    Soft plaque
    Fibrous plaque
    Calcified plaque
    Mixed plaque
    Depth of calcium (deep vs. superficial)

- Dissection

    Severity of lumen compromise
    Length of dissection

atheroma.[5,7,8,9] Mild lesions are characterized by intimal thickening ≤ 0.30 mm. Advanced lesions appear as large echogenic masses that encroach upon the lumen. Most IVUS classifications schemes differentiate plaque by composition and echogenicity (Figures 31.4, 31.5): "Soft" plaques are less echogenic than surrounding adventitia due to their high lipid content; "fibrous" plaques have echodensity similar to adventitia *(in vitro* studies demonstrate that increasing echogenicity correlates with fibrous tissue content); and "calcified" lesions are more echogenic than surrounding adventitia. Calcified plaques attenuate transmission of the ultrasound signal and obscure architectural detail of deeper layers ("acoustic shadowing"). As described in Chapter 12, ultrasound is more sensitive than fluoroscopy in detecting and localizing calcium.

D. ADVANTAGES OF IVUS. IVUS allows visualization of the full circumference of the vessel wall and lumen. Further advantages are described in Table 31.2.

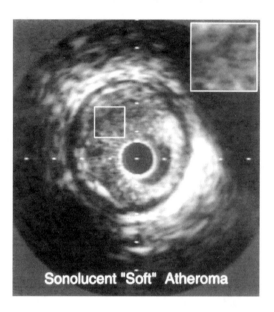

Figure 31.4 Soft, Sonolucent Atheroma

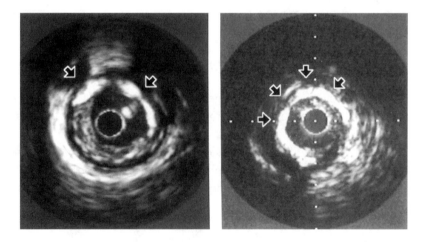

Figure 31.5 Hard, Calcified Atheroma with Acoustic Shadowing

E. LIMITATIONS OF IVUS (Table 31.3)

1. **Non-Uniform Rotational Distortion (NURD).** All available ultrasound devices generate artifacts that can adversely affect image quality. The external motor drive and transducer must rotate in a precise one-to-one relationship to generate accurate images; mechanical transducers exhibit cyclical oscillations in rotational speed, or *non-uniform rotational distortion* (NURD) due to mechanical drag on the catheter drive-shaft. NURD is most evident when the drive-shaft bends in a small radius of curvature (such as tortuous vessel), and is recognized as "stretching" and compression of the image (Figure 31.6).

2. **Ring-Down Artifact.** *Transducer ring-down* arises from acoustic oscillations that obscure the near-field imaging; inability to image structures immediately adjacent to the transducer yields a device with an "acoustic" size larger than its physical size.

3. **Geometric Distortion.** When the ultrasound beam interrogates a plane that is not orthogonal to the vessel wall, a circular lumen appears elliptical. Under some circumstances, it is possible to orient the device in a more coaxial position. Fortunately, the small diameter of the coronary arteries limits the degree of obliquity, minimizing image distortion.

4. **Image Interpretation.** Visual interpretation of IVUS images is dependent upon differences in acoustic impedance of adjacent tissues. Although currently available devices produce remarkably detailed views of the vessel wall, image reconstruction is based upon acoustic reflections, not actual histology. The acoustic properties (echogenicity) of different histologic entities may appear similar:

Table 31.3. Limitations of IVUS

Image artifacts

- NURD (Non-uniform rotational distortion)
- Ring-down artifact
- Geometric distortion

Image interpretation

- Not reliable for evaluation of thrombus
- Similarities in acoustic properties do not necessarily mean similar tissue histology

Cost (see Chapter 1)

For example, a sonolucent lesion may represent intracoronary thrombus or soft atherosclerotic plaque with a high lipid content. The identification of thrombus by IVUS is unreliable and inferior to angioscopy (Chapter 32). Furthermore, IVUS may be unable to distinguish plaque from media because of similar acoustic properties; in some diseased arteries, the media is relatively thick (0.5 to 1.5 mm), but in others it may be thin or absent.

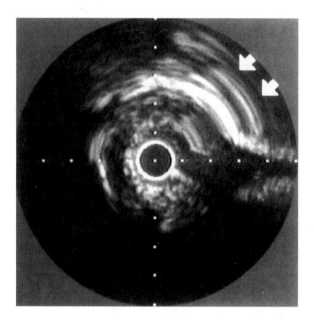

Figure 31.6 Non-Uniform Rotational Distortion (NURD)

F. TECHNIQUE

  1. **Catheter Handling.** IVUS is typically performed with conventional 7 or 8F guiding catheters and a 0.014 inch guidewire. Advancement and retraction of the imaging catheter permits on-line imaging; images recorded on videotape allow off-line analysis and archiving. Although ultrasound devices are reasonably flexible, their handling characteristics are distinctly inferior to modern angioplasty equipment. Interrogation of severely diseased, tortuous, calcified vessels, and distal lesions may be challenging; imaging may be enhanced in these situations by coaxial guiding catheter alignment, excellent guide support, and heavy-duty guidewires. Monorail designs facilitate rapid exchange, but are usually less trackable than over-the-wire devices.

2. **Sheath-Type Systems.** Some IVUS designs employ a thin-walled protective sheath that is advanced into the distal vessel; the transducer is passed freely inside the sheath to image without injuring the vessel wall (Table 31.1). Another advantage of the sheath is the ability to use a motorized pullback device, which may improve reproducibility of serial measurements. The distal lumen is shared by the transducer and guidewire to maximize transducer size and minimize sheath size. An important disadvantage is the need to retract the guidewire during transducer advancement. More recent IVUS catheter designs allow advancement and retraction of the transducer inside the thin-walled sheath without relinquishing guidewire position. A potential disadvantage of the sheath is the development of ischemia when imaging severe lesions (especially before intervention).

3. **Safety.** Serious untoward effects are uncommon.[5] Transient coronary spasm occurs in 5% of patients, but responds rapidly to intracoronary nitroglycerin. The imaging transducer may cause transient ischemia when imaging severe stenoses or small vessels, but usually resolves after catheter withdrawal. Despite the safety of IVUS, any intracoronary instrumentation carries the risk of vessel injury; the necessary personnel and equipment should be immediately available to restore vessel patency.

G. DIAGNOSTIC APPLICATIONS OF IVUS (TABLE 31.4)

1. **Angiographically Unrecognized Disease.** IVUS can detect atherosclerosis at sites that appear angiographically normal (Figure 31.1):[10] this angiographic appearance may be due to compensatory remodeling of the vessel wall (Figure 31.7).[11] The clinical implications of these IVUS observations are unknown.

2. **Lesions of Uncertain Severity.** IVUS provides precise quantitation of stenoses independent of the radiographic projection,[12] and can clarify the severity of angiographically borderline lesions. IVUS can readily characterize ostial and bifurcation lesions, which may be particularly difficult to image by angiography.

Table 31.4. Uses of IVUS: Noninterventional Applications

- Detection of unrecognized atherosclerosis

- Assessment of borderline lesion

- Identification of allograft vasculopathy

3. **Cardiac Allograft Vasculopathy.** Identification of cardiac allograft atherosclerosis is important and clinically challenging since most patients do not experience angina (Figure 31.8). Many centers now routinely perform IVUS at the time of annual catheterization.[13]

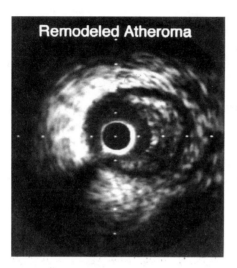
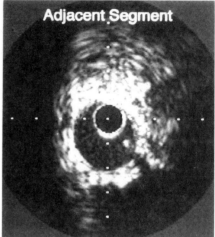

Figure 31.7 Coronary Remodeling

There is a large plaque with expansion of the adventitia (left), resulting in a lumen diameter virtually identical to an adjacent segment (right).

H. **INTERVENTIONAL APPLICATIONS OF IVUS (Table 31.5).**   Many high-volume centers routinely use IVUS to assist in decision-making during interventional procedures. There is no question that IVUS can provide useful information for the interventional cardiologist. However, further studies are needed to determine if IVUS is essential, or simply "nice to have."

1. **Characterize Plaque for Device Selection.** IVUS is extremely useful for characterizing plaque distribution, composition, and calcification; these characteristics have important implications for proper device selection (Figure 31.9). For example, PTCA of calcified lesions often results in suboptimal lumen enlargement and frequent dissection at the interface between calcified plaque and

Table 31.5. Uses of IVUS: Interventional Applications

Definite uses

- Precise vessel sizing for device sizing

- Precise characterization of plaque for device selection

- Assess severity of borderline lesions

- Understanding mechanisms of lumen enlargement

Possible uses

- Predict complications

- Predict restenosis

- Guide "optimal" stenting or atherectomy

Not useful

- Unreliable identification of thrombus

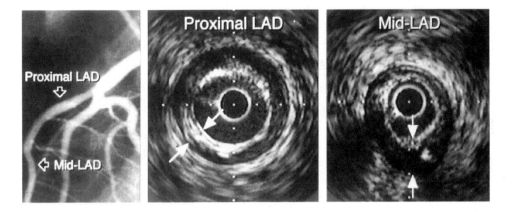

Figure 31.8 Angiographic Underestimation of Atherosclerosis in a Heart Transplant Patient

Although the angiogram is relatively normal, diffuse disease narrows the entire LAD.

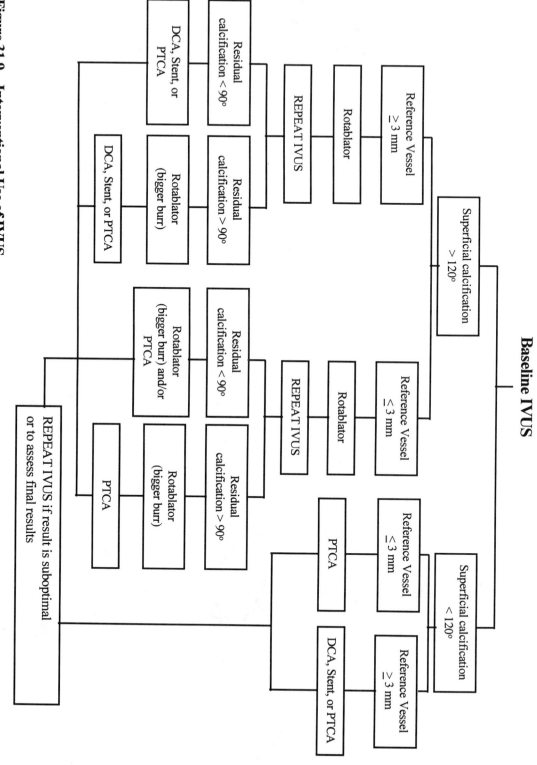

Figure 31.9. Interventional Use of IVUS

normal vessel wall; in contrast, Rotablator atherectomy is very effective at pulverizing superficial (but not deep) calcium and enlarging lumen dimensions without dissection (Figure 31.10). However, a clear need for IVUS has not yet been demonstrated; further studies are needed to determine if IVUS-guided intervention will improve immediate and long-term outcome compared to angiography-guided therapy.

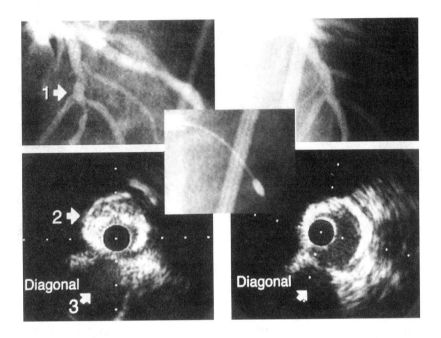

Figure 31.10 Angiography and IVUS Before and After Rotablator

The target lesion (arrow 1) appears more severe by ultrasound (arrow 2). Following Rotablator, there is calcium ablation without injuring the relatively normal wall on the diagonal side of the artery.

2. **Mechanism of Lumen Enlargement.** IVUS is very useful for identifying the mechanisms of lumen enlargement after all devices. IVUS has shown that dissection represents the most common mechanism of luminal enlargement after PTCA (Figure 31.11), but stretching of the vessel wall constitutes the principal or exclusive mechanism in some patients;[4,15] lumen enlargement from plaque "compression" or redistribution is an unusual mechanism of PTCA effect. In contrast to balloon angioplasty, plaque removal is the primary mechanism of luminal enlargement after DCA

(Figure 31.12); however, tissue removal is incomplete since 40-60% of the cross-sectional area of the target lesion is still occupied by plaque.[17,18] IVUS has also shown that Rotablator works by plaque ablation (Figure 31.11),[19] ELCA results in dissection and minimal vessel expansion without plaque ablation, and stenting results in the greatest lumen enlargement and virtually eliminates elastic recoil.

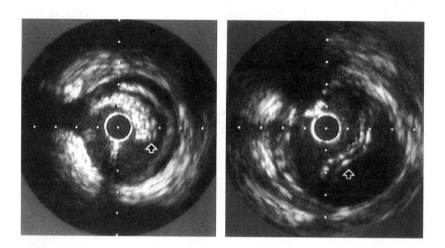

Figure 31.11 Complex Dissection After PTCA

A deep dissection (black arrow, left) is associated with a large intimal flap (black arrow, right).

3.   **Precise Quantitative Measurements.** Therapeutic decisions often hinge upon assessment of lumen dimensions, stenosis severity, diameter of the "normal" reference diameter, and the gain in lumen diameter after intervention. Precise quantitation of vascular dimensions represents an important application of IVUS. Angiographic and IVUS studies after PTCA reveal a poor correlation of final lumen diameter. Since angiographically "normal" segments often have occult atherosclerosis, [10] this could lead to undersizing of devices by angiography. However, there are no prospective data to document a need for device sizing by IVUS, either to improve safety or reduce late cardiac events.

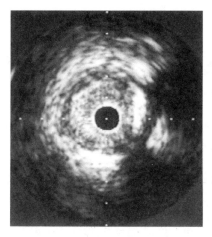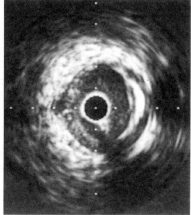

Figure 31.12 IVUS Before and After DCA

Although the angiogram shows an eccentric lesion, IVUS demonstrates a concentric plaque (left). There is little residual plaque after DCA (right).

4. **Guide Directional Atherectomy.** The improved spatial perspective by IVUS could theoretically assist in orienting the AtheroCath (Figure 31.12), but in practice, the precise orientation of the IVUS image remains a difficult challenge. Careful ultrasound interrogation before atherectomy can identify anatomic landmarks such sidebranches, which can be used to help orient the IVUS image. Some operators use sequential ultrasound examinations between passes to determine the extent of plaque removal and assess the need for additional cuts. Ultrasound can also be used to determine the normal vessel diameter and appropriate device size. With currently available DCA devices, the depth and extent of calcification can dramatically affect the efficiency of plaque removal: Although fluoroscopic calcification has been considered a contraindication to directional atherectomy, IVUS suggests that lesions with deep calcification can undergo successful atherectomy. In contrast, the presence of superficial calcification, which may not be detectable by fluoroscopy,[16] precludes successful tissue removal by DCA; Rotablator atherectomy is useful in these situations. "Optimal" DCA involves the use of atherectomy and adjunctive PTCA to achieve final diameter stenoses < 15%. Although the Optimal Atherectomy Restenosis Study (OARS) suggested that IVUS can be used to achieve optimal results, the Balloon vs. Optimal Atherectomy Trial (BOAT) demonstrated that similar results could be achieved without IVUS. Preliminary experience with an integrated ultrasound-DCA catheter (GDCA) suggests the feasibility of ultrasound-guided DCA, but further studies are needed.

5. **Coronary Stent Deployment (Chapter 26).** IVUS studies have demonstrated that despite excellent angiographic appearance, some stents are incompletely apposed to the vessel wall (Figure 31.13) and/or asymmetrically expanded. A single-center, retrospective analysis suggested that the level of systemic anticoagulation may be safely reduced if optimal stenting is confirmed by IVUS (Table 31.6); these IVUS observations have led to the routine use of high-pressure balloons to fully deploy stents. While IVUS-guidance can further lumen dimensions after routine anatomic high-pressure balloon inflations,[24] results from the AVID (Angiography vs. Intravasular ultrasound-Directed Stent Placement) trial have not shown a beneficial effect on 30-day clinical event rate (longterm results are pending).[25] Other randomized studies (STARS, Stent Anticoagulation Regimen Study) are in progress to determine the value of IVUS as an adjunct to stenting, and for identifying suitable patients for low-intensity anticoagulation regimens (Chapter 26).

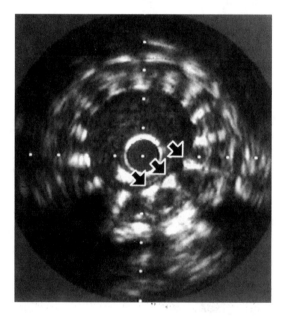

Figure 31.13 Suboptimal Stent Deployment

After deployment of a Palmaz-Schatz stent at 18 atmospheres, several stent struts are not opposed to the vessel wall (black arrows); subsequent inflations with a larger balloon resulted in optimal stent deployment.

Table 31.6. IVUS Criteria for Optimal Stent Deployment

Stent Result	Gap*	CSA Index**	Symmetry Index***
Inadequate	> 0.3 mm	< 0.6	< 0.5
Marginal	0.1 - 0.3 mm	0.6 - 0.8	0.5 - 0.7
Optimal	< 0.1 mm	≥ 0.8	> 0.7

* Gap = Maximum distance between stent strut (or coil) and underlying

** CSA Index = ratio of minimal cross-sectional area (CSA) or stent/CSA or normal reference vessel (average CSA proximal and distal to stent)

*** Symmetry Index = ratio of stent minor diameter/stent major diameter

6. **Characterize Dissection After Intervention.** IVUS confirms single or multiple dissections in 40-80% of lesions after successful PTCA,[8] which typically occur at the junction between hard and soft plaque (Figures 31.2, 31.11). IVUS can also determine the depth and extent of dissection, which may range from superficial intimal disruption to extensive peri-adventitial dissection. IVUS can also determine the true longitudinal extent of a dissection, and can assist in determining how many stents are needed and where they should be placed. The superiority of IVUS compared to other imaging modalities is certain; however, prospective studies have not yet demonstrated better early or late outcome in patients undergoing IVUS-guided intervention.

I. **COMPARISON OF IVUS, ANGIOSCOPY AND DOPPLER FLOW.** Doppler coronary flow measurements and angioscopy represent alternative modalities now commonly used during interventional procedures. The relative value of each of these modalities is summarized in Table 31.7.

J. **NEW INTRAVASCULAR IMAGING DEVICES.** Future technical advances in IVUS technology include 0.014-0.018 inch IVUS guidewires; combination devices incorporating IVUS imaging and percutaneous revascularization (PTCA, DCA); and refinements in signal processing to allow more definitive correlation with the tissue histology. Software enhancements will permit routine longitudinal and 3-dimensional image reconstruction.

K. **SUMMARY AND RECOMMENDATIONS.** There is no question that IVUS provides a great deal of information about vessel dimensions and plaque morphology that cannot be achieved by other imaging modalities. However, the fact that this information can be used to select a certain type or size of device does not necessarily confirm that such a selection will lead to fewer complications or better long-term outcome. Furthermore, routine use of IVUS for all interventional cases can lead to

Table 31.7. Comparison of Imaging and Doppler Techniques

	Digital Angiography	Angioscopy	IVUS	Doppler Flowire
Vessel lumen detail	+	++++	++	-
Vessel wall detail	-	-	++++	-
Vessel dimensions	++	-	++++	-
Coronary flow	++	-	+	++++
Borderline lesions	+	++	+++	++++
Ostial lesions	+	-	+++	++
Detect diffuse disease	+	+++	++++	-
Suboptimal results	+	+++	+++	+++
Clot vs dissection	±	++++	+++	-
Continuous record	-	-	-	+++
Predict complications	+	Possible	Possible	+++
Predict restenosis	±	-	Possible	Possible
Microvascular disease	-	-	-	+++
Cause ischemia	-	+++	++	-

Abbreviation: IVUS = intravascular ultrasound

- = no value

± = limited value

+ - ++++ = increasing value

substantial increases in cost, particularly in large volume centers. Nevertheless, the following recommendations may be useful for the majority of interventional cardiologists:

- Experience in the performance and interpretation of IVUS is strongly recommended.
- For operators who perform only PTCA, IVUS can be useful for:
  ‣ Studying "borderline" lesions, to determine the need for intervention.
  ‣ Balloon sizing in questionable situations.
- For operators who perform PTCA and all other interventional devices, IVUS can be useful for:
  ‣ Studying borderline lesions, to determine the need for intervention.

- ▸ Device sizing in questionable situations.
- ▸ Detailed assessment of fluoroscopically-calcified vessels to guide therapy.
- ▸ Assessment of "suboptimal" results to distinguish dissection from "residual plaque," and to guide subsequent therapy.
- ▸ Suboptimal results after stenting to determine the need for further high-pressure inflations with a larger balloon.

* * * * *

REFERENCES

1. Zir LM, Miller SW, Dinsmore RE, Gilber JP, Harthorne JW. Interobserver variability in coronary angiography. Circulation 1976;53:627-632.

2. Vlodaver Z, Frech R, van Tassel RA, Edwards JE. Correlation of the antemortem coronary angiogram and the postmortem specimen. Circulation 1973;47:162-168.

3. White CW, Wright CB, Doty DB, Hirtza LF, et al. Does visual interpretation of the coronary arteriogram predict the physiologic importance of a coronary stenosis? N Engl J Med 1984;310:819-24.

4. Waller BF: "Crackers, breakers, stretchers, drillers, scrapers, shavers, burners, welders, and melters": The future treatment of atherosclerotic coronary artery disease? A clinical-morphologic assessment. J Am Coll Cardiol 1989;13:969-87.

5. Nissen SE, Gurley JC, Grines CL, Booth DC, et al. Intravascular ultrasound assessment of lumen size and wall morphology in normal subjects and coronary artery disease patients Circulation 1991;84:1087-1099.

6. St. Goar FG, Pinto FJ, Alderman EL, Fitzgerald PJ, et al. Detection of coronary atherosclerosis in young adult hearts using intravascular ultrasound, Circulation 1992;86:756-763.

7. Fitzgerald PJ, St. Goar FG, Connolly AJ, Pinto JF, et al. Intravascular ultrasound imaging of coronary arteries. Is three layers the norm? Circulation 1992;86:154-158.

8. Tobis JM, Mallery J, Mahon D, Lehmann K, et al. Intravascular ultrasound imaging of human coronary arteries in vivo. Analysis of tissue characterizations with comparison to in vitro histological specimens. Circulation 1991;83:913-926.

9. Nissen SE, Tuzcu EM, De Franco AC. Coronary intravascular ultrasound: Diagnostic and interventional applications. In: Topol EJ ed. Update to Textbook of Interventional Cardiology, W B Saunders, Philadelphia, PA, pages 207-222, 1994.

10. Nissen SE, De Franco AC, Raymond RE, Franco I, et al. Angiographically unrecognized disease at "normal" reference sites: a risk factor for sub-optimal results after coronary interventions. Circulation 1993;88:I-412A.

11. Glagov S, Weisenberg E,Zarins CK et al. Compensatory enlargement of human coronary arteries. N Engl J of Med 1987;316:1371-1375.

12. White CJ, Ramee SR, Collin TJ, Jain A, Mesa JE. Ambiguous coronary angiography: clinical utility of intravascular ultrasound. Cathet Cardiovasc Diagn 1992;26:200-203.

13. Tuzcu EM, Hobbs H, Rincon G , Bott-Silverman C , et al. Occult and frequent transmission of atherosclerosis coronary disease with cardia transplantation. Circulation 1995; 91:1706-1713.

14. Nissen SE, Grines CL, Gurley JC, Sublett K, et al. Application of a new phased-array ultrasound imaging catheter in the assessment of vascular dimensions: In vivo comparison to cineangiography. Circulation 1990;81:660-666.

15. DeFranco AC, Tuzcu E, Abdelmeguid A, Lincoff AM, et al. Intravascular ultrasound assessment of PTCA results: Insights into the mechanisms of balloon angioplasty. J Am Coll Cardiol 1993,21:485A.

16. Tuzcu EM, Berkalp B, De Franco AC, Ellis SG, et al. Dilemma of Diagnosing Coronary Calcification: Angiography vs. Intravascular Ultrasound. J Am Coll Cardiol 1995, (in press).

17. Popma JJ, Mintz GS et al. Clinical and angiographic outcome after directional coronary atherectomy. A qualitative and quantitative analysis using angiography and intravascular ultrasound. Am J Cardiol 1994;72:55E-64E.

18. DeFranco AC, Tuzcu EM, Moliterno DJ, et al. "Directional" coronary atherectomy removes atheroma more effectively from concentric than eccentric lesions: intravascular ultrasound predictors of lesional success. J Am Coll of Cardiol 1995;25:137A.

19. Kovach JA, Mintz GS, Pichard AD, Kent KM, et al. Sequential intravascular ultrasound characterization of the mechanism of rotational atherectomy and adjunct balloon angioplasty. J Am Coll Cardiol 1993;22:1024-1032.

20. Donohue TJ, Kern MJ, Aguirre FV, Bach RG, et al. Assessing the hemodynamic significance of coronary artery stenoses: analysis of translesional pressure velocity relations in patients. J Am Coll Cardiol 1993;22:449-458.

21. Kern MJ, Bach RG, Donohue TJ, Caracciolo EA, Aguirre FV. Coronary Stenoses with Low Translesional Gradient and Abnormal Flow Reserve. Cathet Cardiovas Diagn 1994;32:354-58.

22. Kern MJ, Donohue TJ, Aguirre FV, Bach RG, et al. Clinical Outcome of Deferring Angioplasty in Patients with a Normal Translesional Flow-Velocity Measurements. J Am Coll Cardiol 1995;25:178-187.

23. Patrick W. Serruys. Personal communication, Results of the Doppler Endpoints Balloon Angioplasty Trial Europe (DEBATE trial).

24. Russo RJ, Teirstein PS. Angiography versus intravascular ultrasound-directed stent placement. J Am Coll Cardiol 1996;March Special Issue.

25. Goldberg SL, Hall P, Nakamura S, et al. Is there a benefit from intravascular ultrasound when high-pressure stent expansion is routinely performed prior to ultrasound imaging? J Am Coll Cardiol 1996;March Special Issue.

32

CORONARY ANGIOSCOPY

Brian Annex, MD
Barry Kaplan, MD
Robert D. Safian, MD

Although early coronary angioscopes were limited by their large diameters and inflexibility,[1] new flexible catheters with advanced fiberoptics now permit direct visualization of the luminal surface of virtually all native coronary arteries and bypass grafts. Several studies confirm the superiority of angioscopy to contrast angiography in detecting and differentiating plaque, dissection, and thrombus.[2-4] Because optimal use of new devices and adjunctive pharmacotherapy requires accurate detection of thrombus and other intraluminal details,[5,6] angioscopy and other imaging modalities may play an increasingly important role in guiding interventional therapy (Table 32.1).

A. **THE TECHNIQUE OF CORONARY ANGIOSCOPY.** The most widely used angioscope in the United States is the Baxter-Edwards coronary angioscope (Figure 32.1). The system is a monorail design, is compatible with virtually all 8F guiding catheters and 0.014-inch guidewires, and consists of a high intensity light source, a fiberoptic imaging bundle with over 2000 individual fibers, a video monitor for on-line imaging, and a videotape recorder for image archiving, storage, and retrieval. Despite its flexibility, advancement of the angioscope up to the lesion requires good guiding catheter support and the use of an extra-support guidewire. A blood-free field is obtained by gently inflating the occlusion cuff on the angioscope and simultaneously injecting warm heparinized saline (or Lactated Ringers solution) through the irrigation port via a power injector. Special care must be taken to avoid overinflation of the occlusion cuff, since the highly compliant material can rapidly expand to 6 mm in diameter and induce vessel injury. During slow and gentle cuff inflation, simultaneous viewing of the fluoroscopic image (to watch for balloon overinflation) and video monitor (to identify when a blood-free field has been achieved) is required. In general, imaging time (i.e., cuff inflation) should be limited to 45-90 seconds to minimize myocardial ischemia. In most cases, the angioscope can be safely advanced through the lesion, and excellent images can be obtained during pullback. However, if loosely adherent thrombus is identified, the angioscope should not be advanced through the lesion because of the risk of distal embolization. Once imaging is complete, the occlusion cuff is deflated and the angioscope removed.

B. **INDICATIONS FOR CORONARY ANGIOSCOPY (Table 32.2)**

1. **Guiding Saphenous Vein Graft Interventions.** Percutaneous interventions in saphenous vein grafts are limited by a high incidence of complications and restenosis.[7] Although there are no large scale clinical trials demonstrating a clear benefit of angioscopy in vein graft lesions, we frequently use angioscopy to guide therapeutic strategies based on its superior ability (compared to angiography) to detect intraluminal thrombus, friable plaque, and post-procedural dissection.[8,9] If thrombus is identified by angioscopy, we perform transluminal extraction atherectomy (TEC);

Table 32.1. Comparison of Imaging and Doppler Techniques

	Digital Angiography	Angioscopy	IVUS	Doppler Flowire
Vessel lumen detail	+	++++	++	-
Vessel wall detail	-	-	++++	-
Vessel dimensions	++	-	++++	-
Coronary flow	++	-	+	++++
Borderline lesions	+	++	+++	++++
Ostial lesions	+	-	+++	++
Detect diffuse disease	+	+++	++++	-
Suboptimal results	+	+++	+++	+++
Clot vs dissection	±	++++	+++	-
Continuous record	-	-	-	+++
Predict complications	+	Possible	Possible	+++
Predict restenosis	±	-	Possible	Possible
Microvascular disease	-	-	-	+++
Cause ischemia	-	+++	++	-

Abbreviation: IVUS = intravascular ultrasound
- = no value
± = limited value
+ - ++++ = increasing value

if angioscopy confirms thrombus removal, the vein graft is stented. [10] If significant thrombus persists, a larger TEC cutter or PTCA (in conjunction with intragraft lytic therapy) is used; stenting in the presence of thrombus is contraindicated due to the risk of subacute thrombosis.[11,12] If angioscopy confirms the original lesion does not contain thrombus, stenting is perform without TEC. Loose friable material in vein grafts identifies a high risk population for transient or sustained no-reflow.[13,14]

2. **Evaluation of Suboptimal Results.** Evaluation of the "hazy" or suboptimal result after percutaneous intervention may be the most valuable role for angioscopy, [15] given its ability to distinguish between thrombus, dissection, and plaque. [15,16] If thrombus is identified, treatment strategies might include systemic or intracoronary thrombolytic therapy, local delivery of heparin or urokinase, or TEC atherectomy. In contrast, if haziness is caused by an obstructive dissection

flap, stenting or directional atherectomy is indicated; thrombolytic drugs would not be useful, and might increase the risk of complications.

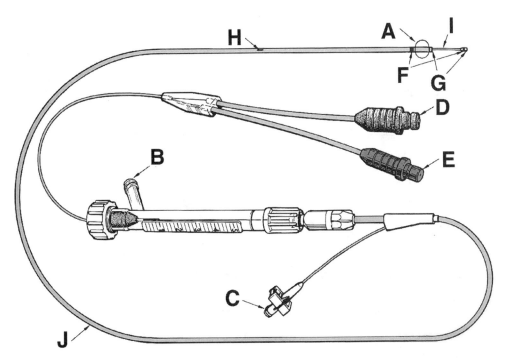

Figure 32.1 The ImageCath Coronary Angioscope

A. Balloon. B. Flush Port. C. Balloon Inflation Port. D. Video Connector. E. Light Connector. F. Radiopaque Markers. G. Tip of Shaft and Imaging Core. H. Guidewire Exit. I. Moveable Imaging Core. J. Catheter Shaft.

3. **Post-Interventional Assessment.** Angioscopic evaluation after stent placement may be used to determine the adequacy of stent expansion, [17] and the nature of residual filling defects. Such filling defects could be due to thrombus, which is treated with thrombolytic drugs and longterm anticoagulation, or residual plaque or dissection protruding through stent struts, which is treated by additional stenting. Angioscopy has also been used to evaluate the effects of laser angioplasty and atherectomy, [9,18,19] and remains the gold-standard for evaluating the efficacy of thrombus removal.

4. **Assessment of Borderline Lesions.** In some cases, angioscopy can be used to assess lesions of intermediate severity, particularly when associated with typical symptoms or other objective signs of ischemia. However, other modalities such as Doppler flow analysis (Chapter 33) and

Table 32.2. Indications for Angioscopy

- Guiding Saphenous Vein Bypass Graft Interventions

- Evaluation of suboptimal results

- Post-intervention assessment

- Assessment of borderline lesions

- Identification of "culprit" lesions

- Predicting the outcome after intervention

intravascular ultrasound (Chapter 31) are probably superior to angioscopy for this purpose, since they provide objective physiologic data (Doppler) or quantitative analysis (ultrasound), which cannot be derived from angioscopy.

5. **Identification of Culprit Lesions.** Given the high incidence (43-80%) of thrombus in de novo unstable lesions,[20] and angioscopy's ability to detect thrombus (and the yellow lipid-rich plaques frequently associated with thrombus[21,22]), angioscopy may be useful for identifying the "culprit" lesion in patients with multivessel disease and unstable or post-infarction angina.

6. **Predicting Outcome after Intervention.** While angioscopic thrombus may be associated with a higher incidence of restenosis after percutaneous intervention,[24] angioscopy's ability to predict acute or longterm outcome is controversial: In one study, plaque color, lesion ulceration, and thrombus were not predictive of PTCA success or complications.[25] Yet, in another report, angioscopic (but not IVUS) findings were important predictors of 1-year outcome using a variety of devices.[26]

D. **LIMITATIONS OF ANGIOSCOPY (Table 32.3).** Angioscopy provides qualitative morphologic information, but in contrast to Doppler analysis and IVUS, does not provide quantitative analysis of flow or lumen dimensions. Angioscopy is also suboptimal for imaging aorto-ostial lesions (due to difficulty ensuring a blood-free imaging field) and proximal LAD or circumflex lesions (due to the need for transient occlusion of the left main coronary artery). Furthermore, blood flow from adjacent sidebranches may obscure the imaging field and preclude image analysis. Currently available angioscopy catheters lack steerability, limit the field of view, and lack some sensitivity and specificity for detecting endoluminal lesions;[27] steerable designs are under investigation.

E. **COMPLICATIONS (Table 32.4).** In general, angioscopy is a safe adjunct to other percutaneous interventions. Complications are unusual and appear to be related to operator experience.[28] In a

Table 32.3. Limitations of Angioscopy

- Does not provide quantitative data

- Inability to reliably image aorto-ostial lesions

- May lead to transient ischemia or hemodynamic instability

- Not safe for imaging lesions at the origin of the LAD or LCX

multicenter registry of 1746 procedures, angiographic complications included dissection (due to the guidewire, occlusion cuff, or imaging bundle) in 2.8% and abrupt closure in 1.0%. Coronary artery perforation due to rupture of the occlusion cuff has been reported in one patient.[29] Improper technique can also lead to air emboli from the flush solution. Although severe angiographic complications are unusual, 9% of lesions treated with PTCA may require a "touch-up" balloon inflation after angioscopy to smooth out the final result. [30] Angioscopy of degenerated vein grafts has been shown to induce transient or sustained no-reflow in nearly 50% of lesions, and identifies a high-risk subgroup for sustained no-reflow after further intervention. [13] Although cuff inflation lasting more than 60 seconds can induce transient myocardial ischemia, the overall incidence of major ischemic complications is < 1%. [28]

Table 32.4. Complications of Angioscopy

Angiographic Complications (%)[13,20]	
Dissection *	2.8
Abrupt closure **	1.0
No-reflow***	45
Clinical Complications (%)[20]	
Death	0.1
MI	0.2
CABG	0.5
VF	1.7

Abbreviations: MI = In-hospital q-wave myocardial infarction; CABG = emergency coronary bypass grafting; VF = ventricular fibrillation
* Dissection due to occlusion cuff, guidewire, or imaging bundle
** Managed by stents or emergency CABG
*** Degenerated vein grafts

* * * * *

REFERENCES

1. Sherman TC, Litvack F, Grundfest W, et al. Coronary angioscopy in patients with unstable angina pectoris. N Eng J Med 1986;315:913-919.

2. Litvack F, Grundfest WS, Lee ME, et al. Angioscopic visualization of blood vessel interior in animals and humans. Clin Cardiol 1985;8:65-70.

3. Grundfest WS, Litvack F, Sherman T, et al. Delineation of peripheral and coronary detail by intraoperative angioscopy. Ann Surg 1985;202:394-400.

4. Sanborn TA, Rygaard JA, Westbrook BM, et al. Intraoperative angioscopy of saphenous vein and coronary arteries. J Thorac Cardiovasc Surg 1986;91:339-343.

5. King SB III. Role on new technologies in balloon angioplasty. Circulation 1991;84:2574-2579.

6. Forrester JS, Eigler N, Litvack F: interventional Cardiology: The decade ahead. Circulation 1991;84:942-944.

7. Schweiger MJ, Roccario E, Weil T. Treatment of patients following bypass surgery: a dilemma for the 1990s. Am Heart J 1992;123:268-272.

8. White CJ, Ramee SR, Collins TJ, et al. Percutaneous angioscopy of saphenous vein coronary bypass grafts. J Am Coll Cardiol 1993;21:1181-1185.

9. Annex, BH, Larkin TJ, O'Neill WW, et al. Evaluation of thrombus removal by transluminal extraction coronary atherectomy by percutaneous coronary angioscopy. Am J Cardiol 1994;74:606-609.

10. Annex BH, Ajluni SC, Larkin TJ, et al. Angioscopic guided interventions in a saphenous vein bypass graft. Cathet Cardiovasc Diagn 1994;31:330-333.

11. Nath FC, Muller DWM, Ellis SG, et al. Thrombosis of a flexible coil coronary stent: frequency, predictors and clinical outcome. J Am Coll Cardiol 1993;21:622-627.

12. Hermann HC, Buchbinder M, Clemen MW, et al. Emergent use of balloon-expandable coronary artery stenting for failed percutaneous transluminal coronary angioplasty. Circulation 1992;86:812-819.

13. Kaplan BM, Safian RD, Grines CL, et al. Usefulness of adjunctive angioscopy and extraction atherectomy before stent implantation in high-risk aorto-coronary saphenous vein grafts. Am J Cardiol 1995;76:822-824.

14. Tilli FV, Kaplan BM, Safian RD, Grines CL, O'Neill WW. Angioscopic plaque friability: A new risk factor for procedural complications following saphenous vein graft interventions. J Am Coll Cardiol (in-press).

15. White CJ, Ramee SR, Collins TJ, et al. Percutaneous coronary angioscopy: Applications in interventional cardiology. J Interven Cardiol 1993;6:61-67.

16. Sassower MA, Abela GS, Koch JM, et al. Angioscopic evaluation of periprocedural and postprocedural abrupt closure after percutaneous coronary angioplasty. Am Heart J 1993;126:444-450.

17. Teirstein PS, Schatz RA, Rocha-Singh KJ, et al. Coronary stenting with angioscopic guidance. J Am Coll Cardiol 1992;19:223A.

18. Nakamura F, Kvasnicka J, Uchida Y, et al. Percutaneous angioscopic evaluation of luminal changes induced by excimer laser angioplasty. Am Heart J 1992;124:1467-1472.

19. Eltchaninoff H, Cribier A, Koning R, et al. Comparative angioscopic findings after rotational atherectomy and balloon angioplasty. J Am Coll Cardiol 1995;25:95A.

20. Waxman S, Mittleman MA, Manxo K, Saaower M, et al. Culprit lesion morphology in subtypes of unstable angina as assessed by angioscopy. Circulation 1995;92:I-79.

21. Waxman S, Saaower M, Mittleman MA, Nesto RW, et al. Characterization of the culprit lesion underlying thrombus: Insights from angioscopy. Circulation 1995;92:I-353.

22. Uchida Y, Nakamura F, Tomaru T, Mortia T, et al. Prediction of acute coronary syndromes by percutaneous coronary angioscopy in patients with stable angina. Am Heart J 1995;130:195-203.

23. Silva JA, Escobar A, Collins TJ, Ramee SR, White CJ. Unstable angina. A comparison of angioscopic findings between diabetic and nondiabetic patients. Circulation 1995;92:1731-1736.

24. Bauters C, Lablanche JM, McFadden E, Hamon M, Bertrand ME. Angioscopic thrombus is associated with a high risk of angiographic restenosis. Circulation 1995;92:I-401.

25. Waxman S, Mittleman MA, Saaower M, Kowalker W, Nesto RW. Can angioscopy predict initial procedural success of PTCA in acute coronary syndromes? Circulation 1995;92:I-785.

26. Feld S, Ganim M, Vaughn WK, Kelly R, et al. Utility of angioscopy and intravascular ultrasound in predicting outcome following coronary intervention. Circulation 1995;92:I-18.

27. Uretsky BF, Denys BG, Counihan P, et al. Accuracy of angioscopy in diagnosing endoluminal lesions. J Am Coll Cardiol;1994:23:407A.
28. Lablanche, JM, Geschwind H, Cribier A, et al. Coronary angioscopy safety survey: European multicenter experience. J Am Coll Cardiol 1995;25:154A.
29. Wolff, MR, Resar JR, Stuart RS, et al. Coronary artery rupture and pseudoaneurysm formation resulting from percutaneous coronary angioscopy. Cathet Cardiovasc Diagn 1993;28:47-50.
30. Alfonso F, Hernandez R, Goicolea J, et al. Angiographic deterioration of the previously dilated coronary segment induced by angioscopic examination. Am J Cardiol 1994;74:604-606.

33

INTRACORONARY DOPPLER BLOOD FLOW MEASUREMENTS

Terry T. Bowers, MD
Robert D. Safian, MD

A. INTRODUCTION TO CORONARY FLOW RESERVE. Myocardial blood flow is regulated by changes in vascular resistance at the level of the coronary arteriole (Table 33.1). As myocardial O_2 demand increases (e.g., exercise), there is a decrease in resistance (coronary vasodilatation) and an increase in blood flow. Coronary flow reserve (CFR), defined as the ratio of hyperemic-to-resting blood flow velocity,[8] is typically > 2. In the presence of a flow-limiting epicardial stenosis, the distal microvasculature dilates to preserve resting basal blood flow;[7] however, maximal hyperemic flow is impaired and CFR is < 2. CFR and other blood flow measurements can be safely, easily, and reliably obtained in the cath lab with the use of the Cardiometrics FloWire, a flexible, steerable 0.014" or 0.018" guidewire with a tip-mounted piezoelectric Doppler crystal (Figure 33.1).[2-4] Ultrasound Doppler signals are transmitted from the tip of the FloWire to the FloMap Instrument, where they are converted to a spectral display on the monitor (Figure 33.2). Preliminary data suggest that the Doppler wire may be of adjunctive value in a variety of clinical and interventional settings (see Section C, below).[8-14]

B. APPROACH TO DOPPLER BLOOD FLOW

1. **Doppler Systems (Table 33.2).** Older 3F Doppler catheters have been largely replaced by the Cardiometrics FloWire.

Table 33.1. Determinants of Coronary Vascular Resistance

Physiologic	Pharmacologic
Autoregulation	Norepinephrine
Increased myocardial O_2 consumption	Papaverine
Sympathetic stimulation	Dipyridamole
	Serotonin
	Vasopressin
	Acetylcholine
	Nitroglycerin
	Adenosine
	EDRF (Nitric Oxide)

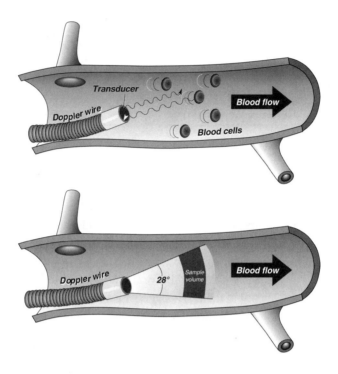

Figure 33.1 Coronary Blood Flow: Doppler Measurements

The ultrasound beam (28°) provides a large sample volume, which ensures measurement of peak flow velocity with minimal dependence on guidewire position. The sample volume is 5 mm and 4 mm from the tip of the 0.018-inch and 0.014-inch FloWire, respectively.

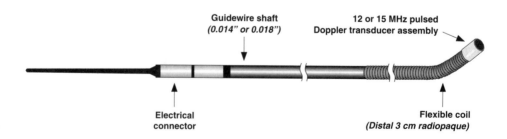

Figure 33.2 Doppler FloWire Construction

Courtesy of Cardiometrics, Inc.

Table 33.2. Doppler Systems for Coronary Blood Flow Velocity Measurements

Device	Size	Crystal Position	Display	Range Gate (mm)	Doppler Signal Analysis	Frequency Shift	Validation Study (Ref.#)
Numed™	3F (1.0 mm)	Side-mounted	Chart recorder	1-10	Zero-cross	20 MHZ	64,65
Millar™	3F (1.0 mm)	End-mounted	Chart recorder	1-10	Zero-cross	20 MHZ	66
Flowire*™	0.018" 0.014"	End-mounted	On-line Spectral Display	5.2	Fast fourier transform	12 MHZ	67

*   Cardiometrics

2. **Coronary Blood Flow Data.** Spectral flow velocity data, along with ECG and arterial blood pressure recording, are displayed in real time on the FlowMap monitor. In addition to coronary flow reserve — the parameter used to assess the functional significance of a lesion before and after intervention — other blood flow measurements can be obtained including the beat-to-beat phasic average peak velocity (APV), diastolic-to-systolic velocity ratio (DSVR), APV trend over 1.5-90 minutes, and the proximal-to-distal translesional velocity ratio. The "normal" range of Doppler-derived flow velocity variables has been defined (Table 33.3),[3,4,16-22] but interpretation of each variable must be considered in the context of other Doppler variables, angiographic features, and clinical characteristics of the patient.[2,3] One possible limitation to the use of Doppler is that it measures changes in coronary blood flow velocity rather than volumetric flow. However, if the cross-sectional area of the artery remains constant between basal and hyperemic conditions, changes in flow velocity parallel changes in volumetric flow. Administration of intracoronary nitroglycerin can be used to minimize differences in vessel dimensions between basal and hyperemic conditions, and improve the reliability of CFR measurements. [15]

   a. **Coronary Flow Reserve (CFR).** CFR is defined as the ratio of hyperemic-to-baseline coronary blood flow velocity. Values > 2 are normal, while values < 2 suggest the presence of a functionally-significant epicardial obstruction. Several pharmacologic agents can be used to induce maximum (hyperemic) flow velocity (Table 33.4). In our cath lab, intracoronary adenosine is the preferred vasodilator because of its short duration of action, ease of use, and proven safety. CFR is the most useful of all the Doppler measurements; it is used primarily to assess the physiologic significance of a stenosis and the functional status of the distal microvascular bed before and after coronary intervention.

   b. **Blood Flow Velocity.** The instantaneous peak velocities are used to derive the average peak velocity, mean velocity, and time-area relationship (integral) of diastolic and systolic velocity averaged over two cardiac cycles. The diastolic to systolic velocity ratio (DSVR)

Table 33.3. Doppler-Derived Flow Velocity Parameters

Variable	Normal Reference Range	Reference
Average Peak Velocity (APV)		3,4,16
Basal	≥ 20 cm/sec	
Hyperemic	≥ 30 cm/sec	
Diastolic/Systolic Mean Velocity Ratio (DSVR)		3,4,16,17
LAD	> 1.7	
LCX	> 1.5	
RCA	> 1.2*	
Proximal/Distal Mean Velocity Ratio (PDR)†	< 1.7	3,4,16-18
Distal Coronary Flow Reserve (CFR)	≥ 2.0	19-22

*   Normal CFR > 1.4 in distal RCA or PDA
†   Also called Translesional Velocity Gradient (TVG)

Table 33.4. Drugs for Maximal Vasodilations

Drug	Dose	Duration	Reference
Adenosine			20,68,69
IC	RCA 6-10 mcg (bolus) LAD/LCX 12-20 mcg (bolus)	20-45 seconds	
IV	100-150 mcg/kg/min	45 seconds after drip discontinued	
Papaverine			70
IC	5-10 mg	45-150 seconds	
IV	*	*	
Dipyridamole			71
IV	0.56 mg/kg over 4 mintues	Peak 4-minutes Duration 20-40 minutes	

*   Intravenous infusion is not recommended because of a slow systemic excretion; drug accumulation may lead to systemic hypotension.

and average peak velocity (APV) are displayed continuously on the monitor and updated every 2 seconds.

c. **Limitations of Translesional Velocity Gradients and Coronary Flow Reserve**. The application of intracoronary Doppler velocimetry demands an in-depth understanding of the limitations of the technique (Table 33.5).[2,24,25] Importantly, abnormalities of the microcirculation may decrease CFR and confound its interpretation. CFR may also be sensitive to changes in hemodynamic conditions, such as tachycardia (increases CFR), hypertension (decreases CFR), and increased contractility (increases CFR); fractional flow reserve (FFR), defined as the ratio of distal hyperemic APV-to-mean aortic pressure, may be independent of hemodynamic changes and particularly useful in the presence of hemodynamic changes.[26] CFR may be less useful for assessing the functional significance of a residual stenosis in acute MI patients treated with PTCA because of the known impairment of CFR in this setting. [27] Since conditions associated with impaired microcirculation have little regional variability, normal CFR in a vessel without an epicardial stenosis reliably excludes small vessel disease as a cause of decreased CFR in a vessel with a significant epicardial stenosis.

C. **CLINICAL APPLICATIONS.** Because of the limited ability of quantitative angiography and translesional pressure gradients to assess lesion morphology and stenosis severity,[1-11] several techniques are now commonly used as adjuncts to coronary angiography, including angioscopy (Chapter 32), intravascular ultrasound (Chapter 31), and Doppler blood flow measurement. These techniques should not be viewed as competitive technologies; rather, each provides complementary information that may be extremely useful during angiography and intervention (Table 33.6). The current standard for the physiologic assessment of coronary artery disease in the cath lab is coronary flow reserve, which has both clinical and interventional applications (Table 33.7).

1. **Clinical Applications**
   a. **Syndrome X.** The "gold standard" for the diagnosis of Syndrome (myocardial ischemia due to impaired coronary microcirculation) is the finding of abnormal CFR in the presence of angiographically "normal" epicardial arteries.[30] Since significant aortic stenosis and other causes of severe left ventricular hypertrophy can also cause angina and a low CFR,[31-33] they should be excluded before making a diagnosis of Syndrome X.

   b. **Cardiac Transplantation.** CFR may be useful in identifying rejection and diffuse coronary atherosclerosis (i.e., transplant arteriopathy),[34] and may help guide therapeutic intervention in cardiac transplant patients.

   c. **Bypass Surgery.** Saphenous vein grafts can normalize CFR;[35,36] differences in resting phasic blood flow between internal mammary and venous conduits may have implications for longterm patency.

Table 33.5. Technical and Anatomic Factors: Impact on Doppler Data

Factor	Potential Effect
Doppler Wire Technical Considerations	
1. Inappropriate on-line IPV tracking	APV and DSVR may be falsely low; CFR and TVG calculated from APV may be erroneous.
2. Inappropriate ECG gating from QRS	False diastolic and systolic time intervals; Erroneous DSVR.
3. Unstable phasic Doppler signal	APV may be falsely low.
4. Doppler probe not positioned to assess peak flow velocity	APV may be falsely low.
Translesional Velocity Gradient (TVG, PDR) may be influence by:	
1. Ostial lesions	No proximal valve to assess lesion.
2. Single unbranched conduits	TVG may be falsely low.
3. Tortuous vessels	Unable to obtain reliable distal peak velocity.
4. Diffuse distal disease	Falsely low TVG secondary to falsely elevated distal velocity.
5. Tandem/sequential lesions	Falsely low TVG secondary to falsely elevated distal velocity (distal lesional flow acceleration).
6. Eccentric lesions	Falsely high TVG secondary to falsely elevated proximal velocity (acceleration at lesional flow convergence).
Coronary Flow Reserve (CFR) may be influence by:	
1. Abnormal microcirculation (hypertrophy, diabetes, connective tissue disease, prior myocardial infarction, (Syndrome X)	May falsely lower CFR.
2. Sequential lesions	Distal CFR is the result of the combined physiologic effect of all lesions.
3. Changes in vasomotor tone	May falsely lower CFR.
4. Submaximal vasodilator dose	May falsely lower CFR.
5. Transient increase in distal flow	May falsely lower CFR.
6. Varying Doppler wire position between baseline and hyperemic assessment	May falsely lower CFR.
7. Varying hemodynamic conditions	May falsely lower CFR

Table 33.6. Comparison of Imaging and Doppler Techniques

	Digital Angiography	Angioscopy	IVUS	Doppler Flowire
Vessel lumen detail	+	++++	++	-
Vessel wall detail	-	-	++++	-
Vessel dimensions	++	-	++++	-
Coronary flow	++	-	+	++++
Borderline lesions	+	++	+++	++++
Ostial lesions	+	-	+++	++
Detect diffuse disease	+	+++	++++	-
Suboptimal results	+	+++	+++	+++
Clot vs dissection	±	++++	+++	-
Continuous record	-	-	-	+++
Predict complications	+	Possible	Possible	+++
Predict restenosis	±	-	Possible	Possible
Microvascular disease	-	-	-	+++
Cause ischemia	-	+++	++	-

Abbreviation: IVUS = intravascular ultrasound
- = no value
± = limited value
+ - ++++ = increasing value

    d. **Myocardial Infarction.** CFR has been used to study flow dynamics in the acute[37,38] and recovery [39] periods after myocardial infarction, and may predict recovery of microcirculatory and contractile function.[40,41]

2. **Interventional Applications**
    a. **Intermediate Lesions.** CFR is a reliable means of assessing the physiologic significance of intermediate or borderline lesions.[8-14,18-22] CFR can often identify the "culprit" lesion in patients with multivessel coronary disease who present with "unstable" angina without ECG changes, and can be used to identify borderline lesions requiring intervention. Normal translesional velocity gradient and/or CFR suggest the presence of non-flow-limiting obstruction(s); intervention may be safely deferred in such lesions.[28,29]

Table 33.7. Applications of Coronary Blood Flow Velocity

Clinical Applications

- Intermediate lesions

- Identify Syndrome X

- Identify transplant arteriopathy

- Bypass grafts

- Myocardial infarction

Interventional Applications

- Assess suboptimal results

- Predict complications (trending)

- Assess no-reflow

- Monitor UK infusions

- Dynamic turbulence

b. **"Suboptimal" Results.** Coronary blood flow velocity may be used to assess the results of percutaneous intervention; normalization of average peak velocity and diastolic-to-systolic velocity ration (DSVR) have been reported after successful PTCA,[3,4] DCA,[42] ELCA,[42] Rotablator,[43] and stent implantation.[44,45] In contrast, normalization of CFR after PTCA is unusual, although immediate Palmaz-Schatz stenting of "successfully" dilated lesions may normalize CFR.[45,49-51] These data suggest that in addition to further lumen enlargement, another potential use of stenting is to improve flow abnormalities after PTCA. "Suboptimal" results after intervention, characterized by intraluminal haziness, moderate residual stenosis, or non-flow-limiting dissection may be ideal indications for Doppler flow assessment, to determine the need for further intervention. Preliminary data from the Doppler Endpoint Balloon Angioplasty Evaluation (DEBATE) study suggest that distal flow velocity measurements after PTCA can predict recurrent ischemia and restenosis.[52] The Doppler wire can be used as an alternative to a conventional PTCA guidewire.[53]

c. **Complications ("Trending") (Table 33.8).** The FloMap can be placed in "trend mode" to record continuous coronary blood flow velocity over time; "trending" is most commonly used following coronary intervention to identify angiographically-inapparent flow impairment due to dissection, vasospasm, platelet aggregation, or changes in vasomotor tone.[54-57] It is possible that post-intervention "trending" can be used to identify patients with unstable flow patterns

Table 33.8. Continuous Doppler-Flow Velocity Patterns (Trending)

Pattern	Cause
Abrupt flow acceleration	Transient spasm
Abrupt flow cessation	Vasovagal reaction
Abrupt flow deceleration	Abrupt closure
Cyclical flow variations	Abrupt closure/thrombus

who may benefit from stents or new antiplatelet agents.[59]

d. **Urokinase Infusions.** Repeat angiographic studies are usually required to identify vessel patency after prolonged (8-48 hours) infusions of intracoronary urokinase for the revascularization of chronic total occlusions. In these situations, continuous monitoring with a Doppler wire may indicate restoration of distal flow, obviating the need for repeat angiography.

e. **No-Reflow.** In our laboratory, patients at risk for "no-reflow" are monitored during intervention to assess the utility of intracoronary verapamil for restoring flow. Doppler flow velocity may also be used to distinguish inapparent residual stenosis from microvascular dysfunction after primary PTCA for acute MI.[60,61]

f. **Dynamic Turbulence.** A new application of the "trend" mode is measurement of dynamic flow velocity for the assessment of stenosis severity.[62] Mechanical pull-back of the Doppler guidewire from the distal to proximal artery may result in transient high velocity recordings, reflecting turbulent flow. Preliminary data suggest that turbulent blood flow may lead to underestimation of CFR in 20% of patients after PTCA.[63] Proponents of this technique believe that dynamic assessment will complement instantaneous assessment of DSVR and CFR.

* * * * *

REFERENCES

1. Benchimol A, Stegall HF, Gartlan JL. New method to measure phasic coronary blood velocity in man. Am Heart J 1971;81:93-101.
2. Doucette JW, Corl PD, Payne HM, et al. Validation of a Doppler guidewire for intravascular measurement of coronary artery flow velocity. Circulation 1992;85:1899-1911.
3. Segal J, Kern MJ, Scott NA, King III SB, et al. Alterations of phasic coronary artery flow velocity in humans during percutaneous coronary angioplasty. J Am Coll Cardiol 1992;20:276-286.
4. Ofili EO, Kern MJ, Labovitz AJ, St. Vrain JA, et al. Analysis of coronary blood flow velocity dynamics in angiographically normal and stenosed arteries before and after endoluminal enlargement by angioplasty. J Am Coll Cardiol 1993;21:308-316.
5. Marcus ML, Chilian WM, Kanatuka H, Dellsperger KC, et al. Understanding the coronary circulation through studies at the microvascular level. Circulation 1990;82:1-7.
6. Bone RM, Rubio R. Coronary circulation, in Berne R, Sperelakis N, (eds): Handbook of Physiology, Section 2: The Cardiovascular System, Volume 1, The Heart. Baltimore, Williams & Wilkins CO, 1979, pp 873-952.
7. Wilson RF, Laxson DD. Caveat Emptor: A clinician's guide to assessing the physiologic significance of arterial stenoses. Cathet Cardiovasc Diagn 1993;29:93-98.
8. Gould KL, Lipscomb K, Hamilton GW. Physiologic basis for assessing critical coronary stenosis. Am J Cardiol 1974;33:87-94.
9. Gould KL, Lipscomb K, Calvert J. Compensatory changes of the distal coronary vascular bed during progressive coronary constriction. Circulation 1975;51:1085-1094.
10. Kirkeeide R, Gould KL, Parsel L. Assessment of coronary stenoses by myocardial imaging during coronary vasodilation. VII. Validation of coronary flow reserve as a single integrated measure to stenosis severity accounting for all its geometric dimensions. J Am Coll Cardiol 1986;7:103-113.
11. Gould KL, Kirkeeide R, Buchi M. Coronary flow reserve as a physiologic measure of stenosis severity. Part I. Relative and absolute coronary flow reserve during changing aortic pressure. Part II. Determination from arterographic stenosis dimensions under standardized conditions. J Am Coll Cardiol 1990;15:459-474.
12. Demer L, Gould KL, Kirkeide RL. Assessing stenosis severity: Coronary flow reserve, collateral function, quantitative coronary arteriography, position imaging, and digital subtraction angiography: a review and analysis. Prog Cardiovasc Dis 1988;30:307-322.
13. Gould KL. Identifying and measuring severity of coronary artery stenosis: quantitative coronary arteriography and position emission tomography. Circulation 1988;78:237-245.
14. Wilson RF, Marcus ML, White CW. Prediction of the physiologic significance of coronary arterial lesions by quantitative lesion geometry in patients with limited coronary artery disease. Circulation 1987;75:723-732.
15. Shammas NW, Thondapu V, Gerasimou EM, Antonio J, et al. Effect of pretreatment with nitroglycerin on coronary flow reserve measured using bolus intracoronary adenosine. Circulation 1995;92:I-264.
16. Ofili EO, Lasovitz AJ, Kern MJ. Coronary flow velocity dynamics in normal and diseased arteries. Am J Cardiol 1993;71:3D-9D.
17. Kajiya F, Ogasawara Y, Tsujioka K, et al. Analysis of flow characteristics in post-stenotic regions of the human coronary artery during bypass graft surgery. Circulation 1987;76:1092-1100.
18. Donohue TJ, Kern MJ, Aguirre FV, Bach RG, et al. Assessing the hemodynamic significance of coronary artery stenosis. Analysis of translesional pressure-flow velocity relations in patients. J Am Coll Cardiol 1993;22:449-458.
19. Kern MJ, Aguirre FV, Bach RG, Caracole EA, Donohue TJ. Translesional pressure-flow velocity assessment in patients: Part I. Cathet Cardiovasc Diagn 1994;313:49-60.
20. Kern MJ, Deligonul, Tatineni S, Serota H, et al. IV adenosine continuous infusion and low dose bolus administration for determination of coronary vascular reserve in patients with and without coronary artery disease. J Am Coll Cardiol 1991;18:718-729.
21. Miller DD, Donohue TJ, Younis LT, Bach RG, et al. Correlation of pharmacologic Technesium 99m-Sestamibi

myocardial perfusion imaging with post-stenotic coronary flow reserve in patients with angiographically intermediate coronary artery stenoses. Circulation 1994;89:2150-2160.

22. Joye JD, Schulman DS, Lesorde D, Farah T, et al. Intracoronary Doppler guide wire versus stress single-photon emission computer tomographic thallium 201 imaging in assessment of intermediate coronary stenoses. J Am Coll Cardiol 1994;24:940-947.

23. Gadallah S, Thaker KB, Kawanishi D, Rashtian M, et al. Comparison of the hyperemic response to intracoronary and intravenous adenosine by intracoronary Doppler flow recording. Circulation 1995;92:I-326.

24. White CW, Wilson RF, Intracoronary Doppler Ultrasound in Nanda P (ed): Doppler Ultrasound. Philadelphia, Lea & Febiger, 1994, pp 403-412.

25. McGinn AL, White CW, Wilson RF. Interstudy variability of coronary flow reserve. Influence of heart rate, arterial pressure and ventricular preload. Circulation 1990;81:1319-1330.

26. De Bruyne B, Bartunek J, Stanislas US, et al. Feasibility and hemodynamic dependency of invasive indexes of coronary stenosis. Circulation 1995;92:I-324.

27. Claeys MJ, Vrints CJ, Bosmans JM, Cools F, et al. Coronary flow reserve measurement during coronary angioplasty in the infarct related vessel. Circulation 1995;92:I-326.

28. Kern MJ, Donohue TJ, Aguirre FV, Bach RG, et al. Clinical outcome of deferring angioplasty in patients with normal translesional pressure-flow velocity measurements. J Am Coll Cardiol 1995;25:178-187.

29. Lesser JT, Wilson RF, White CW. Physiologic assessment of coronary stenosis of intermediate severity can facilitate patient selection for coronary angioplasty. Coronary Art Dis 1990;1:697-705.

30. Cannon RO III, Camici PG, Epstein SE. Pathophysiological dilemma of Syndrome X. Circulation 1992;85:883-892.

31. Marcus ML, Doty DB, Hirratzka LF, Wright CB, Enpthan CE. Decreased coronary reserved a mechanism of angina pectoris in patients with aortic stenosis and normal coronary arteries. N Eng J Med 1982;37:1362-1366.

32. Houghton JL, Prisant LM, Carr AA, van Dohlen TW, Frank MJ. Relationship of left ventricular mass to impairment of coronary vasodilator reserve in hypertensive heart disease. Am Heart J 1991;21:1107.

33. Cannon RO, Bonow RO, Bacharach SL, et al. Left ventricular dysfunction in patients with angina pectoris, normal epicardial coronary arteries, and abnormal vasodilator reserve. Circulation 1985;71:218-226.

34. McGinn AL, Wilson RF, Olisan MT et al. Coronary vasodilator reserve following human orthotopic cardiac transplantation. Circulation 1988;78:1200-1209.

35. Wilson RE, Wilson ML, White CW. Effects of coronary bypass surgery and angioplasty on coronary blood flow and flow reserve. Prog Cardiovasc Dis 1988;31:95-114.

36. Wilson RE, White CW. Does coronary bypass graft surgery restore normal CFR. The effect of diffuse atherosclerosis and focal obstruction lesions. Circulation 1987;76:563-571.

37. Stewart RE, Bowers TR, Ponto R, Miller DD, et al. Coronary Doppler flow velocity and PET myocardial blood flow are highly correlated and predict post-infarction perfusion in patients with TIMI-3 flow. J Am Coll Cardiol 1995;25:427A.

38. Aguirre FV, Donohue TJ, Bach RG, Caracole EA, et al. Coronary flow velocity of infarct-related arteries: Physiologic differences between complete (TIMI III) and incomplete (TIMI 0,I,II) angiographic coronary perfusion. J Am Coll Cardiol 1995;25:401A.

39. Ishihara M, Sato H, Tateishi H, Kawagoe T, Shimatani Y, et al. Time course of impaired coronary vasodilatory reserve after reperfusion in acute myocardial infarction. J Am Coll Cardiol 1995;25:2008A.

40. Wakatsuk T, Nakamura M, Tsundoa T, Ui K, Degawa T, Yamaguchi T. Coronary angioplasty predicts recovery of regional wall motion in acute myocardial infarction. J Am Coll Cardiol 1995;25:161A.

41. Kim HS, Tahk SJ, Shin JH, Kim W, Cho YK, et al. Coronary flow reserve in infarct related artery and myocardial viability in patients with recent myocardial infarction. Circulation 1995;92:I-600.

42. Segal J. Applications of coronary flow velocity during angioplasty and other coronary interventional procedures. Am J Cardiol 1993;71:17D-25D.

43. Bowers TR, Stewart RE, O'Neill WW, Reddy VM, et al. Plaque pulvariation during Rotablator atherectomy: does it impair coronary flow dynamics? J Am Coll Cardiol 1995;25:96A.

44. Bach R, Kern MJ, Bell C, et al. Clinical application of coronary flow velocity for stent placement during coronary

angioplasty. Am J Heart 1993;125:873-880.

45. Bowers TR, Safian RD, Stewart RE, Benzuly KH, et al. Normalization of CFR after stenting, but not after PTCA. J Am Coll Cardiol 1996 (in-press).

46. Larman DJ, Serruys PW, Suryapranata H, et al. Inability of coronary blood flow reserve measurements to assess the efficacy of coronary angioplasty in the first 24-hours in unselected patients. Am Heart J 1991;122:631-639.

47. Wilson RF, Johnson MR, Marcus ML, Aylward PEG, et al. The effect of coronary angioplasty on coronary flow reserve. Circulation 1988;77:873-885.

48. Kern MJ, Deligonul U, Vandormael M, Labovitz A, et al. Impaired coronary vasodilator reserve in the immediate post coronary angioplasty period: Analysis of coronary artery flow velocity indexes and regional cardiac venous efflux. J Am Coll Cardiol 1989;13:860-872.

49. Kern MJ, Aguirre FV, Donohue TJ, Bach RG, et al. Impact of residual lumen narrowing on coronary flow after angioplasty and stent: Intravascular ultrasound Doppler and imaging data in support of physiologically-guided coronary angioplasty. Circulation 1995;92:I-263.

50. Verna E, Gil R, Di Mario C, Sunamura M, Gurne O, Porenta G. Does coronary stenting following balloon angioplasty improve distal coronary flow reserve? Circulation 1995;92:I-536.

51. Haude M, Baumgart D, Caspari G, Erbel R. Does adjunct coronary stenting in comparison to balloon angioplasty has an impact on Doppler flow velocity parameters? Circulation 1995;92:I-547.

52. The D.E.B.A.TE. Study Group. Are flow velocity measurements after PTCA predictive of recurrence of angina or of a positive exercise stress test early after balloon angioplasty? Circulation 1995;92:I-264.

53. The D.E.B.A.T.E. Study Group. Doppler guide wire as a primary guide wire for PTCA. Feasibility, safety, and continuous monitoring of the results. Circulation 1995;92:I-263.

54. Eichhorn E, Grayburn PA, Willard JE, Anderson HV, et al. Spontaneous alterations in coronary blood flow velocity before and after coronary angioplasty in patients with severe angina. J Am Coll Cardiol 1991;17:43-52.

55. Anderson HV, Kirkeeide RL, Stuart Y, Smalling RW, et al. Coronary artery flow monitoring following coronary interventions. Am J Cardiol 1993;71:62D-69D.

56. Kern MJ, Donohue TJ, Bach RG, Aguirre FV, Bell C. Monitoring cyclical coronary blood flow alterations following coronary angioplasty for stent restenosis using a Doppler guidewire. Am Heart J 1993;125:1159-1160.

57. Kern MJ, Aguirre FV, Donohue TJ, Bach RG, et al. Continuous coronary flow velocity monitoring during coronary interventions: Velocity trend patterns associated with adverse events. Am Heart J 1994;128:426-34.

58. The D.E.B.A.T.E. Study Group. Cyclic flow variations after PTCA are predictive of immediate complications. Circulation 1995;92:I-725.

59. Anderson HV, Revana M, Rosales O, Brannigan L, et al. Intravenous administration of monoclonal antibody to the platelet GP IIb/IIIa receptor to treat abrupt closure during coronary angioplasty. Am J Cardiol 1992;69:1373-1376.

60. Yaniyama Y, Iwakure K, Ito H, Takiuchi S, et al. Coronary flow velocity pattern in patients with TIMI flow grade 2: Its relation to residual coronary stenosis and microvascular dysfunction. Circulation 1995;92:I-149.

61. Nemoto T, Kimure K, Shimizu T, Mochida Y, et al. Coronary artery flow velocity waveform in acute myocardial infarction with angiographic no-reflow. Circulation 1995;92:I-325.

62. Geschwind HJ, Melnik L, Kvasnicka J, Dupouy P. Dynamic detection of coronary stenosis by Doppler-tipped guidewire. J Am Coll Cardiol 1995;25:336A.

63. Ferrari M, Werner GS, Nargang L, Figulla HR. Turbulent flow as a cause for underestimating the coronary flow reserve. Circulation 1995;92:I-77.

64. Wilson RF, Laughlin DE, Ackell PH, Chilian WM. Transluminal subselective measurement of coronary blood flow velocity and vasodilator reserve in man. Circulation 1985;72:82-92.

65. White CW, Marcus ML, Wilson RF. Methods of measuring coronary flow in humans. Prog Cardiovasc Dis 1988;31:79-94.

66. Sibley DH, Millar HD, Hartley CJ, Whitlow PL. Subselective measurement of coronary blood flow velocity using a steerable Doppler catheter. J Am Coll Cardiol 1986;8:1332-1340.

67. Vanyi J, Bowers TR, Jarvis G, White CW. Can an intracoronary Doppler wire accurately measure changes in coronary blood flow velocity? Cathet Cardiovasc Diagn 1993;29:240-246.

68. Zijlstra F, Juilliere Y, Serruys PW, Roelandt JRTC. Value and limitations of intracoronary adenosine for the assessment of coronary flow reserve. Cathet Cardiovasc Diagn 1988;15:76-80.
69. Wilson RF, Wych K, Christensen BV, Zimmer S, Laxson DD. Effects of adenosine on human coronary arterial circulation. Circulation 1990;82:1595-1606.
70. Wilson RF, White CW. Intracoronary papaverine: An ideal vasodilator for studies of the coronary circulation in conscious humans. Circulation 1986;73:444-452.
71. Ranhosty A, Kempthorne-Rawson J. Intravenous Dipyridamole Thallium Imaging Study Group. The safety of intravenous dipyridamole thallium myocardial perfusion imaging. Circulation 1990;81:1205-1209.

34 ADJUNCTIVE PHARMACOTHERAPY

Sandeep Khurana, M.D.
Gerald C. Timmis, M.D.
Mark Freed, M.D.

ANALGESIA AND SEDATION

Premedication to ease anxiety and discomfort without compromising patient cooperation and ventilation is usually achieved by combination of an analgesic and sedative. Popular combinations include a narcotic such as hydromorphone HCl (Dilaudid, 0.2-0.5 mg IV) and a short-acting benzodiazepine like midazolam (Versed, 0.25-0.5 mg IV) or diazepam (Valium, 2-5 mg IV). Other useful narcotics include morphine sulfate (1-2 mg IV), fentanyl (Sublimase, 1-2 mcg/kg IV), and meperidine (Demerol, 25-50 mg IV). Fentanyl, an extremely potent narcotic, is not associated with significant hypotension or nausea at low doses; but may cause excessive respiratory depression. Demerol is contraindicated in patients who have received monoamine oxidase (MAO) inhibitors within 14 days due to unpredictable and potentially fatal reactions; these can manifest either as respiratory depression, hypotension and coma, or as paradoxical agitation, seizures, hypertension and hyperpyrexia. Severe reactions should be treated with IV hydrocortisone (100-250 mg IV); when hypertension and hyperpyrexia coexist, chlorpromazine (25 mg IV Q 6-8 hrs) may be of additional value. Demerol should be used cautiously, if at all, in patients with renal failure due to the risk of seizures from toxic accumulation of the metabolite normeperidine. Infiltration of warm xylocaine pre-heated to 37-43°C may reduce the discomfort of local anesthesia.[1,2]

CONTRAST REACTIONS

A. **PROPHYLAXIS AGAINST CONTRAST REACTIONS.** Prophylactic medical therapy is recommended for all patients with a history of urticaria, bronchospasm, or anaphylaxis after previous exposure to radiocontrast agents. No regimen is fully protective. However, premedication started at least 12 hours before contrast exposure has been shown to reduce the risk of recurrent anaphylaxis from 40% to less than 10%.[3,4] "Standard" prophylaxis includes a corticosteroid (prednisone 40-60 mg, solumedrol 40-60 mg IV, hydrocortisone 100 mg IV), and an antihistamine, Benadryl (25-50 mg) given 18, 12, and 6 hours prior to the procedure; most regimens now omit H_2 blockers or use it as an option. Intravenous hydrocortisone (100 mg) and Benadryl (25-50 mg) may also be administered intravenously just prior to the case. In patients with a previous anaphylactic reaction to contrast, it may be prudent to withhold β-blockers the morning of the case in the event a β-agonist (e.g., epinephrine) is required

Table 34.1. Contrast Reactions: Presentation, Onset, and Treatment

Type	Presentation	Onset	Treatment
Minor	Nausea, burning sensation, flushing, mild urticaria without hives, minor bradycardia or vasovagal episodes.	Usually occurs within minutes of exposure	Requires intervention infrequently. Treatment is supportive, including observation and cool compresses; oral benadryl and atropine (0.5-1.0 mg IV) are occasionally needed.
Moderate	Persistent nausea with vomiting, anaphylactoid reaction (urticaria with hives and tongue swelling), bradycardia or vasovagal episodes that persist or produce hypotension.	Usually occur within minutes to hours of exposure.	Usually requires intervention. Treatment includes IV fluids, Benadryl (50 mg IV), steroids (e.g. hydrocortisone 100 mg IV), centrally-acting antiemetics (e.g., Compazine 2 mg IV followed by a 25 mg rectal suppository), and atropine (0.5-2.0 mg for bradycardia or vasovagal reactions). Anaphylactoid reactions are also treated with epinephrine (0.1-0.5 mg of a 1:1,000 dilution subcutaneously every 5-15 minutes as necessary).
Severe	Anaphylaxis (bronchospasm, laryngeal edema and/or profound hypotension.	May occur immediately with a single contrast injection.	Life-threatening and requires aggressive attention. Epinephrine (1-5cc of a 1:10,000 solution via IV or ET tube every 5 min as needed), steroids (e.g., hydrocortisone 100mg IV followed by solumedrol 125 mg IV), Benadryl (50 mg IV), and possible intubation. Bronchodilator treatments (e.g., Albuterol aerosol 2.5 mg nebulized mist every 1-2 hrs) might be of benefit.

to treat a recurrent episode. When emergency angiography is performed in a non-prophylaxed patient, IV premedications are given, a low-osmolar contrast agent is used, and biplane angiography is performed to minimize dye load.

B. TREATMENT OF CONTRAST REACTIONS (Table 34.1)

PREVENTION OF ABRUPT CLOSURE (Table 34.2)

A. ANTIPLATELET THERAPY

1. **Aspirin (ASA).** Preprocedural administration of aspirin reduces the risk of abrupt coronary occlusion after PTCA by 50-75% and is standard therapy for all coronary interventional procedures.[5,6] Other beneficial cardiovascular effects include the primary prevention of coronary

Table 34.2. Pharmacotherapy for Coronary Intervention

Drug	Effect on		Indication and Dose
	Abrupt Closure	**Restenosis**	
Aspirin	↓	-	*Elective PTCA:* 325 mg/d at least one day prior to procedure; continue indefinitely. Urgent PTCA: 4 chewable baby aspirins (total: 325 mg).
Dipyridamole	-	-	Not routinely used.
Ticlopidine	↓	-	*Aspirin-intolerant or aspirin-allergic patient*: 250 mg po bid started 3-5 days prior to intervention. Also used for many stent protocols.
ReoPro	↓/-	↓	*High-risk PTCA or atherectomy*:* 0.25 mg/kg IV bolus and 10 mcg/min IV infusion x 12 hrs. Low-dose heparin and early sheath removal to minimize bleeding.
Heparin	↓	-	*All cases:* Intraprocedural bolus (~ 10,000 units IV) and supplements to maintain HemoTec ACT at 250-300 sec or HemoChron ACT at 300-350 sec. (Higher ACTs may confer some additional benefit but bleeding is increased.) Suboptimal angiographic outcome (thrombus, severe dissection, impaired flow): IV infusion (10-15 U/kg/hr) to maintain PTT at 60-90 sec x 12-48 hrs.
Coumadin	-	-	*Suboptimal stent result:* 10 mg po daily x 2-4 d; maintenance 1-5 mg/day to maintain INR at 2-3 (or higher in select cases)..
LMW Heparin	↓/-	-	Not routinely used.
Intracoronary lytics	↓/-	-	*Dissolution of intracoronary thrombus:* Urokinase (75,000-500,000 units i.c.), SK (250,000 units i.c.), or tPA (10-20 mg i.c.) over 5-45 min.
Dextran	-	-	Rarely used.
Nitrates	-	-	*Prevent/reverse coronary artery spasm or ischemia unrelated to balloon inflation:* Nitroglycerin 100-200 mcg i.c. or IV bolus; maintenance infusion of 10-20 mcg/min, increasing at 10-40 mcg/min increments every 3-5 min. until clinical effect or BP < 100 mm Hg.
β-blockers	-	-	*Possibly to delay/prevent onset of balloon-induced ischemia:* Propranolol - oral: 20-80 mg bid-tid; IV: 5 mg. Metoprolol - oral: 50-100 mg bid; IV: 5 mg. Esmolol: 500 mcg/kg over 1 min; infusion of 25-100 mcg/kg/min. May need to repeat bolus..

Drug	Effect on		Indication and Dose
	Abrupt Closure	**Restenosis**	
Calcium antagonists	-	$\downarrow$/-	***Possibly to delay/prevent onset of balloon-induced ischemia:*** Nifedipine: 0.1 mg i.c.; diltiazem: 10-30 mg IV bolus & infusion of 15 mg over 30-60 min; nicardipine: 0.2 mg i.c. ***Coronary spasm:*** nifidipine: 10 mg sublingual ***No-reflow:*** Verapamil: 100 mcg/min i.c. up to 1 mg; diltiazem: 0.5-2.5 mg slow i.c. up to 5-10 mg
Pressors	-	-	***Norepinephrine (Levophed):*** initial dose: 8-12 mcg/min; titrate to desired BP. Usual maintenance: 2-4 mcg/min. ***Phenylephrine (neosynephrine):*** Initial dose: 0.1-0.18 mg/min; as BP stabilizes, rate to 0.04-0.06 mg/min.

$\downarrow$ Most data suggest a decreased incidence

- No effect or unknown effect

$\downarrow$/- Possible decreased incidence; data inconclusive

* Interim analysis from EPILOG trial suggest possible benefit in patients not at hish risk; not FDA-approved for this indication at the present time.

artery disease;[7] improved outcome in chronic stable angina,[8,9] unstable angina,[10-12] and acute MI;[13] maintenance of saphenous vein graft patency after coronary bypass surgery;[14] and reduction in stroke.

a. **Dose.** Although the optimal dose, timing, and duration of administration are unknown, it is customary to administer 325 mg of ASA at least one day before elective PTCA and continue it indefinitely. If urgent PTCA is required in patients who have not been receiving aspirin, 4 chewable baby aspirins (81 mg each) are given prior to the case. For the aspirin-allergic patient, ticlopidine (250 mg orally twice daily starting at least 3 days prior to intervention) can be used (see A2, below)[15]; other antiplatelet drugs such as dipyridamole, sulfinpyrazone, and dextran have not been studied and are not routinely recommended. Patients with unstable angina syndromes may be resistant to aspirin, but the impact of higher doses has not been studied. Newer slow-release oral and transdermal aspirin preparations may selectively inhibit platelet aggregation without inhibiting the syntheses of prostacyclin (PGI_2), a potent vasodilator and platelet inhibitor; it is unknown whether these preparations offer any advantage over conventional ASA.

    b. **Limitations.** Although aspirin inhibits the thromboxane A2-mediated platelet aggregation, it does not prevent platelet aggregation caused by thrombin, catecholamines, ADP, serotonin, or shear-stress. Thrombin generation and platelet activation may persist in some patients despite "adequate" aspirin and heparin therapy[16] but is difficult to detect in routine clinical settings such as PTCA and unstable angina.

2. **Ticlopidine** is a more potent antiplatelet agent than aspirin whose primary mechanism of action appears to be inhibition of ADP-mediated fibrinogen binding to the platelet GP IIb/IIIa receptor.[17,80] Ticlopidine also inhibits platelet aggregation in response to collagen, thrombin, and shear-stress,[18] and may enhance the antiaggregatory effects of prostacyclin[19] and promote deaggregation of thrombin-activated platelets.[20,21]

    a. **Dosing and Administration.** Ticlopidine (250 mg BID) should be administered for at least 3 days prior to the procedure to maximize its antiplatelet effect. Some data suggest that an oral loading of 500 mg PO BID may expedite the onset of antiplatelet effect,[22] which may confer some benefit in emergency situations. After ticlopidine is stopped, the antiplatelet effects gradually resolve over 1-2 weeks.[21]

    b. **Side Effects.** The most serious side effect of ticlopidine is neutropenia, which occurs in 1-2% of patients after 4 weeks of use and is almost always reversible; complete blood counts are, therefore, recommended every 2-4 weeks during the first few months of therapy. Nausea, vomiting and diarrhea are common and can be minimized by the administration of ticlopidine with food; skin rash and elevated transaminases are rare. Longterm administration of ticlopidine lowers plasma fibrinogen and increases cholesterol.

    c. **Clinical Use.** In a randomized trial of PTCA, ticlopidine (250 mg BID) resulted in fewer ischemic complications than the combination of aspirin and dipyridamole (2% vs. 5%).[15] Ticlopidine is recommended in the aspirin-allergic or intolerant patient; it is also widely used, but not yet approved, as an adjunct to stent implantation (Chapter 26). A randomized study of aspirin alone, aspirin and ticlopidine, and aspirin and Coumadin is underway to identify the best anticoagulation regimen after successful stenting (STARS, STent Anticoagulation Regimen Study). Ticlopidine has been shown to decrease vascular death and nonfatal MI in unstable angina,[23] and decrease the incidence of stroke in patients with carotid artery TIA's.[24] **Clopidogrel**, an analogue of ticlopidine, is currently undergoing clinical investigation in the CAPRIE (Clopidogrel vs. Aspirin in Patients at High Risk of Ischemic Events) trial.

    d. **Combination Therapy**. In patients with coronary artery disease, the combination of aspirin (50 mg/day) and ticlopidine (250 mg twice daily) demonstrated synergy in platelet inhibition.[25]

3. **Dipyridamole.** Compared to ASA alone, dipyridamole has not been shown to offer additional protection against abrupt closure.[26] One retrospective study reported that patients given IV dipyridamole had fewer ischemic complications;[27] in contrast, a randomized trial of dipyridamole (75 mg po QID) failed to demonstrate benefit.[26] Dipyridamole is not recommended for coronary interventions.

4. **Platelet Glycoprotein IIb/IIIa Receptor Antagonists.** Drugs that only block a single mediator or mechanism of platelet aggregation have had limited or no success at preventing abrupt closure or restenosis. Recently, advances in biotechnology have led to the development of potent inhibitors of the platelet glycoprotein IIb/IIIa (GP IIb/IIIa) receptor, the final common mediator of platelet aggregation in response to all possible agonists.

    a. **ReoPro**

        1. **Acute Closure and Restenosis.** The chimeric monoclonal antibody c7E3 (abciximab, *ReoPro*™, manufactured by Centocor and distributed by Eli Lilly and Company) has now been tested in several large-scale, placebo-controlled randomized trials. In the EPIC trial (Evaluation of c7E3 Fab in the Prevention of Ischemic Complications),[28] 2099 patients undergoing PTCA or atherectomy for unstable angina, acute MI, or high-risk coronary lesion morphology were randomized to receive bolus + maintenance infusion of ReoPro, bolus dose only, or placebo; all patients were also treated with aspirin (325 mg QD) and IV heparin during and for ≥ 12 hours after the procedure. Compared to placebo, patients receiving ReoPro bolus + infusion had 35% and 23% reductions in ischemic endpoints at 30-days and 6-months, respectively (Table 34.3); these benefits were observed in all patient subgroups. In addition, ReoPro reduced the need for target vessel repeat revascularization at 6 months. In the EPILOG trial, patients undergoing elective PTCA randomized to ReoPro (and low- or standard-dose heparin) had a lower incidence of death or MI (CPK 3x normal) at 30-days compared to placebo (plus standard-dose heparin) (Table 34.4). This benefit was observed without an increase in major bleeding events (1.8% vs. 3.1% for placebo + heparin group; p = NS). Because of these results, the main trial was stopped prematurely in December 1995. Enrollment was also stopped prematurely in the European CAPTURE trial (ReoPro vs. conventional medical therapy 18-24 hrs. prior to PTCA for medically-refractory unstable angina) due to a significant reduction in the combined endpoint of in-hospital death, MI, or emergency CABG in ReoPro-treated patients.

        2. **Bleeding Complications.** In the EPIC trial, ReoPro bolus + infusion resulted in ≥ 2-fold increases in major and minor bleeding events and transfusions compared to placebo. Independent predictors of major bleeding complications included older age, female gender, low body weight, ReoPro therapy, and increasing duration and complexity of the procedure. For patients receiving ReoPro, major bleeding occurred most often at the femoral access site (72%), was usually evident within 36 hours of treatment, and was transient and not associated with long-term events. Importantly, the incidence of intracranial hemorrhage, need for surgical intervention for major bleeding, and CABG-related major blood loss were similar between placebo and ReoPro-treated groups.

Table 34.3. EPIC Trial: 30-Day and 6-Month Outcomes

Event	Placebo[1] (n=696)	ReoPro	
		Bolus[2] (n=695)	Bolus + infusion[3] (n=708)
	Number of patients (%)		
30-DAY ENDPOINT*	89 (12.8)	79 (11.4)	59 (8.3)[+]
Components of 30-d endpoint			
Death	12 (1.7)	9 (1.3)	12 (1.7)
Acute MI in survivors	60 (8.6)	43 (6.2)	37 (5.2)
Urgent intervention	54 (7.8)	44 (6.4)	28 (4.0)
6-MONTH ENDPOINT**	241 (35.1)	224 (32.6)	189 (27.0)[+]
Components of 6-mo. endpoint			
Death	23 (3.4)	18 (2.6)	22 (3.1)
MI	72 (10.5)	55 (8.0)	48 (6.9)
Repeat TLR	141 (20.9)	133 (19.7)	99 (14.4)[+]
CABG	74 (10.9)	67 (9.9)	65 (9.4)

Abbreviations: MI = myocardial infarction, TLR = target lesion revascuarlization, CABG = coronary artery bypass grafting

* Death from any cause, nonfatal MI, CABG or repeat percutaneous intervention for acute ischemia, insertion of a stent for procedural failure, placement of an IABP to relieve refractory ischemia.
** Death, nonfatal MI, or need for PTCA or CABG.
+ $p < 0.01$ compared to placebo
1. Bolus + infusion of placebo.
2. 0.25 mg/kg 10-60 minutes prior to intervention.
3. 0.25 mg/kg 10-60 minutes prior to intervention followed by an infusion of 10 mcg/min for 12 hours.

To determine if weight-adjusted heparin could improve the safety profile of ReoPro while maintaining its clinical efficacy, the PROLOG pilot trial was conducted. One-hundred-three PTCA patients treated with ReoPro were randomized to standard-dose heparin (100 units/kg

Table 34.4. EPILOG Trial: Results at 30-Days from Interim Analysis of 1500 Patients

Event + (%)	Placebo+ Standard heparin[1]	ReoPro + Low-dose heparin[2]
Death	0.8	0.4*
Death + MI (> 3 x CPK)	8.1	2.6*
Death + MI (> 5 x CPK)	5.7	1.6*
Major bleeding	3.1	1.8
Stroke (hemorrhagic)	0	0.2

* $p < 0.001$ compared to placebo
1. Standard heparin: 100 U/kg/hr
2. ReoPro (0.25 mg/kg 10-60 min. prior to intervention followed by an infusion of 10 mcg/min for 12 hrs.) plus low-dose heparin (70 U/kg/hr).

bolus; additional boluses to achieve ACT of 300 seconds) or low-dose heparin (70 units/kg; no additional boluses prior to intervention). Patients in each group were further randomized to delayed sheath removal (heparin for ≥12 hours; sheaths removed 4 to 6 hours after discontinuation of heparin and ReoPro) or early sheath removal (heparin discontinued at end of PTCA; sheaths removed 4 to 6 hours later during the ReoPro infusion). Guidelines for timing of sheath removal included PTT 45 seconds or ACT ≤ 150 seconds; strict bed rest and limb immobilization for 6 hours after ReoPro infusion; and C-clamp or other mechanical compression device to achieve hemostasis during ReoPro infusion. Overall, the incidence of major bleeding unrelated to CABG was 1.9% (10.6% in the EPIC trial). In addition, minor bleeding and blood transfusions were lower in the low-dose heparin/early sheath removal group (bleeding: 20% vs. 3.9%; transfusions: 8% vs. 0%). These very encouraging results were supported in EPILOG, in which ischemic complications were reduced in patients receiving ReoPro + low-dose heparin *without* an increase in major bleeding events (ReoPro/low-dose heparin 1.8% vs. placebo/standard-dose heparin 3.1%, p=NS).

3. **Cost.** Results from the economic substudy of the EPIC trial are shown in Table 34.5. ReoPro was associated with a cost savings of $622 per patient due to fewer in-hospital ischemic complications, which was offset by a cost of $521 due to bleeding complications. Although ReoPro cost $1350, 6-month costs were comparable due to a 20% reduction in repeat revascularization and hospitalization in patients receiving ReoPro.

4. **Ongoing Clinical Trials (Table 34.6)**

Table 34.5. EPIC Trial: Estimated Costs of Baseline and Follow-Up Hospitalizations

Estimated Cost	ReoPro Bolus + Infusion	Placebo	Net (Cost)/Savings with Bolus + Infusion Treatment
Baseline Hospitalization	$ 13,401	$ 13,467	$ 66
ReoPro cost*	1,350	0	(1,350)
Follow-Up Hospitalization	3,392**	4,531	1,139
TOTAL	$18,143	$ 17,998	$ (145)

*   Typical per patient cost of approximately $1,350 at 1995 net wholesale price of $450/vial. Lilly Price Lists, 1995.
**   p = 0.034

Table 34.6. Ongoing Clinical Trials of ReoPro

Trial	Design
CAPTURE**: Chimeric 7e3 Fab AntiPlatelet antibody trial in Unstable angina Refractory to standard therapy	A randomized, placebo-controlled, multicenter trial enrolling 1,400 patients with refractory unstable angina. Evaluating the safety and efficacy of pretreatment with ReoPro when administered 18-24 hours prior to angioplasty.
EPILOG*: Evaluation of PTCA to Improve Longterm Outcome by c7E3 GP IIb/IIIa Receptor Blockade	*Main trial:* A double-blind, placebo-controlled, multicenter, 3-arm trial in which patients undergoing PTCA are randomized to: 1) ReoPro + low-dose weight-adjusted heparin; 2) ReoPro + standard-dose weight-adjusted heparin; and 3) placebo + standard-dose weight-adjusted heparin. This study excludes patients with unstable angina or acute MI. Recommendations for sheath management, transfusion guidelines, and nursing care are included. Six month angiographic follow-up will be performed in a subset of patients. *Stent substudy:* 1000 patients assigned to 1) PTCA + ReoPro; 2) Stent + placebo; or 3) Stent + ReoPro.
Readministration Trial	Evaluating the safety of repeat injections of ReoPro in patients with stable coronary artery disease.
RAPPORT: ReoPro in Acute MI and Primary PTCA Organization and Randomized Trial	To compare ReoPro versus placebo in acute MI patients undergoing primary PTCA.

.*   Main trial prematurely stopped in December 1995 after a review of the first 1500 patients revealed a significant reduction in ReoPro-treated patients for thecombined endpoint of death and MI (CK elevation) at 30-days.

**   Trial prematurely stopped in December 1995 after interim analysis revealed a significant reduction the the combined endpoint of in-hospital death, MI, or emergency CABG.

5. **Conclusions**. Bolus + infusion of ReoPro reduces acute ischemic complications and repeat target lesion revascularization in patients undergoing high-risk PTCA or atherectomy (EPIC trial). Interim analyses also indicate that ReoPro can reduce ischemic complications in patients undergoing elective PTCA (EPILOG trial), as well as in-hospital ischemic complications in patients undergoing PTCA for medically-refractory unstable angina (CAPTURE trial). Results from EPILOG suggest that these favorable clinical effects can now be achieved without an excess of major bleeding complications. Analyses of cost-effectiveness and longterm follow-up are forthcoming. This exciting antiplatelet agent is likely to play an increasingly important role in coronary intervention; ongoing investigation will determine its role an adjunct to stenting and thrombolytic therapy; and for the treatment of refractory intraprocedural thrombus ("Rescue ReoPro"). Detailed prescribing information, including indications, dosage, administration, drug interactions, adverse events, femoral artery access site hemostasis, and laboratory monitoring can be found on in Chapter 41.

b. **Integrelin.** Integrelin (manufactured by COR Therapeutics, distributed by Shering-Plough) is a synthetic cyclic heptapeptide antagonist of the platelet GPIIb/IIIa receptor. (Integrelin shares homology with a venom isolated from the southeastern pygmy rattlesnake, and has the ligand-mimetic KGD sequence). Like c7E3, Integrelin is administered intravenously and achieves rapid and profound inhibition of platelet aggregation. Unlike c7E3, its action is short, highly specific for the fibrinogen-GPIIb/IIIa receptor, and does not inhibit the binding of fibronectin and vonWillebrand Factor to GPIIb/IIIa.

To test its ability to reduce ischemic complications (and possibly restenosis) after PTCA, 150 patients were entered into the Integrelin to Manage Platelet Aggregation to Prevent Coronary Thrombosis (IMPACT) Pilot trial (Table 34.7). Compared to placebo, there was a trend toward fewer ischemic complications in patients receiving integrelin. In the larger IMPACT II trial, there appeared to be a paradoxical reduction in adverse outcome for elective but not high-risk patients.[81] There was no difference in major bleeding (Integrelin 5.2% vs. placebo 4.8%) or blood transfusions (Integrelin 5.8% vs. placebo 5.2%) between the Integrelin and placebo arms, but an increase in minor bleeding was seen (Integrelin 13% versus 9.3% with placebo). The PURSUIT trial is testing two dosing regimens of Integrelin infused for 72 hrs in 10,000 patients with unstable angina. The primary end-point of the study is death or MI at 30 days.

c. **Other Antiplatelet Agents.** Other promising agents under investigation include oral (Xemlofiban, Searle) and intravenous (Tirofiban, Merck & Co.) inhibitors of the platelet GPIIb/IIIa receptor, thromboxane receptor and synthetase antagonists (Ridogrel), serotonin antagonists (Ketanserin), prostacyclin analogues (Ciprostene), and platelet GPIb receptor antagonists.

B. ANTITHROMBOTIC AGENTS

1. **Heparin.** Intravenous heparin is always employed during PTCA and reduces the risk of abrupt closure. In the cath lab, heparin effect is measured by the activated clotting time (ACT), which is the time it takes for whole blood to form a firm, grossly-apparent clot in response to a potent procoagulant (kaolin or diatomaceous earth).

   a. **HemoTec vs. HemoChron Devices.** The ACT may be measured by the HemoTec or HemoChron devices:[29] The HemoTec ACT (HemoTec, Inc., Englewood, Colorado) uses kaolin to activate clotting and optically senses the "drop time" of a mechanical plunger. The HemoChron ACT (Interventional Technidyne Corp., Edison, New Jersey) uses diatomaceous earth (4% Celite) in a pre-warmed rotating glass tube to activate clotting; a magnet placed at the bottom of the tube is displaced when the clot achieves a certain degree of "firmness." A "therapeutic" ACT depends on which system is used: For the same heparin concentration, a higher ACT is obtained using the HemoChron compared to the HemoTec system. The ACT

Table 34.7. IMPACT Trial Results

Trial	Endpoint (%) [+]
IMPACT I Pilot (N = 150)	
Placebo	12.2
Integrelin bolus + 4-hr infusion[1]	9.6
Integrelin bolus + 12-hr infusion[2]	5.9*
IMPACT II (N = 4010)	
Placebo	11.4
Integrelin bolus + low-dose infusion[3]	9.2**
Integrelin bolus + high-dose infusion[4]	9.9

+   IMPACT I: death, MI, stenting, emergency PTCA or CABG
      IMPACT II: death, MI, or need for urgent intervention within 30 days
*   p = 0.18 vs. placebo
**   p = 0.063 vs. placebo
1,2 Bolus: 90 mcg/kg IV; infusion: 1.0 mcg/kg/min.
3   Bolus: 135 mcg/kg IV; infusion: 0.5 mcg/kg/min x 20-24 hrs.
4   Bolus: 135 mcg/kg IV; infusion: 0.75 mcg/kg/min x 20-24 hrs.

provides a relatively crude estimate of heparin effect;[36] ACT varies when arterial or venous blood are sampled.[30]

b. **"Therapeutic" ACT.** There are no objective standards to identify a "therapeutic" level of anticoagulation during PTCA. Therapeutic values during PTCA have been empirically derived from 1) the early cardiac surgery experience (i.e., ACT needed to prevent microemboli in the bypass circuit), and 2) from observations that ischemic complications after PTCA were increased in patients with an ACT < 250 sec (HemoTec),[33] but were rare (0.3%) when the final ACT was > 300 seconds. It is customary to keep the HemoChron ACT at 300-350 seconds and the HemoTec ACT 250-300 seconds; however, some interventionalists aim for higher values. ACT is usually sampled 3-5 minutes after a heparin bolus. The average heparin dose required to achieve an ACT > 300 seconds has been shown to vary with the anginal syndrome: 17,700 units for stable angina; 18,300 units for unstable angina; and 26,600 units for patients with acute myocardial infarction.[34] Although retrospective studies suggests an inverse relation between ACT and ischemic complications, ACTs ≥ 400 seconds have been associated with more bleeding complications.

c. **Heparin Protocol at William Beaumont Hospital (Figure 34.1).**

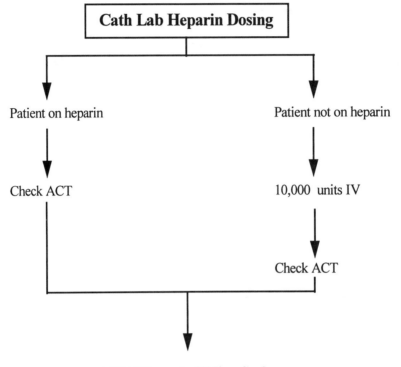

ACT / Heparin Sliding Scale:

ACT > 300 sec: no heparin; recheck ACT in 20 min

ACT 280-299 sec: 2000 units; recheck ACT in 5 min

ACT 250-279 sec: 5000 units; recheck ACT in 5 min

ACT 225-249 sec: 7000 units; recheck ACT in 5 min

ACT 200-224 sec: 8000 units; recheck ACT in 5 min

ACT < 200 sec: 10,000 units; recheck ACT in 5 min

Figure 34.1. ACT/Heparin Sliding Scale

d. Post-procedural Heparin:
The use of heparin after percutaneous therapy varies greatly among interventionalists. Since data are limited, therapy is largely empiric:

- **For elective PTCA and a good angiographic result**, data from the Beaumont Outpatient Angioplasty Trial (BOAT) demonstrate the safety of no further heparin, early sheath removal and patient discharge within 24 hours.[35]

- **For elective PTCA with a suboptimal result** (50% residual stenosis; significant dissection), the issue is stent vs. "prolonged" anticoagulation. In the pre-stent era, prolonged heparin (IV ± subcutaneous) or Coumadin was the rule; now, however, most would favor stenting (more reliable, more predictable, no bleeding) (Chapter 26).

- **For "unstable" angina and non-elective PTCA with a good angiographic result,** the issue of optimal heparin and timing of sheath removal is controversial. The ongoing HAPI (Heparin After Percutaneous Intervention) trial, a multicenter randomized prospective study of various heparin/sheath strategies, should help clarify this issue. In this trial, 1650 patients are being randomized into one of three arms:
  1. Heparin infusion at 13 u/kg/hr for 12-24 hrs, then sheaths out, then home.
  2. Heparin stopped after the procedure, sheaths out when ACT < 140, heparin restarted at 13 u/kg/hr for 12 hrs, then home.
  3. No heparin after procedure, sheaths out when ACT < 140, then home.

Post-procedural heparin infusions require meticulous monitoring to maintain the delicate balance between thrombotic and bleeding risks. Activated PTT's correlate with "therapeutic" heparin levels (0.2-0.4 units per ml) and provide a good estimate of bleeding risk. Bedside aPTT monitoring (Biotrack 512 portable aPTT machine, Ciba-Corning Diagnostics, Medfield, MA) yields immediate and accurate results, and has improved the maintenance and safety of therapeutic anticoagulation after coronary intervention. Prolonged heparin infusions are adjusted to maintain an ACT between 160-200 seconds or an aPTT of 2.0-2.5 times control values (i.e., 60-90 sec.) based on blood samples obtained at least twice daily. Since a rebound in thrombin generation[37] and increased risk of abrupt closure[38] may be temporally associated with discontinuation of heparin infusions, heparin should be discontinued at a time of the day when emergency revascularization is feasible.

e. Limitations. Heparin must bind with antithrombin III to exert its anticoagulant effect (i.e., catalyze the inactivation of thrombin and activated factor Xa). Despite its clinical efficacy, heparin's antithrombotic activity is limited by its: 1) inability to inactivate clot-bound thrombin;[39] 2) neutralization by platelet factor IV from platelet-rich thrombi; and 3) inactivation by fibrin II monomers, which are formed by the action of thrombin on fibrinogen. Accordingly, "therapeutic" concentrations of heparin, even when supplemented by intracoronary antithrombin III,[40] may not prevent propagation of a thrombus.[41]

f.   **Heparin-induced Thrombocytopenia** (platelet count <150,000/mm³). The incidence, time course, and clinical features of heparin-induced thrombocytopenia (HIT) and the more ominous heparin-associated thrombotic thrombocytopenia (HATT)[42] are shown in Table 34.8. Platelet transfusions should be avoided in the setting of heparin-induced thrombocytopenia because of the risk of thrombotic complications. An infusion of the prostacyclin analog Iloprost (Berlex laboratories), titrated to eliminate in-vitro heparin-induced platelet activation (infusion rates of 10 - 48 ng/kg/min), was successful in preventing a recurrence in 11 patients with confirmed HATT requiring a rechallenge with heparin during cardiovascular surgery.[42,43] Anticoagulation with defibrinating viper venoms like Ancrod or Reptilase, and with the heparinoid Org 10172, has also been performed when such patients require anticoagulation.[43] Low molecular weight heparin, which may reduce[44,45] but not eliminate[46] the risk of HIT, is also contraindicated in patients with a prior history of HATT.

2.   **Low Molecular Weight (LMW) Heparin.** LMW heparins are fragments of commercial grade heparin and are usually administered by subcutaneous injection. In contrast to unfractionated heparin, LMW heparins have less anti-thrombin activity and do not prolong the aPTT; their anticoagulant effect is mediated predominantly by inhibition of Factor Xa. LMW heparins have been used to prevent deep venous thrombosis and pulmonary embolism.[49] Preliminary studies during coronary intervention suggest no benefit over unfractionated heparin. Enoxaparin, a LMW heparin, failed to reduce angiographic or clinical restenosis in a randomized trial.[50]

3.   **Direct Thrombin Inhibitors (Hirudin and derivatives).** Hirudin, the naturally occurring anti-thrombin isolated from leech saliva, is an extremely potent and specific inhibitor of thrombin.[51,52] Unlike heparin, hirudin does not require Antithrombin III for its anticoagulant effect; in addition, hirudin forms a highly stable noncovalent complex with *circulating and clot-bound thrombin*, and is not inhibited by platelet factor 4. Hirudin[53] and hirulog[56,60] have been safely administered as alternatives to heparin in patients undergoing PTCA. In one report, hirulog was as effective as heparin in decreasing ischemic complications, and was associated with less bleeding (3.8% vs 9.8%; p < 0.001);[54] in addition, hirulog was associated with fewer ischemic complications than heparin for high-risk patients with post-infarct angina (9.1% vs. 14.2%; p=0.04). In the Hirudin European Trial versus Heparin in the Prevention of Restenosis after PTCA (HELVETICA),[55] 1141 patients undergoing PTCA for unstable angina were randomized to heparin or one of two hirudin regimens (all hirudin-treated patients received an intraprocedural dose of 40 mg followed by an IV infusion for 24 hrs; these patients were then randomized to subcutaneous hirudin or placebo for 72 hrs.): Hirudin reduced early ischemic events, but failed to decrease restenosis. A higher incidence of intracranial hemorrhage was noted in 3 different trials of hirudin and thrombolytics (GUSTO IIa,[57] TIMI 9A,[58] HIT-III[59]); current studies are attempting to define the optimal dose, timing, and route of administration of these agents.

4.   **Other Antithrombin Agents.** Other promising agents under investigation include argatroban,

Table 34.8. Features of Heparin-Induced Thrombocytopenia[42,45,47,48]

Heparin-Induced Thrombocytopenia		
	Type I	Type II (Heparin-associated thrombotic thrombocytopenia; HATT)
Incidence	10%	Rare
Mechanism	Direct platelet aggregating effect of heparin	Autoantibody (IgG or IgM) directed against platelet factor IV-heparin complex
Onset	Early (1-5 days)	Later (> 5 days); may occur sooner if prior heparin exposure
Platelet count	> 50,000/mm³ but < 150,000 mm³	< 50,000/mm³
Duration	Transient; often improves even if heparin is continued	Requires discontinuation of ALL heparin; gradual recovery in platelet count over 1-5 days in most patients
Clinical course	Benign	Recalcitrant venous and arterial thromboses and thromboembolism; may be fatal

recombinant tissue factor pathway inhibitor, recombinant tick anticoagulant peptide (Corvas International), and recombinant activated protein C.

C. **FIBRINOLYTICS (Chapters 5 and 9).** Despite well-documented efficiency in acute MI, lytic therapy has not had a favorable impact on unstable angina (TIMI 3A and 3B trials).[61,62] In fact, the TAUSA (Thrombolysis and Angioplasty in UnStable Angina) trial suggested a possible *detrimental* effect when intracoronary urokinase was given prophylactically to patients undergoing PTCA for rest angina[63]. In contrast, observational studies suggest that intracoronary lytics may help dissolve thrombus that forms during or after or during coronary intervention (Chapter 9). Urokinase is commonly used for this purpose, in doses ranging from 75,000-500,000 units over 15-45 minutes through the guiding catheter, an infusion wire, or the central lumen of a balloon;[64-66] rt-PA (10-20 mg)[67] and Streptokinase (250,000 units)[68] also appear to be effective. Intracoronary lytics should be avoided when a dissection is present; subintimal hemorrhage may extend the dissection and prevent intimal/medial sealing during prolonged balloon inflations.[69] Prolonged urokinase infusions may be useful adjuncts to PTCA of chronic total occlusions (Chapter 16). The promising results with ReoPro are in sharp contrast to the disappointing results with thrombolytic agents in PTCA for unstable angina, suggesting a prominent role for platelet-mediated thrombus in unstable angina.

D. **DEXTRAN.** Dextran is rarely used today in percutaneous interventional cardiology. Despite its theoretical benefits, critical survey of the clinical literature does not show any benefit compared to placebo; it is also associated with anaphylaxis, hypotension, and pulmonary hemorrhage.[70,71]

PREVENTING ISCHEMIA DURING ANGIOPLASTY

A. **NITROGLYCERIN** is commonly used to treat periprocedural chest pain (IV bolus 100-200 mcg ± IV infusion 10-100 mcg/min) and coronary spasm (intracoronary bolus 100-200 mcg; 10-40 mcg per minute IV). Nitrates do not, however, prevent or delay the onset of ischemia *during* balloon inflation. IV nitrates should be used judiciously in patients with hypotension, volume depletion, or right ventricular dysfunction; preload reduction may exacerbate hypotension and predispose to abrupt closure.[72] There are some data to suggest that nitrates may induce a "heparin-resistant state."

B. **BETA-BLOCKERS** have been used by some operators to delay the onset or severity of chest pain, ST segment changes, and myocardial lactate production during PTCA; however, clear clinical benefit has not been demonstrated. In contrast, β-blockers are very useful for intraprocedural hypertension and tachycardia not related to hypovolemia; propranolol (1 mg IV bolus repeated q 1-2 min. up to 3-5 mg), metoprolol (5 mg IV bolus), or the ultra-short-acting b-blocker esmolol (Chapter 41) may be used for this purpose.[73]

C. **CALCIUM CHANNEL ANTAGONISTS.** Oral calcium blockers are frequently given prior to PTCA to decrease myocardial oxygen consumption during balloon inflation.[74] (Some data indicate an increased mortality risk for certain patients receiving short-acting oral agents on a long-term basis.) Intracoronary nifedipine (0.1 mg),[75,76] IV diltiazem (10-30 mg bolus, followed by 15 mg over 30-60 minutes),[77] and intracoronary nicardipine (0.2 mg) have also been used for this purpose.[78] Intracoronary calcium blockers are also highly effective in reversing no-reflow (Chapter 21). Caution must be used when the combination of calcium blockers (verapamil or diltiazem) and β-blockers are administered during or after PTCA since symptomatic hypotension may occur in > 50% of patients.[79] The use of oral nifedipine in unstable angina has been associated with increased mortality.

TREATMENT OF PERIPROCEDURAL HYPOTENSION

Severe hypotension after PTCA greatly increases the risk of abrupt closure of the target lesion. If blood pressure does not respond immediately to a rapid infusion of saline and discontinuation of nitrates, the systemic circulation must be supported pharmacologically and mechanically (IABP or CPS) while the cause is sought and corrected. A variety of pressors have been used for this purpose, including neosynephrine, norepinephrine, dopamine, metaraminol, and dobutamine (Chapter 41).

* * * * *

REFERENCES

1. Davidson JAH, Boom SJ. Warming lignocaine to reduce pain associated with injection. BMJ 1992;305:617-8.
2. Mader TJ, Playe SJ, Garb JL. Reducing the pain of local anesthetic infiltration: warming and buffering have a synergistic effect. Annals of Emergency Medicine 1994;23(3):550-4.
3. Lasser EC, et al. Pre-Treatment with Corticosteroids to alleviate reactions to intravenous contrast material. N Engl J Med 1987;317:845-849.
4. Lang DM, Alpern MB, Visintainer PF, et al. Increased risk for anaphylactoid reaction from contrast media in patients on β-adrenergic blockers or with asthma. Ann Intern Med 1991;115:270-276.
5. Schwartz L, Bourassa MG, Lespérance J, et al. Aspirin and Dipyridamole in the prevention of restenosis after percutaneous transluminal coronary angioplasty. N Engl J Med 1988;318:1714-1719.
6. Mufson L, Black A, Roubin G, et al. A randomized trial of aspirin in PTCA: Effect of high vs. low dose aspirin on major complications and restenosis. J Am Coll Cardiol 1988;11:236A.
7. Levine MN, Hirsh J, Landefeld S, Raskob G. Hemorrhagic complications of long-term anticoagulant therapy. Chest 1992;102(suppl):352S-363S.
8. Ridker PM, Manson JE, Gaziano JM, Buring JE, et al. Low-dose aspirin therapy for chronic stable angina: A randomized, placebo-controlled clinical trial. Ann Intern Med 1991;114:835-839.
9. Chesebro JH, Webster MWI, Smith HC, Frye RI, Holmes DR, et al. Antiplatelet therapy in coronary disease progression: Reduced infarction and new lesion formation. Circulation 1989:80 (suppl II):II-266.
10. Lewis HD Jr, Davis JW, Archibald DG, Steinke WE, Smitherman TC, et al. Protective effects of aspirin against acute myocardial infarction and death in men with unstable angina: Results of a Veterans Administration Cooperative Study. N Engl J Med 1983;309:396-403.
11. Cairns JA, Gent M, Singer J, Finnie KJ, Froggatt GM, Holder DA, Jablonsky G,et al. Aspirin, sulfinpyrazone, or both in unstable angina. N Engl J Med 1985:313:1369-1375.
12. Theroux P, Quimet H, McCans J, Latour JG, Joly P, et al. Aspirin, heparin, or both to treat acute unstable angina. N Engl J Med 1988;319:1105-1111.
13. ISIS-2 Collaborative Group: Randomized trial of intravenous streptokinase, oral aspirin, both or neither among 17,187 cases of suspected acute myocardial infarction: ISIS-2. Lancet 1988;318:349-360.
14. Henderson W, Goldman S, Copeland J, Moritz TE, Harker L. Antiplatelet or anticoagulant therapy after coronary artery bypass surgery: A meta-analysis of clinical trials. Ann Intern Med 1989;III:743-750.
15. White CW, Chaitman B, Knudtson ML, et al. Antiplatelet agents are effective in reducing the acute ischemic complications of angioplasty but do not prevent restenosis: results from the ticlopidine trial. Coronary Artery Dis 1991;2:757.
16. Chronos NA, Patel D, Sigwart U, et al. Intracoronary activation of human platelets following balloon angioplasty despite aspirin and heparin: a flow cytometric study. Circulation 1994;90 (Part 2):I-181.
17. Di Minno G, Cerbone AM, Mattioli PL. Turco S, et al. Functionally thrombasthenic state in normal platelets following the administration of ticlopidine. J Clin Intest 1985;75:328-338.
18. Cattaneo M, Lombardi R, Bettega D et al. Shear-induced platelet aggregation is potentiated by desmopressin and inhibited by Ticlopidine. Arteriosclerosis and Thrombosis 1993;13:393-397.
19. Dembinska-Kiec A, Virgolini I, Rauscha F, et al. Ticlopidine and platelet function in healthy volunteer, Thrombosis Research 1992;65:559-570.
20. Cattaneo M, Akkawat B, Kinlough-Rathbone RL, et al. Ticlopidine facilitates the deaggregation of human platelets aggravated by thrombin. Thrombosis and Hemostasis 1994,71(1):91-94.
21. Heptinstall S, May JA, Glenn JR, Sanderson HM, et al. Effects of Ticlopidine administered to healthy volunteers on platelet function in whole blood. Thrombosis and Haemostasis 1995;74(5):1310-5.
22. Khurana S, Westley S, Mattson J, Safian RD. Is it possible to expedite the antiplatelet effect of Ticlopidine? 1996 Transcatheter Therapeutics (TCT-VIII) meeting Washington Hospital, Washington D.C.
23. Balsano F, Rizzon P, Violi F, et al. Antiplatelet treatment with ticlopidine in unstable angina: A controlled multicenter clinical trial. Circulation 1990;82:17.
24. Hass WK, Easton JD, Adams HP et al. A randomized trial comparing ticlopidine hydrochloride with aspirin for the prevention of stroke in high-risk patients. Ticlopidine Aspirin Stroke Study Group. N Engl J Med 1989;321:501.
25. de Caterina R, Sicari R, Bornane W et al. Benefit/risk profile of combined antiplatelet therapy with Ticlopidine and Aspirin Thrombosis and Haemostasis 1991;65:(5):504-510.
26. Lembo NJ, Black AJR, Roubin GS et al. Effect of pretreatment with aspirin versus aspirin plus dipyridamole on frequency

and type of acute complications of percutaneous transluminal coronary angioplasty. Am J Cardiol 1990;65:422-426.

27. Danchin N, Juilliere Y, Kettani C, Buffet P, et al. Effect of early acute occlusion rate of adjunctive antithrombotic treatment with intravenously administered dipyridamole during percutaneous transluminal coronary angioplasty. American Heart Journal 1994;127:494-8.

28. The EPIC Investigators. Use of a monoclonal antibody directed against the platelet glycoprotein IIb/IIIa receptor in high-risk coronary angioplasty. N Engl J Med 1994;330:956-61.

29. Ferguson JJ. All ACTs are not created equal. Texas Heart Inst J. 1992;19:1-3.

30. Rath B, Bennett DH. Monitoring the effect of heparin by measurement of activated clotting time during and after percutaneous transluminal coronary angioplasty. Br Heart J. 1990;63:18-21.

31. Hattersly PG. Activated coagulation time of whole blood. JAMA 1966;196:436-440.

32. Bull BS, Huse WM, Bauer FS, Korpman RA: Heparin therapy during extracorporeal Circulation. The use of a dose-response curve to individualize heparin and protamine dosage. J Thorac Cardiovascular Surg 1975;69:685-689.

33. Ferguson JJ, Dougherty KG, Gaos CM et al. Relation between procedural ACT and outcome after PTCA. J Am Cardiol Coll 1994;23:1061-5.

34. Neuenschwander C, Attenhofer C, Kiowski W, et al. Activated clotting times and heparin need during coronary angioplasty in acute myocardial infarction and angina pectoris. Circulation 1993;88(4):I-1107.

35. Freidman HZ, Cragg DR, Glazier SM et al. Randomized prospective evaluation of prolonged versus abbreviated intravenous heparin therapy after coronary angioplasty. J Am Coll Cardiol 1994, 24(5):1214-9.

36. Dougherty KG, Gaos CM, Bush HS, Leachman R, Ferguson JJ. Activated clotting times and activated partial thromboplastin times in patients undergoing coronary angioplasty who receive bolus doses of heparin. Catheterization and Cardiovascular Diagnosis 1992;26:260-263.

37. Granger CB, Miller JM, Bovill EG, GA, et al. Rebound increase in thrombin generation and activity after cessation of intravenous heparin in patients with acute coronary syndromes. Circulation 1995;91:1929-1935.

38. Gabliani G, Deligonul U, Kern MJ, et al. Acute closure occlusion occurring after successful percutaneous transluminal coronary angioplasty: Temporal relationship to discontinuation of anticoagulation. Am Heart J 1988;116:696.

39. Chesebro JH, Badimon L, Fuster V. Importance of antithrombin therapy during coronary angioplasty. J Am Coll Cardiol 1991;17:96B-100B.

40. Schachinger V, Allert M, Kasper W et al. Adjuvant intracoronary infusion of antithrombin III during PTCA: Results of a prospective, randomized trial. Circulation 1994;90:2258-2266.

41. Mabin TA, Holmes DR Jr., Smith HC et al. Intracoronary thrombus: Role in coronary occlusion complicating PTCA. JACC 1985;3:198-202.

42. Becker PS, Miller VT. Heparin-induced thrombocytopenia. Stroke 1989;20:1449-1459.

43. Kappa J, Fisher C, Todd B, Stenach N, Bell P, Campbell F, Ellison N, Addonizio VP. Intraoperative management of patients with heparin-induced thrombocytopenia. Ann Thorac Surg 1990;49:714-23.

44. Warkentin TE, Levine MN, Hirsh J, Horsewood P, et al. Heparin-induced thrombocytopenia in patients treated with low-molecular-weight heparin or unfractionated heparin. N Engl J Med 1995;332:1330-5.

45. Aster RH. Heparin-induced thrombocytopenia and thrombosis. New Engl J Med 332(20):1374-e.

46. Eichinger S, Kyrle PA, Brenner B, et al. Thrombocytopenia associated with low-molecular-weight heparin. Lancet 1991;1:1425-6.

47. Warkentin TE, Hayward CPM, Boshkov LK, Santos AV, et al. Sera from patients with heparin-induced thrombocytopenia generate platelet-derived microparticles with procoagulant activity: An explanation for the thrombotic complications of heparin-induced thrombocytopenia. Blood 1994;84:3691-3699.

48. Amiral J, Bridey F, Wolf M, et al. Antibodies to macromolecular platelet factor 4-heparin complexes in heparin-induced thrombocytopenia: a study of 44 cases. Thromb Haemost 1995;73:21-8.

49. Fareed J, Hoppensteadt DA, Walenger JM. Current perspectives on low molecular weight heparins. Seminars in Thromb Heamostasis 1993;19(Suppl I):I-11.

50. Faxon DP, Spiro TE, Minor S, Coté G, Douglas J, Gottlieb R, Califf R, et al. Low molecular weight heparin in prevention of restenosis after angioplasty. Circulation 1994;90:908-914.

51. Lefkovits J, Topol E. Direct thrombin inhibitors in cardiovascular medicine. Circulation 1994;90:1522-1536.

52. Heras M, Cheseboro JH, Webster MWI et al. Hirudin, heparin, and placebo during deep arterial injury in the pig: the in vivo role of thrombin in platelet-mediated thrombosis. Circulation 1990;82:1476-1484.

53. Van den Bos AA, Deckers JW, Heyndrckx GR, et al. Safety and efficacy of recombinant hirudin (CGP 39 393) versus heparin in patients with stable angina undergoing coronary angioplasty. Circulation 1993;88(I):2058-2066.

54. Bittl JA, Strony J, Brinker JA, Ahmed WH, et al. Treatment with bivalirudin (Hirulog) as compared with heparin during coronary angioplasty for unstable or post-infarction angina. N Engl J Med 1995;333:764-9.

55. Serruys PW, Herrman JPR, Simon R, Rutsch W, Bode C, et al. A Comparison of Hirudin with heparin in the prevention of restenosis after coronary angioplasty. N Engl J Med 1995;333:757-63.

56. Topol EJ, Bonan R, Jewitt D, Sigwart U, Kakkar VV, et al. Use of a direct antithrombin, Hirulog, in place of heparin during coronary angioplasty. Circulation 1993;87:1622-1629.

57. The Global Use of Strategies to Open Occluded Coronary Arteries (GUSTO) IIa Investigators. Randomized trial of intravenous heparin versus recominant hirudin for acute coronary syndromes. Circulation 1994;90:1631-1637.

58. Antman EM, for the TIMI 9A Investigators. Hirudin in acute myocardial infarction, Safety report from the thrombolysis and thrombin inhibition in myocardial infarction (TIMI) 9A trial. Circulation 1994;90:1624-1630.

59. Neuhaus KL, Essen R.v, Tebbe U, Jessel A, Heinrichs H, Mäurer W, et al. Safety Observations from the pilot phase of the randomized r-Hirudin for improvement of thrombolysis (HIT-III) study. Circulation 1994;90:1638-1642.

60. Fuchs J, Cannon CP, TIMI 7 Investigators. Hirulog in the treatment of unstable angina, results of the Thrombin Inhibition in Myocardial Ischemia (TIMI) 7 Trial. Circulation 1995;92:727-733.

61. The TIMI IIIA Investigators. Early effects of tissue-type plasminogen activator added to conventional therapy on the culprit coronary lesion in patients presenting with ischemic cardiac pain at rest, results of the Thrombolysis in Myocardial Ischemia (TIMI IIIA) Trial. Circulation 1993;87:38-52.

62. The TIMI IIIB Investigators. Effects of tissue plasminogen activator and a comparison of early invasive and conservative strategies in unstable angina and non-Q-wave myocardial infarction. Results of the TIMI IIIB Trial. Circulation 1994;89:1545-1556.

63. Ambrose JA, Almeida OD, Sharma SK, Torre SR, Marmur JD, Israel DH, et al. Adjunctive thrombolytic therapy during angioplasty for ischemic rest angina, results of the TAUSA Trial. Circulation 1994;90:69-77.

64. Goudreau E, DiSciascio G, Vetrovec GW, et al. The role of intracoronary urokinase in combination with coronary angioplasty in patients with complex lesion morphology. J Am Coll Cardiol 1990;15:154A.

65. Cohen BM, Buchbinder M, Kozina J, et al. Rethrombosis during angioplasty in myocardial infarction and unstable syndromes: Efficacy of intracoronary urokinase and redilation. Circulation 1988;78 (Suppl II):II-8.

66. Schieman G, Cohen BM, Kozina J, et al. Intracoronary urokinase for intracoronary thrombus accumulation complicating percutaneous transluminal coronary angioplasty in acute ischemic syndromes. Circulation 1990;82:2052-2060.

67. Intracoronary t-PA Registry Investigators. Clinical experience with intracoronary tissue plasminogen activator: Results of a multicenter registry. Catheterization and Cardiovascular Diagnosis 1995;34:196-201.

68. Ambrose JA. Thrombolysis as an adjunct to angioplasty. Am J Cardiol 1993;72:34G-39G.

69. Spielberg C, Schnitzer L, Linderer T, et al. Influence of catheter technology and adjunct medication on acute complications in percutaneous coronary angioplasty. Cathet and Cardiovasc Diagn 1990;21:72-76.

70. Swanson KT, Dogs, Dextran, and Dilitation: A story of empiricism run wild. Cath and Cardiovasc Diag 1994;32:203-205.

71. Taylor MA, DiBlasi SL, Bender RM, Santoian EC, Cha SD, Dennis CA. Adult respiratory distress syndrome complicating intravenous infusion of low-molecular weight dextran. Catheterization and Cardiovascular Diagnosis 1994;32:249-253.

72. Brown KJ, Prcela L, Kerrick et al. Analysis of hypotension in percutaneous coronary intervention patients. Circulation 1994;90(Part 2)I-205.

73. Johansson SR, Lamm C, Bondjers G, et al. Role of beta-adrenergic blockers after percutaneous transluminal coronary angioplasty. Am J Cardiol 1990;66:915-920.

74. Kern MJ, Walsh RA, Barr WK, et al. Improved myocardial oxygen utilization by diltiazem in patients. Am Heart J 1985;110:986-990.

75. Kern MJ, Deligonul U, Labovitz A, et al. Effects of nitroglycerin and nifedipine on coronary and systemic hemodynamics during transient coronary artery occlusion. Am Heart J 1988;115:1164.

76. Serruys PW, van den Brand M, Brower RW. Hugenholtz PG. Regional cardioplegia and cardioprotection during transluminal angioplasty. Which role for nifedipine? Eur Heart J 1984;4(suppl C):115.

77. Kern MJ, Pearson A, Woodruff R, et al. Hemodynamic and echocardiographic assessment of the effects of diltiazem during transient occlusion of the left anterior descending coronary artery during percutaneous transluminal coronary angioplasty. Am J Cardiol 1989;64:849-855.

78. Hanet C, Rousseau MF, Vincent MF, et al. Myocardial protection by intracoronary nicardipine administration during percutaneous transluminal coronary angioplasty. Am J Cardiol 1987;59:1035-1040.

79. Mager A, Strasberg B, Rechavia E, et al. Clinical significance and predisposing factors to symptomatic bradycardia and hypotension after PTCA. Am J Cardiol 1994;74:1085-1088.

80. Maffrand JP, Herbert JM. Effect of clopidogrel and ticlopidine on the binding of [^{3}H]-2 Methyl-Thio-ADP to RAT platelets. Thromb Haemost 1993;69:637(abstract 342).

81. Tcheng JE. Effects of Integrelin™, A competitive platelet integrin glycoprotein IIb/IIIa inhibitor, in preventing ischemic complications of percutaneous coronary intervention. (Manuscript submitted for publication).

35 CATHETER-BASED TECHNIQUES OF LOCAL DRUG DELIVERY

Raymond G. McKay, M.D.

A. RATIONALE FOR LOCAL DRUG DELIVERY. Local delivery of therapeutic agents directly to the site of coronary intervention is currently under active investigation as a new technique to modulate the normal arterial response to mechanical injury.[1,2] All forms of percutaneous intervention result in a complex sequence of cellular responses resulting from mechanical trauma and subsequent exposure of intramural components to circulating blood. In some cases, these cellular responses may result in adverse clinical outcomes. Abrupt closure may result from increased platelet deposition with subsequent intracoronary thrombus formation. Similarly, late restenosis may result from transformation of normally-quiescent, medial smooth muscle cell into a phenotype that proliferates, migrates to the neointima and secretes extracellular matrix.

One theory why systemic pharmacologic therapy has been unsuccessful in limiting the biological consequences of balloon injury is that patients are unable to tolerate the high systemic drug concentrations which are needed for prolonged periods of time. As a result, strategies designed to achieve a local therapeutic drug effect at the site of intervention without the risk of systemic side effects have been developed including intraluminal local drug delivery catheters, drug-coated metallic stents, endovascular and extravascular drug-eluting polymers, periadventitial drug pumps, cell-targeting techniques designed to locally activate intravenously-administered agents, and gene therapy. The theoretic goals of local drug delivery extend beyond the obvious control of thrombosis and restenosis. There may also be a role for the deposition of angiogenic growth factors designed to promote neovascularization and for agents designed to selectively alter vasomotor tone.

B. MECHANISMS OF INTRAMURAL DRUG DEPOSITION. A catheter-based, locally administered drug would have to exert its therapeutic effect by either acting intraluminally during the time of catheter deployment, or by persisting after deposition into the arterial wall. Three different mechanisms of intramural deposition are possible with various catheter delivery systems - passive diffusion, active bulk transfer, or facilitated diffusion. In passive diffusion techniques, drugs are infused via catheters into a closed intraluminal space and allowed to bathe the arterial wall, with intramural deposition occurring by simple diffusion down a concentration or electrochemical gradient. With active bulk transfer, agents are introduced directly into the wall by hydrostatic pressure or other physical means. With facilitated diffusion, agents are intramurally distributed by means of a substrate-carrier complex that may undergo translational or rotational diffusion.

C. PHARMACOKINETIC CONSIDERATIONS. The field of catheter-based drug delivery is currently in its infancy. Based upon in-vitro and animal studies, the list of possible agents which might have a local therapeutic effect is enormous and includes antiplatelet, antithrombin, thrombolytic, calcium blocking agents, steroids, antiproliferative agents, specific growth factor inhibitors, antisense oligonucleotides, and many others. Apart from not knowing which drug should be used, the specific dose, optimal time of administration, and the necessary intramural residence time has not been established for any given agent. Moreover, the efficiency of delivery, depth of intramural penetration, and wash-out from the arterial wall is presumably different for each agent depending upon its molecular weight, charge, lipophilicity, ability to bind to specific receptors, and affinity for macrophage ingestion. The inherent differences in individual drug pharmacokinetics are further complicated by differences in local delivery catheter designs. All of the systems which have been developed to-date vary with respect to efficiency and homogeneity of drug deposition, degree of vascular disruption, ability to simultaneously deliver drug and dilate vascular stenoses, and ability to maintain coronary perfusion during drug delivery.

One of the most important aspects of the pharmacokinetics of locally delivered drugs is their intramural residence time. Some agents may exert a therapeutic effect with only a short intramural residence time. Alternatively, given the time course of platelet deposition, smooth muscle cell division, smooth muscle cell migration, and extracellular matrix production following balloon injury, other agents may require an intramural residence time of days to weeks in order to achieve a beneficial impact. Without binding of an intramurally delivered drug, the agent may quickly wash-out from the arterial wall because of diffusion and convection within the wall into surrounding tissues, vasa vasorum, adventitial lymphatics, and the arterial lumen.[3] Although fluid flux through the arterial wall is relatively slow in a normal artery, it may be significantly accelerated following endothelial denudation. Similarly, the presence of plaque neovascularization in an atherosclerotic vessel may also impact the dynamics of drug wash-out.

A number of catheter-based techniques of increasing drug persistence at the angioplasty site are currently under active investigation.[1-3] These strategies have included the use of drugs contained within non-diffusible, biodegradable microparticles, liposomes, gold microparticles, endoluminal polymer "paving" techniques, stents as well as thermally-mediated drug delivery.

D. CATHETER-BASED LOCAL DRUG DELIVERY TECHNIQUES

1. **The Double-Balloon Catheter (Figure 35.1).** The earliest approach to local drug delivery was the use of the double-balloon catheter.[4-9] The double-balloon catheter (USCI, Billerica, MA) consists of a standard angioplasty shaft with two latex balloons, separated by 2 cm, mounted on its distal end. The catheter has four lumens, one for a central guidewire, two for inflating/deflating the balloons, and a fourth for drug infusion. When the catheter is deployed in an artery over a guidewire and the two balloons are inflated, drug may be infused into the closed space between the inflated balloons. The arterial wall is thus bathed in a local intraluminal reservoir of drug, and intramural penetration occurs by passive diffusion or as a result of applied hydrostatic pressure.

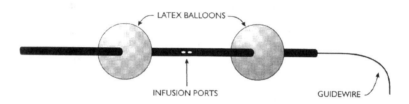

Figure 35.1 The Double-Balloon Catheter

Drugs are infused into the closed space between two inflated balloons.

The double-balloon catheter has been used in several animal models for the delivery of horseradish peroxidase[4] and therapeutically active compounds including heparin,[5] r-hirudin,[6] and t-PA.[7] In addition, at least three groups have also reported successful in vivo gene transfer with the double-balloon catheter.[8,9] Intramural penetration of agents with this device has been documented with low infusion pressures. In one study, the depth of penetration of horseradish peroxidase was shown to be related to infusion pressure, with complete penetration of the arterial media at 300 mmHg.[4] In a second study, infusion pressures of 150 mmHg were both atraumatic and sufficient for uptake of deoxyribose nucleic acid plasmids into the arterial wall, with significant injury noted for pressures greater than 500 mmHg.[9]

Local delivery of heparin to porcine carotid vessels with the double-balloon catheter has recently been shown to reduce intimal hyperplasia 28 days following balloon angioplasty.[5] In a similar model, local r-hirudin delivery with this device has also been shown to reduce early platelet deposition and macroscopic mural thrombus formation following balloon injury in comparison to systemic hirudin or heparin therapy.[6]

The specific advantages of the double-balloon catheter include its ability to atraumatically and homogeneously deliver agents at low pressure, and its ability to limit the site of drug therapy while minimizing systemic exposure. Disadvantages of the catheter, however, include the need for prolonged dwell times with total arterial occlusion, loss of drug from sidebranches that originate from the site of drug administration, and inability to dilate vascular stenoses.

2. **The Wolinsky Perforated Balloon™ Catheter (Figure 35.2).** The Wolinsky perforated balloon catheter (USCI, Billerica, MA) consists of a triple lumen shaft with a distal balloon made of polyethylene terephthalate.[10,11] The balloon has 28 laser-drilled holes which are 25 microns in diameter and arranged in longitudinal rows. During balloon inflation, drug is infused into the balloon and is intramurally deposited by bulk transfer through the balloon's pores.

The perforated balloon catheter has been utilized to deliver a large number of agents including horseradish peroxidase,[11] heparin,[12] t-PA,[13] methotrexate,[14] doxorubicin,[5] colchicine,[6] thiol protease inhibitor,[17] angiopeptin,[18] antisense oligonucleotides to c-myc,[19] and multiple other gene products.[20,21] In all cases, successful intramural delivery of the agent has been reported. In a series of reports studying horseradish peroxidase and fluoresceinated heparin, the depth of penetration of infused fluid was shown to correlate with both the infusion pressure and the duration of infusion.[11] Following local delivery, intramural persistence of agents has been reported up to 48 hours for heparin,12 up to 72 hours for c-myc oligomers,[19] and up to two weeks for methotrexate.[14]

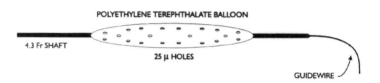

POLYETHYLENE TEREPHTHALATE BALLOON

4.3 Fr SHAFT

25 μ HOLES

GUIDEWIRE

Figure 35.2 The Wolinsky™ Perforated Balloon

Drugs are infused via 28 laser-drilled holes in the balloon surface which are 25 microns in diameter and arranged in longitudinal rows.

Recent studies with local delivery of c-myc oligonucleotides to porcine coronary arteries have demonstrated significant inhibition of neointimal hyperplasia following balloon injury.[19] In spite of successful intramural deposition, however, use of the device to deliver multiple other agents has demonstrated no beneficial therapeutic effect. Studies with heparin, methotrexate, doxorubicin, colchicine, TPI, and angiopeptin have all failed to demonstrate any reduction in neointimal thickening in a variety of animal models. Similarly, studies with heparin, t-PA, and aurin tricarboxylic acid have failed to show any local inhibition of thrombus formation.

The disappointing results from the perforated balloon catheter may be related to the fact that drug delivery with the device may traumatize the angioplasty site from high-pressure fluid jets that emanate from the balloon pores.[13,14,15,22,23,24,25] A minimum pressure of approximately 2 atm is required to fully inflate the balloon and position it against the arterial wall. A higher pressure, ranging between 2 to 5 atm, is usually required for intramural drug deposition. Histologic examination following local delivery of agents at even higher pressures (i.e., between 5 to 10 atms) has demonstrated variable tissue trauma, ranging from disruption of the internal elastic lamina, to medial dissection with medial necrosis, to frank arterial perforation. In addition, vascular damage may be further accentuated from obstructed pores which suddenly regain function at high delivery pressures, resulting in the explosive release of fluid. The disruption of the arterial wall caused by the device may therefore result in a nidus for increased platelet deposition and thrombus formation, as well as an increased proliferative response.

Attempts to limit vascular trauma from the perforated balloon catheter have involved varying the quantity and concentration of solute delivered and changing the design of the catheter. Infusion of smaller quantities of a more concentrated solution may be less traumatic and possibly more efficient than infusion of larger volumes of a lower concentration.[25] Similarly, in-vitro studies have demonstrated that the "jet streaming" effect of a drug infusion at any infusion pressure is significantly diminished by increasing the number of pores in the perforated balloon surface.

3. **The Microporous Balloon Catheter.** The microporous balloon catheter (Cordis Corporation, Miami Lakes, FL) is a variant of the perforated balloon catheter in which therapeutic agents are locally delivered using a membrane balloon containing thousands of pores less than 1 micron in diameter. This catheter theoretically allows for the delivery of drug via bulk transfer at low pressure without significant jet effects. A recent study with horseradish peroxidase has demonstrated successful drug delivery to the inner layers of the arterial wall with catheter-induced injury confined to the endothelium.[26] Additional animal studies have demonstrated successful delivery of heparin and low molecular weight heparin with the device.[27,28]

4. **The Transport™ Catheter.** The Transport Catheter (Scimed Life Systems, Maple Grove, MN) is a triple lumen catheter with a 3.2 Fr shaft and dual balloons located within one another mounted on its distal tip. One lumen is utilized for inflation of an inner conventional balloon used for lesion dilation, a second lumen is used for drug infusion through an outer porous balloon, and the third lumen is for a coronary guidewire. The catheter is available in 2.5-4.0 mm balloons. The outer porous balloon contains 36-48 infusion holes depending upon the balloon size. All infusion holes are 250 microns in diameter and are placed circumferentially and centrally within a 10 mm mid section of the outer balloon. Following lesion dilation with the inner dilating balloon, drug may be infused at 1-3 atm through the outer porous balloon.

    Preliminary studies in patients with the Transport catheter have demonstrated successful local delivery of t-PA to thrombus-containing stenoses.[29] In the United States, the Transport catheter is currently under investigational use for the local delivery of urokinase to treat intracoronary thrombus and studies in acute myocardial infarction patients are planned.

5. **The Hydrogel-Coated Balloon (Figure 35.5).** The hydrogel-coated balloon (Boston Scientific, Watertown, MA) consists of a standard polyethylene balloon coated with a hydrogel polymer (Hydroplus™). The hydrogel coating consists of an interlacing network of polyacrylic acid chains which are adhered to the balloon surface. When the hydrogel comes in contact with an aqueous environment, water is absorbed by the hydrogel and the lattice begins to swell and form a stable matrix of polymer and water. Any agents that are dissolved in the water will also be incorporated into this matrix. The thickness of the coating ranges from 5 microns when dry to 25 microns when fully saturated with water.

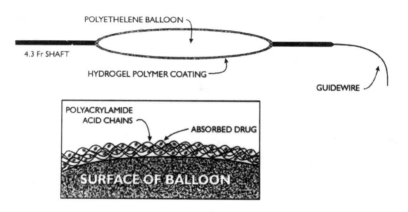

Figure 35.3 The Hydrogel-Coated Balloon

Drugs are absorbed by a hydrogel coating adhered to the balloon surface.

Intramural drug delivery is achieved with the hydrogel system during balloon inflation when the hydrogel polymer comes in contact with the arterial intimal surface. Hydrogel compression during balloon inflation results in pressurized diffusion of a given agent from the polymer directly into the vessel wall.

The hydrogel balloon has been used in the in-vivo delivery of horseradish peroxidase,[30] heparin,[31] urokinase,[32] PPACK,[33] antisense oligonucleotides[34] and various other genes. In all cases, homogeneous intramural penetration of drug has been demonstrated without disruption of the vessel architecture. The in-vivo delivery of heparin[31] and urokinase[32] in the porcine model has been shown to significantly decrease platelet deposition following balloon injury. Similarly, porcine studies involving hydrogel delivery of heparin[31] and antisense oligomers to c-myb have demonstrated a significant decrease in smooth muscle cell proliferation one week following local delivery.

Pharmacokinetic studies with the hydrogel-coated balloon involving the delivery of heparin, antisense oligonucleotides and urokinase have demonstrated that between 2 to 33% of the drug on the balloon surface is intramurally deposited during balloon inflation.[31,32,34] Studies with horseradish peroxidase have also demonstrated that the depth of drug delivery into the arterial wall is proportional to the balloon inflation pressure and inflation time.[30] Following local delivery, heparin has been noted to persist in the arterial wall for as long as 48 hours[31] and antisense oligomers have been detected for at least 24 hours.[34]

Preliminary trials in patients with urokinase-coated hydrogel balloons have also demonstrated efficacy of this system in treating intracoronary thrombus and thrombus-containing stenoses. In one recent study involving 80 patients, locally delivered urokinase resulted in lysis of intracoronary thrombus and/or reversal of abrupt thrombotic closure without evidence of distal embolization or no reflow.[36]

The major advantage of the hydrogel system is that it results in homogenous, atraumatic drug delivery at the same time that an arterial lesion is being dilated. Deficiencies of the catheter, however, include the rapid washoff of drug from the balloon surface, the relatively small amount of drug which can be loaded into the hydrogel coating, and the need for complete vessel occlusion during drug delivery.

6. **The Dispatch™ Catheter (Figure 35.4).** The Dispatch Catheter (Scimed Life Systems, Maple Grove, MN) consists of a 4.4 Fr catheter shaft with a 20 mm polyolefin copolymer, spiral inflation coil wrapped around a non-porous urethane sheath on its distal tip. When the spiral coil is inflated, it forms both an internal lumen that allows for distal coronary perfusion through the inner sheath, and a series of isolated spaces in between the catheter's coils, urethane sheath, and arterial wall. Drug is administered through a separate infusion port and is delivered locally through slits in the shaft of the catheter into the protected spaces between the coils of the device. The arterial wall is thus bathed in drug which is isolated from blood flowing through the inner urethane sheath.

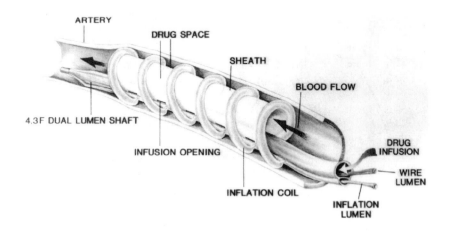

Figure 35.4 The Dispatch™ Catheter

Inflation of the catheter's spiral coil creates an internal lumen for distal coronary perfusion and a series of isolated spaces for drug delivery.

Successful in-vivo delivery of methylene blue, horseradish peroxidase, heparin, hirudin, urokinase, t-PA, and several genes has been accomplished with the Dispatch catheter in several animal models.[37,38] In the case of heparin, the amount of intramurally deposited drug has been shown to be proportional to the drug infusion time and the concentration of infused drug, with intramural persistence for at least one week.[37] Preliminary heparin delivery studies in the porcine model have also demonstrated successful inhibition of platelet deposition following balloon injury. With respect to urokinase, successful intracoronary deposition of the drug has been demonstrated with persistence at the infusion site for over 5 hours.[38] In comparison to systemic urokinase therapy or conventional guiding catheter infusion, urokinase delivery with the Dispatch catheter resulted in 10 to 100 fold greater intramural deposition.

The Dispatch catheter was approved for drug delivery in patients by the United States Food and Drug Administration in December 1993. Since that time, some cases have been reported in which the catheter was used for periods as long as 24 hours without significant alteration of coronary blood flow or ventricular function.[39] Preliminary patient studies have also demonstrated the efficacy of the Dispatch catheter in treating intracoronary thrombus during percutaneous revascularization with infusions of limited quantities of urokinase.[40-43]

Unlike other local drug delivery systems, the specific advantage of the Dispatch catheter is that it allows for prolonged localized drug delivery at an angioplasty site with simultaneous perfusion of the artery. Preliminary animal and patient studies, however, have also clearly illustrated several limitations of the device. First, the catheter may result in significant ischemia from sidebranch occlusion by the device's coils. Second, the catheter was not designed to dilate a coronary stenosis. As a result, deployment of the catheter within an undilated lesion may result in incomplete expansion of the inner urethane sheath with inadequate distal perfusion. Inflation of a device which is oversized by > 0.5 mm may likewise result in incomplete expansion of the inner urethane sheath and inadequate distal perfusion. All of these problems may severely limit the time of drug infusion, which generally is 20-30 minutes to allow passive diffusion into the wall. The long duration required for passive drug infusion is another limitation of the device.

7. **The Channel™ Balloon (Figure 35.5).** The Channel Balloon (Boston Scientific, Watertown, MA) consists of a standard polyethylene terephthalate balloon mounted on a triple lumen shaft. Surrounding the dilatation portion of the balloon are 18 channels which run longitudinally along the surface of the balloon and serve as conduits for delivering agents. Each channel contains one 75 micron pore which connects to a drug infusion port which is independent of the balloon inflation port. When the balloon is inflated at normal pressures through the inflation port (i.e., < 8 atm), drug can be infused at lower pressures (i.e., at 2-4 atm) through the drug infusion port. The infused drug exits the balloon through the pores in the channels and bathes the arterial wall at low pressures.

Successful in-vivo delivery of horseradish peroxidase,[44] heparin,[44] low molecular weight heparin,[45] urokinase,[46] and several genes[47] have been accomplished with the Channel balloon in several animal models. Intramural drug deposition has been shown to correlate with drug infusion pressure and balloon/artery ratio.[46] Local delivery of heparin with the Channel balloon to a Dacron graft in a porcine arteriovenous shunt has been shown to significantly reduce platelet deposition and mural thrombus formation.[48]

The major advantage of the Channel balloon is that successful drug delivery can be achieved with low pressure, atraumatic drug infusions during simultaneous angioplasty of an arterial stenosis. The disadvantages of the catheter include a non-homogenous distribution of drug related to the location of the channels on the balloon surface, and the need for arterial occlusion during drug administration.

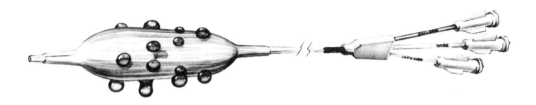

Figure 35.5 The Channel™ Balloon

Drugs are infused into 18 channels which run longitudinally along the surface of the balloon.

8. **The Infusasleeve™ (Figure 35.6).** The Kaplan-Simpson Infusasleeve (Localmed, Sunnyvale, CA) is a multi-lumen catheter that is designed to track over a standard dilating balloon catheter and serve as an adjunctive device for the local delivery of therapeutic agents. The Infusasleeve has a proximal infusion port, a main catheter or body, and a distal infusion region with multiple sideholes. The central lumen of the Infusasleeve accommodates a standard angioplasty balloon catheter and angioplasty guidewire. Following positioning of the standard angioplasty balloon within the coronary vasculature, the drug infusion region of the Infusasleeve is positioned along the angioplasty catheter shaft. Drug can then be infused either proximal to, or directly over the angioplasty balloon during low pressure balloon inflation (i.e., up to 2 atm) to approximate the Infusasleeve directly adjacent to the arterial wall.

Previous animal studies with the Infusasleeve have demonstrated successful intramural delivery of horseradish peroxidase,[49] heparin,[50] and urokinase,[51] with intramural deposition related to balloon inflation and drug infusion pressure. Localized delivery of heparin to peripheral vessels in the porcine model has successfully inhibited platelet deposition following balloon injury.[50]

Preliminary studies in patients in Germany and Italy have demonstrated safe use of the Infusasleeve with local delivery of heparinized saline.[52] In 12/94, the device was approved for use in patients in the United States by the Food and Drug Administration and was released for general use in 1995. Clinical testing in patients with acute myocardial infarction is planned.

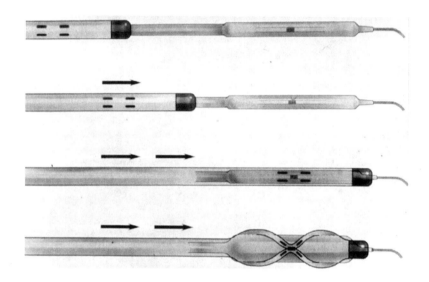

Figure 35.6 The Infusasleeve™

The delivery sleeve is positioned along the shaft of a standard angioplasty catheter for local drug infusion.

9. **The Iontophoresis Catheter (Figure 35.7).** Local drug delivery by iontophoresis is based on the concept that an electrical field can be used as a driving force to intramurally deliver charged agents at an angioplasty site.[53] The iontophoresis system (CorTrak Medical, Roseville, MN) consists of a standard angioplasty catheter shaft with a microporous membrane balloon mounted on its distal end. The middle portion of the membrane balloon, which is contact with the arterial wall during balloon inflation, contains millions of submicron pores for drug delivery. The proximal and distal ends of the membrane balloon are devoid of these pores, minimizing drug loss into the blood stream during iontophoresis. Located under the microporous membrane balloon is an electrode (e.g., Ag/AgCl) which wraps around the catheter shaft. This electrode is connected to a power source, with a return electrode placed on the skin surface. When the membrane balloon is inflated at low pressure (i.e., 1 atmosphere) and an electric current is applied by the power source, charged drug

molecules inside the balloon flow through the balloon pores into the arterial wall in response to the voltage differential between the catheter electrode and return electrode.

Successful in-vivo delivery of hirudin[54] and heparin[.56] has been accomplished with the iontophoresis catheter in both pigs and rabbits. Iontophoretic delivery resulted in tissue concentrations as much as 80 times greater than passive delivery for hirudin, and as much as 13 times greater for heparin. Local iontophoretic delivery of heparin in the porcine model has also

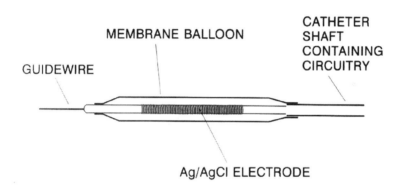

Figure 35.7 The Iontophoresis Catheter

Drugs are delivered through a membrane balloon in response to a voltage differential between the Ag/AgCl catheter electrode and a return electrode.

been shown to significantly decrease platelet deposition following balloon injury.[55] In all studies to-date, iontophoretic drug delivery has been atraumatic and homogenous.

E. DRUG DELIVERY CATHETERS APPROVED FOR CURRENT CLINICAL USE

1. **Medical-legal Implications.** Currently, the United States Food and Drug Administration has approved only the Dispatch catheter and the Infusasleeve for local intracoronary drug infusions. Approval for these devices has been given for *intraluminal* delivery of therapeutic agents, without specific certification for intramural deposition of drugs. The Hydrogel-coated balloon has also been approved for use, although the hydrogel coating has been specified as a lubricous surface rather than a drug delivery vehicle. The Transport catheter is currently in investigational use under the supervision of an IDE. Submissions to the FDA for investigational use of the microporous balloon, the Channel balloon, and the iontophoresis catheter are also expected in the near future.

2. **The Hydrogel-coated Balloon.** The hydrogel-coated balloon is currently available in 0.5 mm sizes from 2.0 to 4.0 mm in diameter. Drugs may be loaded onto the hydrogel balloon surface either by immersion of the inflated balloon into a concentrated drug solution or by "painting" the balloon surface with known aliquots of the drug. Using the immersion technique, in-vitro studies have demonstrated maximum drug loading onto the hydrogel with immersion times as short as 60 seconds. The amount of fluid (and drug) absorbed by the hydrogel coating is proportional to the balloon surface area and amount of hydrogel available for binding. Relatively larger quantities of drug on the balloon surface can be achieved with "painting" of the balloon surface with small aliquots of a drug solution using a sterile pipette, allowing for drying of the surface in between drug applications.

In our laboratory, urokinase-coated hydrogel balloons are currently used for treatment of thrombus-containing coronary stenoses. Balloons are loaded with urokinase by inflating the balloon to 2 atm pressure, immersing the inflated balloon for 60 seconds in a solution of Abbokinase (Abbott Laboratories, North Chicago, IL) (50,000 units/ml), and deflating the balloon while still in solution. The amount of urokinase absorbed on the balloon surface is approximately 240 units for a 2 mm balloon, 320 units for a 2.5 mm balloon, 420 units for a 3.0 mm balloon, 550 units for a 3.5 mm balloon, and 700 units for a 4.0 mm balloon. The balloon is subsequently positioned over an 0.014" angioplasty guidewire through a standard 8 Fr guiding catheter and inflated at the site of thrombus. Balloon sizing is chosen to achieve a balloon:artery ratio of 1:1. Ideally, balloon inflation should be maintained as long as possible (i.e, 2-4 mins), depending upon the clinical response to coronary occlusion during catheter use. Following single use, subsequent inflations of the balloon require "reloading" of the hydrogel with urokinase.

All hydrogel studies have demonstrated significant wash-off of drug from the balloon surface when the drug-coated balloon is exposed to the intact circulation. For this reason, rapid deployment of the balloon to the site of drug delivery is recommended. Use of a protective sleeve to prevent drug washoff is also under investigation.

3. **The Dispatch™ Catheter.** The Dispatch catheter is manufactured with 3.0, 3.5, and 4.0 mm coil sizes, and is deployed within a coronary artery with a 1:1 coil/artery ratio. The catheter is prepared by flushing the central lumen with heparinized saline, flushing the drug infusion port with heparinized saline, and performing a standard negative prep of the coil inflation port to purge the catheter of air. The catheter is placed over an 0.014" angioplasty guidewire through a standard 8 Fr guiding catheter and positioned at the drug infusion site, usually after the PTCA with a standard dilatation catheter has relieved the atherosclerotic obstruction. The coils are inflated with a 50:50 mixture of saline and contrast with a standard indeflator. Inflation of the coils is nominal at 6 atm, with quarter sizing noted at 12 atm. In its inflated state, the catheter's coils exert the equivalent of 2 atm of radial force on the arterial wall. Contrast injection through the guiding catheter can be used to assess distal coronary perfusion and possible sidebranch obliteration by the catheter's inflated coils.

Following deployment of the catheter and inflation of the device's coils, drug is infused via the drug infusion port using an IMED pump and an infusion rate of 0.5 cc/min. Pressure within the drug infusion port can be measured by connecting a three-way stopcock in series between the IMED infusion pump and the Dispatch catheter, and connecting the side arm of the stopcock to a pressure transducer. This infusion pressure should not exceed 300-400 mmHg at the specified volumetric flow rate. In the event that the fit of the Dispatch catheter within the artery is too "tight" to allow the specified infusion rate of 0.5 cc/minute without exceeding the pressure limit of 300-400 mmHg, the catheter's coils should be deflated from the initial 6 atmospheres to the highest pressure which allows a flow rate of 0.5 cc/minute with a pressure of less than 300-400 mmHg.

In the event that the patient is unable to tolerate initial deployment of the Dispatch catheter because of inadequate distal perfusion or sidebranch occlusion, the Dispatch catheter may be repositioned or removed and the lesion predilated with a 2.5 mm conventional angioplasty balloon. Following predilatation, the Dispatch may be repositioned at the target site with a second attempt at drug infusion.

In our laboratory, the Dispatch catheter is utilized to treat intracoronary thrombus and thrombus-containing stenoses with localized infusions of urokinase. Abbokinase (Abbott Laboratories, North Chicago, IL) is mixed at 30,000 units/cc, and a total of 450,000 units are infused over a 30 minute period. Larger quantities of urokinase and longer infusion times may be utilized for patients with persistent thrombus.

4. **The Infusasleeve™.** The Infusasleeve is intended for use in conjunction with standard angioplasty catheters. The Infusasleeve is initially prepared for use by flushing the device's central lumen with heparinized saline or the drug solution to be delivered. The standard angioplasty catheter is then inserted with its balloon in the deflated state through the proximal end of the Infusasleeve and advanced until the balloon portion of the angioplasty catheter has exited the Infusasleeve's distal end. The drug infusion region of the drug sleeve is thus positioned proximal to the angioplasty balloon. The combined angioplasty catheter-Infusasleeve device is then positioned over a 0.014" angioplasty guidewire through a standard 9 Fr guiding catheter to the intracoronary location. Following lesion dilation with the angioplasty balloon, the Infusasleeve may be positioned along the angioplasty catheter shaft to the location intended for drug delivery. Drugs may be infused through the drug sleeve proximal, distal or at the site of the angioplasty balloon. The flow rate for drug infusion is directly related to infusion pressure, and measures 5 ml/min for 10 psi, 15 ml/min for 30 psi, and 25 ml/min for 50 psi. Infusion pressures above 50 psi are undergoing clinical evaluation. In our laboratory, drug infusion is accomplished with the use of a Monarch™ inflation syringe (Merit Medical, Salt Lake City, Utah).

F. **CONCLUSIONS.** The field of catheter-based drug delivery is currently in its earliest stages of development. Multiple drug delivery catheters are being designed and tested, and will probably be available for investigational and clinical use in the next several years. Comparative studies are needed to assess the relative merits of the different systems under development with respect to efficiency of drug delivery, effect on vessel architecture, homogeneity of drug deposition, ability to simultaneously dilate vascular stenoses, and limit ischemia from vessel and sidebranch occlusion. Beneficial therapeutic effects on platelet deposition and smooth muscle cell physiology have been documented with several drugs in animal models, and preliminary patient studies have demonstrated successful treatment of intracoronary thrombus. However, additional information is needed on the pharmacokinetics and therapeutic benefit of individual drugs. Moreover, the eventual success of this field may critically depend upon the success of strategies to prolong intramural drug residence time. Although promising, the ultimate impact of local drug delivery on thrombotic closure and restenosis remains uncertain at the present time.

* * * * *

REFERENCES

1. Riessen R, Isner JM. Prospects for site-specific delivery of pharmacologic and molecular therapies. J Am Coll Cardiol 1994;23:1234-44.
2. Lincoff AM, Topol EJ, Ellis SG. Local drug delivery for the prevention of restenosis: Fact, Fancy and Future. Circulation 1994;90:2070-2083.
3. Wilensky RL, March KL, Gradus-Pizlo I, et al. Methods and devices for local drug delivery in coronary and peripheral arteries. Trends Cardiovasc Med 1993;3:163-170.
4. Goldman B, Blanke H, Wolinsky H. Influence of pressure on permeability of normal and diseased muscular arteries to horseradish peroxidase. Atherosclerosis 1987;65:215-225.
5. Lopez-Sendon J, Sobrino N, Gamallo C, Lorenzo A, et al. Locally delivered heparin reduces intimal hyperplasia and lumen stenosis following arterial balloon injury in swine. European Heart Journal 1993;14(supplement):191 (abstract).
6. Meyer BJ, Fernandez-Ortiz A, Mailhac A, Falk E, et al. Local delivery of r-hirudin by a double-balloon perfusion catheter prevents mural thrombosis and minimizes platelet deposition after angioplasty. Circulation 1994;90:2474-2480.
7. Jorgensen B, Tonnesen KH, Bulow L, et al. Femoral artery recanalisation with percutaneous angioplasty and segmentally enclosed plasminogen activator. Lancet 1989;1:1106-8.
8. Nabel EG, Plautz G, Nabel GJ. Site-specific gene expression in vivo by direct gene transfer into the arterial wall. Science 1990;249:1285-8.
9. Nabel EG, Yang Z, Liptay S, et al. Recombinant platelet-derived growth factor B gene expression in porcine arteries reduces intimal hyperplasia in vivo. J Clin Invest 1993;91:1822-9.
10. Wolinsky H, Thung SN. Use of a perforated catheter to deliver concentrated heparin into the wall of the normal canine artery. J Am Coll Cardiol 1990;15:475-81.
11. Wolinsky H, Lin CS. Use of the perforated balloon catheter to infuse marker substances into diseased coronary artery walls after experimental postmortem angioplasty. J Am Coll Cardiol 1991;17:174B-178B.
12. Gimple LW, Gertz SD, Haber HL, Ragosta M, et al. Effect of chronic subcutaneous or intramural administration of heparin on femoral artery restenosis after balloon angioplasty in hypercholesterolemic rabbits. A quantitative angiographic and histopathological study. Circulation 1992;86:1536-46.
13. Gellman J, Enger CD, Sigal SL, True LD, et al. The successful application of a local infusion angioplasty catheter in a rabbit model of focal femoral atherosclerosis. J Am Coll Cardiol 1990;15:164A (abstract).
14. Muller DWM, Topol EJ, Abrams GD, Gallagher K, Ellis SG. Intramural methotrexate therapy for prevention of neointimal thickening after balloon angioplasty. J Am Coll Cardiol 1992;20:460-466.
15. Franklin SM, Kalan JM, Currier JW, Mejias Y, Cody C, Haudenschild CC, Faxon DP. Effects of local delivery of doxorubicin or saline on restenosis following angioplasty in atherosclerotic rabbits. Circulation 1992;86:I-52 (abstract).
16. Wilensky RL, Gradus-Pizlo I, Marck KL, Sandusky GE, Hathaway DR. Efficacy of local intramural injection of colchicine in reducing restenosis following angioplasty in the atherosclerotic rabbit model. Circulation 1992;86:I-52 (abstract).

17. Wilensky RL, March KL, Hathaway DR. Restenosis in an atherosclerotic rabbit model is reduced by thiol protease inhibitor. J Am Coll Cardiol 1991;17:286A (abstract).

18. Hong MK, Bhatti T, Mathews BJ, Stark KS, et al. Locally delivered angiopeptin reduces intimal hyperplasia following balloon injury in rabbits. Circulation 1991;84:II-72 (abstract).

19. Shi Y, Fard A, Galeo A, Hutchinson HG, et al. Transcatheter delivery of c-myc antisense oligomers reduces neointimal formation in a porcine model of coronary artery balloon injury. Circulation 1994;90:944-951.

20. Flugelman MY, Jaklitsch MT, Newman KD, Casscell W, et al. Low level in vivo gene transfer into the arterial wall through a perforated balloon catheter. Circulation 1992;85:1110-7.

21. Chapman GD, Lim CS, Gammon RS, et al. Gene transfer into coronary arteries of intact animals with a percutaneous balloon catheter. Circ Res 1992;71:27-33.

22. Stadius ML, Collins C, Kernoff R. Local infusion balloon angioplasty to obviate restenosis compared with conventional balloon angioplasty in an experimental model of atherosclerosis. Am Heart J 1993;126:47-56.

23. Lambert CR, Leone JE, Rowland SM. Local drug delivery catheters: functional comparison of porous and microporous designs. Cor Art Dis 1993;4:469-475.

24. Herdeg C, Oberhoff M, Baumbach A, Kamenz J, et al. Application of porous balloon catheter with two different injection pressures: differences in outcome. European Heat Journal 1994:15 (Supplement):561 (abstract).

25. French BA, Mazur W, Finnigan JP, Carter Grinstead W, et al. Gene transfer into intact porcine coronary arteries via infusion balloon catheter: influences of delivery volume and pressure. Circulation 1992;86:I-799 (abstract).

26. Lambert CR, LeoneJ, Rowland S. The microporous balloon: A minimal trauma local drug delivery catheter. Circulation 1992;86:I-381 (abstract).

27. Thomas CN, Robinson KA, Cipolla GD, Jones M, King SB. In-vivo local delivery of heparin to coronary arteries with a microporous infusion balloon. J Am Coll Cardiol 1994;23:187A (abstract).

28. Lincoff AM, Furst JG, Penn MS, Lee P, MacIssac AI, Chisolm GM, Topol EJ, Ellis SG. Efficiency of solute transfer by a microporous balloon catheter in the porcine coronary model of arterial injury. J Am Coll Cardiol 1994;23:18A (abstract).

29. Cumberland DC, Gunn J, Tsikaderis D, Arafa S, Ahsan A. Initial clinical experience of local drug delivery via a porous balloon during percutaneous coronary angioplasty. J Am Coll Cardiol 1994;23:186A (abstract).

30. Fram DB, Aretz TA, Azrin MA, Mitchel JF, et al. Localized intramural drug delivery during balloon angioplasty using hydrogel-coated balloons and pressure-augmented diffusion. J Am Coll Cardiol 1994;23:1570-7.

31. Azrin MA, Mitchel JF, Fram DB, Pedersen CA, et al. Decreased platelet deposition and smooth muscle cell proliferation following intramural heparin delivery with hydrogel-coated balloons. Circulation 1994;90:433-441.

32. Mitchel JF, Azrin MA, Fram DB, Hong MK, et al. Inhibition of platelet deposition and lysis of intracoronary thrombus during balloon angioplasty with urokinase-coated hydrogel balloons. Circulation 1994:90:1979-88.

33. Nunes GL, Hanson SR, King SB, Sahatjian RA, Scott NE. Local delivery of a synthetic antithrombin with a hydrogel-coated angioplasty balloon inhibits platelet-dependent thrombosis. J Am Coll Cardiol 1994;23:1578-83.

34. Azrin MA, Mitchel JF, Pedersen C, Curley TM, et al. Inhibition of smooth muscle cell proliferation in-vivo following local delivery of antisense oligonucleotides to c-myb during angioplasty. J Am Coll Cardiol 1994;23:396A (abstract).

35. Riessen R, Rahimizadeh H, Blessing E, Takeshita S, et al. Arterial gene transfer using pure DNA applied directly to a hydrogel-coated angioplasty balloon. Hum Gene Ther 1993;4:749-58.

36. Mitchel JF, Hirst JA, Kiernan FJ, Fram DB, et al. Local, intracoronary thrombolysis using urokinase-coated hydrogel balloons. Circulation 1994;90(4):I-493 (abstract).

37. Fram DB, Mitchel JF, Azrin MA, Schwedick MW, et al. Local heparin delivery in porcine coronary arteries with the Dispatch catheter: delivery, washout and effect on platelet deposition following balloon angioplasty. Circulation 1994;90(4):I-493 (abstract).

38. Mitchel JF, Fram DB, Palme DF, Foster R, et al. Enhanced local thrombolysis with urokinase using the Dispatch catheter. Circulation 1995;91:785-793.

39. Camenzind E, di Mario C, de Jaegere P, de Feyter P, et al. Left ventricular and coronary hemodynamics during local drug delivery with a new infusion catheter: First experience in humans. European Heat Journal 1994;15 (Supplement):561 (abstract).

40. McKay RG, Fram DB, Kiernan FJ, Hirst JA, et al. Localized thrombolysis of intracoronary thrombus using a new drug delivery system - The Dispatch catheter. Cathet Cardiovasc Diagn 1994;33:181-188.

41. Mitchel JF, McKay RG. Treatment of acute stent thrombosis with local drug delivery systems. Cathet Cardiovasc Diagn 1995;34:149-154.

42. Mitchel JF, Fram DB, Palme DF, Foster R, et al. Enhanced intracoronary thrombolysis using the Dispatch catheter. Circulation 1994;90(4):I-493 (abstract).

43. Mitchel JF, Fram DB, Hirst JA, Kiernan FJ, et al. Local dissolution of intracoronary thrombus with urokinase using the Dispatch catheter: clinical studies. J Am Coll Cardiol 1995;25:347A (abstract).

44. Hong MK, Wong SC, Farb A, Mehlman MD, et al. Feasibility and drug delivery efficiency of a new balloon angioplasty catheter capable of performing simultaneous local drug delivery. Cor Art Dis 1993;4:1023-1027.

45. Hong MK, Wong SC, Haudenschild CC, Mehlman MD, et al. Local delivery with low molecular weight heparin by the Channelled balloon during simultaneous angioplasty in atherosclerotic rabbit iliac arteries. Circulation 1994;90(4):I-157 (abstract).

46. Mitchel JF, Fram DB, Azrin MA, Bow L, et al. Localized intracoronary delivery of urokinase with the Channelled balloon: pharmacokinetics of drug delivery and washout. J Am Coll Cardiol 1995;25:347A (abstract).

47. Feldman LJ, Steg PG, Zheng LP, Barry JJ, et al. Efficient percutaneous adenovirus-mediated arterial gene transfer using a channelled angioplasty balloon. Circulation 1994;90(4):I-20 (abstract).

48. Thomas CN, Barry JJ, King SB, Scott NA. Local delivery with heparin with a PTCA infusion balloon inhibits platelet-dependent thrombosis. J Am Coll Cardiol 1994;23:4A (abstract).

49. Kaplan AV, Kermode J, Grant G, Klein E, et al. Intramural delivery of marker agent in ex vivo and in vivo models using a novel drug delivery sleeve. J Am Coll Cardiol 1994;23:187A (abstract).

50. Moura A, Lam JYT, Hebert D, Letchacovski G, et al. Local heparin delivery decreases the thrombogenicity of the balloon-injured artery. Circulation 1994;90(4):I-449 (abstract).

51. Azrin MA, Mitchel JF, Bow LM, Alberghini TV, et al. Local delivery of urokinase to porcine coronary arteries using the Localmed infusion sleeve. J Am Coll Cardiol 1995;25:347A (abstract).

52. Kaplan AV, Vandormael M, Bartorelli A, Hofman M, et al. Local delivery at the site of angioplasty with a novel drug delivery sleeve: Initial clinical series. J Am Coll Cardiol 1995;25:286A (abstract).

53. Chien YW, Banga AK: Iontophoretic delivery of drugs: Overview of historical development. J Pharm Sci 1989;78:353-354.

54. Fernandez-Ortiz A, Meyer BJ, Mailhac A, Falk E, et al. A new approach for local intravascular drug delivery. The iontophoretic balloon. Circulation 1994;89:1518-1522.

55. Mitchel JF, Azrin MA, Schwedick MW, Bow LM, et al. Local delivery of heparin with a novel iontophoretic catheter - quantitative heparin delivery and effect on platelet deposition following balloon angioplasty. Circulation 1994;90(4):I-492 (abstract).

56. Mitchel JF, Azrin MA, Fram DB, Feroze H, et al. Localized intracoronary delivery of heparin with iontophoresis. J Am Coll Cardiol 1995;25:285A (abstract).

PERCUTANEOUS INTERVENTIONS ON PERIPHERAL AND VISCERAL VASCULAR DISEASE

36

Phillip J. Bendick, Ph.D.
Daniel Diffin, M.D.
Krishna Kandarpa, M.D., Ph.D.

Patients with coronary artery disease frequently have symptomatic lower extremity atherosclerotic disease. [1,2] Historically the treatment for patients with severe ischemia has been bypass surgery;[3,4] however, the development of endovascular interventional techniques has broadened the indications and utilization of peripheral revascularization. [5-7] The purpose of the diagnostic workup of patients with peripheral vascular disease is to identify the specific sites of obstruction and to determine if patients are suitable candidates for percutaneous and/or surgical intervention.

A. PATHOPHYSIOLOGY

The pathophysiology of lower extremity atherosclerotic disease is similar to coronary artery disease; the disease progresses slowly, and symptoms of ischemia develop when diameter stenosis >60%. [8] As the severity of obstruction increases, there is a gradual progression of limb claudication; when multiple arterial segments have significant obstructive disease, chronic ischemia may cause progressive rest pain, ulceration, gangrene, and limb loss.

It is helpful to consider peripheral vascular obstruction in three anatomic zones (Figure 36.1):[1]

1. **Inflow Tract.** The abdominal aorta and common and external iliac arteries make up the inflow tract to the lower extremities. Diffuse atherosclerosis is often present throughout the infrarenal aorta; the most severe lesions are typically found at the aortic bifurcation involving the origin of the common iliac arteries, or at the iliac bifurcation involving the origin of the external and internal iliac arteries. Aorto-iliac disease usually causes claudication in the hips and buttocks, but may extend into the thighs and calves with further exertion. Femoral artery pulses may or may not be diminished, depending on the degree of proximal obstructive disease. [2]

2. **Outflow Tract.** The outflow tract extends from the inguinal ligament to just below the knee, and consists of the common femoral, superficial femoral, and popliteal arteries (the femoropopliteal system). The common femoral artery and the mid segment of the popliteal artery are often spared; the superficial femoral artery may be involved throughout its length, and the most critical lesions frequently occur near the adductor hiatus. [3]

3. **Runoff Bed.** The runoff bed consists of the anterior tibial artery, posterior tibial artery and peroneal artery (the trifurcation vessel system) in the lower leg. The proximal segments of these vessels are

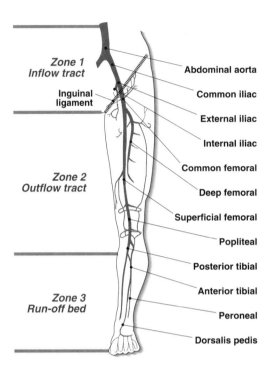

Zone 1
Inflow tract

Inguinal
ligament

Zone 2
Outflow tract

Zone 3
Run-off bed

Abdominal aorta

Common iliac

External iliac

Internal iliac

Common femoral

Deep femoral

Superficial femoral

Popliteal

Posterior tibial

Anterior tibial

Peroneal

Dorsalis pedis

Figure 36.1 Arterial Circulation of the Lower Extremity

Zone 1: In-flow tract (abdominal aorta, common iliac artery, and external iliac artery).
Zone 2: Out-flow tract, extends from the inguinal ligament to the knee (common femoral artery, superficial femoral artery, and popliteal artery).
Zone 3: Run-off bed (anterior tibial artery, posterior tibial artery, and peroneal artery).

frequently diseased, limiting distal runoff to the foot. Diabetic patients comprise a unique population: One-third of diabetics with peripheral atherosclerotic lesions have disease limited to the lower leg trifurcation vessels; one-third have disease limited to the aortoiliac or femoro-popliteal vessels; and one-third have multiple segmental disease involving the inflow, outflow and runoff systems. [9,.10] Isolated trifurcation vessel lesions in diabetic patients are often not amenable to surgical bypass; small diameter balloon catheters provide an alternative endovascular approach. In non-diabetic patients the distribution of lesions is isolated to the inflow or outflow tracts in 50%; multiple segment disease involving the runoff vessels is present in the other 50%.

B. DIAGNOSIS AND PATIENT EVALUATION

1. **Lower Extremity.** The clinical history will determine the likelihood of ischemia and the degree of functional impairment; the quality of pulses will help localize the site(s) of obstruction, but is unreliable for estimating disease severity. [11]

a. **Ankle-Brachial Index.** Objective data are provided by the ankle-brachial index (ABI), defined as the ratio of systolic pressure in the ankle to the upper arm (Table 36.1). [12-14] Brachial systolic pressure should be measured in both arms; the higher value is used to calculate the right and left ABI. Ankle systolic pressures are measured with a standard adult blood pressure cuff (12 x 23 cm bladder) wrapped snugly around the ankle, with the lower edge of the cuff just above the malleoli. While using a Doppler pencil probe to monitor the signal from the posterior or anterior tibial artery, inflate the cuff to 30 mmHg above systolic pressure to temporarily occlude flow; as the cuff is slowly deflated (2 - 4 mmHg per second), the pressure at which a Doppler flow signal is heard is recorded as the ankle systolic pressure.

b. **Duplex Ultrasound.** Further noninvasive evaluation is provided by duplex ultrasound, which allows direct real-time ultrasound imaging of obstructive lesions and simultaneous assessment of hemodynamic significance by Doppler. The entire peripheral arterial tree from the abdominal aorta to the tibial arteries can be surveyed if necessary (Figures 36.1, 36.2). The Doppler flow signals can be subjectively graded (Table 36.2) and stenosis severity can be estimated using Doppler velocity spectra (Table 36.3). [15-18]

2. **Carotid.** Duplex ultrasound evaluation of atherosclerotic disease is also possible in the cerebrovascular circulation (Figure 36.3). The North American Symptomatic Carotid Endarterectomy Trial (NASCET) and Asymptomatic Carotid Artery Stenosis (ACAS) studies showed benefit for surgical management of symptomatic patients with carotid stenosis > 60% and asymptomatic patients with carotid stenosis > 70%. It is important to emphasize that there are very few established objective criteria for duplex ultrasound in carotid disease. At present, the most sensitive indicator is the absolute peak velocity at end-diastole at the site of stenosis; velocity >100 cm/sec suggests a high likelihood of severe stenosis, and further workup with angiography is warranted (Table 36.4).

Table 36.1. Correlation of Ankle-Brachial Index (ABI) with Clinical Presentation and Severity of Obstructive Lesions

ABI	Symptoms	Disease Severity
> 1.30	Indeterminate	Medial wall calcification; nondiagnostic
0.90 - 1.25	Asymptomatic	No hemodynamically significant lesions
0.60 - 0.90	Claudication	Single segment stenosis or well-collateralized occlusion
0.30 - 0.60	Claudication	Multiple segment disease
0.15 - .030	Resting pain	Multiple segment total occlusions
< 0.15	Impending tissue loss	Multiple segment total occlusions

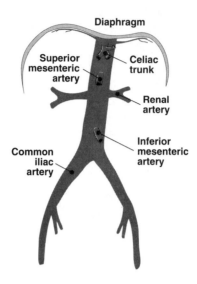

Figure 36.2 The Abdominal Aorta and Branches

Table 36.2. Qualitative Assessment of Doppler Flow Signals

Flow Pattern	Characteristics	Significance
Normal	Multiphasic flow signal with a brisk, well-defined high pitched systolic peak; lower pitched signals during diastole; transient reversal of flow during early diastole.	No significant obstruction
Damped	Slow systolic upstroke with a poorly defined systolic peak; slowly diminishing flow from systole through diastole, with antegrade flow during the entire cardiac cycle.	Significant proximal obstructive
Absent	No flow signal	Total vessel occlusion; absent collateral reconstitution.
Hyperemia	Sustained hyperemic flow throughout diastolic	Markedly diminished peripheral vascular resistance; characteristic of an arterio-venous fistula or arterial conduit supplying a distal runoff bed with significant inflammatory reaction (e.g., cellulitis).

Table 36.3. Doppler Velocity Spectrum Diagnostic Criteria for Grading Severity of Stenosis

Diameter Stenosis (%)	Spectrum Characteristics
< 20	No increase in V_p relative to proximal arterial segment; minimal spectral broadening.
20 - 49	>30% increase in V_p relative to proximal artery segment; V_p <125 cm/sec; spectral broadening throughout pulse cycle.
50 - 75	>100% increase in V_p relative to proximal arterial segment; V_p <125 cm/sec; spectral broadening throughout pulse cycle.
< 75	Spectrum similar to 50-75% diameter stenosis, with end-diastolic velocity > 100 cm/sec.

Abbreviations: V_p = Peak systolic velocity

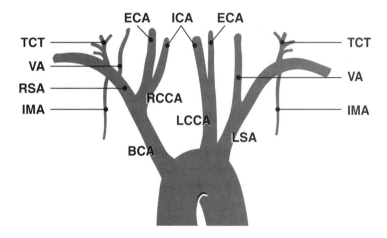

Figure 36.3 Arch of the Aorta and Great Vessels

BCA = brachiocephalic (innominate) artery; LCCA = left common carotid artery; LSA = left subclavian artery; RSA = right subclavian artery; RCCA = right common carotid artery; ICA = internal carotid artery; ECA = external carotid artery; VA = vertebral artery; IMA = internal mammary artery; TCT = thyrocervical trunk.

3. **Renal and Mesenteric Arteries.** The renal arteries, celiac axis and superior mesenteric artery (SMA) may all be evaluated at their origin from the abdominal aorta (Table 36.4).[19] The Doppler flow signal from the aorta just above the renal artery is used as a reference signal to determine the Renal/Aortic Ratio (RAR); absolute velocities are used in the celiac trunk and SMA. Patients should be fasting for at least eight hours prior to an abdominal vascular examination. Normal resting flow waveforms in the renal arteries and celiac axis are those of low distal vascular

resistance, with good antegrade flow throughout diastole. In contrast, distal vascular resistance is relatively high in the SMA in the fasting state, resulting in a Doppler waveform that has a very sharp systolic peak and minimal antegrade flow in late diastole. Following a caloric challenge, (e.g., 16 oz. Ensure) vascular resistance in the gut decreases sharply, with an attendant increase in end diastolic flow velocity. In the normal mesenteric circulation, the SMA end diastolic velocity should at least double (compared to fasting) within 30 minutes of a caloric challenge.

4. **Subclavian Artery.** A systolic pressure difference $\geq$ 20 mmHG between the two arms suggests significant subclavian artery obstruction; reversal of flow in the ipsilateral vertebral artery is diagnostic for hemodynamically significant subclavian stenosis. Direct evaluation of the subclavian artery by duplex ultrasound will show post-stenotic turbulence for subtotal lesions, or a damped flow waveform indicative of collateral reconstitution (Table 36.2).

C. **PERCUTANEOUS ANGIOPLASTY TECHNIQUES.** Non-surgical approaches to percutaneous vascular interventions include angioplasty (PTA), intra-arterial thrombolysis (PIAT), stents, and atherectomy. Each technique has its own limitations; they should be considered complementary tools for averting or limiting the extent of vascular bypass surgery. Clinical indications for percutaneous intervention are similar to those for bypass grafting; optimal treatment is dependent on clinical and angiographic data and target lesion location (Table 36.5).[20-36]

1. **Adjunctive Medication.** Aspirin should be given at least 24 hours before PTA; Nifedipine 10 mg SL and intra-arterial Nitroglycerin (NTG) 100-200 mcg are recommended before crossing target lesions in the renal artery and infrapopliteal vessels, to minimize spasm. Heparin 5,000 units IV should be administered after the lesion has been crossed with a guidewire. After intervention, sheath removal should be performed when the ACT is <175 sec; post-procedure heparin (PTT 2.0-2.5 times control for 12-24 hrs) is recommended for renal and infrapopliteal PTA, severe dissection, and in slow-flow states. Aspirin should be prescribed for at least 6 months in all patients; Persantine 75 mg PO TID may be added if desired.

Table 36.4. Duplex Ultrasound Diagnostic Criteria for the Renal and Mesenteric Arterial System[19]

Arterial System	Duplex Criteria*
Carotid artery	Absolute Peak Velocity > 100 cm/sec at end-diastole at the lesion site.
Renal artery	Renal/Aortic Ratio (RAR) > 3.5, and Peak Systolic Velocity > 180 cm/sec.
Celiac trunk	Peak Systolic Velocity > 200 cm/sec.
Superior mesenteric artery (SMA)	Peak Systolic Velocity > 275 cm/sec; failure to increase post-prandial end-diastolic velocity by at least two-fold compared to fasting velocity (within 30 minutes).

* Significant stenosis is defined as renal artery stenosis > 60%; iliac or SMA stenosis > 70%

Table 36.5. Indications and Contraindications for Peripheral Vascular Intervention

Target Vessel	Indications	Relative Contraindications	Absolute Contraindications
Aorta[20,21]	• Short stenoses of infrarenal aorta without other aortic disease • Buttock or lower extremity claudication or impotence	• Stenoses > 4cm in infrarenal aorta • Stenoses resulting in blue-toe syndrome • Stenoses 2-4 cm in length associated with diffuse infrarenal atherosclerosis	• Total occlusion of aorta • Stenoses associated with abdominal aortic aneurysm
Peripheral Artery[20,21]	• Intermittent claudication • Critical limb ischemia (rest pain, ulceration, gangrene, poor wound healing) • Improve inflow or outflow, before or after vascular bypass surgery • Bypass graft stenosis or anastomotic lesion • Impending amputation (to improve the level)	• Ulcerated plaque with atheroemboli • Long total occlusions (iliac > 4 cm, SFA > 10 cm), unless converted to shorter occlusions by thrombolysis • Long segment of infrapopliteal disease • Heavy, eccentric calcification • Lesion in or adjacent to an essential collateral	• Mild-moderate stenosis with no significant pressure gradient (>10mm Hg at rest, >20 mm Hg after priscoline • Stenosis immediately adjacent to an aneurysm • Embolic occlusions (3)ions
Renal Artery[22-34]	• Renovascular Hypertension: correction of a stenosis > 50%, resting pressure gradient > 10mm Hg or occlusion associated with refractory hypertension or documentation of renovascular hypertension • Renal Insufficiency: deterioration of renal function or asymmetric decrease in renal size, and renal artery stenosis > 50% • Recurrent pulmonary edema: due to bilateral renal artery stenosis • Renal transplant arterial stenosis or bypass stenosis producing hypertension, azotemia, or both	• Long occlusion • Stenosis associated with renal artery aneurysm • Atherosclerotic stenoses involving ostia (some authors recommend initial angioplasty, others advocate primary stenting) • Stenosis in renal artery arising from severely diseased or aneurysmal aorta	• Irreversible renal dysfunction • Hemodynamically insignificant stenosis • Medically unstable patient • Renal size < 6 cm
Visceral/Mesenteric[35,36]	• Chronic mesenteric ischemia (unexplained weight loss with postprandial pain and chronic nausea, vomiting, diarrhea) with significant stenoses or occlusion of two or more visceral vessels or acute symptoms in a patient who is not a surgical candidate. At this time surgery remains the first line of treatment.	• Stenoses >3 cm or ostial lesions of the superior mesenteric or celiac arteries • Occlusions of visceral vessels • Acute mesenteric ischemia	

2. **Vascular Access.** Arterial access should be achieved as close as possible to the target lesion (Table 36.6). Retrograde punctures are made with Seldinger or single wall techniques (Figure 36.4); antegrade puncture is most commonly performed with a single wall technique (Figure 36.5). Axillary and brachial artery punctures are typically performed with a single wall technique using a Potts-Cournand needle; alternatively, a micropuncture set may cause less arterial spasm (Figure 36.6). Placement of an appropriate arterial sheath facilitates exchange of catheters and guidewires.

   a. **Catheterization of Contralateral Femoral Artery.** This route often provides a better angle for reaching iliac artery branches, for dilating distal iliac and proximal femoral artery lesions, for thrombolytic therapy of occluded femoro-popliteal grafts, and for gaining access to distal femoral artery branches when the ipsilateral antegrade approach is difficult. Catheterization is performed by retrograde puncture of the contralateral femoral artery, initially advancing a guidewire up the iliac, then using a Cobra catheter, Simmons sidewinder, or internal mammary artery catheter to direct the wire down the opposite iliac artery (Figure 36.7). A stiff teflon-coated guidewire (Amplatz or Rosen guidewire) may be used to further advance the catheter around the bifurcation; an alternative technique is to use a flow-directed balloon catheter.

   b. **Left Axillary Artery Puncture.** This approach is used when there is no femoral artery access, and if there is no stenosis in the subclavian or axillary arteries (Figure 36.8). This approach may be useful for gaining access to sharply angulated lesions at the origin of the renal or mesenteric arteries:

Table 36.6. Site of Vascular Access for Peripheral Vascular Interventions.

Arterial Approach	Target Lesion Location
Retrograde femoral*	Aorta, common iliac, proximal external iliac, renal, visceral
Antegrade femoral*	Superficial femoral, profunda femoral, popliteal, infrapopliteal
Contralateral femoral (retrograde)[+]*	Internal iliac and its branches, distal external iliac, common femoral; can be used for fem-pop vessels if antegrade approach is not feasible
Left brachial [++]	Indicated if femoral access is not feasible
Left axillary [+++]	Indicated if all other routes are not available

*   Arterial puncture is over the femoral head
+   Internal mammary, Simmons sidewinder, or Cobra catheter may be used to hook the contralateral iliac artery
++   Nifedipine 10mg SL may be given to prevent spasm
+++   Puncture over the humeral head

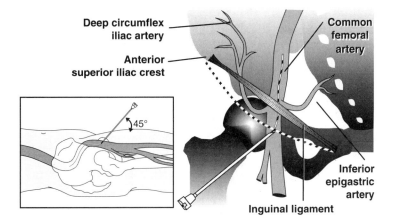

Figure 36.4 Common Femoral Artery: Retrograde Puncture

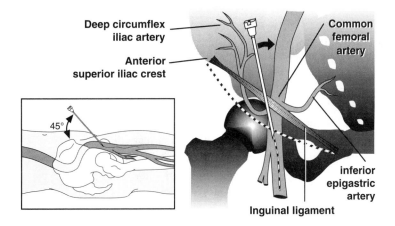

Figure 36.5 Common Femoral Artery: Antegrade Puncture

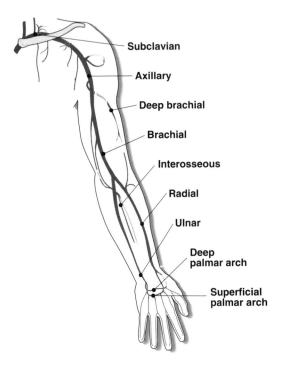

Figure 36.6 Arterial Circulation of the Upper Extremity

1. Abduct the left arm and place hand under the patient's head.
2. Obtain baseline axillary, brachial, radial, and ulnar pulses.
3. Locate the puncture site of the axillary artery along the lateral axillary fold over the proximal humerus so that the underlying bone provides support during compression.
4. Administer local anesthesia carefully and avoid deep penetration; an axillary hematoma may compress the brachial plexus.
5. The axillary artery is easily displaced; fix the artery firmly at the intended puncture site with left index and middle fingers on either side of the pulse.
6. The axillary artery should be entered at an angle of 45°, followed by insertion of an appropriate guidewire. Use of a micropuncture kit, vascular sheath (5-7FR), and vasodilators will minimize spasm.

3. **Crossing the Lesion.** Diagnostic angiography should be performed using appropriate catheters (Figure 36.9) and radiographic views (Table 36.7) to delineate the lesion and major branch vessels.[37] After baseline angiography, the lesion should be crossed with a soft-tip floppy straight

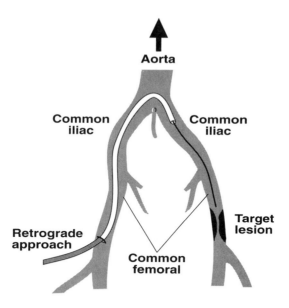

Figure 36.7 Peripheral Angioplasty: Contralateral Femoral Artery Approach

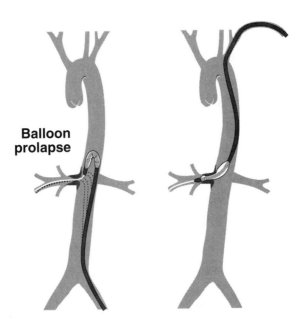

Figure 36.8 Peripheral Angioplasty: Axillary Artery Approach

Application	Name	Tip shape
Aortography Venacavography Pulmonary arteriography *(with tip deflector wire)*	Pigtail	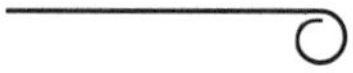
Pulmonary arteriography	Grollman	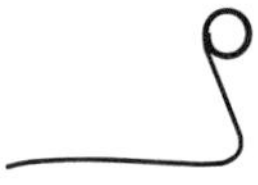
Iliac and antegrade femoral angiography	Straight-flush	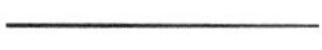
	Multipurpose (curve)	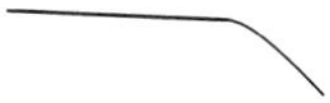

Inferior mesenteric
    artery; hooking
    contralateral iliac
	IMA (single hook)	

Left gastric arteriography	LGA	
Visceral and extremity	Cobra C1-C3 C2 and C3 have wide primary curves, for adults	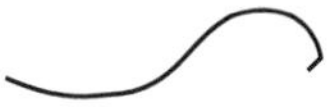
Selective renal arteriography	Renal Curve Right Judkins Coronary Simmons Sidewinder	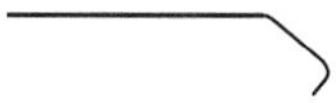
Aortic arch and subclavian	Modified Headhunter Simmons Sidewinder	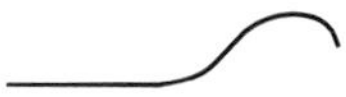

Visceral and cerebral
    selective arteriography
    *(shape must be reformed
    in the artery)*
	Simmons Sidewinder
	1: narrow aorta
	2: normal aorta
	3: wide aorta
	4: elongated aorta
	    (numbered by increasing
	    radius of primary curve)
		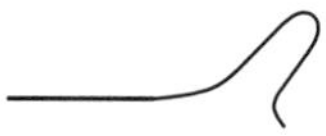

Figure 36.9 Peripheral Angioplasty: Catheter Selection

Table 36.7. Radiographic Views for Peripheral Angiography and Intervention[37]

Vessel	Radiology Film-Screen	Cine/DSA
Carotid bifurcation	Lateral and AP (with head turned to opposite extreme)	AP/oblique or lateral
Aortic arch (to open arch)	AP and RPO	AP and LAO
Aortic arch (for brachiocephalic vessels)	45° RPO with head turned, chin raised, shoulders dropped down	45° LAO
Origins of mesenteric vessels	Lateral aorta	Lateral
Origin of renal arteries	Left: 15° RPO Right: 15° LPO	Left: 15° LAO* Right: 15° RAO*
Common iliac bifurcation	Ipsilateral posterior oblique	Right: 15-30° LAO* Left: 15-30° RAO*
Common femoral bifurcation	Contralateral posterior oblique	Right: 15-30° RAO* Left: 15-30° LAO*

Abbreviations: DSA = digital-subtraction angiography; AP = anteroposterior; RPO = right posterior oblique; LPO = left posterior oblique; LAO = left anterior oblique; RAO = right anterior oblique
* Varying degrees of cranial and caudal angulation may be necessary

wire, a hi-torque floppy wire, an angulated glidewire, or a TAD (tapered attenuated diameter) wire. For subtotal stenoses, it may be useful to advance a guiding catheter just proximal to the lesion and cross the lesion with the guidewire. If necessary, the guiding catheter can be advanced across the lesion and the initial guidewire exchanged for a heavy-duty wire; PTA can then be performed as indicated.

4. **Balloon Catheter Selection.** Balloon size is estimated by measuring the diameter of the reference artery distal to the target lesion; if based on cut-film, the balloon will be oversized by 10-15% due to geometric magnification. Measurements can also be obtained from DSA images; typical balloon sizes are given in Table 36.8. The balloon may be positioned using anatomic landmarks, DSA road-mapping, or external markers (such as a hemostat). The balloon should be inflated using an inflation device with 50% contrast for 30-60 seconds; if the "waist" persists despite 2-3 inflations, consider a larger balloon or higher inflation pressures. Repeat angiography and transluminal pressure gradients may be used to assess the final result.[38]

5. **Special Considerations for Renal Artery Angioplasty.** Long-acting antihypertensive medications should be discontinued; short acting drugs should be substituted. Vascular surgery back-up is recommended for renal artery interventions. Guiding catheters (7-9F) facilitate selective angiography, wire manipulations, catheter exchanges, PTA, and stent placement, if necessary; high pressure polyethylene balloons are useful. Blood pressure and renal function must be closely monitored before, during, and after the procedure.

Table 36.8. PTA and Balloons Size

Target Vessel	Balloon Diameter (mm)*
Common or External iliac artery	6 - 10
Common or Superficial femoral artery	4 - 6
Popliteal artery	3 - 5
Tibial or Peroneal artery (below trifurcation)	< 4**
Renal artery	4 - 8

*   Balloon length varies from 2-10 cm; use the shortest balloon to straddle the lesion, and kissing balloons for bifurcation lesions.
**   Coronary balloons may be useful.

D.   **RESULTS OF PTA.** There is no universally accepted definition of PTA success; success may be defined angiographically (residual stenosis <15-20%), hemodynamically (residual pressure gradient 0 mmHg at rest or <10 mm Hg after priscoline), or clinically (increase in ABI >0.15, limb salvage, relief of claudication, or improvement in hypertension or renal function.[39] In most older studies, early or technical failures were not included when reporting long-term patency;[40] different end-points and definitions of success make it difficult to compare different studies.

1.   **Renal Artery PTA.** Renal angioplasty is technically more difficult than iliac or peripheral angioplasty; failures usually result from inability to cross the lesion or elastic recoil. Slightly oversized balloon may reduce the incidence of restenosis.[41] Several large series[25,41-45] reported angiographic success in 79-96% (Table 36.9) and a favorable blood pressure response in 80-90%. If a good initial result is obtained, the renal arteries may remain patent in 70-93% of patients for up to 6 years. Procedural success and long-term results are dependent upon lesion location, morphology and underlying pathology: Fibromuscular dysplasia is associated with excellent initial and long-term results; atherosclerotic stenoses are associated with a higher incidence of restenosis (Table 36.10).[24,25,27,33,46-48] Procedural success has been reported in 75-100% of non-ostial stenoses;[24,25,27,30-36,38-40,49-51] total occlusions or ostial stenoses have lower success rates, with success in 25% in one study.[6] Some interventionalists recommend primary stenting in ostial lesions,[52,53] but further study is needed. Restenosis occurs in approximately 15% of non-ostial lesions;[53] these patients may be treated with repeat PTA, with similar initial and long-term results.

2.   **Aortoiliac PTA (Table 36.11).** PTA of the aorta and iliac arteries has high success rates and a lower incidence of restenosis;[54-56] initial procedural success rates are 83-100% in the aorta and 73-100% in iliac arteries. Long-term patency at 5 years is 70-92% and 32-92%, respectively.

3.   **Iliofemoral PTA.** Results are best in the ilio-femoral system, with initial success in of 90-95% and 3-year patency of 75-80% (Table 36.12).[22,57-61] For focal subtotal stenoses of the common iliac artery in patients with claudication, 3-year patency is 90%.[57] Total iliac occlusions and stenoses > 10 cm in length lead to poor technical results and are not suitable for PTA.[58,61]

Table 36.9. Results of Percutaneous Renal Artery Angioplasty

Series	No.	Initial Success (%)	Long-Term Patency (%)	Follow-up (months)
Tegtmeyer[41] (1984)	149	94	93*	72
Sos[25] (1983)	101	79	-	-
Colapinto[42] (1982)	68	85	81	36
Puijlaert[44] (1981)	54	96	70	-
Schwarten[45] (1981)	70	93	71	6
Katzen[43] (1979)	17	94	75	12

Abbreviation: - = not reported
*   Includes successful redilatations

Table 36.10. Long-term Outcome After Renal Artery Angioplasty for Renovascular Hypertension

Series	Follow-up (m)	Etiology	Outcome (%)		
			Cured	Improved	No Response
Sos[25,33]	16	Fibromuscular Dysplasia	59	33	8
		Atherosclerotic	27	60	13
Tegtmeyer[24,46,47]	39	Fibromuscular Dysplasia	37	63	0
		Atherosclerotic	25	55	20
Miller[27]	6	Fibromuscular Dysplasia	85	15	0
		Atherosclerotic	25	58	17
Lossino[48]	60	Fibromuscular Dysplasia	57	21	21
		Atherosclerotic	12	51	37

Table 36.11. Results of Aortoiliac Angioplasty[54-56]

Target Vessel	Success (%)	Long-Term Patency (%)		
		1-year	2-year	3-year
Aorta	83 - 100	83 - 100	83 - 96	70 - 92
Iliac artery	73 - 100	63 - 100	58 - 95	32 - 92

4. **Femoropopliteal PTA.** Results in the femoral and popliteal arteries are consistently worse than in the aortoiliac arteries, with higher rates of early failure and restenosis (Table 36.12). For femoro-popliteal disease, initial success is achieved in 85%; 3-year patency is approximately 60%.[21,58,60,62,63] The best results are in focal stenoses or total occlusions <3 cm in length with good distal runoff; 3-year patency for this group is 75%.[63,64] In contrast, PTA of occlusions ≥ 9 cm in length with poor distal run off is associated with 3-year patency of 20-25%.[64,65] Although long-term patency is significantly decreased when PTA is performed for limb salvage as opposed to claudication, PTA alone will provide adequate inflow for limb salvage in 34%; PTA combined with bypass surgery may result in limb salvage in 71% of patients. Factors favorably influencing long-term outcome include proximal, focal stenoses in patients with claudication; adverse factors include distal lesions, total occlusion, poor distal run-off, and symptoms of critical ischemia.[21,40,54-56] Long-term success is most influenced by distal run-off.

5. **Infrapopliteal PTA (Table 36.13).** Until recently, PTA angioplasty at or below the popliteal trifurcation has been reserved for patients with critical ischemia (rest pain or tissue necrosis) or for patients with disabling claudication who were poor surgical candidates.[66-69] This reluctance to perform infrapopliteal PTA was based on early reports, which showed a high incidence of serious complications, and the belief that such complications frequently resulted in amputation of the affected limb. However, improvements in guidewire and balloon catheter technology, combined with better use of adjunctive medication has limited the frequency of serious complications. Technical success is approximately 95%; 1-year patency is 75-80%. In selected cases, PTA may be a useful adjunct for salvaging critically ischemic limbs.[70] There are limited data on the long term success of PTA in the infrapopliteal trifurcation vessels; the availability of modified coronary angioplasty catheters has increased the utilization of this technique.[71,72]

6. **Cerebral PTA.** Preliminary data from the North American Cerebral PTA Registry (NACPTAR) indicate clinical success in 76% (angiographic success in 83%); stroke and death occurred in 10% and 3%, respectively.[73]

E. **COMPLICATIONS OF PTA.** The overall incidence of complication is 5-10%; only 2-2.5% require treatment.[49,50,74] For renal artery angioplasty, the incidence of complications is 2-13%.[24,25,27,50] Major complications include thrombotic occlusion and distal embolization, which usually respond to low dose (60,000 IU/hr) Urokinase for 12-24 hrs. For femoro-popliteal PTA, major complications requiring

Table 36.12. Impact of Target Vessel Location and Morphology on PTA Success

Characteristic	Immediate Success (%)	3-Year Patency (%)
All lesions:		
Iliofemoral	90	75
Femoropopliteal	85	60
Ideal lesion*		
Iliofemoral	95	90
Femoropopliteal	90	75
Poor lesion**		
Iliofemoral	-	-
Femoropopliteal	70	20

Abbreviations: - = not available
*   Ideal lesion = focal stenosis, good runoff; claudication
**   Poor lesion = occlusion length > 9 cm, poor run-off; limb salvage

emergency surgery occur in 3% of patients. Procedure related mortality is 0.1-0.5%,[49] but may be as high as 6% in elderly patients with critical ischemia.[51] Minor complications such as hematoma usually respond to prolonged compression.

F. **NEW DIRECTIONS IN PERCUTANEOUS VASCULAR INTERVENTIONS.** PTA remains the mainstay of vascular intervention. Intravascular stents, thrombolytic therapy and atherectomy represent important advances, whose precise applications await definition.

1. **Intravascular Stents.** Suboptimal results after PTA are due to elastic recoil and/or extensive dissection. The only intravascular stent approved by the FDA is the Palmaz Stent (Johnson & Johnson, Warren, NJ) in the iliac arteries. The Schneider Wallstent (Schneider Stent Division, Pfizer, Minneapolis, MN) has gained acceptance in Europe and is in clinical trials in the U.S. for iliac and femoral intervention.

   a. **Indications for Stenting.** Possible indications for stenting include eccentric lesions or total occlusions in the renal or iliac arteries; ostial renal artery stenoses; residual gradient > 10 mm Hg or stenosis > 30% post PTA; renal artery stenosis; and dissection or restenosis after PTA.[52,74-79]

Table 36.13.   Results of Infrapopliteal Angioplasty[67-69]

Series	No	Success (%)			Complications (%)	
		Technical	Early	Late	Major	Minor
Bull[69] (1992)	168	83	77	67	11	8
Brown[67] (1988)	12	75	66	50	17	-
Schwarten[68] (1988)	98	97	88	86	2	1

Abbreviation: - = not reported

b.   **Contraindications.** Co-existing aneurysmal disease requiring surgical intervention; heavily calcified stenoses; noncompliant arteries; and extravasation of contrast following PTA are contraindications to peripheral stenting. Specific contraindications to renal artery stenting include non-functional kidney or size < 6 cm; diffuse intrarenal vascular disease; renal artery diameter <4 mm; and contraindications to anticoagulation.[75]

c.   **General Technique.** If stent placement is indicated, a vascular sheath or guiding should be positioned at the lesion; after the stent is positioned and delivered by balloon inflation, a larger balloon at higher pressure may be used if necessary. Medications are the same as those for PTA; post-procedure aspirin is recommended for 6 months. Some authors favor heparin for 24 hrs post procedure and Coumadin for four weeks after renal artery stenting.[53,75]

d.   **Results (Table 36.14).** Procedural success in the iliac and renal arteries is > 95%;[81-85] iliac artery patency at 5-years is 93% with stents and 70% for PTA.[81] The incidence of complications is approximately 5-10%, including renal failure; hematoma or pseudoaneurysm at the puncture site; systemic or intracranial hemorrhage due to anticoagulation (required in renal stents); and branch artery occlusion.[75] There are now several small studies of stenting innominate, subclavian, and carotid arteries with angiographic success rates > 90% and a low incidence of complications;[86-88] long-term follow-up studies are pending. Preliminary studies of stent-endoluminal grafts are also encouraging.[89] Stent-endografts are also under investigation for percutaneous treatment of abdominal aortic aneurysms[90] and dissection.[91]

2.   **Peripheral Intra-Arterial Thrombolysis (PIAT).** Peripheral Intra-Arterial Thrombolysis (PIAT) consists of direct intra-arterial infusion of fibrinolytic agents to restore blood flow to an ischemic limb due to thrombotic or embolic occlusion (Figure 36.10). Adjunctive thrombolytic therapy can convert a long occlusion to a short occlusion or discrete stenosis, thus limiting the extent of surgical revascularization or making the lesion more amenable to percutaneous intervention. Although no

Table 36.14. Stents for Peripheral Vascular Disease

Series	Target Lesion	No.	Stent	Success (%)	Comments
Henry[83] (1995)	Femoral, Popliteal	126	PS	99.6	RS 13%; 4-year patency 88% for upper SFA, 44% for lower SFA and popliteal; 4-year patency 39% for total occlusions
White[84] (1995)	Renal	98	BE	99	SAT 1.4%; RF 2.7%; Vasc 2.7%; ARS 28%
Bacharach[85] (1995)	Renal	116	NR	-	DUS patency 79% (9.5m); AP = 70% (9m)
Sullivan[86] (1995)	Subclavian, Innominate	33	PS	94	DE 6%; VAO 3%; Vasc 12%
Yadav[129]	Carotid	96	PS+GR	99	SAT 0%; no MI, or death; minor stroke 5%; RS 4.5%
Iyer[87] (1995)	Carotid	55	BE	100	SAT 0%
Dietrich[88] (1995)	Carotid	55	PS	94.5	Death 1.8%; TIA 3.6%; Vasc 18%; direct carotid puncture technique in 44%
Dietrich[89] (1995)	SFA	47	PS-ELG	98	Graft migration 4.3%; thrombosis 12.8%; Vasc 4.3%; 10 month patency 75%

Abbreviations: PS = Palmaz stent; GR = Gianturco-Roubin stent; BE = balloon expandable stent; PS-ELG = Palmaz stent-endoluminal graft (PTFE); DE = distal embolization ; VAO = vertebral artery occlusion; Vasc = vascular injury; SAT = subacute thrombosis; RF = renal failure; ARS = angiographic restenosis; DUS = duplex ultrasound; AP = angiographic patency; - = not reported

thrombolytic agent has received FDA approval for peripheral vascular use, Urokinase is currently the most commonly used agent for PIAT because it offers distinct advantages over Streptokinase (shorter infusion time, fewer complications)[92,93] and tissue plasminogen activator (lower cost, fewer hemorrhagic complications).[94,95]

a. **Indications .** Potential indications for PIAT include acute claudication or limb-threatening ischemia from thrombotic or embolic occlusion;[96-99] usual contraindications include recent stroke, internal bleeding, recent cardiopulmonary resuscitation, uncontrolled hypertension (diastolic blood pressure > 125 mm Hg), or severe coagulopathy.

b. **Technique.** The puncture site should be carefully chosen to allow the most direct access to the suspected lesion (Table 36.6). After baseline angiography, the thrombus is probed with a guidewire; acute thrombus usually allows easy passage of a guidewire, but chronic thrombus may be resistant. After entering the lesion, a multi-sidehole catheter is passed over the guidewire, and a transthrombus bolus of Urokinase is administered, using a pulsed-spray

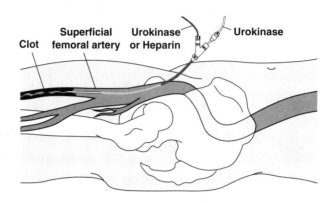

Figure 36.10   Peripheral Intra-Arterial Thrombolysis (PIAT)

technique.[99] Typically, a bolus of Urokinase (150-250,000 IU) is given over a twenty minute period, followed by a slow infusion of Urokinase (4,000 IU/minute for 2 hrs; then 2,000 IU/minute for 2 hrs; and then 1,000 IU/minute for 24-72 hrs). For patients without sensorimotor defects, the transthrombus bolus may be followed by low-dose infusion of Urokinase at 1,000 IU/hr.[100] Intravenous heparin is started as soon as the thrombus is crossed with a wire using a bolus of 70 u/kg, followed by infusion at 600-1,000 u/hr. The aPTT should be maintained at 2.0-2.5 times control. Angiography is repeated at 4 and 12 hrs, and every 12 hrs thereafter; lysis is terminated for successful recanalization, bleeding complication, or failure. Underlying stenotic or occlusive lesions should be treated promptly with PTA, atherectomy, or surgical revascularization.[98,100]

c.   **Results in PIAT.** Initial success rates are 60-95%;[99,101] duration of treatment varies with dose, thrombolytic agent (r-TPA <UK < SK), and rates of infusion. Long-term patency correlates with correction of the underlying stenosis;[97,98,102,103] 2-year patency is 80%.[91] Grafts with no identifiable stenosis have long-term patency of only 10%.[104] A prospective, randomized comparison of PIAT and surgical revascularization for patients with acute lower limb ischemia showed similar better 1-year survival (84% vs. 58%) for PIAT.[105]

d.   **Complications of PIAT[105-109].** The most common complication of PIAT is bleeding at the puncture site in 3%-20%. Intracranial hemorrhage occurs in 0.1-0.5%, and acute MI occurs in 8% of PIAT patients. Distal embolization occurs in 12% after PIAT, but acute limb ischemia occurs in only 2%; this is more common in patients with popliteal aneurysms. Other complications of PIAT include compartment syndrome in 2%; pericatheter thrombus in 5%;[91] oliguria and increased creatinine in <3%; and chills and rigors in 25% of patients.

Table 36.15. Comparison of PTA and Atherectomy for Peripheral Vascular Disease

Technique	Success (%)	Complications (%)	Patency* (%)
Balloon	90	8 - 12	70
Atherectomy	90	20 - 30	15 - 45

*   Patency at 2-3 years

3.   **Atherectomy (Table 36.15).** Mechanical atherectomy is undergoing extensive evaluation; [110-115] 4 devices have received FDA approval in the peripheral vessels: DCA, TEC, the Kensey catheter, and Rotablator. With the exception of the Kensey catheter, all depend on the ability to pass a guidewire through the lesion. Initial success after directional atherectomy is 95% for femoro-popliteal stenoses in patients with claudication; 2-year patency is only 45% and major complications occur in 5%. Directional atherectomy is not useful for distal vessels, long total occlusions or for limb salvage. Despite early enthusiasm for directional atherectomy, several large series suggest worse results compared to PTA.[39,116-118] However, it may be useful for specific indications, such as ulcerated atheromas causing "Blue-toe syndrome"; extensive dissections which are not amenable to intravascular stents; and stenoses in vein grafts.[119,120] The rotational atherectomy devices have achieved initial success rates of 80%, with 6-month patency of 40% and 2--year patency of only 15%; 8% of patients require urgent surgery for perforation or distal embolization. Similar to all other angioplasty techniques, the worst results are observed in long occlusions in the femoro-popliteal system for limb salvage.

4.   **Laser Ablation Techniques.** Hot-tip laser assisted balloon angioplasty and excimer laser angioplasty are rarely used; immediate results and long-term patency are worse than PTA.[121-128]

* * * * *

REFERENCES

1. Graor RA, Whitlow P. Coronary artery disease associated with peripheral vascular disease. In Young JR, Graor RA, Olin JW, et al (Eds). Peripheral Vascular Diseases. Mosby, St Louis, 1991;201-213.

2. Glover JL, Bendick PJ, Dilley RS, et al. Efficacy of balloon catheter dilatation for lower extremity atherosclerosis. Surgery 1982;91:560-565.

3. Rutherford RB. Evaluation and Selection of Patients for Vascular Surgery. In Rutherford RB (Ed). Vascular Surgery, Third Edition. WB Saunders, Philadelphia, 1989;10-16.

4. Smith RB, Fulenwider JT. Reversed Autogenous Vein Graft for Lower Extremity Occlusive Disease. In Ernst CB, Stanley JC (Eds). Current Therapy in Vascular Surgery. BC Decker, Toronto, 1987;206-210.

5. Veith FJ. The Impact of Nonoperative Therapy on the Clinical Management of Peripheral Arterial Disease. In Yao JST, Pearce WH (Eds). Technologies in Vascular Surgery. WB Saunders, Philadelphia, 1991;402-411.

6. Graor RA, Gray BH. Interventional Treatment of Peripheral Vascular Disease. In Young JR, Graor RA, Olin JW, et al (Eds). Peripheral Vascular Diseases. Mosby, St Louis, 1991;111-133.

7. Salles-Cunha Sx, Andros G. Preoperative Duplex Scanning Prior to Infrainguinal Revascularization. In Pearce WH, Yao JST (Eds). Surg Clin of NA 1990;70:41-59.

8. Strandness DE Jr, Sumner DS. Hemodynamics for Surgeons. Grune & Stratton, New York, 1975.

9. Bendick PJ, Glover JL, Kuebler TJ, et al. Progression of Atherosclerosis in Diabetics. Surgery 1983;93:834-838.

10. Krajewski LP, Olin JW. Atherosclerosis of the Aorta and Lower Extremity Arteries, In Young JR, Graor RA, Olin JW, et al. Peripheral Vascular Diseases. Mosby, St Louis, 1991;179-200.

11. Strandness DE Jr. Noninvasive Vascular Laboratory and Vascular Imaging. In Young JR, Graor RA, Olin JW, et al. Peripheral Vascular Diseases. Mosby, St Louis, 1991;39-69.

12. Yao JST. Hemodynamic Studies in Peripheral Arterial Disease. Br J Surg 1970;57:761-770.

13. Bridges RA, Barnes RW. Segmental Limb Pressures. In Kempczinski RF, Yao JST (Eds). Practical Noninvasive Vascular Diagnosis, Second Edition. Year Book Medical Publishers, Chicago, 1987;112-126.

14. Binnington HB. Segmental Limb Pressures, Doppler Waveforms, and Stress Testing. In Hershey FB, Barnes RW, Sumner DS (Eds). Noninvasive Diagnosis of Vascular Disease. Appleton Davies, Pasadena, California, 1984;16-23.

15. Jager KA, Ricketts HJ, Strandness DE Jr. Duplex Scanning for the Evaluation of Lower Limb Disease. In Bernstein EF (Ed). Noninvasive Diagnostic Techniques in Vascular Disease. Mosby, St Louis, 1985;619-631.

16. Kohler TR, Nance DR, Cramer M, et al. Duplex Scanning for Diagnosis of Aortoiliac and Femoropopliteal Disease: A Prospective Study. Circulation 1987;76:1074-1080.

17. Strandness DE Jr. Duplex Scanning in Vascular Disorders. Raven Press, New York,1990;121-145.

18. Bandyk DF. Postoperative Surveillance of Infrainguinal Bypass. In Pearce WH, Yao JST (Eds). Surg Clin NA 1990;70:71-85.

19. Vascular Technology, Vol II of Vascular Registry Review and Vascular Educational Program, 1995. Society of Vascular Technology, Lanham, MD.

20. Standards of Practice Committee of the Society of Cardiovascular and Interventional Radiology. Guidelines for Percutaneous Transluminal Angioplasty. Radiology 1990; 177: 619-626.

21. Schwarten DE, Tadavarthy SM, Casta–eda-Zu–iga WR. Aortic, iliac, and peripheral arterial angioplasty. Castaneda-Zuniga WR. Tadavarthy SM (eds). Interventional Radiology. 2ed. Williams & Wilkins, Baltimore, 1992; 378-421.

22. Becker GJ, Katzen BT, Dake, MD. Noncoronary Angioplasty. Radiology, 1989;170:921-940.

23. Pickering TG. Diagnosis and evaluation of renovascular hypertension: indications for therapy. Circulation 1991; 83: I-147--I-154.

24. Tegtmeyer Cj, Kellum CD, Ayers A. Percutaneous transluminal renal angioplasty of renal arteries: Results and long term follow-up. Radiol 1984; 153: 77-84

25. Sos TA, Pickering TG, Sniderman K, et al. Percutaneous transluminal renal angioplasty for renovascular hypertension due to atherosclerosis and fibromuscular dysplasia. N Engl J Med 1983; 309 274-279.

26. Gerlock AJ, MacDonnell RC Jr, Smith CW, et al. Renal transplant arterial stenosis: Percutaneous transluminal

angioplasty. Am J Roentgen 1983; 140: 325-331.

27. Miller GA, Ford KK, Braun SD, et al. Percutaneous transluminal angioplasty vs. surgery for renovascular hypertension. Am J Roentgen 1985; 144: 447-450.

28. Kuhlman U, Greninger P, Gruntzig A, et al. Long term experience in percutaneous transluminal dilation of renal artery stenosis. Am J Med 1985; 79: 692-698.

29. Martin LG, Casarella WJ, Gaylord GM. Azotemia caused by renal artery stenosis: treatment by percutaneous angioplasty. Am J Roentgen 1988; 150: 839-844.

30. Pickering TG, Sos TA, Saddekni S, et al. Renal angioplasty in patients with azotemia and renovascular hypertension. J Hypertension 1986; 4: s667-s669.

31. Pickering TG, Sos Ta, Vaughan ED, Case DB, Sealey JE, Harshfield GA, Laragh JH. Predictive value and changes of renin secretion in hypertensive patients with unilateral renovascular disease undergoing successful renal angioplasty. Am J Med 1984; 76: 398-404.

32. Martin EC, Mattern RF, Baer L et al. Renal angioplasty for hypertension: predictive factors for long term success. Am J Roentgen 1981; 137:921-924.

33. Sos TA. Angioplasty for the treatment of azotemia and renovascular hypertension in atherosclerotic renal artery disease. Circulation 1991; 83: I-162--I-166.

34. Pickering TG, Devereux RB, James GD, et al. Recurrent pulmonary edema in hypertension due to bil;ateral renal artery stenosis: treatment by angioplasty or surgical revascularization. Lancet 1988; 9: 551-552.

35. Sniderman, KW. Transluminal Angioplasty in the Management of Chronic Intestinal Ischemia. In DE Strandness and A Van Breda (eds), Vascular Diseases: Surgical and Interventional Therapy. New York: Churchill Livingstone, 1994. pp. 803-809.

36. Roberts L, Wertman DA, Mills SR, et al: Transluminal Angioplasty of the superior mesenteric artery: an alternative to surgical revascularization. Am J Roentgen 141: 1039, 1983.

37. Kandarpa, K. Handbook of Cardiovascular and Interventional Radiologic Procedures, 1st ed. Little, Brown and Company, Boston, 1989.

38. Kaufman SL, Barth KH, Kadir S. et al. Hemodynamics measurements in the evaluation and follow-up of transluminal angioplasty of the iliac and femoral arteries. Radiol 1982; 142: 329-336.

39. Becker GJ. Femoropopliteal Angioplasty, Atherectomy, Stents. Second International Symposium on Cardiovascular and Ind Interventional Radiology. Harvard Medical School/Brigham and Women's Hospital, Vol. 1, 1994: 53-65.

40. Johnston KW. Femoral and popleteal arteries: reanalysis of results of balloon angioplasty. Radiol 1992; 183: 767-771.

41. Tegtmeyer CJ, Kellum CD, Ayers C. Percutaneous Transluminal Angioplasty of the Renal Artery: Results and Long-Term Follow-up. Radiol 1984;153:77-84.

42. Colapinto RF, Stronell RD, Harries-Jones EP, et al. Percutaneous Transluminal Dilatation of the Renal Artery: Follow-up Studies on Renovascular Hypertension. Am J Roentgen 1982;139:727-732.

43. Katzen BT, Chang J, Knox WG. Percutaneous Transluminal Angioplasty with the Gruntzig Balloon Catheter: A Review of 70 Cases. Arch Surg 1979;114:1389-1399.

44. Puijlaert CBAJ, Boomsma JHB, Ruijs JHJ, et al. Transluminal Renal Artery Dilatation in Hypertension: Technique, Results and Complications in 60 Cases. Urol Radiol 1981;2:201-210.

45. Schwarten DE. Percutaneous Transluminal Renal Angioplasty. Urol Radiol 1981;2:193-200.

46. Tegtmeyer CJ, Sos TA. Techniques of Renal Angioplasty. Radiol 1986; 161: 577-586.

47. Tegtmeyer CJ, Selby JB. Percutaneous Transluminal Angioplasty of the Renal Arteriea. In WR Castenada-Zuniga and SM Tadavarthy (eds), Interventional Radiology (2nd ed). Baltimore: Williams & Wilkins 1992.pp364-377.

48. Losinno, F, Zuccala, A; Busato, F: Zuccali. Renal artery angioplasty for renovascular hypertension and preservation of renal funtion: long-term angiographic and clinical follow-up. Am J Roentgen 1994;16.2:853-7.

49. Gardiner GA, Meyerovitz MF, Stokes KR, Clouse ME, Harrington DP, Bettmann MA. Complications of transluminal angioplasty. Radiol. 1986; 159: 201-208.

50. Werbull H, et al. Complications after percutaneous transluminal angioplasty in the iliac, femoral and popliteal arteries. J Vasc Surg, 5: 681-686, 1987.

51.   Plecha FR, et al. The early results of vascular surgery in patients 75 years of age and older: an analysis of 3259 cases. J Vasc Surg, 2: 767-774, 1985.

52.   Thomson, KR. Longterm Results of Renal Artery Stenting: the Australian Experience. Harvard Medical School/Brigham and Women's Hospital Second International Symposium on Cardiovascular and Interventional Radiology. 1994, Vol I, 892-6.

53.   Sos, Thomas. Renal Angioplasty: Optimal Techniques, Long-term Results. Harvard Medical School/Brigham and Women's Hospital Second International Symposium on Cardiovascular and Interventional Radiology. 1994, Vol. I, 75-75N.

54.   Capek P, Mclean GK, Berkowitz HD. Femoropopliteal angioplasty: Factors influencing long-term success. Circulation 1991; 83: I-70-I-80.

55.   Rholl KS and von Breda A, Percutaneous Intervention for Aortoiliac Disease. In: <u>Vascular Diseases: Surgical and Interventional Therapy.</u> 1994, Churchill Livingston, New York.

56.   Gallino A, Mahler F, Probst P, Nachbur B. Percutaneous transluminal angioplasty of the arteries of the lower limbs: a 5-year follow-up. Circulation 1984; 70: 619-623.

57.   van Andel GJ, van Erp WF, Krepel VM et al. Percutaneous Transluminal Dilatation of the Iliac Artery: Long-Term Results. Radiol 1985;156:321-323.

58.   Johnston KW, Rae M, Hogg S, et al. 5-year Results of a Prospective Study of Percutaneous Transluminal Angioplasty. Ann Surg 1987;206:403-413.

59.   Wilson SE, Wolf GL, Cross AP. Percutaneous Transluminal Angioplasty Versus Operation for Peripheral Arteriosclerosis: Report of a Prospective Randomized Trial in a Selected Group of Patients. J Vasc Surg 1989;9:1-9.

60.   Rutherford RB, Durham J. Percutaneous Balloon Angioplasty for Arteriosclerosis Obliterans: Long-Term Results. In Yao JST, Pearce WH (Eds). Technologies in Vascular Surgery. W.B. Saunders, Philadelphia, 1992;329-345.

61.   Colapinto RF, Stronell RD, Johnston KW. Transluminal Angioplasty of Complete Iliac Obstructions. Am J Roentgen 1986;146:859-862.

62.   Schwarten DE. Clinical Anatomical Considerations for non-operative therapy in Tibial disease and the results of Angioplasty. First International Symposium on Cardiovascular and Interventional Radiology., Harvard Medical School/Brigham and Women's Hospital , 1992: pp 196-205.

63.   Berkowitz HD, Spence RK, Frieman DB, et al. Long-Term Results of Transluminal Angioplasty of the Femoral Arteries. In Dotter CT, Gruntzig A, Schoop W, et al. (Eds). Percutaneous Transluminal Angioplasty. Springer-Verlag, Berlin 1983;207-214.

64.   Jeans WD, Armstrong S, Cole SE, et al. Fate of Patients Undergoing Transluminal Angioplasty for Lower Limb Ischemia. Radiol 1990;177;559-564.

65.   Rutherford RB, Patt A, Kumpe DA. The Current Role of Percutaneous Transluminal Angioplasty. In Greenhalgh KM, Jamieson CW, Nicolaides AN (Eds). Vascular Surgery: Issues in Current Practice. Grune & Stratton, London, 1986;229-244.

66.   Adar R, Critchfield GC, Eddy DM. A Confidence Profile Analysis of the Results of Femoro-Popliteal Percutaneous Transluminal Angioplasty in the Treatment of Lower-Extremity Ischemia. J Vasc Surg 1989;10:57-67.

67.   Brown KT, Schoenberg NY, Moore, ED, Saddekni S. Percutaneous transluminal angioplasty of infrapopliteal vessels: preliminary results and technical considerations. Radiol 1988; 169: 78-78.

68.   Schwarten DE Cutcliff WB. Arterial occlusive disease below the knee: treatment with percutaneous transluminal angioplasty performed with low profile catheters and steerable guide wires. Radiol 1988; 169: 71-74.

69.   Bull PG, Mendel H, Hold M, Schlegl A, Denck H, Distal popliteal and tibioperoneal tibioperoneal transluminal angioplasty: long-term follow-up. J Vasc Interv Radiol 1992; 3: 15-53.

70.   Schwarten DE. Clinical and Anatomical Considerations for Nonoperative Therapy in Tibial Disease and the Results of Angioplasty. Circulation 1991;83:86-90.

71.   Horvath W, Oertl M, Haidinger D. Percutaneous Transluminal Angioplasty of Crural Arteries. Radiol 1990;177:565-569.

72.   Tamura S, Sniderman KW, Beinart C, et al. Percutaneous Transluminal Angioplasty of the Popliteal Artery and its Branches. Radiol 1982;143:645-648.

73. The North American Cerebral Percutaneous Transluminal Angioplasty Register (NACPTAR) Investigators. Update of the immediate angiographic results and in-hospital central nervous system complications of cerebral peructaneous transluminal angioplasty. Circulation 1995;92:I-382.

74. Rutherford RB, Becker GJ. Standards for evaluating and reporting the results of surgical and percutaneous therapy for peripheral arterial disease. Radiol 1991; 181: 277-281.

75. Saeed M. Aortoiliac and Renal Artery Stenting. In: Kandarpa K and Aruny J, (eds). Handbook of Interventional Radiologic Procedures, 2nd edition. Boston: Little Brown, 1996. pp. 103-114.

76. Richter GM, Roeren T, Brado M, Noeldge G. Renal Artery Stents: Long-term results of a European trial. Society of Cardiovascular and Interventional Radiology Meeting Abstracts, J. Vasc Interv Radiol, 4: 47, 1993.

77. Becker GJ, Palmaz JC, Rees CR, et al. Angioplasty-induced dissections in human iliac arteries: management with Palmaz balloon-expandable intaluminal stents. Radiol 1990; 176:31-38.

78. Rees CT, Palmaz JC, Garcia O, et al. Angioplasty and stenting of completely occluded iliac arteries. Radiol 1989; 172:953-959.

79. Williams JB, Watts PW, Nguyen VA, Peterson CL. Balloon Angioplasty with intraluminal stenting vs the initial treatment modality in aortoiliac occlusive disease. Am J Surg 1994; 168:202-204.

80. Rees CR, Palmaz JC, Becker GJ, et al. Palmaz stent in atherosclerotic stenoses involving the ostia of the renal arteries. Preliminary report of a Multi-center study. Radiol 1991; 181:507-514.

81. Richter GM, Noeldge, G, Roeren, T et al. Further Analysis of the Randomized Trial: Primary iliac stenting vs. PTA. Harvard Medical School (BWH 2nd Intl'l Symposium of CVIR. 1994, vol 1, 52-52 L.

82. Palmaz JC, Laborde JC, Rivera FJ, et al. Stenting of the iliac arteries with the Palmaz stent: experience from a multicenter trial. Cardiovasc Interven Radiol 1992; 15:291-297.

83. Henry M, Amor M, Henry I, Ethevenot G, et al. Placement of Palmaz-Schat in femoropopliteal arteries: A 6-year experience. Factors influencing restenosis and longterm results. Circulation 1995;92:I-58.

84. White CJ, Ramee SR, Collins TJ, Jenkins JS, et al. Stent placement for unfavorable renal artery stenosis. Circulation 1995;92:I-129.

85. Bacharach JM, Olin JW, Sullivan TM, Childs MB, Piedmonte M. Renal artery stents: Early patency and clinical followup. Circulation 1995;92:I-128.

86. Sullivan TM, Bacharach JM, Childs MB. PTA and primary stenting of the subclavian and innominate arteries. Circulation 1995;92:I-383.

87. Iyer SS, Yadav S, Vitek J, Wadlington V, et al. Technical approaches to angioplasty and stenting of the extracranial carotid arteries. Circulation 1995;92:I-383.

88. Diethrich EB, Lopez JR, Galarza L. Stents for vascular reconstruction in the carotid artereis. Circulation 1995;92:I-383.

89. Diethrich EB, Papazoglou CO, Lopez JR, Lopez-Galarza L. Endoluminal grafts for aneurysm exclusion and intraluminal bypass in the superficial femoral arteries. Circulation 1995;92:I-377.

90. Gomes AS, Moore WS, Quinones-Baldrich WJ, Yoon HC, Vescera CL. Tr3eatment of abdominal aortic aneurysm with the EVT-EGS endograft. Circulation 1995;92:I-127.

91. Slonim SM, Dake MD, Semba CP, Razavi MK, et al. True lumen obliteration in complicated aortic dissection: Endovascular management. Circulation 1995;92:I-127.

92. Belkin M, Belkin B, Buckman CA, et al. Intra-arterial fibrinolytic therapy: efficacy of streptokinase vs urokinase. Arch Surg 1986; 121: 769-773.

93. Van Breda A, Groar RA, Katzen BT, et al. Relative Cost-effectiveness of Urokinase versus Streptokinase in the Treatment of Peripheral Vascular Disease. J Vasc Interv Radiol 1991; 2: 77-87.

94. Graor RA, Olin J,Bartholomew JR, et al. Efficacy and Safety of Intraarterial local infusion of Streptokinase, Urokinase and tissue Plasminogen Activator for peripheral arterial occlusion: a retrospective review. J Vasc Med Biol;1990:310-5.

95. Meyerovitz MF, Goldhaber SZ, Reagan K, et al., Recombinant Tissue-type Plasminogen Activator versus Urokinase in Peripheral Arterial and Graft Occlusions: A Randomized Trial. Radiol 1990; 175:75-78.

96. McNamara TO. Thrombolysis as an Alternative Initial Therapy for the Acutely Ischemic Limb. Sem Vasc Surg 1992;

5: 89-98.

97.   Gardiner GA, Koltun W, Kandarpa K, et al: Thrombolysis of occluded femoropopliteal grafts. Am J Roentgen 1986; 147:621-626.

98.   Sullivan KL, Gardiner GA, Kandarpa K, et al. Efficacy of Thrombolysis in Infrainguinal Bypass Grafts. Circulation 1991; 83:: I-99 - I-105.

99.   Valji K,Roberts AC, Davis GB, Pulsed Spray thrombolysis of arterial and bypass graft occlusions. Am J Roentgen 1991;156: 617-21.

100. McNamara TO. Thrombolysis Treatment for Acute Lower Limb Ischemia. In: Strandness DE and Van Breda A (eds). Vascular Diseases: Surgical and Interventional Therapy. New York: Curchill-Livingstone, 1994. pp 355-378.

101. McNamara TO, Bomberger RA: Factors affecting initial and six month patency rates after intra-arterial thrombolysis with high dose urokinase. Am J Surg 1986; 152:709-712.

102. Hoch JR, Tullis MJ, Acher CW et al. Thrombolysis vs. surgery as the initial management for native artery occlusion: efficacy,safety and cost. Surgery, 1994;116:649-56.

103. Durham JD, Rutherford RB. Assessment of long-term efficacy of fibrinolytic therapy in the ischemic extremity. Sem Intervent Radiol 1992; 9:166-173.

104. Belkin M, Donaldson MG, Whittemore AD, et al. Observation of the use of thrombolytic agents for thrombotic occlusion of infrainguinal vein grafts. J Vasc Surg 1990; 11:289-96.

105. Ouriel K, Shortell CK, DeWesse JA, Green, RM, Francis CW, Azodo MV, Gutierrez OH, Manzione JV, Cox C, Marder VJ. A comparison of thrombolytic therapy with operative revascularization in the initial treatment of acute peripheral arterial ischemia. J Vasc Surg 1994; 19:1021-30.

106. McNamara TO, Goodwin SC, and Kandarpa K. Complications of thrombolysis. Seminars in Interventional Radiol. 1994;II: 134-144.

107. Smith CM, Yellin AE, Weaver FA, et al. Thrombolytic therapy for Arterial occlusion: a mixed blessing. Am J Surg 1994;116: 649-56; discussion 656-7.

108. Galland RB, Earnshaw JJ, Baird RN et al. Acute limb deterioration during intra-arterial thrombolysis. Br J Surg 1993; 80: 1118-20.

109. Kandarpa K. Regional Intraarterial Thrombolysis. In: Kandarpa K and Aruny J.(eds) Handbook of Interventional Radiological Procedures. Boston: Little Brown, 1996. pp. 59-68.

110. Queral LA, Criado FJ, Patten P et al. Long-term Results of Simpson Atherectomy. In Yao JST, Pearce WH (Eds). Technologies in Vascular Surgery. W.B. Saunders, Philadelphia, 1992;366-372.

111. Simpson JB, Selmon MR, Robertson GC et al. Transluminal Atherectomy for Occlusive Peripheral Vascular Disease. Am J Cardiol 1988;61:96G-101G.

112. Ahn SS, Eton D, Mehigan JT. Preliminary Clinical Results of Rotary Atherectomy. In Yao JST, Pearce WH (Eds). Technologies in Vascular Surgery. W.B. Saunders, Philadelphia, 1992;388-401.

113. Snyder SO, Wheeler JR, Gregory RT et al. Kensey Catheter: Early Results with a Transluminal Endarterectomy Tool. J Vasc Surg 1988;8:541-543.

114. Wholey MH, Smith JAM, Godlewski BS, et al. Recanalization of Total Arterial Occlusions with the Kensey Dynamic Angioplasty Catheter. Radiol 1989;172:95-98.

115. Ahn SS, Auth D, Marcus D, et al. Removal of Focal Atheromatous Lesions by Angioscopically Guided High-Speed Rotary Atherectomy: Preliminary Experimental Observations. J Vasc Surg 1988;7:292-300.

116. Dorros G, Lewin RF, Sachdev N, et al: Percutaneous atherectomy of occlusive peripheral vascular disease: Stenoses and/or occlusions. Cathet Cardiovasc Diagn 1989 18:1-6.

117. McLean GK. Percutaneous peripheral atherectomy. J Vasc Interv Radiol1993; 4:465-480.

118. Johnson DE, Hinohara T, Selmon MR, et al: Primary peripheral arterial stenoses and restenoses excised by transluminal atherectomy: A histopathological study. J Am Coll Cardiol 1990 15:410-425.

119. Dolmatch BL, Rholl KS, Moskowitz LB, et al. Blue toe syndrome: Treatment with percutaneous Atherectomy. Radiol 1989; 172:799-804.

120. Katzen BT, Becker GJ, Benenati JF, et al. Long-term follow-up of directional atherectomy in the femoral and popliteal arteries. (abstr). J Vasc Interv Radiol 1992; 3:38-39.

121. Rosenthal D. Hot-tip Laser Angioplasty: A Three Year Follow-up Study. In Yao JST, Pearce WH (Eds). Technologies in Vascular Surgery. W.B. Saunders, Philadelphia, 1992, pg. 357-365.

122. Rosenthal D, Pesa FA, Gottsegen WL, et al. Thermal Laser Balloon Angioplasty of the Superficial Femoral Artery: A Multicenter Review of 602 cases. J Vasc Surg 1989;14:152-159.

123. White RA, Grundfest WS. Lasers in Cardiovascular Disease. Year Book Medical Publishers, Chicago, 1987.

124. Choy DSJ. History of Lasers in Medicine. Thorac Cardiovasc Surg 1988;36:114-117.

125. Litvack F, Grundfest WS, Adler L, et al. Percutaneous Excimer-Laser and Excimer-Laser-Assisted Angioplasty of the Lower Extremities: Results of Initial Clinical Trial. Radiol 1989;172:231-235.

126. McCarthy WJ, Vogelzang RL, Nemcek AA Jr et al. Excimer Laser-Assisted Femoral Angioplasty: Early Results. J Vasc Surg 1991;13:607-614.

127. McCarthy WJ, Vogelzang RL, Pearce WH et al. Excimer Laser Treatment of Femoral Artery Atherosclerosis. In Yao JST, Pearce WH (Eds). Technologies in Vascular Surgery. W.B. Saunders, Philadelphia, 1992;346-356.

128. Perler BA, Osterman FA, White RI et al. Percutaneous Laser Probe Femoropopliteal Angioplasty: A Preliminary Experience. J Vasc Surg 1989;10:352-357.

129. Yadav S, Roubin G, Iyver S, et al. Immediate and Late Outcome after Carotid Angioplasty (PTA) and Stenting. J Am Coll Cardiol 1996;March Special Issue.

37

BALLOON VALVULOPLASTY

Gregory Pavlides, MD
Robert D. Safian, MD

PERCUTANEOUS BALLOON MITRAL VALVULOPLASTY

Patients with mild-to-moderate mitral stenosis (i.e., valve area > 2.0 cm²) are asymptomatic or have only mild dyspnea; treatment consists of prophylaxis for rheumatic fever and infectious endocarditis; warfarin for atrial fibrillation or embolism; and β-blockers for exercise-induced dyspnea. In contrast, patients with "critical" mitral stenosis (i.e., valve area < 1.0 cm²) usually present with incapacitating dyspnea; as pulmonary hypertension and right heart failure supervene, orthopnea and paroxysmal nocturnal dyspnea dominate the clinical picture. Atrial fibrillation eventually develops in 80% of these patients and may be complicated by systemic thromboembolism in 20%. Percutaneous balloon mitral valvuloplasty (PBMV), first introduced by Inoue in 1984 and later used by others,[1-6] is now considered the treatment of choice for selected patients with critical mitral stenosis. Antegrade transseptal[7-15] and retrograde transarterial left atrial catheterization techniques have been described.[16-18]

A. **MECHANISM OF MITRAL VALVULOPLASTY.** Closed surgical commissurotomy and PBMV increase orifice diameter and leaflet mobility by separating fused commissures and fracturing calcified nodules.[26-29] In contrast to open surgical commissurotomy (i.e., performed under direct vision using circulatory arrest and cardiopulmonary bypass), PBMV and closed commissurotomy have little or no impact on subvalvular thickening or chordal involvement. In bioprosthetic valves, where the mechanism of stenosis is calcification and fibrosis of the cusps rather than commissural fusion, balloon dilatation may result in severe mitral regurgitation; surgery is preferred in these patients.[30-33]

B. **PREPROCEDURAL EVALUATION.** Once the diagnosis of mitral stenosis is established, 2-D and transesophageal echocardiography (TEE) are recommended to assess the extent of mitral valve thickening, calcification, leaflet mobility, subchordal disease, and mitral regurgitation. Findings by 2-D echocardiography can be used to generate an "echo score," which has important prognostic impact on the immediate and longterm results after PBMV (Table 37.1).[8] TEE is particularly useful in evaluating left atrial thrombus, especially in patients with atrial fibrillation: Patients with cavitary thrombus should be treated with anticoagulants for 2 - 3 months prior to valvuloplasty (due to the risk of systemic embolization). Persistent thrombus is a contraindication to PBMV, although small numbers of patients with thrombus limited to the left atrial appendage have undergone PBMV with TEE guidance.[19-22] A prior history of embolism in the absence of thrombus on TEE is not a contraindication to PBMV.[23-25]

C. **TECHNIQUE.** Diagnostic right and left heart catheterization and left ventriculography should be performed prior to PBMV, to assess the severity of mitral stenosis (i.e, transmitral gradient from

Table 37.1. Mitral Valve Echo Score Based on Morphologic Features *

Grade	Definition

Leaflet Mobility

1	Highly mobile valve; only leaflet tips restricted
2	Normal mobility (mid portion and base of leaflet)
3	Valve moves forward in diastole, mainly from the base
4	No forward movement of leaflets in diastole

Leaflet Thickening

1	Leaflets normal in thickness (4-5mm)
2	Mid portion of leaflets normal; thickening of margins (5-8mm)
3	Moderate thickening of entire leaflet (5-8mm)
4	Marked thickening of leaflet (>8 mm)

Subvalvular Disease

1	Minimal thickening just below mitral leaflets
2	Thickening of chordal structures extending up to one-third of the chordal length
3	Thickening extends to distal third of the chords
4	Extensive thickening and shortening of all chordal structures to papillary muscles

Calcification

1	Single area of increased echo brightness
2	Scattered areas of brightness confined to leaflet margins
3	Brightness extends into mid portion of leaflets
4	Extensive brightness throughout the leaflets

* Echo score is determined by adding the individual scores for leaflet mobility, leaflet thickening, subvalvular disease, and calcification

simultaneous LV and pulmonary capillary wedge pressure recordings) and mitral regurgitation. The two general approaches to PBMV are the antegrade transvenous approach and the retrograde transarterial approach.

1. **Antegrade Transvenous Approach (Inoue Technique; Single or Double-Balloon Technique).** This approach requires transseptal left heart catheterization:

   a. **Technique of Transseptal Left Heart Catheterization.** An 8F sheath is introduced into the right femoral vein and exchanged for a modified 8F Mullins sheath and dilator, which is advanced over a 0.032-inch J-guidewire into the superior vena cava. The guidewire is removed, a Brockenbrough needle is advanced to within a few mm of the tip of the dilator, and the needle is then flushed and connected to a transducer for continuous pressure monitoring (Figure 37.1). There are several techniques for crossing the interatrial septum; the easiest is to orient the arrow on the Brockenbrough handle to 5 o'clock while monitoring the position of the needle in the AP projection. In this position, as the sheath, dilator, and needle are

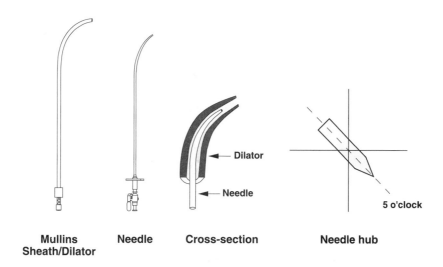

Figure 37.1 Catheters Used for Transseptal Catheterization

A. Mullins sheath and dilator.
B. Brockenbrough needle and stylet.
C. Correct position of needle inside the dilator.
D. Orientation of arrow on needle hub. When hub maker is approximately 5:00, the tip of the needle is in correct position.

withdrawn along the shadow of the spine, the needle tip will descend over the top of the aortic knob, and then drop into the fossa ovalis. Further slight pullback and then gentle re-advancement of the Mullins sheath and dilator will usually produce a "catching" sensation, indicating that the tip is in the fossa ovalis. This position can be confirmed by further imaging in a standard 30° RAO projection, which should demonstrate that the needle is directed toward the atrial side of the AV groove. Similarly, fluoroscopy can be employed in the lateral projection (Figure 37.2). In some cases, a high left atrial pressure may result in flattening and posterior displacement of the fossa ovalis. If the fossa cannot be easily identified as described above, the needle can be oriented more posteriorly by turning the arrow to 6 o'clock. In some cases, it may be necessary to repeat the entire approach after adding an extra bend to the tip of the Brockenbrough needle. In particularly difficult cases, transesophageal echo may be useful for identifying the fossa ovalis.   Once proper position is achieved, the Mullins sheath and dilator are gently advanced into the fossa (which may result in transient pressure damping), and the Brockenbrough needle is advanced across the atrial septum to the left atrium, which is usually associated with a slight "popping" sensation. In general, the AP and RAO projection result in mild foreshortening of the atrial septum and left atrium; it is therefore preferable to advance the needle into the left atrium in a 60°-90° LAO projection. Transseptal

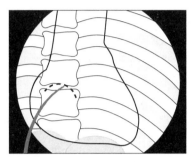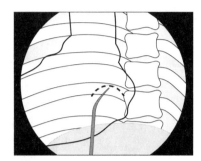

Figure 37.2 Transseptal Puncture

Orientation of needle in antero-posterior (A) and left lateral (B) view. The dotted line represents the limbus of the fossa ovalis.

catheterization described above is safe: Perforation leading to tamponade has been reported in 1.3%; mortality is less than 0.1%.[34]

b. **Inoue Technique.** The Inoue balloon catheter is a 12F, 70-cm long polyvinyl chloride catheter with two central coaxial lumens. The inner lumen allows pressure measurement and passage of a guidewire, and the outer lumen is for balloon inflation. Balloon size is based on patient height: balloon size in mm = height (cm; rounded to the nearest 0) divided by 10, and added to 10. The stainless steel guidewire is inserted into the left atrium through the Mullins sheath until the coiled tip touches the superior wall of the left atrium. After dilating the groin and atrial septum, the Inoue balloon is carefully advanced over the guidewire into the left atrium and across the mitral valve. The distal balloon is partially inflated and then is pulled back and anchored in the mitral valve; full balloon inflation is completed to dilate the mitral valve. After deflating the balloon, left atrial pressure is remeasured; if an inadequate result is obtained, the balloon can be advanced and inflated to larger size (the Inoue balloon diameter is adjustable within 4 mm). When the dilation process is complete, the balloon catheter is removed and final measurements obtained.

c. **Single or Double-balloon Technique.** Following transseptal catheterization, heparin is administered, and a balloon-tipped floatation catheter is advanced through the Mullins sheath into the left atrium, left ventricle, and the ascending aorta. One (single balloon technique) or two (double balloon technique) 0.035" J wires are then advanced through the balloon-tipped catheter into the aorta, after which the interatrial septum is dilated with an 8 mm balloon. After septostomy, one (25 mm) or two (18,20 mm) balloons are advanced across the mitral valve and inflated using a hand-held syringe (Figure 37.3). The final balloon size depends on the patient's size; for patients with a small body habitus (< 60 kg), it is reasonable to start with a single 25 mm balloon, with further increases depending on hemodynamics. A single 25 mm balloon has an inflated area of 4.9 cm^2, combined use of 15-mm and 20-mm balloons inflate to 5.51 cm^2, and two 18-mm balloons inflate to 5.78 cm^2 ; PBMV is most effective using inflated balloons > 4.9 cm^2. Following dilation, the balloons are removed and the floatation catheter is advanced to the left atrium for repeat pressure measurements.

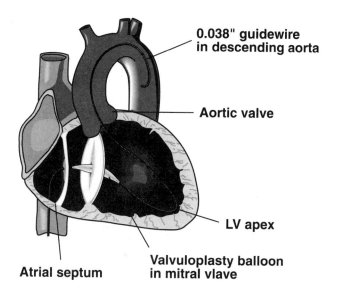

0.038" guidewire in descending aorta

Aortic valve

LV apex

Valvuloplasty balloon in mitral vlave

Atrial septum

Figure 37.3 Percutaneous Balloon Mitral Valvuloplasty (PBMV)

2. **Retrograde Transarterial Approach.** The left ventricle is entered retrograde with a pigtail catheter via the right femoral artery and exchanged for a special steerable left atrial catheter. The steering wire is retracted and a J is formed in the left ventricular apex. To enter the left atrium, the 45° LAO and 45° RAO projections are used. Ventriculography in these views can define the mitral valve plane and facilitate cannulation of the left atrium. After the guide wire enters the left atrium, the left atrial catheter is exchanged for a pigtail catheter to obtain pressure measurements and calculation of mitral valve area. The pigtail catheter is exchanged for a standard valvuloplasty balloon catheter using a single or double balloon technique.

D. RESULTS

1. **Hemodynamics Results (Tables 37.2, 37.3).** PBMV produces immediate improvement in hemodynamic and clinical status in the majority of patients.[9-12,14,15,17,25,35-44] In general, there is a 50-70% decrease in transmitral gradient and a 50-100% increase in mitral valve area (Figure 37.4). Approximately 10% of patients have persistent mitral valve area < 1.0 cm^2. Valve areas are smaller after PBMV with single balloons than double balloons, and results with the Inoue balloon are similar to the double balloon technique (Table 37.3).[10,42-44] Several reports confirm the effectiveness of PBMV after previous surgical commissurotomy[45-48] (although symptom recurrence is more frequent at 6 months),[45-47] and for pregnant women with mitral stenosis.[25,49-53]

2. **Complications (Table 37.4).** Serious complication include death (0-1.6%), thromboembolic events (0-6.5%), and severe mitral regurgitation requiring valve replacement (0.9%-3%); transient heart block and pericardial tamponade occur infrequently (<5%) with the transseptal techniques. [34] While a left-to-right shunt is detected in 20% of patients immediately after transseptal PBMV, the shunt ratio is usually < 1.5 and decreases over the next 6 months in the majority of cases.[55-58]

3. **Longterm Results (Tables 37.5, 37.6).** In general, improvements in hemodynamic and clinical status persist in the majority of patients.[11,15,17,35,39,40,42,59-61] However, restenosis, defined as a loss of $\geq 50\%$ of the original gain in mitral valve area, develops in 7-24% of patients within 5 years. Factors adversely affectiving longterm outcome include high echo score, elevated left ventricular end diastolic pressure, and higher NYHA functional class; predicted 5-year event-free survival is 60-84% and 13-41% in patients with ≤ 1 risk factor and ≥ 2 risk factors, respectively.[8] Total survival and event-free survival at 2 years were 98% and 79% for patients with an echo score ≤ 8, and 72% and 39% for patients with echo score > 8. In another study, independent predictors of event-free survival at 2 years were echo score, change in valve gradient, and change in left ventricular end-diastolic pressure.[62]

Table 37.2. Immediate Results of PBMV

Series	Technique	N (pts)	MVA (cm²) Pre	Post	MVG (mm Hg) Pre	Post
Chen [5] (1995)	I	4832	1.1	2.1	18	5
Arora [35] (1994)	2,I	600	0.8	2.2	27	4
Block [36] (1994)	1,2	570	0.9	2.0	16	6
Vahanian [25] (1994)	2,I	790	1.1	2.1	15	6
Stephandis [37] (1994)	R	154	1.0	2.2	16	6
Feldman [38] (1993)	I	260	1.0	1.8	14	6
Pan [39] (1993)	2,I	350	1.0	2.1	18	7
NHLBI [10] (1992)	1,2	738	1.0	2.0	14	6
Cohen [11] (1992)	1,2	146	1.0	2.1	14	6
Abascal [12] (1992)	1,2	130	0.9	1.8	16	6
Stephanadis [17] (1992)	R	86	0.9	2.1	16	5
Hung [40] (1991)	I	219	1.0	2.0	13	6
Ruiz [41] (1990)	2	276	0.9	2.4	16	5
Vahanian [9] (1989)	1,2	200	1.1	2.2	16	6
Nobuyoshi [14] (1989)	I	106	1.4	2.0	12	7

Abbreviations: MVA = mitral valve area; MVG = transmitral valve gradient; I = Inoue technique; 1 = single balloon technique; 2 = double balloon technique; R = retrograde (transarterial) technique

Table 37.3. Immediate Results and Technqiue of PBMV

Series	N (pts)	Technique	MVA (cm²)		MVG (mmHg)	
			Pre	Post	Pre	Post
Park[10]	59	I	0.9	1.9	-	-
(1993)	61	2	0.9	2.0	-	-
Ribeiro[42]	9	I	0.8	1.8	-	-
(1993)	9	2	0.8	1.9	-	-
NHLBI[43]	114	1	0.9	1.7	14	7
(1992)	591	2	1.0	2.0	14	6
Bassand[44]	161	2	1.0	2.0	13	5
(1991)	60	I	1.1	2.0	12	5

Abbreviations: MVA = mitral valve area; MVG = transmitral valve gradient; I = Inoue technique; 1 = single balloon technique; 2 = double balloon technique; R = retrograde (transarterial) technique; - = not reported

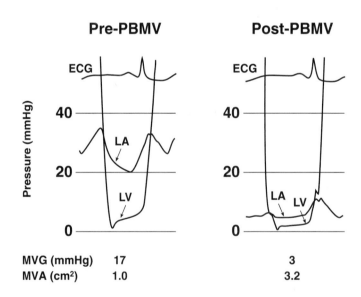

	Pre-PBMV	Post-PBMV
MVG (mmHg)	17	3
MVA (cm²)	1.0	3.2

Figure 37.4 PBMV: Immediate Hemodynamic Results

PBMV results in a decrease in mitral valve gradient (MVG) and an increase in mitral valve area (MVA). Pressure in the left atrial atrium (LA) decreases; there is no change in the left ventricular (LV) diastolic pressure.

Table 37.4. Complications of PBMV

Series	N (pts)	Death (%)	Emb/CVA (%)	Perf/Tamp (%)	MR (%)
Chen[15] (1995)	4832	0.1	0.5	0.8	0.4
Arora[35] (1994)	600	1.0	0.5	1.3	1.0
Block[36] (1994)	570	0.5	1.0	1.0	1.4
Vahanian[25] (1994)	810	0.5	3.6	0.9	3.5
Stephanadis[37] (1994)	155	0.6	0	0	1.3
Feldman[38] (1993)	260	1.1	0.7	0.7	2.7
NHLBI[10] (1992)	737	1.6	1.7	0.4	-
Cohen[11] (1992)	146	1.0	2.0	4.0	2.7
Stephanadis[17] (1992)	86	0	0	0	1.2
Bassand[44] (1991)	232	0	6.5	2.6	-
Ruiz[41] (1990)	285	0.7	1.4	4.9	-
Hung[40] (1991)	219	0.5	1.4	0	6.0
Vahanian[9] (1989)	200	0	4	-	-
Noboyoshi[14] (1989)	106	0	0	2	4

Abbreviations: Emb/CVA = embolic event or stroke; Perf/Tamp = cardiac perforation or tamponade; MR = severe mitral regurgitation; - = not reported

Table 37.5. Clinical Follow-up After PBMV

Series	N (pts)	F/U (months)	Restenosis (%)	RePBMC (%)	MVR (%)	Death (%)
Chen[15] (1995)	4832	32	5.2	0.4	-	-
Arora[35] (1994)	600	37	1.7	0.3	0.2	-
Chan[59] (1994)	253	20	23.5	3.6	10.3	3.9
Pan[39] (1993)	350	38	11.7	0.6	5.1	1.7
Chen[60] (1992)	85	60	6.8	1.1	4.7	-
Cohen[11] (1992)	146	36	18	4.1	12.4	22.1
Stephanadis[17] (1992)	84	24	15.4	-	3.6	-

Abbreviations: F/U = follow-up interval; RePBMC = repeat PBMC; MVR = mitral valve replacement; - = not reported

Table 37.6. Hemodynamic Follow-up after PBMV

Series	N (pts)	F/U (Year)	Technique	MVA (cm²) Pre	MVA (cm²) Post	MVA (cm²) F/U
Chen[18] (1995)	-	2.6	I	1.1	2.1	1.8
Park[52] (1993)	-	1	I,2	0.9	1.9	1.7
Chen[57] (1992)	85	5	I	1.1	2.0	1.8
Block[58] (1992)	41	2	1,2	1.1	1.8	1.6
Stephanadis[9] (1992)	26	2	R	0.9	2.0	1.9

Abbreviations: F/U = follow-up interval; I = Inoue technique; 1 = single balloon technique; 2 = double balloon technique; R = retrograde (transarterial) technique; MVA = mitral valve area; - = not reported

4. **Predictors of Early Outcome.** Clinical, echocardiographic, hemodynamic and procedural factors associated with a less successful immediate outcome include:[8,10-12,39,63-69]

Advanced age (only 50% of patients > 65 years achieve a final valve area > 1.5 cm²) [77,78]

- Rhythm other than sinus
- High echo score (although some patients with high scores have good results)
- Mitral valve calcification (Mitral valve area after PBMV was smaller in calcified than noncalcified valves (1.8 vs 2.1 cm²)
- Treatment with smaller balloons

Factors not affecting the results of PMBV include severity of mitral stenosis[71] and mild-to-moderate mitral or aortic regurgitation.[72,73] Elevated pulmonary artery pressure has been variably associated with an adverse outcome.[74-76]

5. **Comparison of Different Techniques and Surgical Commissurotomy.** Selection of the technique used for mitral valvuloplasty is based primarily on personal experience and available equipment. In appropriate hands, all techniques are effective and safe.[10,42-44,79-83] In studies comparing double balloons to the Inoue technique, final valve area was slightly larger after double balloons (2.0-2.2 cm² vs. 1.7-2.0 cm²), but the degree of mitral regurgitation and intracardiac shunting were similar. (There are no studies that directly compare transarterial and transseptal techniques.) PBMV and surgical techniques (closed[84-86] and open commissurotomy[86]) have been shown to achieve similar early results, although in one report, mitral valve area at 3 years was greater in patients treated with PBMV (2.4 vs. 1.8 cm²).[86]

PERCUTANEOUS BALLOON AORTIC VALVULOPLASTY

Aortic stenosis (AS) in adults is most commonly caused by degenerative calcification of a congenital bicuspid valve. Characterized by a long latent period during which progressive stenosis and left ventricular (LV) hypertrophy occur, patients with severe AS may remain asymptomatic for years. However, once symptoms develop, prognosis is poor: Life-expectancy for those with angina, syncope, and heart failure is 5-, 3-, and 2-years, respectively.

Percutaneous balloon aortic valvuloplasty (PBAV) was first performed in children and adults with aortic stenosis,[87] and later applied to adults with degenerative calcific aortic stenosis.[88,91] Although PBMV has become a viable alternative to surgical commissurotomy for select patients with mitral stenosis, PBAV has not become a viable alternative to aortic valve replacement (AVR) in adults. AVR is the standard treatment for adults with symptomatic aortic stenosis and is typically associated with marked hemodynamic improvement, regression of LV hypertrophy, enhanced LV performance, and increased survival;[94,96] perioperative mortality rates are 1.5-5% but may be as high as 15-40% for emergency operations or in patients with severe LV dysfunction and shock.[97]   The impact of advanced age per se is somewhat controversial; some studies of AVR in patients > 70 years reported perioperative mortality rates of 12-33%, [98,99] but contemporary studies report perioperative mortality rates < 10%.[100,101]   Actuarial 1- and 5-year survival rates are 83% and 67% for octogenarians treated with isolated AVR for aortic stenosis, which is similar to the actuarial survival of octogenarians without aortic stenosis.[100]

A. **MECHANISM OF AORTIC VALVULOPLASTY.** Post mortem and intraoperative studies indicate that the mechanisms of PBAV include fracture of calcified nodules, separation of fused commissures (rheumatic aortic stenosis), and simple stretching of valve leaflets. Although leaflet mobility and orifice dimensions improve, valve leaflets remain severely deformed, calcified, and stenotic.[102]

B. **PREPROCEDURAL EVALUATION.**   Adults with clinical evidence of aortic stenosis should undergo 2-D echocardiography to evaluate valve function and morphology, and left ventricular performance.   Right and left heart catheterization, coronary angiography, and aortography are recommended to assess the extent of coronary artery disease and aortic insufficiency.

C. **TECHNIQUE.** The two potential approaches for PBAV are the retrograde arterial approach and the antegrade transvenous approach:

1. **Retrograde Arterial Approach (Figure 37.5).** The most common approach to PBAV is the retrograde femoral arterial approach. (A retrograde brachial approach may also be used if femoral arterial access cannot be achieved.) To perform PBAV using the retrograde femoral approach:

    - Place an 8F sheath in the left femoral vein for right heart catheterization, cardiac output determination, and central access in the event a temporary pacemaker is needed.

    - Place an arterial monitoring line in the left femoral or radial artery.

    - Perform left heart catheterization via the right femoral artery (or brachial artery) using a 7F angled pigtail catheter and a long (30-cm) 8F introducing sheath; heparin (3000-5000 units) should be administered intravenously after arterial access is obtained. Simultaneous LV and systemic pressures may be obtained via the pigtail catheter and arterial sidearm, or by using an 8F double-lumen pigtail catheter, which permits pressure measurements in close proximity to the aortic valve; special care must be taken to adequately flush the proximal lumen, since a damped pressure will falsely overestimate the transaortic valve gradient and degree of aortic stenosis.

    - Cross the aortic valve with the pigtail catheter using a 0.038-inch straight guidewire. After baseline hemodynamic measurements are obtained, a 280-cm 0.038-inch J-guidewire should be placed in the left ventricle; a large curve should be fashioned on the distal end of the guidewire to conform to the shape of the apex.

    - Exchange the 8F arterial sheath and pigtail for a 12F introducing sheath and a 20 x 5 mm valvuloplasty balloon. Position the balloon across the aortic valve, and inflate the balloon with dilute contrast using a hand-held syringe. If blood pressure allows, balloon inflations of 30-60 seconds are desirable.

- After 2-4 inflations, the valvuloplasty balloon is exchanged for the pigtail catheter for repeat hemodynamic assessment. Once the desired result is achieved (generally a 50% reduction in gradient), the procedure is terminated. Vascular sheaths may be removed when the ACT is less than 140 seconds.

2. **Antegrade Transvenous Approach.** The antegrade transvenous approach requires transseptal left heart catheterization, as described for balloon mitral valvuloplasty. This techniques should be reserved for operators experienced in transseptal techniques and in circumstances where retrograde crossing of the aortic valve is impossible.

3. **Single vs. Multiple Balloon Techniques.** PBAV may be performed using single or multiple balloons; multiple balloon techniques seem to achieve slightly larger valve areas, but no difference in late outcome. In most patients, the simplest approach is the single balloon technique using a 20 mm balloon; if necessary, larger or multiple balloons may be used.[103]

D. RESULTS

1. **Hemodynamic Results (Table 37.7).** PBAV results in a 50-70% decrease in aortic valve gradient, and a 40-60% increase in aortic valve area (Figure 37.6). Despite these results, all patients still have severe AS. The hemodynamic results are similar for retrograde or antegrade approaches, and for single or multiple balloons.[103-110]

2. **Complications (Table 37.8).** Major clinical complications are not infrequent and include death (2.6-10.4%), cerebrovascular events (0.4-4.6%), cardiac perforation (0-1.8%), myocardial infarction (0.3-1.6%), severe aortic insufficiency (0-1.6%), and vascular injury requiring blood transfusion and/or vascular repair (7.5-27%).[103,104,106-108,111,112] Procedure-related mortality is more common in acutely decompensated patients with severe LV dysfunction. Cardiac perforation may be caused by the guidewire or balloon catheter. Sudden hemodynamic collapse during the procedure is usually due to cardiac tamponade or aortic valve disruption,[113-116] while worsening congestive heart failure immediately after PBAV is usually due to aortic insufficiency.[117,118] Other reported complications include transient complete heart block,[119] mitral valve rupture,[120,121] and bacterial endocarditis.[122]

3. **Longterm Results (Table 37.9).** In contrast to balloon mitral valvuloplasty, the longterm results of PBAV are poor. Available studies of 1-3 year follow-up report a high incidence of late cardiac events, including death in 30-60%, aortic valve replacement in 7-27%, and repeat balloon valvuloplasty in 4-22%.[103,106,108,111] Acute and longterm results of repeat PBAV are similar to initial PBAV.[123-125]

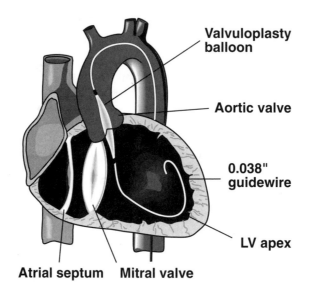

Figure 37.5 Percutaneous Balloon Aortic Valvuloplasty (PBAV)

Table 37.7.   Immediate Hemodynamic Results of PBAV

Series	N (pts)	Approach	AVA (cm²)		AVG (mm Hg)	
			Pre	Post	Pre	Post
Block[104] (1994)	375	All	0.50	0.90	61	27
Cribier[105] (1993)	406	S,R	0.55	0.97	72	29
Safian[103] (1991)	225	S,R	0.60	0.90	67	33
NHLBI[106] (1991)	674	All	0.5	0.8	65	31
Mansfield[107] (1991)	492	All	0.50	0.82	60	30
Lewin[108] (1989)	125	M,R	0.60	1.00	87	32

Abbreviations: S = single balloon; M = multiple balloons; R = retrograde approach; A = antegrade approach; AVA = aortic valve area; AVG = transaortic valve gradient

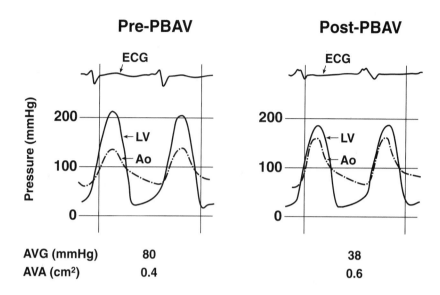

Figure 37.6 PBAV: Immediate Hemodynamic Results

PBAV results in a decrease in aortic valve gradient (AVG) and an increase in aortic valve area (AVA). Left ventricular (LV) pressure decreases, and aortic (AO) pressure increases.

4. **Predictors of Late Outcome.** The poor longterm results of PBAV are secondary to several factors, including persistent severe aortic stenosis despite successful dilation, a high incidence (30-60%) of early restenosis, the presence of concomitant severe coronary artery disease, and associated noncardiac comorbid diseases. The most important determinants of event-free survival are those associated with baseline LV performance,[126-131] not improvement in valve area. In a study of 205 valvuloplasty patients, event-free survival correlated with baseline LV ejection fraction, LV systolic pressure, aortic systolic pressure, and percent reduction in valve gradient; baseline pulmonary wedge pressure was inversely related to outcome.[126] Although overall event-free survival at 2-years was 25%, it was only 4% in patients with all 3 baseline adverse predictors. Patients with severe LV dysfunction who underwent PBAV had Longterm results similar to those of untreated aortic stenosis. [126]

Table 37.8. Complications of PBAV

Series	N (pts)	Death (%)	CVA (%)	Perf (%)	MI (%)	AI (%)	Vasc (%)
Block[104] (1994)	308	5.0	2.0	0.3	0.5	0	9.0
Safian[103] (1991)	225	3.1	0.4	1.2	0.5	0.8	7.5
Isner[112] (1991)	492	2.6	-	1.8	-	0.8	-
NHLBI[106] (1991)	672	3.0	4.6	1.0	1.0	1.0	27
Mansfield[107] (1991)	492	7.5	2.2	1.8	0.2	1.0	11
Cribier[111] (1990)	334	4.5	1.4	0.6	0.3	0	13.1
Lewin[108] (1989)	125	10.4	3.2	0	1.6	1.6	9.6

Abbreviations: CVA = stroke; Perf = cardiac perforation; MI = myocardial infarction; AI = severe aortic insufficiency; Vasc = vascular injury requiring surgical repair or blood transfusion; - = not reported

Table 37.9. Clinical Follow-up After PBAV

Series	N (pts)	F/U (months)	Death (%)	AVR (%)	reBAV (%)
Safian[103] (1991)	225	24	40	27	22
NHLBI[109] (1991)	648	36	60	13	4
Cribier[111] (1990)	300	16	30	19	17
Lewin[108] (1989)	125	12	42	7	8

Abbreviations: F/U = follow-up interval (months); AVR = aortic valve replacement; reBAV = repeat BAV

5. **Comparison of Balloon Valvuloplasty and Aortic Valve Replacement (Table 37.10).** There are no prospective randomized studies of PBAV and AVR. However, a single center observational study reported the superiority of AVR in octogenarians with symptomatic aortic stenosis: In-hospital mortality rates were similar, but event-free survival at 22 months was 78% in AVR patients but only 6.5% in PBAV patients.[132]

E. **RECOMMENDATIONS.** Available data are compelling: Aortic valve replacement is the preferred treatment for virtually all adults with symptomatic aortic stenosis. Octogenarians with aortic stenosis should not be denied the opportunity for valve replacement based on age alone. Nevertheless, there may be selected patients for whom PBAV may be considered:

1. **Severe LV Dysfunction.** Some adult patients with aortic stenosis have severely depressed ejection (EF < 25%), but LV dysfunction may be explained by one or more factors such as critical aortic stenosis and afterload mismatch, previous myocardial infarction, coexisting hypertensive heart disease, advanced mitral regurgitation, or an undefined cardiomyopathy. Although patients with left ventricular dysfunction due to critical aortic stenosis and after mismatch will improve after aortic valve replacement, it is difficult to identify these patients using standard clinical criteria. In contrast, patients with aortic stenosis and left ventricular dysfunction secondary to causes after than after mismatch may not have improvement in left ventricular performance after aortic valve replacement. In patients with aortic stenosis and severe LV dysfunction, PBAV may be used to identify a subgroup of patients who are likely to improve after AVR. In such patients, significant improvement in LV ejection fraction is observed in 40-50% of patients 3 months after PBAV; [133] however, PBAV should not be considered definitive treatment since the late clinical outcome of these patient is poor.[134,135] However, patients who demonstrate improvement in LV ejection fraction after PBAV should be considered for AVR, to improve survival. The role of PBAV in improving mitral regurgitation associated with aortic stenosis is controversial; some studies suggest a benefit,[136] but others do not.[137]

2. **Low-Gradient, Low-Output State.** Symptomatic patients with aortic stenosis, a low cardiac output, and a low transaortic valve gradient are at high risk for AVR and have a poor Longterm prognosis. In these patients, PBAV may identify a subgroup of patients with hemodynamic and clinical improvement, who might then be considered for AVR.[138]

3. **Cardiogenic Shock.** PBAV may be a life-saving procedure in select patients with aortic stenosis and cardiogenic shock. However, because in-hospital mortality is high and Longterm prognosis is poor, patients who survive hospitalization should be strongly considered for AVR, or rarely cardiac transplantation.[139-145]

Table 37.10. Comparison of PBAV and AVR[132]

	PBAV (n=46)	AVR (n=23)
Age (yrs)	80	78
Preop AVG (mm Hg) *	105	107
In-hospital death (%)	6.5	8.7
Follow-up** (%)		
Death	52	13
AVR	35	0
EFS	6.5	78
Total survival		
1 yr.	75	83
2 yr.	47	83
3 yr.	33	75

Abbreviations: AVR = aortic valve replacement; AVG = transaortic valve gradient; EFS = event free survival
* Doppler gradient
** Follow-up at 22 months

4. **Preoperative Palliation Before Noncardiac Surgery.** PBAV may be considered in some patients with aortic stenosis who require urgent noncardiac surgery.[146-148] In these patients, PBAV results is significant hemodynamic improvement, similar to that observed in other patients treated with PBAV. In spite of this hemodynamic improvement, there are no data to suggest that routine PBAV will improve the perioperative risks of noncardiac surgery. In fact, in one study of 48 patients with severe aortic stenosis, careful monitoring of anesthesia resulted in no major complications, despite the need for vascular, orthopedic, abdominal, and other forms of surgery without preoperative PBAV. [149] We empirically proceed with valvuloplasty in patients with overt heart failure or systolic blood pressures < 100 mmHg, who require urgent noncardiac surgery.

* * * * *

REFERENCES

1. Inoue K, Owaki T, Nakamura T, et al. Clinical Application of transvenous mitral commissurotomy by a new balloon catheter. J Thorac Cardiovas Surg. 1984;87:394-402.

2. Lock JE, Khalilulah M, Shrivastava S, et al. Percutaneous Catheter Commissurotomy in rheumatic mitral stenosis. N Engl J Med 1985;313:1515-1518.

3. Al Zaibag MA, Kasab SA, Ribeiro PA, et al. Percutaneous double-balloon mitral valvuloplasty for rheumatic mitral valve stenosis. Lancet 1986;1:757-761.

4. McKay RG, Lock JE, Keane JF, et al. Percutaneous mitral valvuloplasty in an adult patient with calcific rheumatic mitral stenosis. J Am Coll Cardiol 1986;7:1410-1415.

5. Palacios IF, Lock JE, Keane JF, et al. Percutaneous transvenous balloon valvuloplasty in a patient with severe calcific mitral stenosis. J Am Coll Cardiol 1986;7:1416-1419.

6. Babic UU, Pejac P, Djurisic Z, et al. Percutaneous transarterial balloon valvuloplasty for mitral valve stenosis. Am J Cardiol 1986;57:1101-1104.

7. Brockenbrough EC, Braunwald E. A new technique for left ventricular angiocardiography and transseptal left heart catheterization. Am J Cardiol 1960;6:1062.

8. Palacios IF, Block PC, Wilkins GT, et al. Follow-up of patients undergoing percutaneous mitral balloon valvotomy. Analysis of factors determining restenosis. Circulation 1989;79:573-579.

9. Vahanian A, Michel PL, Cormier B, et al. Results of percutaneous mitral commissurotomy in 200 patients. Am J Cardiol 1989;63:847-852.

10. The National Heart, Lung, and Blood Institute Balloon Valvuloplasty Registry Participants Multicenter Experience with Balloon Mitral Commissurotomy: NHLBI Balloon Valvuloplasty Registry report on immediate and 30-day follow-up results. Circulation 1992;85:448-461.

11. Cohen DT, Kuntz RE Gorday SP, et al. Predictors of Longterm outcome after percutaneous balloon mitral valvuloplasty. N Engl J Med 1992;327:1329-1335.

12. Abascal VM, Wilkins GT, O'Shea JP, et al. Prediction of successful outcome in 130 patients undergoing percutaneous mitral valvotomy. Circulation 1990;82:448-456.

13. Palacios IF, Tuzcu ME, Weyman AF, et al. Clinical follow-up of patients undergoing percutaneous mitral balloon valvotomy. Circulation 1995;91:671-676.

14. Nobuyoshi M, Hameishi N, Dimura T, et al. Indications, complications, and short-term clinical out-come of percutaneous transvenous mitral commissurotomy. Circulation 1989;80:782-792.

15. Chen CR, Cheng TO. Percutaneous balloon mitral valvuloplasty by the Inoue technique. A multicenter study of 4832 patients in China. Am Heart J 1995;129:1197-1203.

16. Orme EC, Wray RB, Mason JW. Balloon mitral valvuloplasty via retrograde left atrial catheterization. Am Heart J 1989;117:680-683.

17. Stefanadis C, Stratos C, Pitsaves C, et al. Retrograde nontransseptal balloon mitral valvuloplasty immediate results and Longterm follow-up. Circulation 1992;85:1760-1767.

18. Bahl VK, Juneya R, Thatar D, et al. Retrograde nontransseptal balloon mitral valvuloplasty for rheumatic mitral stenosis. Cathet Cardiovasc Diagn 1994;33:331-334.

19. Yeh K-H, Hung J-S, Wu C-J, Fu M. Safety of inoue balloon mitral commissurotomy in patients with left atrial appendage thrombi. Am J Cardiol 1995;75:302-304.

20. Hung J. Mitral stenosis with left atrial thrombi: Inoue balloon catheter technique. New York: Igakushoin Medical, 1992:280-293.

21. Fu M, Hung J-S, Lee C-B, Cherng W-J. Coronary neovascularization as a specific sign for left atrial appendage thrombus in mitral stenosis. Am J Cardiol 1991;67:1158-1160.

22. Chen WJ, Chen MF, Liau CS, Chung C. Safety of percutaneous transvenous balloon mitral commissurotomy in patients with mitral stenosis and thrombus in the left atrial appendage. Am J Cardiol 1992;70:117-119.

23. Chow WH, Chow TS, Yip A, Cheung KL. Percutaneous balloon mitral valvotomy in patients with history of embolism. Am J Cardiol 1993;71:1243-1244.

24. Kamalesh M, Burger AJ, Shubrooks SJ. The use of transesophageal echocardiography to avoid left atrial thrombus during percutaneous mitral valvuloplasty. Cathet Cardiovasc Diagn 1993;28:320-322.

25. Vahanian A, Acar J. Mitral valvuloplasty: The French Experience. In: Topol EJ, Editor. Textbook of Interventional Cardiology; Philadelphia, WB Saunders, 1994.

26. McKay RG, Lock JE, Safian RD, et al. Balloon dilation of mitral stenosis in adult patients: post morterm and percutaneous mitral valvuloplasty studies. J Am Coll Cardiol 1987;9:723-731.

27. Block PC, Palaeios IF, Jacobs ML, et al. Mechanism of percutaneous mitral valvotomy. Am J Cardiol 1987;59:178-179.

28. Kaplan JD, Isner JM, Karas RH, et al. In vitro analysis of mechanisms of balloon valvuloplasty of stenotic mitral valves. Am J Cardiol 1987;59:318-323.

29. Hogan K, Ramaswamy K, Losordo DW, et al. Pathology at mitral commissurotomy performed with the Inoue catheter: implication for mechanisms and complications. Cathet Cardiovasc Diagn 1994;32(Suppl 2):42-51.

30. Lin PJ, Chang J-P, Chu J-J, Chang C-H. Balloon valvuloplasty is contraindicated in stenotic mitral bioprostheses. Am Heart J 1994;127:724-726.

31. Calvo OL, Sobrino N, Gamallo C, Oliver J. Balloon percutaneous valvuloplasty for stenotic bioprosthetic valves in the mitral position. Am J Cardiol 1987;60:736-737.

32. Cox D, Friedman P, Selwyn A, Lee R, JA B. Improved quality of life after successful balloon valvuloplasty of a stenosed mitral bioprosthesis. Am Heart J 1989;118:839-41.

33. Babic U, Gruijicic S, Vucinic M. Balloon valvuloplasty of bioprosthesis. Int J Cardiol 1991;30:230-2.

34. Roelke M, Smith AJ, Palacios IF. The technique and safety of transseptal left heart catheterization: the Massachusetts General Hospital experience with 1279 procedures. Cathet Cardiovasc Diagn 1994;32:332-339.

35. Arora R, Kalra G, Murty G, et al. Percutaneous transatrial mitral commissurotomy: Immediate and intermediate results. J Am Coll Cardiol 1994;23:1327-32.

36. Block PC, Palacies IF. Aortic and mitral balloon valvuloplasty. The US Experience. In: Topol EJ, Editor. Textbook of Interventional Cardiology; Philadelphia, WB Saunders, 1994.

37. Stephanadis, Toutouzas P. Retrograde nontransseptal mitral valvuloplasty. In: Topol EJ, Editor. Textbook of Interventional Cardiology; Philadelphia, WB Saunders, 1994.

38. Feldman T, Carroll JD, Herrmann HC, Holmes DR. Effect of balloon size and stepwise inflation technique on the acute results of inoue mitral commissurotomy. Cathet Cardiovasc Diagn 1993;28:199-205.

39. Pan M, Medina A, deLexo JS, Hernandez E. Factors determining late success after mitral balloon valvulotomy. Am J Cardiol 1993;71:1181-1185.

40. Hung J, Chern M, Wu J, Fu M. Short and longterm results of catheter balloon percutaneous transvenous mitral commissurotomy. Am J Cardiol 1991;67:854-862.

41. Ruiz CE, Allen J, Lau F. Percutaneous double balloon valvotomy for severe rheumatic mitral stenosis. Am J Cardiol 1990;65:473-477.

42. Park SJ, Kim JJ, Park SW, et al. Immediate and one-year results of PBMV using Inoue and double-balloon techniques. Am J Cardiol 1993;71:938-943.

43. Ribeiro PA, Fawzy ME, Arafat MA, Dunn B. Comparison of mitral valve area results of balloon mitral valvotomy using the inoue and double balloon techniques. Am J Cardiol 1991;68:687-688.

44. Bassand J, Schiele F, Bernard Y, Anguenot T. The double-balloon and inoue techniques in percutaneous mitral valvuloplasty: comparative results in a series of 232 cases. J Am Coll Cardiol 1991;18:982-989.

45. Davidson CT, Bashere TM, Mickel M, et al. Balloon mitral commissurotomy after previous surgical commissurotomy. The NHLBI balloon valvuloplasty registry participants. Circulation 1992;86:91-99.

46. Jang I-K, Block P, Newell J, Tuzcu M, Palacios I. Percutaneous mitral balloon valvotomy for recurrent mitral stenosis after surgical commissurotomy. Am J Cardiol 1995;75:601-605.

47. Serra A, Bonan R, Lefevre T, Barraud P. Balloon mitral commissurotomy for mitral restenosis after surgical commissurotomy. Am J Cardiol 1993;71:1311-1315.

48. Rediker D, Block P, Abascal V. Mitral balloon valvuloplasty for mitral restenosis after surgical commissurotomy. J Am Coll Cardiol 1988;11:252-256.

49. Glantz JC, Pomerantz RM, Cunningham MJ, et al. Percutaneous balloon valvuloplasty for severe mitral stenosis during pregnancy: a review of therapeutic options. Obstet Gyn Surg 1993;48:503-508.

50. Kalra G, Arora R, Kahn J, Nigam M. Percutaneous mitral commissurotomy for severe mitral stenosis during pregnancy. Cathet Cardiovasc Diagn 1994;33:28-30.

51. Lung B, Cormier B, Elias J, Michel P. Usefulness of percutaneous balloon commissurotomy for mitral stenosis during pregnancy. Am J Cardiol 1994;73:398-400.

52. Safian R, Berman A, Sachs B, et al. Percutaneous balloon mitral valvuloplasty in a pregnant woman with mitral stenosis. Cathet Cardiovasc Diagn 1988;15:103-108.

53. Esteves CA, Ramos AIO. Effectiveness of percutaneous balloon mitral valvotomy during pregnancy. Am J Cardiol 1991;68:930-934.

54. Herrmann HC, Lima JA, Feldman T, et al. Mechanisms and outcome of severe mitral regurgitation after Inoue balloon valvuloplasty. J Am Coll Cardiol 1993;22:783-9.

55. Thomas MR, Monaghan MJ, Metealfe JM, et al. Residual atrial septal defects following balloon mitral valvuloplasty using different techniques. A transthoracic and transesophageal study demonstrating an advantage of the Inoue balloon. Eur Heart J 1992;13:496-502.

56. Arora R, Jolly N, Kalra GS, et al. Atrial septal defect after balloon mitral valvuloplasty: a transesophageal echocardiographic study. Angiology 1993;44:217-221.

57. Cequier A, Bonan R, Serra A, et al. Left to right shunting after percutaneous mitral valvuloplasty. Incidence and longterm hemodynamic follow-up. Circulation 1990;81:1190-1197.

58. Casale P, Block PC, O'Shea JP, et al. Atrial septal defect after percutaneous mitral balloon valvuloplasty: Immediate results and follow-up. J Am Coll Cardiol 1990;15:1300-1304.

59. Chan C, Berland J, Cribier A, Rocha P. Results of percutaneous transseptal mitral commissurotomy in patients 40 years and above with those under 40 years of age: Immediate and 5-year follow-up results. Cathet Cardiovasc Diagn 1994;32:223-230.

60. Chen CR, Cheng To, Chen JY, et al. Longterm results of percutaneous mitral valvuloplasty with the Inoue balloon catheter. Am J Cardiol 1992;70:1445-8.

61. Block PC, Palacios IF, Block EH, et al. Late (two-year) follow-up after percutaneous mitral balloon valvotomy. Am J Cardiol 1992;69:537-554.

62. Pavlides GS, Hauser AM, Dudlets PI, et al. The value of transesophageal echocardiography in predicting immediate and Longterm outcome in balloon mitral valvuloplasty. Comparison with transthoracic echocardiography. J Interven Cardiol 1994;7:401-408.

63. Wilkins GT, Weyman AE, Abascal VM, et al. Percutaneous mitral valvotomy: An analysis of echocardiographic variables related to outcome and the mechanism of dilation. Br Heart J 1988;60:299-308.

64. Herrmann HE, Wilkins GT, Abascal VM, et al. Percutaneous balloon mitral valvotomy for patients with mitral stenosis. Analysis of factors influencing early results. J Thorac Cardiovasc Surg 1988;96:33-38.

65. Abascal VM, Wilkins GT, Choong CY, et al. Mitral regurgitation after percutaneous balloon mitral valvuloplasty in adults: Evaluation by pulsed Doppler echocardiography. J Am Cardiol 1988;11:257-263.

66. Come PC, Riley MF, Diver DJ, et al. Noninvasive assessment of mitral stenosis before and after percutaneous balloon mitral valvuloplasty. Am J Coll Cardiol 1988;61:817-825.

67. Reid CL, Chandraratna AN, Kawamishi DT, et al. Influence of mitral valve morphology on double-balloon catheter balloon valvuloplasty in patients with mitral stenosis. Analysis of factors predicting immediate and 3-month results. Circulation 1989;80:515-524.

68. Reid CL, Otto CM, Davis KB, et al. Influence of mitral valve morphology on mitral balloon commissurotomy:

Immediate and six-month results from the NHLBI Balloon Valvuloplasty Registry. Am Heart J 1992;124:657-665.

69. Complications and mortality of percutaneous balloon mitral commissurotomy. A report from the National Heart, Lung, and Blood Institute Balloon Valvuloplasty Registry. Circulation 1992;85:2014-2024.

70. Tuzcu Em, Block PC, Griffin B, et al. Percutaneous mitral balloon valvotomy in patients calcific mitral stenosis: Immediate and Longterm outcome. J Am Coll Cardiol 1994;23:1604-1609.

71. Herrmann HE, Feldman T, Isner JM, et al. Comparison of results of percutaneous balloon valvuloplasty in patients with mild and moderate mitral stenosis. Am J Cardiol 1993;71:1300-1303.

72. Alfonso F, Macaya C, Hernandex R, et al. Early and late results of PBMV for mitral stenosis associated with mild mitral regurgitation. Am J Cardiol 1993;71:1304-1310.

73. Chen CR, Cheng TO, Chen JY, et al. Percutaneous balloon mitral valvuloplasty for mitral stenosis with and without associated aortic regurgitation. Am Heart J 1993;125:128-137.

74. Alfonso F, Macaya C, Hernandez R, et al. Percutaneous mitral valvuloplasty with severe pulmonary artery hypertension. Am J Cardiol 1993;72:325-330.

75. Wisenbaugh T, Essop R, Middlemost S, Skoularigis J. Effects of severe pulmonary hypertension on outcome of balloon mitral valvotomy. Am J Cardiol 1992;70:823-825.

76. Dev V, Shrivastrava S. Time course of changes in pulmonary vascular resistance and the mechanism of regression of pulmonary arterial hypertension after balloon mitral valvuloplasty. Am J Cardiol 1991;67:439-442.

77. Tuzcu EM, Block PC, Griffin BP, et al. Immediate and Longterm outcome of percutaneous mitral valvotomy in patients 65 yeas and older. Circulation 1992;85:963-971.

78. Shapiro LM, Hassanein H, Crowley JJ. Mitral balloon valvuloplasty in patients > 70 years of age with severe mitral stenosis. Am J Cardiol 1995;75:633-636.

79. Kasper W, Wollschlager H, Gerbel A, et al. Percutaneous mitral balloon valvuloplasty: a comparative evaluation of two transatrial techniques. Am Heart J 1992;124:1562-6.

80. Abdullah M, Halim M, Rajedran V. Comparison between single (Inoue) and double balloon mitral valvuloplasty. Immediate and short-term results. Am Heart J 1992;123:1581-1588.

81. Rihal CS, Nishimura RA, Reeder GS, et al. Percutaneous balloon mitral valvuloplasty: Comparison of double and single (Inoue) techniques. Cathet Cardiovasc Diagn 1993;29:183-190.

82. Manga P, Landless P, Gebka M. Comparative results of PBMV using the Trefoil/Biofoil and Inoue balloon techniques. Int J Cardiol 1994;43:21-25.

83. Zhang HP, Gamra H, Allen J, Lau F, Ruiz C. Comparison of late outcome between inoue balloon and double-balloon techniques for percutaneous mitral valvotomy in a matched study. Am Heart J 1995;130:340-4.

84. Shrivastava S, Mathur A, Der V, et al. Comparison of immediate hemodynamic response to closed mitral commissurotomy, single balloon and double balloon mitral valvuloplasty in rheumatic mitral stenosis. J Thorac Cardiovasc Surg 1992;104:1262-7.

85. Turi ZG, Reyes VP, Raju BS, et al. Percutaneous balloon versus surgical closed commissurotomy for mitral stenosis: a prospective randomized trial. Circulation 1991;83:1179-1185.

86. Reyes VP, Raju BS, Wynne J, et al. Percutaneous balloon valvuloplasty compared with open surgical commissurotomy for mitral stenosis. N Engl J Med 1994;331:961-967.

87. Lababidi Z, Wu JR, Walls JT. Percutaneous balloon aortic valvuloplasty. Results in 23 patients. Am J Cardiol 1984;53:194-197.

88. Cribier A, Saoudi N, Berland J, et al. Percutaneous transluminal valvuloplasty of acquired aortic stenosis in elderly patients: An alternative to valve replacement? Lancet 1986;1:63-67.

89. McKay R, Safian RD, Lock J, Mandell V. Balloon dilatation of calcific aortic stenosis in elderly patients: postmortem, intraoperative, and percutaneous valvuloplasty studies. Circulation 1986;74:119-125.

90. Frank S, Johnson A, Ross J. Natural history of valvular aortic stenosis. British Heart J. 1973;35:41-46.

91. Lombard JT, Selzer A. Valvular aortic stenosis. A clinical and hemodynamic profile of patients. Ann Int Med 1987;106:292-298.

92. Turina J, Hess O, Sepulcri F, Kravenbuehl HP. Spontaneous course of aortic valve disease. Eur Heart J 1987;8:471-483.

93. O'Keefe JH, Vlietstra RE, Bailey KR, Holmes DR. Natural history of candidates for balloon aortic valvuloplasty. Mayo Clin Proc 1987;62:986-991.

94. Smith N, McAnulty J, Rahimtoola S. Severe aortic stenosis with impaired left ventricular function and clinical heart failure: Results of valve replacement. Circulation 1978;58:255-264.

95. Kennedy W, Doces J, Stewart D. Left ventricular function before and following aortic valve replacement. Circulation 1977;56(6):944-950.

96. Pantely G, Morton M, Rahimtoola S. Effects of successful, uncomplicated valve replacement on ventricular hypertrophy, volume and performance in aortic stenosis and in aortic incompetence. J Thorac Surg 1978;75:383-391.

97. Magovern J, Pennock J, Campbell D, Pae W. Aortic valve replacement and combined aortic valve replacement and coronary artery bypass grafting: Predicting high risk groups. J Am Coll Cardiol 1987;9:38-43.

98. Copeland J, Griepp R, Stinson E, Shumway N. Isolated aortic valve replacement in patients older than 65 years. JAMA 1977;237:1578-1581.

99. Edmunds H, Stephenson L, Edie R, Ratcliffe M. Open-heart surgery in octogenarians. N Engl J Med 1988;319:131-136.

100. Levinson JR, Akins CW, Buckley MJ, et al. Octogenarians with aortic stenosis: outcome after aortic valve replacement. Circulation 1989;80:I-49-I-56.

101. Fremes S, Goldman B, Ivanov J, Weisel R. Valvular surgery in the elderly. Circulation 1989;80:I77-90.

102. Safian RD, Mandell VS, Thurer RE, et a. Postmortem and intraoperative balloon valvuloplasty of calcific aortic stenosis in elderly patients: Mechanisms of successful dilatation. J Am Coll Cardiol 1987;9:655-660.

103. Safian RD, Kuntz RE, Berman AD. Aortic valvuloplasty. Cardiol Clin 1991;9:289-299.

104. Block P, IF P. Aortic and mitral balloon valvuloplasty: The United States experience. In: Topol EJ, Editor. Textbook of Interventional Cardiology; Philadelphia, WB Saunders, 1994.

105. Letac B, Cribier A. Aortic balloon dilatation as a treatment of aortic stenosis: what are the indications? J Interven Cardiol 1993;6:1-6.

106. NHLBI Balloon Valvuloplasty Registry Participants. Percutaneous balloon aortic valvuloplasty. Acute and 30-day follow-up results in 674 patients from the NHLBI Balloon Valvuloplasty Registry. Circulation 1991;84:2383-2397.

107. McKay RG for the Mansfield Scientific Aortic Valvuloplasty Registry Investigators. Overview of acute hemodynamic results and procedural complications. J Am Coll Cardiol 1991;17:485-491.

108. Lewin R, Dorros G, King J, Mathiak L. Percutaneous transluminal aortic valvuloplasty: acute outcome and follow-up of 125 patients. J Am Coll Cardiol 1989;14:1210-1217.

109. Isner JM, Salem DN, Desnoyers MR, Fields CD. Dual balloon technique for valvuloplasty of aortic stenosis in adults. Am J Cardiol 1988;61:583-589.

110. Block PC, Palacios IF. Comparison of hemodynamic results of anterograde versus retrograde percutaneous balloon aortic valvuloplasty. Am J Cardiol 1987;60:659-662.

111. Cribier A, Gerber L, Letac B. Percutaneous Balloon Aortic Valvuloplasty: The French Experience,. Philadelphia: WB Saunders, 1990. (Eds) Topol,E. Textbook of Interventional Cardiology; vol p.849).

112. Isner JM. Acute catastrophic complications of balloon aortic valvuloplasty. J Am Coll Cardiol 1991;17:1436-1444.

113. Lewin RF, Dorros G, King JF, Seifert PE. Aortic annular tear after valvuloplasty: The role of aortic annulus echocardiographic measurement. Cathet Cardiovasc Diagn 1989;16:123-129.

114. Seifert PE, Auer JE. Surgical repair of annular disruption following percutaneous balloon aortic valvuloplasty. Ann Thorac Surg 1988;46:242-243.

115. Vrolix M, Piessens J, Moerman P, Vanhaecke J, De Geest H. Fatal aortic rupture: An unusual complication of percutaneous balloon valvuloplasty for acquired valvular aortic stenosis. Cathet Cardiovasc Diagn 1989;16:119-122.

116. Lembo NJ, King SB, Roubin GS, Hammami A. Fatal aortic rupture during percutaneous balloon valvuloplasty for valvular aortic stenosis. Am J Cardiol 1987;60:733-736.

117. Dean LS, Chandler JW, Saenz CB, Baxley WA. Severe aortic regurgitation complicating percutaneous aortic valve valvuloplasty. Cathet Cardiovasc Diagn 1989;16:130-132.

118. Sadaniantz A, Malhotra R, Korr KS. Transient acute severe aortic regurgitation complicating balloon aortic valvuloplasty. Cathet Cardiovas Diagn 1989;17:186-189.

119. Plack RH, Porterfield JK, Brinker JA. Complete heart block developing during aortic valvuloplasty. Chest 1989;96:1201-1203.

120. deUbago J, dePrada JAV, Moujir F, Olalla JJ. Mitral valve rupture during percutaneous dilation of aortic valve stenosis. Cathet Cardiovasc Diagn 1989;16:115-118.

121. Farb A, Galloway J, Davis R, Burke A, Virmani R. Mitral valve laceration and papillary muscle rupture secondary to percutaneous balloon aortic valvuloplasty. Am J Cardiol 1992;69:829-830.

122. Cujec B, McMeekin J, Lopez J. Bacterial endocarditis after percutaneous aortic valvuloplasty. Am Heart J 1988;115:178-179.

123. Ferguson J, Garza R. Efficacy of multiple balloon aortic valvuloplasty procedures. J Am Coll Cardiol 1991;17:1430-1435.

124. Kuntz R, Tosteson, Anna, Maitland L, Gordon P. Immediate results and Longterm follow-up after repeat balloon aortic valvuloplasty. Cathet Cardiovasc Diagn 1992;25:4-9.

125. Koning R, Cribier A, Asselin C, Mouton-Schleifer D, Derumeaux G, Letac B. Repeat balloon aortic valvuloplasty. Cathet Cardiovasc Diagn 1992;26:249-254.

126. Kuntz RE, Tosteson AN, Berman AD, et al. Predictors of event-free survival after balloon aortic valvuloplasty. N Engl J Med 1991;325:17-23.

127. Otto K, Mickel M, Kennedy W, et al. Three-year outcome after balloon aortic valvuloplasty: Insights into prognosis of valvular aortic stenosis. Circulation 1994;89:642-650.

128. O'Neill WW. Predictors of Longterm survival after percutaneous aortic valvuloplasty: report of the Mansfield Scientific Balloon Aortic Valvuloplasty Registry. J Am Coll Cardiol 1991;17:193-198.

129. Holmes D, Nichimura R, Reeder G. In-hospital mortality after balloon aortic valvuloplasty: frequency and associated factors. J Am Coll Cardiol 1991;17:189-192.

130. Legrand V, Beckers J, Fastrez M, et al. Longterm follow-up of elderly patients with severe aortic stenosis treated by balloon aortic valvuloplasty. Importance of hemodynamic parameters before and after dilatation. Eur Heart J 1991;12:451-457.

131. Davidson C, Harrison K, Pieper K, Harding M. Determinants of one-year outcome from balloon aortic valvuloplasty. Am J Cardiol 1991;68:75-80.

132. Bernard Y, Etievent J, Mourand J, et al. Longterm results of percutaneous aortic valvuloplasty compared with aortic valve replacement in patients more than 75 years old. J Am Coll Cardiol 1992;20:796-801.

133. Safian R, Warren S, Berman A, et al. Improvement in symptoms and left ventricular performance after balloon aortic valvuloplasty in patients with aortic stenosis and depressed left ventricular ejection fraction. Circulation 1988;78:1181-1191.

134. Berland J, Cribier A, Savin T, Lefebvre E, Koning R, Letac B. Percutaneous balloon valvuloplasty in patients with severe aortic stenosis and low ejection fraction: Immediate results and 1-year follow-up. Circulation 1989;79:1189-1196.

135. Davidson CJ, Harrison K, Leithe M, Kisslo K. Failure of balloon aortic valvuloplasty to result in sustained clinical improvement in patients with depressed left ventricular function. Am J Cardiol 1990;65:72-77.

136. Come P, Riley M, Berman A, Safian R, Waksmonski C, McKay R. Serial assessment of mitral regurgitation by pulsed doppler echocardiography in patients undergoing balloon aortic valvuloplasty. J Am Coll Cardiol 1989;14:677-682.

137. Adams P, Otto C. Lack of improvement in coexisting mitral regurgitation after relief of valvular aortic stenosis. Am J Cardiol 1990;66:105-107.

138. Nishimura R, Holmes D, Michela M. Follow-up of patients with low output, low gradient hemodynamics after percutaneous balloon aortic valvuloplasty: the Mansfield Scientific Aortic Valvuloplasty Registry. J Am Coll Cardiol

1991;17:828-833.

139. Moreno P, Jank I-K, Newell J. The role of percutaneous aortic balloon valvuloplasty in patients with cardiogenic shock and critical aortic stenosis. J Am Coll Cardiol 1994;23:1071-1075.

140. Smedira NG, Ports TA Merrick SH, et al. Balloon aortic valvuloplasty as a bridge to aortic valve replacement in critically ill patients. Ann Thorac Surg 1993;55:914-916.

141. Friedman H, Cragg D, O'Neill W. Cardiac resuscitation using emergency aortic balloon valvuloplasty. Am J Cardiol 1989;63:387-8.

142. Desnoyers M, Salem D, Rosenfield K, Mackey W, O'Donnell T, Isner J. Treatment of cardiogenic shock by emergency aortic balloon valvuloplasty. Ann Int Med 1988;108:833-5.

143. Losordo D, Ramaswamy K, Rosenfield K, Isner J. Use of emergency balloon dilation to reverse acute hemodynamic decompensation developing during diagnostic cardiac catheterization for aortic stenosis (bailout valvuloplasty). Am J Cardiol 1989;63:388-9.

144. Brady S, Davis C, Kussmaul W, Laskey W. Percutaneous aortic balloon valvuloplasty in octogenarians: Morbidity and mortality. Ann Int Med. 1989;110:761-766.

145. Cribier A, Remadi F, Koning R, Rath P, Stix G, Letac B. Emergency balloon valvuloplasty as initial treatment of patients with aortic stenosis and cardiogenic shock. N Engl J Med 1992;326:646.

146. Levine MJ, Berman AD, Safian RD, Diver DJ. Palliation of valvular aortic stenosis by balloon valvuloplasty as preoperative preparation for noncardiac surgery. Am J Cardiol 1988;62:1309-1310.

147. Roth R, Palacios I, Block P. Percutaneous aortic balloon valvuloplasty: Its role in the management of patients with aortic stenosis requiring major noncardiac surgery. J Am Coll Cardiol 1989;13:1039-1041.

148. Hayes SN, Holmes DR, Nishimura RA, Reeder GS. Palliative percutaneous aortic balloon valvuloplasty before noncardiac operations and invasive diagnostic procedures. Mayo Clin Proc 1989;64:753-757.

149. O'Keefe JH, Shub C, Rettke SR. Risk of noncardiac surgical procedures in-patients with aortic stenosis. Mayo Clin Proc 1989;64:400-405.

SPECIAL CONSIDERATIONS FOR CATH LAB PERSONNEL

38

Harold Z. Friedman, M.D.
Alan Bennett
Kevin L. Kelco, B.S.
Kathleen A. Fasing, B.S., RCVT

Percutaneous Transluminal Coronary Angioplasty (PTCA) is performed as an alternative to coronary artery bypass surgery or medical therapy alone for the treatment of obstructive coronary artery disease and has been shown to effectively relieve ischemic symptoms, improve exercise tolerance and functional capacity and shorten hospital stay for patients with unstable angina. Patients well-suited for percutaneous revascularization include: those with lifestyle-limiting angina pectoris who are unresponsive or intolerant to medical therapy; patients at high risk of myocardial infarction or sudden cardiac death by one or more high-grade stenoses which subtend large amounts of viable myocardium; and individuals considered poor operative candidates due to severe co-existing medical illness or absence of suitable bypass conduits.

Patients previously considered unsuitable for PTCA due to their high-risk status are now routinely submitted for percutaneous coronary revascularization due to advances in the design of PTCA hardware, improved operator experience, the proliferation of new interventional technologies. Through technological advances, cath lab personnel duties have become substantially more complex. Patient care involves, in addition to allaying fears and monitoring vital signs, identifying conditions which may result in case postponement, anticipating and reacting to procedural complications, participating in the actual performance of the case, and expertly troubleshooting equipment malfunctions.

This chapter has been written specifically for cath lab personnel with the intention of providing an overview of the organizational framework of the interventional laboratory, identifying specific responsibilities, and detailing patient management strategies and technical considerations involved in the performance of complex coronary interventional procedures. In this regard, overview of patient evaluation, equipment selection, troubleshooting, identification and management of procedure-related complications is presented.

PRE-PROCEDURAL CONSIDERATIONS

A. **STAFF RESPONSIBILITIES.** The cardiac catheterization lab must function as a critical care unit. Greater than 95% of cases performed in the interventional suite are successful, that still means that 1 out of every 20 cases will result in myocardial infarction, emergency CABG, or death. The likelihood of developing a major complication has been associated with specific angiographic and clinical findings, however, anaphylaxis, ventricular tachycardia or fibrillation, pulmonary edema, and shock can occur without warning. In the event of an emergency, every cardiovascular technician should be able to handle any deterioration in patient status, ranging from delivering basic life support to troubleshooting equipment failure. The successful resolution of PTCA-induced acute closure may be entirely dependent upon the ability of the CVT to immediately correct malfunctioning x-ray equipment, enabling the interventional cardiologist to re-wire and treat the occlusion before adverse clinical and hemodynamic consequences ensue.

The catheterization lab can seem a cold and technologically intimidating environment quite alien to most patients. Every CVT should sense the responsibility to soothe patient anxiety and provide communication with waiting family members. Sensitivity to patient comfort and needs often reveal early warning signals of impending complications (e.g., restlessness indicating hypoxia, somnolence indicating hypoventilation, nausea, hives, itching, and rhinorrhea as a precursor to anaphylaxis; bladder discomforts indicating the need for Foley catheterization; lower quadrant abdominal pain and distention suggesting retroperitoneal hemorrhage).

Our experience suggests that a minimum of three technologists with overlapping responsibilities should be routinely assigned to an interventional lab:

1. **Scrub Technician:**
   a. Sterile preparation, iodine debridement and scrub of catheterization site(s).
   b. Placement of ancillary drapes/sterile covers on image intensifier and lead shielding.
   c. Preparation of all necessary sterile materials and case pack.
   d. Assists physician during portions of the procedure by a) passing or exchanging guidewires, b) injection of contrast material, or c) panning of the x-ray table.
   e. Performs CPR.

2. **Circulating Technician:**
   a. Confirms type of interventional procedure and needed equipment before case.
   b. Places ECG patches.
   c. Inserts peripheral IV.
   d. Administers prescribed sedation and other medication and reassures the patient throughout the procedure.
   e. Inspects for hemostasis and stability of vascular sheath access.
   f. Data collection: imaging intensifier angulation, material usage record.
   g. Obtains accessory equipment and supplies during cases.
   h. Monitors aortic and other hemodynamic pressures.
   i. Monitors oxygen saturation through pulse oximetry.
   j. Monitors activated clotting times (ACT) results.
   k. Assures lab equipment quality assurance completed in accordance with Joint Commission on Accreditation of Hospital Organization (JCAHO) guidelines before each case.

l.   In the event of CPR, places metal support under head of table and reminds physician to place table over the main pedestal. (Otherwise, CPR is not effective)

m.   Bags the patient in the event of respiratory failure or CPR.

3.   **Monitoring Technician:**

a.   Confirms the patient's signature for consent.

b.   Acquires pertinent preprocedural laboratory information and baseline demographic data.

c.   Continuously monitors hemodynamic pressures, waveforms, ECG rate, rhythm, and ST segments, and relays data collection to the physicians. Alerts physician if CPR is not effective (pressure generated ≤ 60 mmHg).

d.   Documents any resuscitative efforts which may be occurring during the procedure, and keeps a procedural log.

e.   Logs controlled drugs and duration of radiation exposure.

f.   Inspects equipment before each case and troubleshoots when necessary (see below).

g.   Arranges bed transfers.

h.   Monitors accumulated dose of contrast

i.   Registers deployed devices with manufacturer.

B.   **PATIENT CARE.** Amidst an endless stream of new equipment designs (high-pressure balloons, long-balloons, low-profile balloons, autoperfusion balloons), new devices (atherectomy, lasers, and stents), and new imaging modalities (intravascular ultrasound, angioscopy, Doppler wire), lies the simple truth of commitment to patient care. Attention to the patients, (apostrophte) anxiety level and needs are of primary importance. Successful coordination of the multitude of responsibilities facing the CVT demands organization. A pre-procedural checklist is such an organizational tool and is one of the keys to a safe procedure. By insuring that a pre-procedural checklist has been completed for every interventional patient, the CVT may assist the attending cardiologist by identifying conditions which may require postponement of the procedure (e.g. unexplained leukocytosis, excessive anticoagulation or lack of premedication for dye or drug allergy). Should complications develop, the checklist assures that important details are not overlooked such as type and cross for CABG, documentation of pre-procedural peripheral pulses in the event leg pain develops upon case completion.

Pre-procedural Check List:

- Is there signed consent?
- Does the patient have a functioning IV?
- Are the patients vital signs stable? (temp <37.5°, systolic BP >90mmHg or <200mmHg). If not, notify physician immediately.
- Does the patient have abnormal laboratory values which may indicate a severe medical illness and necessitate postponement of the procedures? (hemoglobin <10 or >17gm/d, WBC >15,000, platelets <100,000, Na^+ >155-160 or <120-125 meq/l, K^+ <3.3 or >6.0 meq/l, creatinine >1.8mg/dl or PT >1.2 x control).
- Has a type and cross-match request been received by the blood bank?
- Is there a recent ECG on the chart?

- Allergies: if a history of dye allergy, was the patient pre-medicated? If not, notify the physician. Note any adverse reaction during previous intervention.
- Has the patient been taking at least one aspirin a day for 24 hours prior to the procedure? If not, notify physician. This is extremely important, as patients not taking aspirin are at increased risk of developing ischemic complications following PTCA.
- If the patient has an elevated (>2.0 gm/dl) creatinine, has he/she been well-hydrated? Does the physician wish to administer Mannitol or loop diuretic?
- Note peripheral pulses, record amplitude and locate with Doppler and mark if needed.
- Insert Foley catheter for complex procedures, prolonged lytic infusions, percutaneous transluminal cardiopulmonary bypass (CPS), or when both groins used for arterial venous access.
- Apply defibrillation pads in acute myocardial infarction patients.
- Assure O_2 delivery, suction and defibrillation is functional.
- Place the patient on pulse oximetry.

C. **SEDATION (Chapter 34).** The drugs used for sedation vary greatly between institutions. Opiates, barbiturates, and benzodiazapines are used commonly. The dose should be titrated according to the patients clinical status. Intravenous drugs should be given slowly over several minutes and never as a bolus. Naloxone and flumazaril must be immediately available to reverse any exaggerated narcotic response. We typically use 3 mg diazepam and 25 mg diphenhydramine IV. This combination avoids the nausea of opiates and reduces contrast reactions. Medication dosage should be reduced or withheld in the setting of:
- Advanced age
- Chronic renal failure
- Respiratory insufficiency or hypoxia.
- Liver disease
- Hypotension
- Mental status depression

D. **ASSESSMENT OF PROCEDURAL RISK AND CASE PREPARATION (Chapter 4).** Patient and lesion characteristics have been identified that increase the risk of percutaneous intervention. An estimate of procedural risk should be ascertained prior to each case. High-risk lesion characteristics refer to morphologic features associated with an increased likelihood of acute closure (e.g. degenerated saphenous vein graft, diffuse disease, thrombus-containing lesions, coronary artery dissection, angulated stenosis). High-risk patient characteristics refer to those features associated with an increased risk of cardiac mortality in the event acute closure develops (e.g. left main coronary artery disease, left ventricular dysfunction, multivessel disease, age greater than 70 years old). High-risk patient characteristics are felt to be more important determinants of overall procedural risk:

Patient Risk	+	Lesion Risk	=	Procedural Risk
High		High		Highest
High		Low		High
Low		High		Intermediate
Low		Low		Low

High-risk patients typically require modifications of patient preparation, drug therapy, and angioplasty technique. All potential complications must be anticipated and prepared for by the CVT team in advance. Additional safety measures to be taken are highlighted in Table 38.1.

INTRAPROCEDURAL CONSIDERATIONS

A. **STAFF RESPONSIBILITIES.** During an interventional case the cardiologist is focused mainly on the angiographic image and the performance of the balloon or device in treating the target lesion. In order that he/she be free to concentrate on this vital task, the technologist must focus on three things:

Table 38.1. Safety Measure for High Risk Procedures

Measure	Rationale
1. Bilateral inguinal prep	Need for IABP, CPS
2. Baseline and continuous 12-lead ECG monitor	Useful for comparison
3. Decrease sedation	Marginal cardiovascular and respiratory reserve
4. R-2 Pads	Immediate cardioversion capabilities
5. Low osmolar contrast	Minimize hypotension/LV dysfunction/arrhythmias
6. PA catheter monitoring	Monitor intravascular volume - Avoid CHF
7. ABG (Arterial Blood Gases)	Maintain optimal oxygenation
8. CCU monitoring post procedure	Quick recognition and treatment of catastrophic complications

1. **Patient Clinical Status.** This includes, but is not limited to, EKG, blood pressure, respirations, arterial oxygen saturation as monitored by pulse oximetry, level of conscious and comfort or discomfort. IV patency should be checked periodically to be sure that medications are truly infusing and not going subcutaneous or running into lines which may have become disconnected under the sterile sheets. Also IV fluid totals should be tracked and drips should not be allowed to run dry (something that can easily happen in long cases in a darkened lab). **The technologist must monitor the contrast bottle and line at all times. Arterial air emboli can be fatal!**

2. **Equipment Operation.** This involves safe and optimum functioning of all devices and accessories. It also requires alertness to the mechanical environment around the patient. The moving C-arm is a powerful motorized device capable of indicting damage to other equipment and to patient and staff as well. It is the technologist who must observe and intervene to prevent collisions with IVAC's, monitors, ventilators, pulling out of IV's, disconnecting EKG leads, etc. A well tuned sense of hearing can also be a valuable asset in the darkened cath lab. An experienced tech can recognize subtle changes in the sound of the X-ray equipment an catch film jams, wrong speeds or fluoro boost selection, and early indications of tube bearings failure. Naturally attention to heat unit alarms, error messages, circuit breaker problems, and collision alarms are all necessary to ensure that the physician has the imaging power he/she needs to do the job.

3. **Completeness of Data.** In any complex interventional case meticulous recording of procedure details is essential. This is particularly true if any of the data acquired is to be used in any cardiology research studies. Obtaining and documenting ACT valves using the in lab Hemochron or similar device, informing the physician if time elapsed since last heparin or ACT reaches 45 minutes, monitoring contrast use and notifying the physician of the accumulated total exceeds 300 ml, all are vital details which have serious implications for patient care if overlooked. Recording of inflation times and pressures, number of atherectomy or laser passes, patient subjective assessment of pain on 1 to 10 scale, angiographic view angle readings all need to be entered into the case's database.

B. EQUIPMENT SELECTION (Chapter 1)

1. **Sheaths.** The majority of PTCA procedures employ 7F or 8F arterial sheaths whereas most atherectomy devices mandate use of 9F to 11F sheaths. Extra-long sheaths can be used to span tortuous femoral and iliac vessels and improve guide catheter movement and torque-control. Floppy-tipped or slippery hydrophilic guidewires are used to steer through highly diseased or tortuous arterial segments. Venous access is also established in most cases with smaller 5F to 8F sheaths, permitting fluid resuscitation, administration of medications, insertion of a temporary pacemaker or pulmonary artery catheter as necessary.

2. **Guide Catheters.** 8F right and left Judkins 4.0 angioplasty guide catheters are selected most often. A 7F guide, or 8F guide with side holes, is selected when vessels appear to be small or when catheter pressure damping occurs. Conversely, large lumen guide (>0.86-inch) may be required if

intracoronary stent placement is likely. An early left main trunk bifurcation might favor a standard catheter with a shortened tip or a 3.5 Judkins curve if the LAD is the target vessel. Left Amplatz and Voda catheters provide superior support compared to Judkins curves. In addition, an enlarged aortic root favors a larger Judkins curve (4.5-6.0) or Amplatz or Voda catheter. Angulated Judkins catheters are selected for anterior and posterior orientations of the left main trunk. The physician's goal in all cases is to optimize coaxial alignment between the catheter tip and long axis of the proximal target vessel segment.

3. **Guidewires.** Several guidewire designs are available, each with different degrees of pushability, flexibility and steerability. Floppy wires are preferred in the vast majority of cases due to their extremely flexible and atraumatic tip; however, stiffer wires have improved steerability and pushability and may be necessary when attempting to cross a complex, high-grade, or total occlusion.

4. **Balloons.** Balloon dilatation catheters come in one of two basic designs; balloon over-the-wire and balloon on-the-wire systems. With balloon over-the-wire systems, both wire and balloon move independently. The principal advantage of this system is the ability to maintain lesion access (i.e. the wire remains across PTCA site throughout the procedure) should acute closure of the PTCA vessel occur or balloon upsizing be required. Balloon on-the-wire systems are "fixed systems," both guidewire and balloon are bonded together and cannot move independently. The principal advantage of this system is derived from its extreme low profile and may be of particular value when over-the-wire systems fail to cross a lesion due to proximal tortuosity, diffuse disease, or high-grade stenosis. In addition, single operators may favor a fixed-wire or monorail (rapid-exchange) system due to their simplicity of use. Long balloons (30-40mm versus 20mm) may be used to treat diffuse coronary disease or lesions located on highly angulated segments. Autoperfusion catheters have sideholes proximal and distal to its balloon and allow passive delivery of aortic blood to the isosemic myocardial bed during balloon inflation. This balloon is of particular value when patients are intolerant of balloon inflations (severe angina, hypotension) or prolonged inflations are required (e.g. tack-up dissections).

C. **SUBOPTIMAL RESULTS.** Major arterial complications develop in 2-4% of elective PTCA cases and may result in acute myocardial infarction, emergency surgery or death. Far more often (15-30%), a patient remains stable, but the angiographic results appears hazy, contains a filling defect or reveals dye staining with or without slow distal dye flow. Reasons for suboptimal results include the presence of a hard atheroma which is resistant to cracking or compression, distal coronary spasm, local vessel dissection and formation of thrombus. Guiding catheter induced coronary trauma, coronary perforation, and embolization of clot or atheroma occur less commonly.

For the CVT, the key is to plan ahead of complications and anticipate physician needs. Attention should be directed to observation of new ECG changes, hypotension and development of chest pain that might otherwise escape early detection. One should anticipate the need for intra-aortic balloon pump support, temporary transvenous pacing, placement of a Swan-Ganz catheter, preparation and administration of new medications or exchange for a different balloon or device. In all such cases, therapy is directed toward restoring normal antegrade blood flow and achieving a <30% residual stenosis by treating spasm (with intracoronary nitrates; Chapter 19), thrombus (lytics, repeat balloon dilatation, TEC atherectomy; Chapter 9), perforation (prolonged balloon inflations; Chapter 22) and dissection (prolonged balloon inflation, directional atherectomy, intracoronary stenting; Chapter 20).

D. MAJOR INTRAPROCEDURAL COMPLICATIONS. Acute complications during angioplasty most frequently involve bradycardia/asystole, ventricular tachycardia/fibrillation, hypotension/shock, and acute allergic reaction. In many cases, the CVT may be the first person to recognize the diagnosis "observe the change in condition" or initiate treatment. The cause and treatment for commonly encountered complications are listed in Table 38.2.

E. SPECIAL PROCEDURES

1. **Directional Coronary Atherectomy (Chapter 28).** Directional Coronary Atherectomy (DCA) is indicated for a subset of complex angioplasty patients. Highly eccentric lesion in a proximal vessel

Table 38.2. Common Intraprocedural Management Problems

Complications	Cause	Treatment
Bradycardia/ Asystole	• Ionic contrast • Hypoxia • Vagal response • AV node ischemia • Bezhold-Jarish	• Cough • Oxygen • IV atropine, fluids • Treatment of ischemia placement • TVP
Ventricular tachycardia/ fibrillation	• Catheter induced • Guidewire induced • Contrast mediated • Ischemia/infarct artery reperfusion	• Remove catheter/wire • Immediate cardioversion/defibrillation • Switch to low osmolar contrast-replace K $\oplus$, mg # is low. • IV lidocaine if persistent • Typically self-limited with reperfusion
Hypotension	• Artifact • Dehydration • Medications • Ischemia/infarction • Pericardial tamponade/perfusion • VT/VF • Dye reaction	• Recalibrates transducer, tighten ring on Y-adapter • Saline IV bolus • D/C nitrates • Pericardiocentesis • Dopamine/Dobutamine • Aramine-Sympathetometics • IABP/CPS
Hives/itchy/ bronchospasm	• Dye allergy	• Diphenhydramine • Hydrocortisone • Epinephrine • ABGs/pulse oximetry • See Chapter ___.

segment is the most common indication. This technique has also been used to excise focal, flow-limiting dissection. In this situation, successful atherectomy may result in stable vessel patency, improved antegrade blood flow and avoidance of emergency bypass surgery. However, it may also perforate the vessel thus most dissection are treated with prolonged balloon inflations or stents. Contraindications to DCA include vessel diameter <2.5mm, marked proximal vessel angulation tortuosity, heavy lesion calcification, and degenerated saphenous vein grafts. The catheter design and function is presented in Chapter 21. Some degree of ischemia commonly occurs during directional atherectomy due to mechanical obstruction of coronary blood flow produced by the cutting device itself or by the large guiding catheter. Coronary artery dissection, thrombosis, perforation and intimal disruption secondary to nosecone trauma have been described. The technologist should have 10% formalin or other preservative available if atherectomy cuttings are to be sent for histologic examination. If collagen study is to be made the specimen must be fast frozen in a liquid nitrogen bath and stored in a carbon dioxide freezer. Availability of these resources must be assured by the technologist before the case begins.

2. **Rotablator Atherectomy (Chapter 27).** Technologist responsibilities in these cases include: 1) Equipment setup and operation; 2) safety concerns particular to this device; and 3) documentation and preservation of device components in the event of a malfunction. Equipment assembly requires an H-cylinder of compressed nitrogen to drive the motor unit. When nitrogen psi falls below 400 the tank should be changed to avoid pressure loss during the procedure. Flow rate should be located at 100 psi. There should be easy access to a burr size comparability chart (perhaps mounted on the rolling device supply cart). This is necessary to ensure selection of a guiding catheter with adequate inner lumen diameter to accept the appropriate burr. A liter bag of heparinized saline or lactated ringers should be evacuated of air and hung in a pressure bag set at least 200 mm Hg. Sterile contrast tubing without an air chamber or Y branches should be selected to avoid air emboi; air bubbles should be flushed out. A high degree of vigilance on the part of the technologist throughout the procedure can be vital in preventing a catastrophic air embolus. Remember the room is semi-dark. The physician is concentrating on the fluoroscopic image to observe wire position, burr performance and coronary response. It is up to the technologist to check frequently the fluid level of the pressurized flush solution and to alert the physician to any danger of air in the system. Other possible complications the technologist should be alert to include the no-reflow phenomenon and bradycardia or asystole during verapamil or adenosine rotablation. For no-reflow (Chapter 21), be prepared for the physician to administer large doses of intracoronary verapamil and anticipate the need to treat any resulting systemic hypotension and/or bradycardia, particularly for target lesions in the RCA or dominant LCx. The technologist should have a pacing electrode, connector cables and an external pulse generator immediately available. The generator should be checked just before the case for battery function. Nothing should be left to chance. During device operation, the technologist should maintain a speed of 160,000 to 190,000 rpm without interruption. Drops in RPM more than 5000 indicate resistance against the lesion, and increases the risk of dissection and large particle formation. The physician should "peck" at the lesion, avoiding drops in RPM which generate excessive heat. The technologist should <u>not</u> increase the PRM in that situation (it will generate more heat), but advise the physician of excessive

deceleration. As with any other medical device, if a malfunction occurs which results in possible injury to the patient, care must be taken to comply with all requirements of the federal government's Safe Medical Devices Act. It is the technologist's responsibility to immediately document the details of any potentially reportable incident immediately and to save all components of the system for further investigation by the hospital's Biomedical Engineering Department. Attention must be paid during cleanup to retrieve wires, burrs, catheters, accessories, etc. so that the biomed specialists can examine everything for possible defects and determine any follow-up action that may be necessary.

3. **Stents.** These devices reduce restenosis, are the treatment of choice for abrupt closure, and may one day be performed on 50% of all patients needing percutaneous intervention. The technologist must distinguish between Gianturco-Roubin and Palmaz-Schatz stents; both are approved by the FDA. If intravascular ultrasound is available, the technologist should be proficient in image processing. Use of the electronic caliper feature in digital cath lab systems is an alternative approach to provide optimal stent sizing and deployment.

4. **Excimer Laser Coronary Angioplasty (ELCA) (Chapter 30).** This procedure may be indicated for long lesions, diffusely diseased coronary segments, ostial narrowings, stenoses resistant to high balloon pressures and calcified lesions that cannot be crossed or dilated with a balloon catheter. These systems are considered "cold" lasers; their mode of action is to transform laser energy into vibrational energy breaking apart chemical bonds in the atheroma. They differ from thermal-laser balloons which rely on heating and welding effects. Safety precautions require that all personnel and patients undergoing laser procedures wear protective eye glasses. The laser system may require specialized CVT maintenance with special attention to power elements, lenses and adjustment of power output based on catheter size and required energy density. Contemporary excimer lasers are elss demanding with respect to routine maintenance old models. Flushing with saline is now considered essential with ELCA to reduce the risk of severe dissection. Adjunctive balloon angioplasty is performed after lasing in >90% of cases. Contraindications to ELCA include severe lesion eccentricity, marked angulation or proximal vessel tortuosity, and true bifurcation lesions. Greater details and clinical results are described in Chapter 30.

5. **Cardiopulmonary Support (CPS) (Chapter 6).** CPS (femoral vein to femoral artery bypass) is specifically designed for hemodynamic support of the patients with severe LV dysfunction or those undergoing PTCA of their only patent vessel. Use of the portable CPS equipment requires a minimum of 20 minutes of preparation and the assistance of a hemoperfusionist thoroughly familiar with the system. Arterial cannulas are 18F and 20F and are selected based on body size. Considerable physician experience is also required to avoid vascular complications. In order to avoid oxygenator induced consumption of the coagulation factors (increased PT, PTT, and decreased fibrinogen, platelets) a bolus of 30,000 units of heparin is typically given and the ACT level maintained at >400 seconds. Frequent monitoring of the ACT and arterial blood gases is required to avoid profound anemia, metabolic acidoses and hypoxemia. Following case completion, the patient is transferred to a specially-designed stretcher with extra thick padding to

increase patient comfort during prolonged immobilization (12-24 hrs) required to achieve hemostasis once CPS cannulae are removed. The ability to be lowered closer to the floor than conventional stretchers and a siderail configuration that does not interfere with positioning of the CPS vascular clamp used following removal of the large cannulae are features necessary in the stretcher utilized with CPS. Distal pulses should be checked frequently. Physicians may request keeping the patient on the stretcher thereby minimizing bed to bed transfers and the risk of accidental or premature dislodgement of cannulae.

6. **Prolonged Urokinase Infusion (Chapter 9).** This form of adjunctive pharmacotherapy has gained increasing popularity and is sometimes used to recanalize occluded saphenous vein grafts and native coronary arteries. A standard 7 or 8F guiding catheter is seated in the target vessel. The guidewire is advanced into the artery as far as possible and a hollow core wire or multiple hole perfusion catheter is advanced until it abuts or enters the occlusion. The angioplasty guidewire is then removed, leaving a conduit through which urokinase is selectively infused. The entire system must be sutured and secured to the patient's leg (Chapter 9). Tape and dressings can be applied to further secure the system since any movement jeopardizes equipment position and procedural success. **Since this is an intracoronary infusion it is essential that absolutely no bubbles are present in the infusion line.** Sterile stopcocks are attached to the infusion system to permit exit of bubbles and contrast injection during follow-up angiography. Forceful flushing is contraindicated because of ongoing clot dissolution and possible embolization. The urokinase infusion protocol typically extends up to a 12-24 hr period. As a result, the patient must remain supine with vascular sheaths in situ for up to 48 hrs. A secure vascular sheath, bladder catheterization and continuous sedation are important patient care considerations. A successful infusion protocol results in partial clot lysis, improved antegrade blood flow and is typically followed by further intervention on any residual stenosis that is seen.

F. **TROUBLESHOOTING.** Frequent technical problems encountered by the CVT include 1) abnormal pressure on monitor, 2) temporary venous pacemaker malfunction, 3) power injection failure, 4) x-ray equipment malfunction and 5) intra-aortic balloon pump malfunction. In every case, as highlighted in Tables 38.3 to 38.6, a systematic step-by-step approach will often identify and solve most simple problems.

POSTPROCEDURAL CONSIDERATIONS

This is a critical period when control of patient care is transferred to the CVT. The technician must confirm the security of vascular sheaths, oxygen supply and IV medication infusions. The patient should be chest

Table 38.3. Pressure Monitoring Problems

Waveform	Assessment	Options
Absent	• Reversed or broken transducers • Disconnected cable • Pressure tubing disconnected, hemostatic valve open • Incorrect zero • Incorrect scale	• Notify M.D. • Secure & clean cable connection • Flush pressure lines. Check for back-bleeding • Recalibrate system
Low Amplitude	• Incorrect scale • Valve/stopcock open Air • Twisted catheter or tip obstructed	• Reset scale • Recalibrate system • Flush pressure lines • Observe catheter tip placement & shaft on fluoroscopy
Overshoot	• Air	• Flush system
Drift	• Transducer setup	• Refill strain gauge membrane with fluid

Table 38.4 Assessment of Temporary Ventricular Pacemaker (TVP) Malfunction

No Pacing Spike
1. Check and clean cable connections.
2. Confirm appropriate generator lead connection (atrial vs ventricular).
3. Check pacing mode (demand/asynchronous).
4. Check pacing rate set (generator > patient).
5. Increase output to maximum.
6. Recheck battery indicator.
7. Replace cable and/or generator.
8. Generator switch on

Spike Without Capture
1. Confirm that catheter position is level with right ventricle apex or right ventricular outflow tract.
2. Increase pacemaker generator output to maximum, determine threshold and set output 2-3 times above this.
3. Observe for signs of perforation: hypotension, chest pain, ST-segment elevation on ECG, hiccoughs, friction rub on auscultation.

Intermittent Capture
1. Confirm catheter position.
2. Check generator settings, reset to increased HR.
3. Recheck threshold.

Failure to Capture
1. Check generator sensing threshold and set 2-3 below this.
2. Check catheter position.

Table 38.5. Simple Causes of Power Injector Failure

1. Improperly loaded injection syringe
2. Syringe compartment latch not secure
3. Trigger cable short circuit
4. Insufficient contrast for programmed injection

Always purge injector syringe and extension tubing of all air before connecting to catheters.

pain free and prepared for stretcher transfer. Concurrently, patient comfort needs must be assessed. Patient anxiety and complaints often reveal warning signs of impending complications (e.g., vessel reocclusion, nausea, hives, itching, and numbness as a precursor to anaphylaxis; lower quadrant abdominal pain and distention signaling retroperitoneal bleeding; leg pain in patients who may develop limb-threatening ischemia within several hrs). Therefore, it is critical that the CVT understand the initial assessment and management of chest pain, rhythm disorders, bleeding and limb pain.

Chest pain is the most worrisome post-procedural complication since it often heralds abrupt vessel closure. Multiple factors must also be considered and ruled out before the patient emergently returns to the interventional lab. Bleeding is relatively uncommon after coronary intervention despite the use of systemic

Table 38.6 Simple Causes of X-Ray Equipment Malfunction

No Image

1. Inappropriate monitor brightness and contrast
2. Accidental activation of reset or "panic" buttons
3. Auto dose exposure mode not on (KV freeze mode is on)
5. Generator error, check message and reset. Check computer room air condition.
6. No file magazine on camera
7. Magazine sensor

No Cine

1. Cine mode not selected on control board
2. Film magazine misaligned, misloaded, or film torn
3. No film
4. "Overspeed" trip activated on camera
5. Loose cable from cine camera to image intensifier
6. Incorrect use of foot pedals for digital cine mode

C-Arm Failure

1. Proximity or safety switch bent, broken, or triggered (check image intensifier, collimator, table base position)
2. Biplane lateral arm out of "park" position
3. Collision of X-ray tube or image intensifier requiring manual override

anticoagulation and large arterial sheaths. If difficulties with vascular sheaths are observed, hematoma formation should be monitored closely. Bleeding may be encountered within the GI tract or the pericardium (as a result of an occult coronary or temporary pacemaker induced perforation). Rhythm disturbances, extremity pain and confusion are additional problems that first present to the CVT. Early recognition, accurate diagnosis, and prompt treatment will have a major impact on patient outcome (Table 38.7).

LABORATORY LOGISTICS AND SAFETY

A. MATERIAL MANAGEMENT

1. **Room Supplies.** It is advisable to stock each lab identically to minimize confusion. Basic items including IV lines, solutions, needles, sutures, standard diagnostic and PTCA catheters, drug cassettes, and emergency medications should always be in similar arrangements. However, inventory consisting of expensive devices and custom catheters should be centralized and dispensed individually for patients. Several computerized systems are available to track and control inventory. A bar code type system has been extremely effective in this regard.

2. **Sterile Packs.** Contents are custom tailored to the specific needs of a particular cath lab and are often dictated by physician preference. The cost of the packaging should be offset by improved operational efficiency. Different packs for brachial cutdown and femoral approaches can be stocked. The identical sterile packs may be used for percutaneous brachial and femoral techniques and contain only disposable items.

3. **Specialty Carts.** These carts are dedicated to a single interventional procedure and contain all possible materials needed to complete that case. Carts are ideal for specialized or less frequently used techniques such as valvuloplasty, laser, atherectomy, and stenting. The carts are extremely portable, easy to use, and consolidate inventory storage. This concept can be extended to include standard supply stock carts.

4. **ACLS Equipment.** The minimum standard equipment for ACLS should be present in each catheterization suite. A cassette system of commonly used drugs facilitates storage and access. The entire cassette chest should be rotated periodically for complete restocking by the pharmacy. In addition a "crash cart" containing defibrillation intubation supplies and ACLS medications must be

Table 38.7. Common Post Procedural Management Problems

Problem	Cause	Assessment
Chest Pain	Ischemia Pericardial perforation Reflux esophagitis Musculoskeletal	Obtain: • Compare pre, intra, and post procedural ECGs. • Pain similar to pain on balloon inflation? Felt on inspiration? • Response to nitrates and antacids. • Palpable tenderness or arthritis? • Check vital signs and pulsus paradox.
Arrhythmia	Nausea/vagal effect AV node (RCA) ischemia Drug effect Hypoxia	• Check ECGs for acute change (as above). • Check medications & dosage. • Check pulse oxygen saturation or ABG
Tachycardia/Hypotension	Ischemia Hypovolemia Drug Effect Congestive failure	• Arouse patient, administration naloxone. • Perform manual BP check. • Ischemia evaluation as above. • Response to saline fluid bolus and trendelenburg position.
Bleeding	Local Retroperitoneal Gastrointestinal Pericardial	• Local compression. • Check vascular sheath, exchange to bigger sheath or remove sheaths • Check ACT, CBC. Consider reversing heparin with protamine • Pericardiocentesis • Surgical evaluation.
Limb Pain	Ischemia Emboli Retroperitoneal hematoma (femoral nerve compression)	• Check for loss of pulse (use Doppler). • Look for livedo riticularis. • Quadriceps weakness? • Check for IABP or possible sheath movement.
Mental Status Change	Stroke Over sedation Hypoxia Hypoglycemia Lidocaine	• Look for focal motor deficits. • Give Naloxone • Check ABG, O_2 SATS, lytes. • Give glucose • Stop lidocaine

present in every room. The contents within this cart, however, are usually sealed as a further quality assurance measure. In addition to the cassette and crash cart system, certain medications should be immediately available at all times. Fresh intravenous preparations of lidocaine, nitroglycerin and dopamine can be mixed daily, labeled, and separately placed on standby infusion pumps in each lab.

5. **Quality Assurance.** The quality assurance process is an integral part of cath lab function and should begin before the patient enters the interventional laboratory. Preparatory to each case, it is mandatory that the monitoring technician complete a "check-out" list ensuring that all appropriate

equipment, medications, and ACLS support devices are ready. The basic list should apply to all cardiac procedures. This check-out list must be completed, signed, and should accompany the patient chart. The key to every emergency situation that develops is being prepared ahead of time.

B. RADIATION PROTECTION. Radiation exposure is a concern to all members of the interventional team. The goal is to limit x-ray exposure to levels as low as reasonably achievable. Table 38.8 includes tips to help minimize an individual's exposure. The importance of utilizing lead shielding, observance of the inverse square law and rotating team member responsibilities in the lab deserve emphasis. Exposure appears to be no higher in biplane systems than monoplane systems provided that total fluoroscopy and cine operation time is the same in both systems. The average radiation dose from the fluoroscopy and cine operation in diagnostic angiography is roughly equal to the average dose during simple PTCA. During angioplasty, fluoroscopy time tends to be longer than during diagnostic angiography whereas cine time, which causes the highest exposure to radiation, is considerably shorter. Film badge monitoring is intended to provide personnel important information about the radiation exposure in the lab. It is in the best interest of both the wearer and institution that this information be as accurate as possible.

Table 38.8. Ways to Reduce Radiation Exposure

1. Keep as far away from the radiographed object (inverse square law).

2. Select the minimum collimation possible.

3. Set image intensifier as close as possible to the patient.

4. Do not reach into the radiation beam with your hands.

5. Use the unit components for "shadowing" as designed.

6. Wear radiation protection clothing at all times (apron, glasses and thyroid shield).

7. Use pulsed fluoroscopy whenever available.

8. Where possible, use cine operation with 12.5 or 30 f/s.

9. During cine film identification, wear lead gloves or apply text to image intensifier.

10. Utilize leaded glass shields between staff and X-ray tube.

* * * * *

39 INTERVENTIONAL CARDIOLOGY SURVEY

The explosive growth of new interventional technologies, imaging modalities, and pharmacotherapy has created an impossible number of combinations to test in randomized trials:

Lesion Characteristics	Lesion Locations	Percutaneous Interventions	Imaging Modalities	Drugs
Calcification	Native coronary	PTCA balloons	None	Antiplatelets
Angulation	Ostial	Conventional	Ultrasound	Antithrombins
Eccentricity	Nonostial	High-pressure	Angioscopy	Lytics
Thrombus	Saphenous vein graft	Long	Doppler	
Proximal tortuosity	Ostial	Cutting		
Long lesion length	Body	Atherectomy		
Ulceration	Distal anastamosis	AtheroCath		
Total occlusion		Rotablator		
Bifurcation		TEC		
		Lasers		
		Excimer		
		Holmium		
		Stents		
		Self-expanding		
		Balloon-expandable		
		Thermal-memory		
Possible Combinations = $511 \times 5 \times 12 \times 4 \times 3 = 551{,}880!$				
511*	5	12**	4	3

* $2^{(n=9)} - 1$

**   Does not take into account device combinations (e.g., Rotablator + Stent)

Efforts to gather clinically-relevant information are frustrated by the fact that "current" journals frequently report results of studies performed 2-3 years ago; that most textbooks are outdated by the time of publication; and that attempts to absorb every statistic and detail presented at every conference and meeting is anything but anxiolytic: "...Interventionalist A at meeting B recommended device C using technique D, drug E, imaging modality F, and contrast agent G for lesion type H ... or was it device D using technique C? .. Or drug F? ... or lesion type K?

In an effort to relieve rather than add to this confusion, we asked 27 leading interventionalists from 7 countries over 100 questions about patient triage, technical pearls and pitfalls, clinical follow-up and more.

This survey helps to identify areas of consensus and controversy among the experts. Cover up the responses and take the survey yourself. We hope you find this exercise both enjoyable and enlightening!

Survey Participants:

Donald Baim, MD	USA
John Bittl, MD	USA
Antonio Colombo, MD	ITALY
John Douglas Jr., MD	USA
David Faxon, MD	USA
Barry George, MD	USA
Cindy Grines, MD	USA
Richard Heuser, MD	USA
David Holmes, MD	USA
Dean Kereiakes, MD	USA
Ferdinand Kiemeneij, MD	NETHERLANDS
Takeshi Kimura, MD	JAPAN
Morton Kern, MD	USA
Spencer King III, MD	USA
Frank Litvack, MD	USA
Bernard Meier, MD	SWITZERLAND
Richard Myler, MD	USA
Masakiyo Nobuyoshi, MD	JAPAN
William O'Neill, MD	USA
Nicolaus Reifart, MD	GERMANY
Timothy Sanborn, MD	USA
Richard Schatz, MD	USA
Patrick Serruys, MD	NETHERLANDS
Ulrich Sigwart, MD	ENGLAND
Paul Teirstein, MD	USA
David Williams, MD	USA
Patrick Whitlow, MD	USA

Average Interventional Experience of 27 Survey Participants:

Device	Total # cases	# Cases 1995 (estimate)
PTCA	4326 (1000-16,400)	286 (50-2150)
DCA	230 (20-900)	32 (0-160)
TEC	47 (0-300)	16 (0-200)
Rotablator	191 (0-1000)	78 (0-300)
ELCA (or other laser ablation)	88 (0-500)	5 (0-36)
Stent J & J Coronary	388 (15-1300)	118 (5-463)
J & J Biliary	61 (0-250)	15 (0-100)
Cook	68 (0-300)	14 (0-100)
AVE Microstent	25*(5-70)	10 (1-20)
Wiktor	14 (0-150)	1 (0-20)
Wallstent	26*(1-50)	10 (1-29)
Support system IABP	251 (20-1000)	25 (2-90)
CPS	15 (0-100)	3 (0-20)
Intravascular Ultrasound	176 (5-800)	79 (0-400)
Angioscopy	36 (0-300)	4 (0-50)
Doppler FloWire	80 (0-1500)	14 (0-200)

*   Physicians outside USA

Q: **What type of results do you expect after** *conventional PTCA* **for the following lesion types:**

Lesion Type	Primary Success (Final stenosis <50%)	Major Complications (Death, Q-MI, CABG)
Eccentric	1.2	1.2
Calcified (moderate-severe	1.4	1.5
Long (>20mm)	1.5	1.3
Ulcerated	1.7	1.5
Thrombus (definite)	2.2	2.3
Total occlusion (chronic)	2.8	1.3
Angulated (>60°)	2.3	2.4
Bifurcation	1.6	1.4
Ostial	1.8	1.7
Proximal tortuously	1.4	1.5
SVG nondegenerated	1.3	1.8
degenerated	2.4	2.9

CODES:

Success	Complications
1: > 90% of cases	1: < 2% of cases
2: > 70-90% of cases	2: > 2-5% of cases
3: < 70% of cases	3: > 5% of cases

Q: **Considering all factors (success, complications, restenosis, cost, user-friendliness, etc), what is your *device of choice* for each of the following lesion types, lesion locations, and angiographic complications:**

Lesion	Device (%)*					
	DCA	ROTA	ELCA	PTCA	TEC	STENT
Eccentric	29	14	0	10	0	48
Calcification (moderate-severe)	0	86	0	5	0	9
Long (>20mm)	0	43	10	33	0	14
Ulcerated	10	5	0	19	5	62
Thrombus (definite)	18	0	0	41	29	11
Total occlusion (chronic) crossed with a guidewire	0	11	6	56	0	28
Angulated (>60°)	0	5	0	65	0	30
Bifurcation	58	5	0	26	0	11
Ostial	26	37	16	0	0	21
Proximal tortuosity	5	0	0	80	0	15
SVG nondegenerated	0	0	0	0	5	95
degenerated	0	0	0	0	29	71
Undilatable	0	80	10	0	0	10
Dissection focal (<10mm)	5	0	0	11	0	84
long (≥10mm)	0	0	0	0	0	100
Elastic recoil	10	5	0	0	0	85
Haziness	14	0	0	36	0	50

Abbreviations: DCA = Directional Coronary Atherectomy, ROTA = Rotablator, ELCA = Excimer Laser Coronary Atherectomy, PTCA = balloon angioplasty, TEC = Transluminal Extraction Catheter

* Numbers refer to percentage of survey participants choosing a particular device for a given lesion type (e.g., 29% indicated that DCA was their device of choice for eccentric lesions).

TRIAGE OF CHEST PAIN:

Q: A 51 year old man in good health develops a chest pain syndrome and corresponding resting EKG as described below. What do you recommend?

Syndrome	Recommendations				
	Medical Therapy; no further testing	Outpatient Stress Test	Outpatient Cath	In-patient Stress	In-patient Cath
Atypical pain, normal EKG	12%	85%	4%	0%	4%
Stable exertional angina, normal EKG	0%	54%	38%	0%	4%
Progressive exertional angina, normal EKG	0%	15%	50%	8%	15%
Prolonged rest angina, normal EKG Single episode 2 d. Ago x 30 min., none since	0%	12%	27%	12%	50%
Several episodes over last few days, pain-free now	0%	0%	4%	0%	96%
Ongoing chest pain unresponsive to nitrates	0%	0%	0%	12%	88%
Ongoing chest pain responsive to nitrates	0%	0%	0%	8%	92%
Prolonged rest angina, ST depression Chest pain & EKG responsive to medicine	0%	0%	0%	4%	96%
Chest pain responsive to medicine, EKG persists.	0%	0%	0%	0	100%
Chest pain & EKG persist despite meds	0%	0%	0%		

CIRCULATORY SUPPORT:

Q: **What support strategy do you use for patients who require percutaneous revascularization with baseline EF = 15-30%:**

46% Standby IABP (arterial access established in contralateral femoral artery)

35% Prophylactic IABP

4% Standby CPS

4% Prophylactic CPS

12% Other

Q: **What support strategy do you use for patients who require percutaneous revascularization with baseline EF < 15%:**

23% Standby IABP (arterial access established in contralateral femoral artery)

50% Prophylactic IABP

8% Standby CPS

12% Prophylactic CPS

4% Other

Q: **What support strategy do you use for patients who require percutaneous revascularization of a single patent vessel:**

15% Standby IABP (arterial access established in contralateral femoral artery)

46% Prophylactic IABP

8% Standby CPS

8% Prophylactic CPS

12% Other

CLINICAL FOLLOW-UP AFTER INTERVENTION:

Q: **For patients who present with symptomatic ischemia, what type of follow-up do you recommend after successful percutaneous intervention:**

31%   Clinical follow-up only; no routine stress test

Routine stress test at:

42%   1 month

46%   3 months

15%   6 months

19%   12 months

4%   Routine catheterization at 6 months

Q: **For patients who present with asymptomatic ischemia, what type of follow-up do you recommend after successful percutaneous intervention:**

35%   Clinical follow-up only; no routine stress test

Routine stress test at:

42%   1 month

42%   3 months

27%   6 months

4%   12 months

4%   Routine catheterization at 6 months

Q: **For patients who present with acute myocardial infarction, what type of follow-up do you recommend after successful percutaneous intervention:**

12%   Clinical follow-up only; no routine stress test

     Routine stress test at:

       4%   predischarge

       8%   1 month

      12%   3 months

       4%   6 months

           12 months

12%   Routine catheterization at 6 months

Q: **What type of stress test do you recommend for the following situations**

CONDITION	STRESS TEST					
	Exercise EKG	Exercise Perfusion	Pharmacologic Perfusion	Exercise Echo	Dobut Echo	Exercise MUGA
Normal EKG able to exercise	79%	13%	0%	8%	0%	0%
unable to exercise	0%	0%	58%	0%	42%	0%
Abnormal EKG able to exercise	12%	72%	0%	16%	0%	0%
unable to exercise	0%	0%	56%	0%	44%	0%
Post-MI able to exercise	24%	56%	4%	12%	0%	4%
unable to exercise	0%	0%	58%	0%	42%	0%

Q：　**How are you currently using c7E3 during percutaneous revascularization (monoclonal antibody to platelet IIb/IIIa receptor)?**

　0%　For all patients

　0%　For all patients with high-risk anatomy and/or unstable ischemic syndromes

　59%　In selected patients with high-risk anatomy and/or unstable ischemic syndromes

　41%　Not using this agent at the present time.

ACTIVATED CLOTTING TIMES (ACT):

Q:　**Which device do you use to measure ACTs?**

　15%　HemoTec

　78%　HemoChron

　7%　Other

Q:　**Which balloon material you routinely use for PTCA for the following situations:**

	PET	Duralyn	POC	PE-600	HDPE	No Preference
Routine PTCA	15%	25%	10%	30%	5%	15%
Post Stent	32%	18%	0%	0%	8%	32%
Post DCA	26%	26%	0%	32%	0%	15%
Post Rotablator	38%	14%	5%	14%	5%	15%
Angulated	30%	25%	10%	20%	0%	15%
Calcified	50%	20%	0%	10%	10%	10%
Length >20 mm	20%	20%	10%	30%	5%	15%

PET = polyethylene terephthalate; POC = polyolefin co-polymer; PE = polyethylene; HDPE = high-density polyethylene

Q: What ACT do you aim for during each of these procedures?

	<300 sec.	300-350 sec.	350-400 sec.	>400 sec.
PTCA Stable angina	9%	91%	0%	0
Unstable angina	9%	70%	22%	0
Acute MI	4%	70%	26%	0
Lytic failure	4%	61%	35%	0
DCA	5%	86%	9%	0
TEC	5%	95%	0%	7
Rotablator	9%	91%	0%	0
ELCA	5%	89%	5%	0
Stent Bailout	9%	65%	26%	0
Elective-native	13%	78%	9%	0
Elective-SVG	13%	74%	13%	0

PTCA TECHNIQUE:

Q: Which inflation technique do you routinely employ?

16%   Oscillating

65%   Incremental (2atm-4atm-8atm) over 30-60 seconds

20%   Rapid (<10 seconds) increase to desired pressure

Q: What is your average time per inflation?

0%	< 30 sec.
15%	30-60 sec.
59%	60-120 sec.
26%	> 120 sec.

Q: What is your total inflation time per balloon

0%	1 min.
41%	1-3 min.
52%	3-5 min.
4%	5-10 min.
4%	10-20 min.
0%	> 20 min.

Q: For multivessel disease amenable to percutaneous intervention, do you routinely:

8%	Stage the procedure over 1-3 days if possible
4%	Stage the procedure over 2-4 weeks if possible
81%	Treat all lesions during the same procedure; stage if suboptimal result for the last lesion
4%	Treat all lesions during the same procedure
4%	Treat only the culprit lesion, then reassess the need for further intervention

Q: **Which contrast agent do you use in the following settings:**

	Ionic, High Osmolar (Reno-76, hypaque)	Ionic, Low Osmolar (Hexabrix)	Nonionoic (Isovue, Omnipaque)
Cath stable angina	44%	22%	33%
unstable angina	33%	30%	37%
acute MI	7%	41%	52%
PTCA stable angina	37%	33%	30%
unstable angina without thrombus	26%	44%	30%
unstable angina with thrombus	26%	41%	33%
acute MI	4%	52%	44%
Stent elective	37%	33%	30%
bailout	26%	44%	30%
DCA	37%	33%	30%
TEC	32%	36%	32%
Rotablator	31%	38%	31%
ELCA	38%	29%	33%
Pulmonary edema	0%	31%	69%
Shock	0%	31%	69%

Q: **A 50-year old male presents to the emergency room with prolonged atypical chest pain and a normal EKG. What type of work-up do you recommend:**

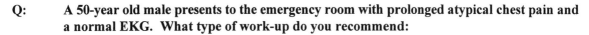

78% Noninvasive work-up; cath if abnormal

7% Cath; noninvasive workup if abnormal

15% Cath; PTCA if abnormal

Q: **How do you manage patients with unstable angina and reversible EKG changes who are currently pain-free?**

11% Immediate cath; defer intervention for 24 hours

48% Immediate cath and intervention (if appropriate)

41% Medical therapy to "cool-off" the patient for 1-3 days followed by cath and intervention

0% Medical therapy to "cool-off" patient for 1-3 days, then noninvasive evaluation & cath if abnormal

TRIAGE & TREATMENT OF ACUTE MI:

Q: **How would you manage each of the following acute ischemic syndromes? (Assume the patient presents within 6 hours, has ST elevation, and that cath lab is immediately available.)**

	Thrombolytic Therapy			Cath/PTCA	Medical - no lytic
	IV SK	IV tPA	other		
Inferior MI BP normal	4%	4%	4%	89%	0%
Hypotension	4%	4%	0%	93%	0%
Anterior MI BP normal	0%	4%	4%	92%	0%
Hypotension	0%	0%	0%	100%	0%
Any MI	0%	0%	0%	100%	0%
Age > 70 years	4%	4%	4%	85%	4%
Previous CABG	4%	4%	4%	88%	0%
Prior MI	4%	4%	4%	88%	0%
Pulmonary edema	4%	0%	4%	92%	0%
Shock	0%	0%	0%	100%	0%

Q: **How do you treat patients with acute inferior MI who are 1 hour away from a PTCA center** *and hemodynamically stable:*

19%   IV SK; transfer only if clinically indicated

50%   IV tPA; transfer only if clinically indicated

19%   lytic therapy and immediate transfer to PTCA center

12%   immediate transfer to PTCA center

Q: **How do you treat patients with acute anterior MI who are 1 hour away from a PTCA center** *and hemodynamically stable*:

8%   IV SK; transfer only if clinically indicated

31%   IV tPA; transfer only if clinically indicated

50%   Lytic therapy and immediate transfer to PTCA center

12%   Immediate transfer to PTCA center

Q: **How do you treat patients with acute** *inferior MI* **who are hemodynamically unstable and 1 hour away from a PTCA center:**

13%   Immediate transfer to PTCA center

13%   IABP and immediate transfer to PTCA center

39%   Lytic therapy and immediate transfer to PTCA center

26%   Lytic therapy, IABP, and immediate transfer

9%   Lytic therapy and IABP; transfer only for continued or recurrent problems

Q: **How do you treat patient with acute anterior** *MI* **who arehemodynamically unstable and 1 hour away from a PTCA center:**

18%   Immediate transfer to PTCA center

14%   IABP and immediate transfer to PTCA center

36%   Lytic therapy and immediate transfer to PTCA center

32%   Lytic therapy, IABP, and immediate transfer

5%   Lytic therapy and IABP; transfer only for continued or recurrent problems

Q: **Which device (or device combination) do you prefer for acute MI?**

69%   PTCA

8%   TEC + PTCA

0%   TEC + stent

0%   DCA

0%   Stent

0%   Laser

23%   Other

Q: **Which intracoronary lytic do you use during rescue angioplasty for failed IV lytic therapy?**

4%   tPA

62%   UK

0%   UK & tPA

0%   UK & SK

0%   SK

0%   Other

35%   None

Q: **What do you recommend after uncomplicated thrombolytic therapy for acute MI?**

26%   Stress test; cath/PTCA if abnormal

44%   Cath all patients; PTCA if appropriate

30%   Cath high-risk patients; stress test for others with cath/PTCA if abnormal

PRIMARY ANGIOPLASTY FOR ACUTE MI:

Q: **Do you perform a pre-discharge stress test after successful PTCA?**

22%   Yes, for all patients

4%   Yes, for patients with poor LV function, multivessel disease, or a suboptimal PTCA result

74%   No

Q: **How do use IABP in the setting of primary angioplasty for acute MI?**

0%   Routine for all patients

33%   All high-risk patients (large MI, CHF, hypotension)

17%   For post-PTCA dissection, thrombus, or slow-flow, **regardless** of clinical/hemodynamic status

50%   For post-PTCA dissection, thrombus, or slow-flow and hemodynamic instability

Q: **Do you routinely prescribe a β-blocker following successful primary infarct angioplasty?**

41%   Yes

4%   For patients with LV dysfunction

56%   No

Q: **Which intracoronary lytic drug (or drug combination) do you prefer for thrombus-containing lesions?**

5%   SK

82%   UK

0%   tPA

0%   SK + UK

0%   SK + tPA

9%   UK + tPA

5%   none

5%   other

Q: **What PTCA technique do you prefer for bifurcation lesions when the branch vessel is > 2.0 mm?**

32%   Kissing balloons

68%   Double guidewire, sequential balloons

CHRONIC TOTAL OCCLUSION:

Q: **What % of chronic total native coronary occlusions that *cannot* be crossed with a guidewire do you treat with prolonged lytic infusion?**

67%   0%

22%   1-10%

7%   11-24%

0%   25-50%

4%   > 50%

Q: **Which i.c. lytic do you use?**

6%   SK

13%   tPA

72%   UK

Q: **What % of chronic total saphenous vein graft occlusions that *cannot* be crossed with a guidewire do you treat with a prolonged lytic infusion?**

44%   0%

19%   1-10%

15%   11-24%

15%   25-50%

7%   > 50%

Q: **Which intragraft lytic do you use?**

6% SK

11% tPA

83% UK

Q: **What is your device of choice for total occlusions that cannot be crossed with a conventional PTCA wire?**

7% Magnum wire

64% Glidewire

0% Ultrasound wire

14% Laser wire

0% LASTAC

0% ROTACS

14% Lytic infusion

Q: **What medical therapy do you recommend following successful recanalization of a chronic total occlusion (i.e., residual stenosis < 35%, no residual thrombus or dissection, TIMI 3 flow)?**

52% IV heparin x 1-3 days

0% Overnight infusion of IV lytic

0% Overnight infusion of IC lytic

0% Dextran

7% Ticlopidine

8% Coumadin x 2-6 weeks

4% c7E3

78% Aspirin

SAPHENOUS VEIN GRAFTS:

Q: **What is your device of choice for nondegenerated SVGs?**

4% PTCA

0% TEC

0% DCA

0% ELCA

0% Rotablator

92% Stent

4% Other

Q: **What is your device of choice for degenerated SVGs?**

4% PTCA

15% TEC

0% DCA

0% ELCA

0% Rotablator

70% Stent

11% Other

Q: **Do you use prophylactic intracoronary verapamil for lesions at high risk for no-reflow?**

37% Yes

63% No

DIRECTIONAL CORONARY ATHERECTOMY:

Q: **What % of your DCA cases require predilation?**

12%	0%
56%	1-10%
16%	11-24%
12%	25-50%
4%	>50%

Q: **What % of your DCA cases require post-dilation?**

0%	0%
8%	1-10%
4%	11-24%
12%	25-50%
76%	>50%

Q: **In what % of your DCA cases do you utilize IVUS?**

32%	0%
20%	1-10%
8%	11-24%
16%	25-50%
24%	>50%

Q: **What final diameter stenosis do you try to achieve with DCA?**

48%	0-5%
48%	5-10%
4%	10-20%
0%	20-30%

ROTABLATOR ATHERECTOMY:

Q: Do you insert a pacemaker prophylactically?

12%   Never

20%   Always

68%   Only when treating a dominant RCA or LCX

Q: What is your final burr-to-artery ratio?

4%   0.4-0.49

4%   0.5-0.59

30%   0.6-0.69

57%   0.7-0.79

4%   0.8-0.89

Q: In general, which Rotablator technique do you prefer?

10%   Use of a single, large burr

90%   Sequential upsizing of burrs

Q: Do you think Rotablator atherectomy facilitates PTCA (i.e., does pretreatment with the Rotablator improve the final result compared to PTCA alone)?

88%   Yes

12%   No

TRANSLUMINAL EXTRACTION ATHERECTOMY (TEC):

Q: What is your final cutter-to-artery ratio?

0%   0.4-0.49

13%   0.5-0.59

56%   0.6-0.69

25%   0.7-0.79

6%   0.8-0.89

Q: **In general, which TEC revascularization technique do you prefer?**

56%   Use of a single, large cutter

44%   Sequential upsizing of cutters

Q: **What is your preferred approach for TEC in degenerated vein grafts:**

0%   TEC alone

25%   TEC alone; Coumadin for 2-4 weeks; then repeat intervention

13%   TEC/PTCA at same time

63%   TEC/stent at same time

EXCIMER LASER CORONARY ANGIOPLASTY:

Q: **What is your final probe-to-artery ratio?**

0%   0.4 - 0.49

20%   0.5 - 0.59

60%   0.6 - 0.69

20%   0.7 - 0.79

0%   0.8 - 0.89

Q: **In general, which ELCA revascularization technique do you prefer?**

60%   Use of a single, large probe

40%   Sequential upsizing of probes

Q: **Have you had experience using the saline infusion technique during ELCA?**

82%   Yes

18%   No

Q: If so, do you think it reduces complications?

100%	Yes
0%	No

STENTS:

Q: In what % of successful *elective stent* cases does your post-stent medical regimen consist of aspirin and ticlopidine without anticoagulants?

4%	0%
23%	1-25%
8%	26-50%
23%	51-75%
42%	76-100%

Q: How many days prior to stenting do you initiate ticlopidine?

42%	begin on day of procedure
19%	1 day
8%	2 days
23%	3-5 days
4%	$\geq$ 6 days

Q: In what % of successful *bailout stent* cases does your post-stent medical regimen consist of aspirin and ticlopidine without anticoagulants?

27%	0%
23%	1-25%
15%	26-50%
12%	51-75%
23%	76-100%

Q: In what % of elective stent procedures do you use IVUS?

8%	Not available
31%	1-10%
12%	11-24%
23%	25-50%
27%	>50%

Q: In what % of bailout stent procedures do you use IVUS?

8%	Not available
31%	1-10%
23%	11-24%
15%	25-50%
23%	>50%

Q: **When do you discharge patients after successful, uncomplicated, elective stenting?**

11%   Same day

59%   Day 2

30%   Day 3-5

0%   ≥ Day 6

Q: **When do you discharge patients after successful bailout stenting?**

0%   Same day

26%   Day 2

59%   Day 3-5

15%   ≥ Day 6

Q: **What is your final post-stent balloon inflation pressure?**

0%   7-10 atm.

0%   11-13 atm.

38%   14-16 atm.

62%   17-20 atm.

0%   >20 atm.

Q: **What stent do you prefer for abrupt closure indications:**

17%   Cook stent

79%   J & J coronary stent

0%   Wallstent

4%   AVE Microstent

0%   Other

INTRAVASCULAR ULTRASOUND:

Q: **In what % of your interventional procedures do you use IVUS?**

7%	Not available
41%	1-10%
26%	11-24%
22%	25-50%
4%	>50%

Q: **How often does IVUS alter your interventional approach?**

30%	<5%
46%	5-10%
12%	10-25%
0%	25-50%
0%	>50%

Q: **Do you think IVUS will become routine for:**

8%	All devices
19%	DCA
0%	TEC
0%	ELCA
35%	Elective stent
15%	Bailout stent
0%	Rotablator
58%	None

ANGIOSCOPY:

Q: **In what % of your interventional procedures do you use angioscopy?**

0%	Not available
100%	0-25%
0%	26-50%
0%	51-75%
0%	76-100%

Q: **How often does angioscopy alter your interventional approach?**

63%	<5%
25%	5-10%
0%	10-25%
0%	25-50%
13%	>50%

Q: **Will angioscopy become routine during interventional procedures?**

5%	Yes
95%	No

DOPPLER FLOWIRE:

Q: **In what % of your interventional procedures do you use the Doppler FloWire?**

34%	Not available
63%	1-25%
0%	26-50%
4%	51-75%
0%	76-100%

Q: **How often does the FloWire alter your interventional approach?**

88% <5%

6% 5-10%

0% 10-25%

6% 25-50%

0% >50%

Q: **Will the FloWire become routine during interventional procedures?**

10% Yes

90% No

Q: **Do you use the FloWire to decide the "significance" of a lesion (i.e., whether to treat medically or revascularize)?**

39% Yes

61% No

40 The Bottom Line

In a hurry? Need to quickly review a topic? Look no further than the bottom line—

1   EQUIPMENT AND TECHNIQUE

PREPROCEDURAL PREPARATION
A. EVALUATION OF THE PATIENT PRIOR TO PERCUTANEOUS INTERVENTION

1. **History.** Specific history should be elicited of MI, CABG, CHF, arrhythmia, valvular disease, complications of previous catheterization or intervention; important noncardiac diseases; allergic reactions to medications and radiographic contrast.

2. **Physical Examination.** Pertinent findings include peripheral edema, venous distension, rales, heart murmur, vascular bruits and pulses, and neurologic status.

3. **Laboratory Studies.** Routine studies include CBC, clotting studies, full chemistry panel, and EKG. Additional studies are useful in select patients (CXR, drug levels, peripheral vascular studies). Review of prior cardiac catheterization is essential.

B. THERAPEUTIC MEASURES

1. **Routine Pre-PTCA Medication.** Aspirin is essential (at least 24 hours prior to PTCA).

2. **Aspirin Allergy.** Desensitization can be performed for aspirin-induced asthma and rhinosinusitis; patients with aspirin-induced angioedema, urticaria, or anaphylaxis should be treated with other antiplatelet agents such as Ticlopidine.

C. INFORMED CONSENT. Must be obtained from all patients; includes discussion of risks, benefits, alternative treatments, need for repeat revascularization.

EQUIPMENT AND TECHNIQUE
A. PROCEDURAL OVERVIEW

1. **Intraprocedural Medication.** Analgesics, sedatives, and narcotics are useful for premedication. Heparin is essential during intervention (ACT 250-350 seconds).

2. **Vascular Access: Femoral Approach.** Modified Seldinger technique (anterior wall puncture) is widely used; important to access the common femoral artery, central venous access is also recommended in most patients.

3. **Pacemaker Insertion.** Routinely recommended for Rotablator of RCA or patients with pre-existing high-degree AV block.

4. **Equipment Setup.** Typical setup includes guiding catheter attached to a multiport manifold

via a Y-adapter and extension tubing; allows contrast injection, pressure monitoring, and manipulation of interventional hardware.

5. **Balloon Sizing.** Attempt to achieve a balloon/artery ratio 0.9-1.1.

6. **Guidewire Shaping.** Guidewire selection is based on coronary anatomy, lesion morphology, and operator preference.

7. **Purging Air From the System.** Air must be purged from the Y-adapter and guiding catheter.

8. **Crossing the Lesion with the Guidewire.** Nitroglycerin IC is recommended before crossing the lesion. The wire should be gently steered into position; forceful manipulation must be avoided.

9. **Balloon Dilatation.** After crossing the lesion with the guidewire, the balloon should be advanced into position and inflated with 25-50% contrast mixture. Inflation times are usually 1-3 minutes.

10. **Evaluation of Acute Angiographic Outcome.** Repeat angiography is recommended after administration of nitroglycerin. A good result is characterized by residual stenosis < 30%, normal flow, and lack of significant dissection.

B. **EQUIPMENT SECTION**

1. **Vascular Sheaths.** Commonly use 6F-8F arterial sheaths; larger sheaths are available for atherectomy, valvuloplasty, and CPS.

2. **Guiding Catheter Selection.** Vast selection, depending on type of device, target vessel, target lesions, and operator preference; guiding catheters must provide reliable pressure monitoring, adequate contrast delivery, coaxial alignment, torque control, kink resistance, and back-up support.

3. **Guidewires.** Vast selection, depending or type of device, lesion morphology, coronary anatomy, and operator preference; important features include torque control, visibility, flexibility and support. Most coronary guidewires are 0.010-0.021 inches in diameter.

4. **Balloon Dilatation Catheters.** Vast selection, depending mostly on operator preference. Balloon catheters are usually classified as over-the-wire, single-operator-exchange, or fixed-wire devices. Characteristics such as balloon material, compliance, creep, burst pressure, and deflated profile are less important than pushability and trackability.

5. **Accessories.** Standard accessories include inflation devices, Y-adapters, guidewire introducers, and torque devices.

6. **Transport and Infusion Catheters.** Useful for exchanging guidewires and for intracoronary drug delivery.

7. **Coatings.** Variety of lubricious coatings for balloons, guides, and guidewires.

8. **Cost.** There is a wide range of costs for interventional devices and accessories; equipment costs for PTCA are less than for other devices.

POSTPROCEDURAL CONSIDERATIONS

A. **TRIAGE AND MONITORING.** Patients are observed for 12-36 hours in a skilled nursing telemetry unit. If the intervention was complicated by acute closure, severe dissection in a large vessel, or prolonged hypotension, observation in a cardiac intensive care unit is preferred..

B. **COMPLICATIONS.** Recurrent chest pain occurs in half of PTCA patients; return to the catheterization laboratory for chest pain and ECG changes. Mild hypotension is usually caused by medications and volume depletion (NPO status, contrast-induced diuresis); hypotension from these causes should respond promptly to saline administration. More serious cause include acute vessel closure, retroperitoneal bleeding, or sepsis.

C. **POST-PTCA PHARMACOTHERAPY.** Final stenosis <30% stenosis, normal flow, no dissection or thrombus: No additional heparin. Suboptimal angiographic result: Prolonged (18-48 hrs) post-procedural heparin may be warranted (Chapters 20, 34).

D. **SHEATH REMOVAL, AMBULATION, & PATIENT DISCHARGE.** Femoral sheaths are removed 4-6 hrs after discontinuing heparin (ACT <140 seconds or PTT < 50 seconds). The majority of uncomplicated PTCA patients are discharged within 24-36 hrs.

2 BRACHIAL AND RADIAL APPROACH

A. **PROCEDURAL OVERVIEW**
   1. **Cutdown Approach to Brachial Artery Access.**
      a. **Technique.** A variety of techniques are available; strict, sterile techniques is essential.
      b. **Brachial Artery Repair.** A variety of techniques are available; interrupted sutures are preferred.
   2. **Percutaneous Approach to Brachial Artery Access.** Use a modified Seldinger or micropuncture technique; 6-8 F sheaths may be inserted.
   3. **Radial Artery Approach**
      a. **Technique.** Confirm normal Allen test; micropuncture technique is preferred. Better catheter engagement from left radial artery.
      b. **Sheath Removal and Hemostasis.** Compression for 30 minutes after sheath removal; restrict movement of wrist for 6 hours.

B. **SPECIAL INDICATIONS FOR BRACHIAL AND RADIAL TECHNIQUES**
   1. **Peripheral Vascular Disease.** Femoral access may be difficult or contraindicated; brachial cutdown may be extremely useful.
   2. **Patient Preference.** Brachial and radial techniques allow more rapid ambulation; may be easier for patients with severe low back pain.
   3. **Need for Uninterrupted Anticoagulation.** Brachial cutdown technique can be used for patients who require uninterrupted anticoagulation.
   4. **Difficult Internal Mammary Artery Cannulation.** Ipsilateral or contralateral brachial approach can be used if femoral approach fails.

5. **Severe Proximal Vessel Tortuosity.** Left brachial approach provides excellent guiding catheter alignment and support.

C. INTERVENTIONAL CONSIDERATIONS

1. **Guide Catheter Selection.** For RCA, use JR (especially from left arm), AL, or multipurpose catheters; for LCA, use JL (left arm), AL, or Voda.
2. **Devices Other Than PTCA.** Virtually all devices can be inserted using brachial cutdown techniques.

D. COMPLICATIONS

1. **Brachial Approach.** Complications are similar to femoral technique, including hematoma (1.3%), retroperitoneal hemorrhage (0.4%), false aneurysm (0.4%), vessel occlusion (0.1%), infection (0.1%), distal embolization (0.1%).
2. **Radial Approach.** Most limited by operator experience; more technical failures than femoral approach but fewer vascular complicati

---

3   SINGLE-VESSEL & MULTIVESSEL ANGIOPLASTY

SINGLE VESSEL PTCA. PTCA is superior to medical therapy for relieving symptoms and improving exercise capacity; CABG is a consideration in patients with proximal LAD disease.

MULTIVESSEL PTCA

A. MULTIVESSEL PTCA IN PATIENTS WITH PRESERVED LV FUNCTION

1. **Randomized Trials.** More than 6000 patients have been randomized in six trials of PTCA vs. CABG; there are important differences between trials with respect to inclusion and exclusion criteria, study design, baseline patient characteristics, study endpoints. In-hospital results: Similar mortality between PTCA and CABG patients; length of hospital stay and MI were higher in CABG patients. Follow-up results: Similar infarct-free survival at 1-year; diabetics treated with PTCA had higher late mortality (BARI Trial); PTCA patients required more revascularization procedures (20% required CABG within 1-3 years after initial PTCA).
2. **Nonrandomized Trials.** Suggest improving outcomes after percutaneous intervention, possibly due to availability of stents. Failure to include new devices in randomized trials of PTCA vs. CABG may have important implications, and may underestimate the long-term benefit of percutaneous therapies.

B. MULTIVESSEL PTCA IN PATIENTS WITH LV DYSFUNCTION. LV dysfunction is an important determinant of outcome, even for patients with single-vessel disease. For multivessel

disease, CABG results in better 5-year survival and less angina than PTCA. However, late outcome is most strongly related to completeness of revascularization, not the mode of revascularization per se.

C. **REVASCULARIZATION STRATEGY**
1. **Complete vs. Incomplete Revascularization.** Completeness of revascularization may be considered in terms of "anatomic" or "functional" revascularization; the optimal strategy is unknown. Complete anatomic revascularization appears to be important for patients with multivessel disease and LV dysfunction; further studies are in progress.
2. **Approach to Moderate Stenoses.** "Anatomically-significant" lesions (50-70% stenosis) may not be "physiologically-significant". Factors favoring revascularization include ischemic ECG changes, wall motion abnormality, Doppler coronary flow reserve < 2.0, and lesion morphology suggesting plaque rupture or thrombus.
3. **Order of Dilatation.** Generally, the most severe stenosis ("culprit") is treated first.
4. **Staging.** A variety of staging strategies are possible, depending on the morphology of the target lesions (presence or absence of thrombus), results of intervention on antecedent lesions (dissection, contrast load, duration of procedure), and whether revascularization is indicated on an elective vs. urgent basis.

D. **SPECIAL SUBSET OF MULTIVESSEL DISEASE**. The treatment of patients with chronic total occlusions which are supplied by another vessel with a critical stenosis is controversial. If possible, PTCA of the occluded vessel should be attempted. If PTCA of the occluded vessel is not feasible, PTCA of the other vessel is feasible with acceptable complication rates; CABG should be considered for such patients when lesion morphology is unfavorable or in the presence of significant LV dysfunction.

HIGH-RISK INTERVENTION

RISK STRATIFICATION. The risk of procedural mortality can be estimated from angiographic and clinical characteristics before the procedure, based on the risk of acute closure (lesion closure factors) and the risk of death if acute closure does occur (patient mortality factors).

RISK REDUCTION
A. **PREPROCEDURAL CONSIDERATIONS**. Patients at moderate-high risk of major complications should be managed at experienced centers with adequate ancillary support staff, new interventional techniques (especially stents), and devices for hemodynamic support (IABP, CPS). Careful attention must be paid to optimizing volume status, ensuring surgical backup, and renal function.

B. **INTRAPROCEDURAL CONSIDERATIONS.** Limiting ischemia is an important consideration. Careful technique must be employed to ensure optimal guiding catheter engagement, proper positioning of the inflated balloon, and adequate imaging of the target vessel to anticipate and manage angiographic complications (filling defects, dissection, sidebranch occlusion, no-reflow). Newer imaging modalities (IVUS, angioscopy, Doppler), adjunctive pharmacotherapy (platelet receptor antagonists, lytic agents, calcium channel blockers), and regional and systemic support systems (perfusion balloons, IABP, CPS) can enhance patient safety.

C. **POSTPROCEDURAL CONSIDERATIONS.** After intervention, patients should be monitored in the appropriate setting. Most patients should be transferred to a telemetry unit; high-risk patients should be monitored in a coronary care unit. Recurrent chest pain with ischemic ECG changes mandates immediate return to the catheterization laboratory. Patients with hypotension should be carefully evaluated for vasovagal reactions, hypovolemia, bleeding, drug-effects, sepsis, and ischemia.

LEFT MAIN DISEASE. PTCA of an unprotected left main is technically feasible (immediate success >90%); in-hospital mortality is 9%, 3-year mortality is 64%. CABG is the treatment of choice for surgical candidates. Elective stenting is under evaluation.

 PTCA IN UNSTABLE ISCHEMIC SYNDROMES

ACUTE MYOCARDIAL INFARCTION. For thrombolytic therapy: Only 33% of all patients are eligible, only 80% of vessels open, and only 55% of vessels achieve TIMI-3 flow. There are no clinical markers to accurately predict reperfusion, and there are high rates of recurrent ischemia and intracranial bleeding.

A. **PRIMARY (DIRECT) PTCA.** Primary PTCA achieves patency in 95-99% of patients, TIMI-3 flow in 94%; low rates of reocclusion, recurrent ischemia, intracranial bleeding; and appears to limit reperfusion injury, cardiogenic shock and myocardial rupture.
   1. **Nonrandomized series.** Difficult to interpret since high risk thrombolytic-ineligible patients were excluded.
   2. **Thrombolytic-ineligible patients.** More often older, female, prior MI, multivessel disease and lower ejection fractions. PTCA is performed with high success rates.
   3. **Cardiogenic shock.** PTCA successful (80%); a survival benefit is apparent.
   4. **Thrombolytic-eligible patients**.
      a. **PAR Registry.** Patency achieved in 99% and TIMI-3 flow in 97%; 6-month patency in 87%..
      b. **Randomized trials.** Demonstrated less recurrent ischemia, reocclusion, reinfarction, stroke, and death in PTCA patients.
   5. **Recommendations.** Primary PTCA should be strongly considered in: Thrombolytic-

ineligible, high risk thrombolytic eligible (anterior MI, age > 70, heart rate > 100, blood pressure < 100 mmHg or Killip Class > 1) and cardiogenic shock. Low risk thrombolytic-eligible patients: Primary PTCA should be considered to reduce recurrent ischemia, reinfarction and length of hospital stay.

B. RESCUE (SALVAGE) PTCA FOR FAILED THROMBOLYSIS

1. **Observational Series**. Rescue PTCA: 90% success, reocclusion 6-30%.
2. **Randomized Trials**. Improved regional wall motion; lower incidence of recurrent ischemia and combined endpoint of death or congestive heart failure.
3. **Recommendation**. Rescue PTCA: Ongoing chest pain, hemodynamic instability, or persistent ST-elevation within 12 hours of symptom-onset.

C. IMMEDIATE PTCA AFTER SUCCESSFUL THROMBOLYSIS (ASYMPTOMATIC)

1. **Randomized Trials**. Higher rate of transfusion, emergency CABG, and death.
2. **Limitations of Studies**. Lack of pre-procedural aspirin and ACTs.
3. **Recommendations**. Avoid PTCA after successful thrombolysis except for ongoing ischemia, hemodynamic instability, or TIMI flow $\leq$ 2.

D. DELAYED PTCA AFTER SUCCESSFUL THROMBOLYSIS (ASYMPTOMATIC)

1. **Randomized Trials**. No difference between invasive and conservative approaches regarding death, reinfarction, LV ejection fraction.
2. **Limitations of Studies**. Lack of aspirin and ACTs; total occlusions were not dilated; 69% of the deaths were unrelated to revascularization (patients never received PTCA or CABG).
3. **Recommendations**. Late revascularization may be warranted: Patients with prior MI, TIMI flow $\leq$ 2, multivessel disease, stenosis > 90% supplying a moderate or large amount of myocardium.

E. DELAYED PTCA OF AN OCCLUDED VESSEL (ASYMPTOMATIC)

1. **Observational Trials**. Improvement in LV volume and ejection fraction after PTCA.
2. **Randomized Trials**. Improved ejection fraction at 6 weeks, but 40% of vessels were reoccluded at 6-months.
3. **Recommendations**. Perform late PTCA: Occluded vessel supplies a large amount of myocardium or there is viable myocardium.

F. PTCA FOR POST MI ISCHEMIA

After thrombolysis, PTCA reduced the incidence of MI, rehospitalization, and the use of anti-ischemic drugs (DANAMI). Patients with post-MI angina or an abnormal stress test should undergo catheterization and mechanical revascularization with PTCA or CABG if a significant lesion is present.

UNSTABLE ANGINA

A. PATHOPHYSIOLOGY
High incidence of thrombus in patients with unstable angina; thrombolytic therapy increases the risk of MI and is not recommended.

B. PTCA AND UNSTABLE ANGINA
Rrest angina with ECG changes: Worse prognosis with medical therapy, but more complications with PTCA and devices. There is no proven benefit for "cooling the patient down" with heparin and aspirin for several days.

C. MEDICAL THERAPY, PTCA, AND CABG
1. **Medical Therapy vs. CABG.** Randomized trials demonstrated similar survival for medicine and CABG; patients with LV dysfunction, 3-vessel disease, or 2-vessel disease with proximal LAD stenosis do better with CABG.
2. **Medical Therapy vs. PTCA.** PTCA allows earlier discharge, fewer readmissions, and less anti-anginal medication (TIMI 3B).
3. **PTCA vs. CABG.** In the BARI trial, 64% of patients had unstable angina, and outcomes with PTCA and surgery were similar.

DEFICIENCIES OF PTCA FOR UNSTABLE ISCHEMIC SYNDROMES

A. REPERFUSION ARRHYTHMIAS.
Ventricular fibrillation and bradyarrhythmias are more common with RCA interventions; we recommend intravenous beta-blockers, low osmolar ionic contrast (ioxaglate), continuous monitoring of O_2 sats, and adequate hydration prior to reperfusion of the RCA.

B. BLEEDING COMPLICATIONS.
PTCA is associated with less intracranial bleeding but more blood transfusion (12-14%). Early sheath removal is recommended.

C. ISCHEMIC COMPLICATIONS.
Recurrent ischemia occurs in 10-15% of PTCA patients, necessitating repeat catheterization, re-PTCA, and increased length of hospital stay and cost.

DEVICES AND DRUGS FOR PATIENTS WITH ACUTE MI OR UNSTABLE ANGINA

A. IABP.
In high risk MI patients, IABP reduced ischemia; no influence on death, recurrent MI, CHF, stroke, or in-hospital reocclusion (PAMI-2). IABPs recommended in patients with LV dysfunction, hypotension, or persistent TIMI flow ≤ 2 after PTCA.

B. DIRECTIONAL CORONARY ATHERECTOMY
1. **Observational Trials.** Increase in abrupt closure, need for CABG and distal embolization.
2. **Randomized trials.** Higher frequency of non-Q-wave MI (CAVEAT).

3. **Recommendations.** We do not recommend routine DCA in the acute or post MI patient, unless the target lesion is well-suited for DCA and is not well-suited for PTCA.

C. **TEC ATHERECTOMY**
1. **Non-randomized series.** TEC can extract thrombus; uncertain value compared to PTCA.
2. **Randomized studies.** In progress (TOPIT).
3. **Recommendations.** Consider TEC for degenerated vein graft or failed thrombolytic therapy with a large thrombus.

D. **ROTABLATOR ATHERECTOMY.** Rotablator is not recommended unless the lesion is rigid and cannot be dilated with a high pressure balloon.

E. **STENTS**
1. **Observational series.** Stenting can be performed with high success and low complication rates.
2. **Randomized trials.** Several trials are in preparation.
3. **Recommendations.** Stents should be avoided in the setting of large thrombi (TEC and UK infusions may be useful adjuncts); stents should not be withheld from acute MI patients who meet other criteria for stenting.

F. **LASER.** Further studies are needed.

G. **THERMAL BALLOON ANGIOPLASTY.** Further studies are needed.

6 LV DYSFUNCTION

BACKGROUND

A. **Historical Results.** Patients with coronary artery disease and LV dysfunction have 4-year survival rates of 35-60% with medical therapy; 72% after CABG. Nonrandomized studies show similar results between PTCA and CABG in patients with LV dysfunction.

B. **Determination of Need for Supported Angioplasty.** Important to estimate the hemodynamic significance of target lesions before intervention (jeopardy score). Several techniques for support are available.

SYSTEMIC SUPPORT

A. **IABP.** Effective device for afterload reduction, increasing coronary perfusion pressure, and decreasing myocardial oxygen consumption. Useful for refractory angina, cardiogenic shock, weaning from CPS. May increase risk of vascular complications in women, elderly.

B. **CPS.** Effective device for maintaining systemic circulation; does not protect the myocardium in cases of acute coronary occlusion. Frequent vascular and bleeding complications, coagulopathy limit its use to < 6 hours. Indicated for circulatory collapse.

C. **Ventricular Assist Devices.** Hemopump results in marked unloading of left ventricle; little clinical experience in cath lab setting.

D. **Left Atrial-Femoral Bypass.** Requires transseptal catheterization. Not widely used.

SYSTEMIC MYOCARDIAL SUPPORT

A. **Autoperfusion Catheters.** Permit passive perfusion of distal myocardial bed during balloon inflation. Typical flow rate = 40-60 cc/min. Useful for prolonged balloon inflation to decrease ischemia and/or hemodynamic dysfunction. Also useful as a "bailout" catheter before emergency CABG.

B. **Active Coronary Hemoperfusion.** Deliver autologous arterial blood to distal coronary bed. Not widely used, but effective at reducing chest pain and ECG changes during balloon inflations.

C. **Perfluorochemicals.** Withdrawn from market in 1995 (Fluosol).

D. **Coronary Sinus Retroperfusion.** Deliver arterial blood to the coronary sinus; can ameliorate ischemia and protect myocardium, but offers no circulatory support. Not useful for interventions on the RCA or LCx.

E. **Pharmacotherapy.** Nitroglycerin, beta blockers, and calcium antagonists can ameliorate ischemia.

7   PATIENT CHARACTERISTICS

YOUNG PATIENTS (Age < 40 years)

A. **BACKGROUND.** Account for 3-6% of patients with coronary artery disease. CABG mortality (0-2%), but higher risk of late graft failure.

B. **PTCA.** Procedural success (86-90%); major complications (0-6%).

C. **FOLLOW-UP.** 3-6 years: RePTCA (32-34%); CABG (5-11%); total survival (98%); return to work (93%).

D. **CONCLUSION.** PTCA may be preferred over CABG for young patients.

ELDERLY PATIENTS (Age 65-75 years)

A. **BACKGROUND.** In the United States, 31 million people are over 65: 25% have symptomatic coronary artery disease now; will increase to 65% in 30 years.

B. **PROCEDURAL RESULTS.** Success: PTCA (82-94%); devices (86-98%). Major complications: PTCA (3-17%); devices (1.6-14%); CABG (2-14%). Elderly have increased risk of vascular complications and death after abrupt closure.

C. **FOLLOW-UP.** 1-year outcome: Survival (95%), MI (5%), CABG (15%), repeat PTCA (20%). 3-year survival (90%).

D. **APPROACH.** Elderly patients with symptomatic coronary artery disease are well treated by PTCA, new devices, and CABG. In-hospital morbidity and mortality may be less with PTCA, but repeat vascularization is common.

ELDERLY PATIENTS (Age ≥ 80 years)

A. **CABG.** In-hospital mortality (5-10%), MI (5%); 5-year survival (60-85%). Late deaths are often due to noncardiac causes (30%).

B. **PTCA.** Success (65-91%); death (0-23%), QMI (0-14%), emergency CABG (0-14%); 3-year survival (80-91%).

C. **CONCLUSION.** PTCA and CABG can be performed with good results in octogenarians; elderly patients should not be denied revascularization on the basis of age alone.

FEMALE PATIENTS

A. **BACKGROUND.** There are gender differences in prevalence, manifestations, and prognosis of coronary artery disease.

B. **PTCA.** Compared to males, females are older, have more diabetes, hypertension, unstable angina, and prior MI. After accounting for these differences, gender has little or no impact on PTCA results.

C. **FOLLOW-UP.** No gender differences in total-and event-free survival.

D. **NEW DEVICES.** No gender differences in procedural success or late outcome; increased risk of complications in females may be due to differences in comorbidity and body surface area.

E. **CONCLUSIONS.** Females have more morbidity and mortality than males, but these differences are related to a higher incidence of comorbid conditions, and not to gender per se.

AFRICAN-AMERICANS

A. **BACKGROUND.** Higher prevalence of risk factors for coronary artery disease.

B. **PERCUTANEOUS INTERVENTION.** Procedural success (76-92%); death (0-4.1%); MI (1.2-7%); emergency CABG (2.4-4.8%).

C. **FOLLOW-UP.** 1-year outcome: Death (1.5%), MI (0.8%), CABG (9%), rePTCA (21%); 5-year outcome: Death (11%), MI (13%), CABG (20%), rePTCA (25%); similar to outcome of non-African-Americans.

D. **CONCLUSIONS.** Results of percutaneous intervention are similar (after correcting for other comorbid conditions).

DIABETICS

A. **BACKGROUND.** Diabetics have greater cardiovascular morbidity and mortality than non-diabetics.

B. CABG. Compared to non-diabetics, diabetics have higher in-hospital mortality (4.2% vs. 1.8%), stroke (3.1% vs. 1.5%), 5-year mortality (26% vs. 13%), and 10-year mortality (50% vs. 28%).

C. PTCA. Procedural success (85-93%) is similar to non-diabetics; death (0.4-3.2%), MI (0.6-1.6%), emergency CABG (1.8-2.3%). Compared to non-diabetics, diabetics have reduced 5-year outcome: Death (7%), MI (19%), CABG (23%), rePTCA (43%), event-free survival(36%).

D. CONCLUSIONS. Immediate procedural success for diabetics and non-diabetics is similar. diabetics have worse longterm outcome.

CHRONIC DIALYSIS PATIENTS

A. BACKGROUND. Coronary artery disease causes 40% of deaths in patients with end-stage renal failure.

B. PTCA. Procedural success (88-92%), death (0-12%), MI (8-12%), emergency CABG (0-8%).

C. FOLLOWUP. 2-year outcome: Late cardiac events (50-80%), restenosis (> 50%); 2-3 fold higher mortality at 1 and 12 months compared to non-dialysis patients.

D. CONCLUSIONS. Percutaneous and surgical revascularization are associated with greater morbidity and mortality in dialysis patients.

CARDIAC TRANSPLANT PATIENTS

A. BACKGROUND. Coronary artery disease is the leading cause of death in transplant patients surviving more than 1 year after surgery; affects 20-40% of allografts within 5 years.

B. PTCA. Success (75-94%).

C. FOLLOWUP. Longterm outcome limited mostly by distal arteriopathy.

D. CONCLUSIONS. Few transplant patients have focal stenoses amenable to PTCA; immediate success rates are acceptable, but longterm outcome is limited by distal arteriopathy.

SILENT ISCHEMIA

A. BACKGROUND. Revascularization may improve anginal status and survival compared to medical therapy alone.

B. PTCA. Success (81-95%), death (< 1%), MI (< 1%), CABG (2%).

C. FOLLOWUP. 3-year outcome: Survival (98%), infarct-free survival (96%).

D. CONCLUSIONS. PTCA is safe and effective in patients with silent ischemia.

8 OVERVIEW OF INTERVENTIONAL DEVICES

A. LIMITATIONS OF INTERVENTIONAL DEVICES

1. **Failure to Cross a Chronic Total Occlusion with a Guidewire.** Precludes use of PTCA, atherectomy, lasers, and stents; investigational devices include ROTACS, ultrasound angioplasty, excimer laserwire, vibrational angioplasty; intracoronary lytic infusion may be useful.

2. **Failure to Cross a Lesion with a Device**. Usually due to tortuosity or severe lesion rigidity or calcification; low profile balloons (tortuosity) or Rotablator, ELCA, low-profile balloons, (rigid) may be useful.

3. **Failure to Dilate or Deploy a Device.** Rigid lesions may be treated with Rotablator, ELCA, hi-pressure balloons, DCA; recoil can be treated with DCA, stents.

4. **Dissection/Abrupt Closure.** 2-10% of PTCA procedures; similar with laser, atherectomy; most important advance is the coronary stent.

5. **Recurrent Ischemia and Restenosis.** Restenosis (30-40%); target lesion revascularization (20%); no change with laser, atherectomy. Stents have lowest incidence of restenosis for de novo lesions > 3 mm.

B. IMPORTANT CONSIDERATIONS IN EVALUATING INTERVENTIONAL DEVICES

1. **Procedural Success.** Many definitions are used; preferred definition is final diameter stenosis <50% without major complication. When multiple devices are used, each may be associated with success or failure.

2. **Assessment of Lumen Enlargement.** Conventional measures include lumen diameter and diameter stenosis; assessment of device efficiency normalizes dimensions for device size and vessel diameter.

3. **Relationship Between Immediate Lumen enlargement and Late Outcome.** Strong relationship between post-procedure lumen diameter and restenosis; other factors are important since more late events and higher restenosis may occur despite better post-procedure lumen enlargement for some devices.

4. **Cost.** All devices are associated with higher cost; length of hospital stay is lowest for PTCA.

5. **Complications.** The incidence of major complications is similar for all devices; nonQ MI is more frequent after DCA and Rotablator. Significance of clinically-silent enzyme rise is controversial.

C. IMPORTANT CONSIDERATIONS IN USING INTERVENTIONAL DEVICES

1. **Facilitated Lumen Enlargement.** Potentially important, but unproven concept behind the common practice of devices and PTCA (facilitated angioplasty) and device combinations (device synergy).

2. **Lesion-Specific Approach to Coronary Intervention.** Certain lesions are better suited for some devices than others: Ostial (Rotablator, ELCA); nondilatable (Rotablator, ELCA); elastic recoil (DCA, stents).

3. **Adjunctive Imaging Techniques.** IVUS: Assess vessel dimensions, extent and distribution of calcium; optimize stents, DCA and MRA. Angioscopy: Distinguish clot from dissection. Doppler flowire: Predict complications, restenosis.

4. **Adjunctive Pharmacotherapy.** Ticlid (stents, ASA-allergy); platelet IIb/IIIa receptor antagonists (high-risk intervention); calcium antagonists (no-reflow); antithrombins are under investigation.

D. NEW INVESTIGATIONAL DEVICES

1. **Hydrolyzer.** Hemodynamic thrombectomy; may be useful for thrombus and degenerated vein grafts; clinical trials in progress.

2. **Angiojet.** Hemodynamic thrombectomy; may be useful for thrombus and degenerated vein grafts; clinical trials in progress.

3. **Therapeutic Ultrasound.** Ablate thrombus and recanalize atherosclerotic vessels; uncertain value; clinical trials in progress.

4. **Radiofrequency/Thermal Angioplasty Devices.** May decrease elastic recoil; uncertain value; clinical trials in progress.

5. **Vibrational Angioplasty.** May be useful for refractory total occlusions that cannot be crossed by a guidewire; clinical studies in progress.

6. **Cutting Balloon Angioplasty.** Facilitate lumen enlargement by "scoring" the vessel wall; uncertain value; randomized trial in progress.

7. **Pullback Atherectomy Catheter.** Cutting and collecting device; minimize distal embolization and no-reflow; uncertain value; clinical trials in progress.

8. **Rotary Atherectomy System.** Rotating auger system; clinical trials are pending.

9. **Low-Speed Rotational Angioplasty Catheter System (ROTACS).** May be useful for refractory total occlusions; clinical studies in progress.

10. **Excimer Laser Guidewire.** May be useful for refractory total occlusions; clinical trials in progress.

9   INTRACORONARY THROMBUS

A. DEFINITION. Angiography is insensitive for detecting intracoronary thrombus compared to angioscopy. However, defects are identified in more than one view, or a total occlusion with convex margins stains with contrast, the specificity approaches 100%.

B. PATHOPHYSIOLOGY. Rupture of lipid-rich plaque initiates intracoronary thrombus formation. PTCA is a powerful thrombogenic stimulus, resembling the injury of spontaneous plaque rupture.

C. PTCA AND THROMBOTIC LESIONS. Thrombus increases the risk of major cardiac events; no drugs or devices have been clearly shown to be beneficial when administered before, during, or after PTCA of a thrombotic lesion.

D. NEW DEVICES AND THROMBOTIC LESIONS. All laser, atherectomy, and stent devices are associated with an increased risk of complications when thrombus is present. TEC and stenting may be useful for thrombotic vein grafts.

E. INVESTIGATIONAL TECHNIQUES. The most promising investigational techniques for thrombus removal are the rheolytic thrombectomy catheters (Cordis Hydrolyzer, POSSIS AngioJet).

F. PHARMACOLOGIC THERAPY OF PRE-EXISTING THROMBUS

1. **Heparin and Aspirin.** A stabilization period of several days using intravenous heparin and aspirin has been advocated. During the procedure, maintain ACT 350-400 seconds. Use of slightly oversized balloons and local infusion of heparin may be associated with reduced thrombosis.

2. **Thrombolytic Therapy.** Although early nonrandomized studies suggested a role for intracoronary thrombolytic therapy when thrombus was present before and after PTCA, recent randomized data demonstrate an adverse outcome when thrombolytic therapy is utilized. Prolonged infusion of urokinase for chronic total occlusions in native vessels or vein grafts.

3. **Novel Antiplatelet and Antithrombin Drugs.** Although the new glycoprotein IIb/IIIa receptor antagonist and antithrombin agents have not been evaluated for coronary thrombosis, they may be useful.

4. **Local Drug Delivery.** Some operators use local drug delivery of heparin or thrombotic agents during PTCA.

G. POST-PTCA THROMBUS. Thrombolytics are not beneficial for angiographic thrombus post-PTCA, unless definite thrombus is confirmed by angioscopy. ReoPro should be considered.

H. STENT THROMBOSIS. Stent thrombosis requires emergency catheterization and PTCA, correction of underlying problems with stent deployment, and lytic therapy or ReoPro, if necessary.

10 BIFURCATION LESIONS

A. DESCRIPTION. Stenosis ≥ 50% involving parent vessel and ostium of its sidebranch; true bifurcation lesions represent 4-6% of target lesions.

B. APPROACH TO BIFURCATION LESIONS

1. **Need for Sidebranch Protection.** Sidebranch occlusion may de due to shifting plaque, dissection, spasm, or thrombosis; branch occlusion is greatest when parent vessel and branch ostium have stenosis > 50% (branch protection is recommended).

2. **PTCA Techniques.**
   a. **Double Guiding Catheter Technique.** Outdated technique, rarely used.
   b. **Single Guiding Catheter Technique.** Most giant lumen 8F guides can accommodate virtually all balloon catheters.
      1. **Double Guidewire, sequential PTCA.** Maintain continuous access to parent vessel and branch; does not prevent snow-plow injury and branch narrowing.
      2. **Kissing Balloon Technique.** Maintain continuous access to parent and branch, minimizes snow-plow injury or branch narrowing.

3. **DCA Techniques.** Good for minimizing shifting plaque; use kissing wire or sequential "cut and retrieve" technique.

4. **Stent Technique.** Bifurcation lesion can be treated with stent on parent vessel and PTCA retrieval of sidebranch if necessary; kissing stents also feasible, but technically demanding.

C. PROCEDURAL RESULTS

1. **PTCA.** Success: Parent vessel (87-100%), branch (76-89%); risk of sidebranch occlusion is 14-34% when sidebranch is diseased.

2. **Directional Atherectomy.** Success: Parent vessel (91-100%), major complications (0-3%); transient sidebranch occlusion (37% of true bifurcation lesions); sidebranch occlusion managed by PTCA or DCA.

3. **Stents.** Low risk of sidebranch occlusion after stenting; most branch occlusions occur after initial PTCA; most are patent 6-months later.

4. **Other Devices.** ELCA, MRA, and TEC are not recommended for true bifurcation lesions; can't protect sidebranch.

5. **Retrieval of Sidebranch Occlusion.** Success depends on severity of branch ostial stenosis and protection of branch by guidewire.

6. **Parent Vessel Closure.** Patency of parent vessel is rarely affected by sidebranch; retrograde propagation of dissection is rare.

7. **Myocardial Infarction, Emergency CABG and Death.** Major complications are related to occlusion of parent vessel, not sidebranch.

11   TORTUOSITY AND ANGULATION

TORTUOSITY

A. **DEFINITION.** Multiple definitions exist; none are uniformly accepted.

B. PROCEDURAL OUTCOME

1. **PTCA.** Success (72-84%); acute closure (6%); ischemic complications and technical failures more frequent.

2. **New Interventional Devices.** Severe tortuosity presents problems for virtually all laser, atherectomy and stent devices. The most flexible atherectomy device is the Rotablator, the most flexible stent is the MicroStent.

C. TECHNICAL CONSIDERATIONS AND APPROACH

1. **Guiding Catheter.** Co-axial alignment and adequate back-up are crucial.

2. **Guidewires.** Guidewires with single-core construction are especially useful. Extra-support and heavy-duty guidewires provide an excellent platform for balloon advancement; pseudolesions are common.

3. **Balloon Catheters.** Deflated profile, shaft-size are less important than trackability and pushability. In general, over-the-wire systems are more trackable than monorail designs; fixed wire devices can be used if other balloons fail.

ANGULATED LESIONS

A. **PTCA.** Contemporary studies report high success (85-95%) and low complication rates (< 3%). Long (30-40 mm) balloons produce less straightening force, and may be useful. Balloon material and compliance have little or no impact on results.

B. **NEW INTERVENTIONAL DEVICES.** Severe angulation is a strong predictor of procedural failure and complications after laser and atherectomy. Stenting may also be associated with suboptimal results due to prolapse of atheroma through stent coils or articulation.

C. **APPROACH.** PTCA with a long (30-40 mm) balloons is preferred over new devices.

12   CALCIFIED LESIONS

A. **LIMITATIONS OF ANGIOGRAPHY.** Angiography is relatively insensitive for identifying the extent and distribution of vascular calcification; IVUS is much more useful.

B. **PTCA**
   1. **Acute Results.** The impact of lesion calcification on PTCA success and complications is controversial; differences reflect the insensitivity of angiography in assessing calcification.
   2. **Dissection.** IVUS studies suggest that dissection frequently occurs at the junction between calcified plaque and non-calcified vessel wall. The incidence and extent of dissection are higher in calcified lesions.
   3. **Restenosis.** No association between lesion calcification and restenosis.
   4. **Technical Requirements.** Most calcified lesions can be dilated at inflation pressures < 10 ATM; for lesions resistant to inflation pressure > 12 ATM, Rotablator should be considered.

C. **NEW INTERVENTIONAL DEVICES**
   1. **Atherectomy**
   a. **Rotablator.** Treatment of choice for lesions with superficial calcification. Procedural success (> 90%), major complications (< 5%).
   b. **DCA.** Success is heavily influenced by proximal vessel calcification (which precludes passage

of the AtheroCath) and superficial calcification (which precludes tissue resection). Future calcium-cutters may improve results.

    c. **TEC.** Not recommended for calcified lesions.

2. **Lasers.** Not as effective as Rotablator for calcified lesions. Plaque fracture, rather than ablation, can improve lesion compliance.

3. **Stents.** Heavy calcification increases the risk of incomplete stent expansion. Stents are contraindicated if a calcified lesion cannot be fully expanded with a high-pressure balloon.

4. **Device Synergy.** Rotablator followed by DCA or stenting may be useful for calcified lesions.

D. TECHNICAL STRATEGY

1. **Superficial and Deep Calcium.** If calcium is present on angiography, IVUS should be used to guide device selection. Rotablator is recommended for superficial calcification; repeat IVUS is useful for assessing the degree of calcium ablation, and guide further intervention with Rotablator (larger burr), PTCA, DCA, or stenting. ELCA is not as effective as Rotablator for calcium ablation.

2. **Deep Calcium Only.** Rotablator is not effective for ablation of deep calcium; other devices such as PTCA, stenting, or DCA are recommended.

13   ECCENTRIC LESIONS

A. LIMITATIONS OF ANGIOGRAPHY. Weak correlation between angiography and IVUS for assessing eccentricity.

B. DEFINITIONS. Various definitions exist; most commonly employed is lumen located in outer quarter of apparent normal lumen by angiography.

C. BALLOON ANGIOPLASTY. Success (79%), major complication (< 4%); eccentricity may be associated with more recoil and suboptimal lumen enlargement.

D. NEW INTERVENTIONAL DEVICES

1. **DCA.** Success (86-95%); outcome is heavily dependent on other associated lesion characteristics (length, calcification, etc).

2. **Rotablator.** Effective for eccentric, calcified lesions.

3. **TEC.** No value for eccentric lesions.

4. **ELCA.** For extremely eccentric lesions, directional ELCA is preferable to conventional ELCA.

5. **Stents.** Virtually all stents are effective for eccentric lesions in vessels ≥ 3 mm.

E. TECHNICAL STRATEGY. Most devices and PTCA can be used for eccentric lesions, particularly if other complex features are absent. Consider Rotablator for calcified lesions and directional ELCA for small vessels.

14   OSTIAL LESIONS

A. **DEFINITIONS**
1. **Aorto-ostial stenosis.** Stenosis involves the aorta and origin of a native coronary artery or vein graft.
2. **Branch-ostial stenosis.** Stenosis involves the origin of a branch arising from another epicardial coronary artery.
3. **Other.** Some studies include proximal vessel location within 3-5 mm of the vessel origin.

B. **RESULTS**
1. **PTCA.** Success (74-100%); major complications (0-13%); restenosis (38-58%). Elastic recoil and suboptimal lumen enlargement are common.
2. **New Devices.** Success (70-90%) for all new devices; compared to PTCA alone, the use of Rotablator, ELCA, or TEC and adjunctive PTCA result in 22-41% gain in lumen diameter (facilitated angioplasty).

C. **TECHNICAL CONSIDERATIONS**
1. **Balloon Angioplasty.** Coaxial alignment, not aggressive vessel intubation is crucial. Sidehole guides are useful to minimize pressure damping and ensure coronary blood flow. Long (30-40 mm) balloons are useful to prevent "watermelon seeding."
2. **New Devices.** Coaxial guiding catheter alignment is imperative. DCA and stenting of ostial lesions are technically challenging.

D. **CASE SELECTION: LESION-SPECIFIC, MULTI-DEVICE THERAPY.** Results of PTCA alone are often suboptimal. For calcified, ostial lesions, consider Rotablator. For noncalcified ostial lesions, Rotablator, DCA, and stents are preferred.

15   LONG LESIONS

A. **BALLOON ANGIOPLASTY**
1. **Standard-length (20 mm) Balloons.** Success (74-97%); variable success rates probably relate to different definitions of "long" lesions. Impact of lesion length on complications and restenosis is controversial.
2. **Long (30-40 mm) Balloons.** Success (85-98%); observational data suggest fewer complications

than with 20 mm balloons.

3. **Tapered Balloon.** Useful for vessels tapering > 0.5 mm over 20 mm.

B. NEW INTERVENTIONAL DEVICES
1. **Atherectomy**
   a. **Rotablator.** Success (70-90%); increasing lesion length is associated with increased risk of non-Q-MI (up to 19%).
   b. **DCA.** Success (79-97%); lower procedural success, more emergency CABG, and higher restenosis rates compared to DCA of focal lesions; lesion length was a predictor of DCA failure in CAVEAT.
   c. **TEC.** Success (93-95%); no advantage over PTCA with long balloons.
2. **Lasers.** Success (87-92%); no relationship between lesion length and ELCA success. Randomized trials (AMRO, ERBAC): No differences in procedural success, complications or restenosis between ELCA and PTCA.
3. **Stents.** Success (> 90%); stent thrombosis (1-3.7%); relationship between number of stents and stent thrombosis is controversial.

C. APPROACH TO LONG LESIONS. PTCA is the preferred approach for most long lesions; Rotablator is recommended for long lesions with superficial calcification.

16 CHRONIC TOTAL OCCLUSIONS

NATIVE CORONARY ARTERY OCCLUSION
A. **PATHOPHYSIOLOGY.** Chronic total occlusions account for 10-20% of all procedures. Acute occlusions are due to thrombus; chronic occlusions consist of dense atherosclerotic plaque with varying degrees of organized thrombus and fibrosis.

B. **INDICATIONS AND BENEFITS**
1. **Indications.** Medically refractory angina, large region of reversible ischemia by noninvasive studies, amenable to percutaneous revascularization.
2. **Proven Benefits.** Relief of angina, improvement in LV function, reduced need for CABG.
3. **Possible Benefits.** Reverse collaterals to other vessels, improve LV remodeling after MI, increase survival.

C. **PTCA**
1. **Procedural Outcome.** Success (47-81%). Predictors of success: Functional occlusion (99% stenosis), occlusion duration < 12 weeks, occlusion length < 15 mm, presence of a tapered stump, no sidebranch at occlusion, absence of "bridging" collaterals.
2. **Complications.** Acute closure (5-10%), MI (0-2%), emergency CABG (0-3%), death (0-1%).

Higher risk of perforation compared to non-total occlusions.

3. **Late Outcome.** Restenosis (40-75%). Asymptomatic: 1-year (76%); 2-years (69%); 3-years (66%); absence of symptoms does not exclude restenosis. Reduced need for CABG by 50-75%.

D. EQUIPMENT SELECTION AND PTCA TECHNIQUE

1. **Guiding Catheter.** Must provide coaxial alignment, excellent back-up support. Voda catheters provide the most support.

2. **Guidewires.** >50% require intermediate or standard guidewires. Use transport catheter (or deflated balloon catheter) for extra support. Glidewires are especially useful for refractory occlusions but cannot be extended. Magnum wire may also be used, but it is not clearly superior to other guidewires.

3. **Balloon Dilatation Catheter.** Over-the-wire systems are preferred because they permit guidewire exchanges, enhanced push and trackability.

4. **Adjunctive Thrombolytic Therapy.** Prolonged (8-24 hours) infusion of intracoronary Urokinase may enhance procedural success if occlusion cannot be crossed with a guidewire.

E. NEWS DEVICES. All FDA-approved atherectomy, laser, and stent devices require that the total occlusion be crossed with a guidewire.

1. **Devices for Occlusions Resistant to PTCA Guidewire.** All are investigational. Excimer laser guidewire and ROTACS may cross 50% of refractory occlusions; therapeutic ultrasound and vibrational angioplasty are also under evaluation.

2. **Devices Used After Crossing Occlusion With a Guidewire.**
   a. **Lasers.** AMRO trial: No difference between PTCA and ELCA; success (65%), late reocclusion (23-33%), restenosis (50%).
   b. **Atherectomy.** DCA, TEC, are rarely indicated for chronic occlusions in native vessels; Rotablator value is uncertain.
   c. **Stents.** Focal occlusions in vessels ≥3 mm are suitable for stenting. Followup studies are in progress.

SAPHENOUS VEIN GRAFT OCCLUSION

A. PATHOLOGY. Etiology of occlusion depends on time interval after CABG: < 1 month: Thrombosis (poor surgical technique or poor distal run-off); 1-12 months: Intimal proliferation; > 12 months: Graft atherosclerosis.

B. PTCA RESULTS. Success (70%); distal embolization (5-15%); late graft occlusion (40-50%). Event-free survival: 1-year (54%), 3-years (34%).

C. NEW DEVICES. Longterm results are discouraging for all devices. Stents offer the most hope for sustained benefit; adjuncts to stenting include TEC, angiojet, and prolonged Urokinase infusion.

D. PROLONGED INTRAGRAFT THROMBOLYSIS. Can successfully recanalize 50-80% of

occluded grafts; mandatory need for more definitive techniques to maintain long-term patency.

17 CORONARY ARTERY BYPASS GRAFTS

A. TREATMENT OPTIONS FOR VEIN GRAFT DISEASE

1. **Repeat CABG.** Risks 2-4 hold higher than initial CABG; 5-year event-free survival (64%), angina-free survival (50%). Some patients are poor candidates for redo CABG (small vessels, poor LV , comorbid problems, no conduits).

   a. **Recurrent Ischemia.** 1-year (17%), 10-years (63%). May be due to new disease in nonbypassed vessels, disease in conduits, progressive disease beyond graft anastomosis.

   b. **Vein Graft Failure.** 1-year (8%); 5-years (38%); and 10-years (75%).

   c. **Repeat Revascularization.** Repeat CABG or PTCA: 5-years (4%); 10-years (19%); 12-years (31%).

2. **PTCA**

   a. **Success and Major Complication Rates.** Success (78-97%); major complications (0-12%).

   b. **Angiographic Complications**

      1. **Distal Embolization.** Vein grafts > 3 years old (2-15%). Most important risk factors are diffuse degeneration, large plaque volume, and graft friability, not thrombus or device type. ReoPro may reduce distal embolization.

      2. **No-reflow.** Vein grafts > 3 years old (5-15%). Most important treatment strategy is intracoronary calcium antagonists.

      3. **Abrupt Closure.** 1-2% of vein graft interventions. Most common etiology is dissection; most important treatment strategy is stenting.

      4. **Perforation.** < 1%; cardiac tamponade is rare.

3. **New Interventional Devices.** Account for 25-35% of vein graft interventions in busy practice.

   a. **Translumunial Extraction Catheter (TEC)**

      1. **Overall Results.** Procedural success: Nonoccluded grafts (80-90%), occluded grafts (60-75%). Distal embolization (2-17%), no-reflow (8.8%), abrupt closure (2-5%), major complications (0.7-11%), restenosis 60-70%).

      2. **Thrombotic Vein Grafts.** More complications and procedural failures than non-thrombotic vein grafts; possible role for TEC and stenting.

   b. **Directional Coronary Atherectomy.** Procedural success (85-97%); major complications (0-7%); restenosis (31-63%); similar results between PTCA and DCA (CAVEAT-II)

   c. **Excimer Laser Angioplasty.** Procedural success (92%); major complications (6.1%); restenosis (52%).No advantage compared to PTCA.

   d. **Stents.** Procedural success (95-100%); major complications (0-4%); restenosis (17-60%); optimal stent techniques will decrease need for oral anticoagulation. Treatment of choice if stenting is feasible.

   e. **Rotablator Atherectomy.** Rarely used in vein grafts at ostium or distal anastomosis; not recommended for lesions in body of vein grafts.

    f.   **Other Atherectomy Devices.** Hydrodyzer, Angiojet are potentially useful for aspiration of clot and debris.

    g.   **Prolonged Low-Dose Intra-graft Urokinase Infusion for Chronically Occluded Saphenous Vein Graft.** Useful for recanalizing occluded grafts; 6-month patency (<50%).

B. **APPROACH TO THE PATIENT WITH PREVIOUS BYPASS SURGERY**
    1. **Graft Age.** Lesion location and morphology are more important than graft age per se.
    2. **Lesion Location.**
        a. **Proximal and Aorto-ostial Lesions.** Procedural success for PTCA and other devices (86-95%); restenosis (47-93%); best results with stents.
        b. **Lesions in the Body of the Graft.** Procedural success (> 90%); major complications (< 5%). Restenosis: Stenting (20-35%); other devices (42-63%); best results with stents.
        c. **Distal Anastomotic Lesions.** PTCA is preferred for most lesions.
    3. **Lesion Morphology**
        a. **Vein Grafts > 3 mm.** Stents are treatment of choice for most focal or tubular lesions.
        b. **Vein Grafts < 3 mm.** PTCA is treatment of choice; no advantages for other devices. Use of stents is under investigation.
        c. **Degenerated Grafts and Chronic Total Occlusions.** Longterm results are disappointing with all percutaneous interventions; consider medical therapy or redo CABG. Potential role for Angiojet, Hydrolyzer (studies pending).
    4. **Acute Myocardial Infarction.** Generally have large clot burden; mechanical techniques are better than lytic therapy.

C. **INTERNAL MAMMARY ARTERY INTERVENTION**
    1. **Technical Considerations.** PTCA is device of choice in most lesions; stenting is feasible.
        a. **Subclavian Artery Tortuosity.** May limit access to IMA; ipsilateral brachial approach is useful.
        b. **IMA Engagement.** Liberal use of nitrates to attenuate vasospasm.
        c. **Equipment Selection.** Low profile balloons are necessary because of tortuosity; long shafts (> 135 cm) and 90 cm guides may be useful.
    2. **Coronary Steal and the IMA.** Stenosis in subclavian artery proximal to IMA may cause coronary ischemia; PTA, stenting are useful.

D. **GASTROEPIPLOIC ARTERY.** Technically difficult; procedural success (50%).

E. **APPROACH TO PTCA OF NATIVE VESSELS VIA BYPASS GRAFTS.** Procedural success (> 90%); results, complications, and restenosis are similar to PTCA of native vessels.

18   PTCA EXOTICA

Various techniques are available to deal with unusual problems in interventional cardiology.

19   CORONARY ARTERY SPASM

A. PATHOPHYSIOLOGY. PTCA and other interventions result in endothelial denudation and loss of EDRF; vessels have more propensity for vasospasm.

B. PTCA. Incidence: Intralesional spasm (1-5%), distal epicardial spasm (16-30%), post-procedural spasm induced by pharmacologic means (15-46%).

C. NEW DEVICES. Incidence: Rotablator (4-36%); ELCA (1.2-16%); DCA (0.8-1.6%). Spasm is more frequent after new devices than PTCA; readily reversible.

D. MANAGEMENT. Most cases respond readily to nitrates, calcium antagonists; low pressure balloon inflations can "break" severe spasm. In tortuous vessels, removal of interventional hardware may ameliorate spasm. Stents, CABG are rarely needed. For refractory spasm, exclude dissection.

E. PREVENTION. Intravenous NTG is reasonable. For Rotablator cases, a "Rotaflush cocktail" of heparin, Verapamil, and NTG is widely used.

F. PTCA FOR VARIANT ANGINA. Rarely necessary.

20   DISSECTION & ACUTE CLOSURE

A. CLASSIFICATION. Established closure (total occlusion, TIMI flow $\leq$ 1); imminent closure (high grade stenosis, TIMI flow = 2); threatened closure (residual stenosis > 50%, TIMI flow = 3).

B. INCIDENCE AND TIMING. Incidence (2-11%). Timing: In-lab (50-80%), out-of-lab (20-50%).

C. CAUSES. Most common is dissection; other causes include thrombus formation, spasm. Angiogram is often unreliable in distinguishing dissection from thrombus; many cases are probably multifactorial.

1. **Dissection.** Small intimal dissections rarely require treatment; patients with acute closure virtually always require treatment.

   a. **Classification.** NHLBI classification is most popular. A,B = minor dissection; C-F = major dissection with 5-fold higher risk of major complications.

   b. **Incidence.** PTCA: Angiography (20-40%); IVUS (60-80%). Saline infusion technique may decrease dissection after ELCA.

   c. **Pathophysiology.** Frequently occur at junction of calcified plaque and non-calcified wall; laser-induced dissection results from acoustic effects.

   d. **Risk Factors for Dissection.** Lesion complexity is important.

   e. **Prognosis After Dissection.** Severe dissection (class C-F) increases the risk of major complications; dissection per se has no impact on restenosis.

D. RISK FACTORS

1. **Acute Closure.** Strongest predictor of acute closure is complex dissection after intervention; pre-procedural variables are weak predictors of acute closure. "Lesion Score" may be useful in some patients.

2. **Cardiac Death After Acute Closure.** Strongest predictor of death after acute closure is the "jeopardy score."

E. PREVENTION OF ACUTE CLOSURE

1. **Antiplatelet Agents.** Preprocedural aspirin reduces acute closure by 50-75%; bolus and infusion of c7E3 causes 35% reduction in major complications after PTCA and DCA; Integrelin showed a non-statistically significant decrease in major complications. Ticlopidine may be useful in aspirin-allergic patients.

2. **Anticoagulants.** ACT is a predictor of acute closure; most recommend heparin to achieve ACT 250-350 seconds. Rebound thrombosis may occur after heparin discontinuation in some patients with acute ischemic syndrome. Hirudin is an effective thrombin-inhibitor; Hirulog was withdrawn from further clinical trials (no advantage compared to hirudin).

3. **IABP.** Uncertain role; may be useful in high-risk acute MI patients.

4. **PTCA Technique.** Over-size balloons (balloon/artery ratio > 1.2) can increase the risk of acute closure and major complications.

F. RECOGNITION OF ACUTE CLOSURE. Clinical presentation: Acute chest pain (90%), ST elevation (75%), hypotension (20%), sudden death (1-10%). Immediate return to the cath lab is recommended.

G. MANAGEMENT OF ACUTE CLOSURE. Stenting is the most important advance in mechanical treatment of acute closure.

1. **Initial Management.** Administer IC NTG to revere spasm; verify ACT > 300 seconds. Repeat PTCA if occlusion can be crossed with guidewire (balloon/artery ratio 1-1.1). Adjunctive Urokinase is reserved for definite thrombus.

2. **Poor Result After rePTCA.**

    a. **Vessel ≥ 3 mm.** Must identify the distal extent of dissection; stenting is treatment of choice. DCA is feasible for focal dissection not associated with dye staining, but stents are more reliable.

    b. **Vessels < 3 mm.** Prolonged inflation (10-30 minutes); DCA is not recommended; stenting is reasonable, but of uncertain benefit.

3. **Refractory Acute Closure.** CABG virtually always needed; "bail-out-catheter" and/or IABP are useful to attenuate ischemia.

4. **In-Hospital Management After Successful Reversal of Acute Closure.** Triage patient to monitored setting; sheaths, heparin overnight. Consider Warfarin if thrombus was present. Low-intensity medical regimens may be sufficient for "perfect" stent results; otherwise, use Warfarin and prolonged heparin.

H. OTHER MANAGEMENT ISSUES

1. **Non-Flow-Limiting Dissection.** Final stenosis < 30%: No treatment. Final stenosis > 50%: Stent if possible (data are controversial about the role of stenting, but most interventionalists would stent these lesions); Final stenosis 30-50%: Data are not available.

2. **Primary Thrombotic Acute Closure.** Less common cause of acute closure, except after DCA (thrombosis may cause 50% of acute closures). Recommend repeat PTCA and adjunctive IC Urokinase. Local drug delivery, platelet IIb/IIIa inhibitors may be useful.

I. **PROGNOSIS.** Acute closure is a serious problem: 5-fold increase in death, 10-25-fold increase in MI, CABG. Impact on restenosis is controversial.

21   NO-REFLOW

A. **DEFINITION.** No-reflow (TIMI flow ≤ 1) and slow-flow (TIMI flow = 2) not explained by dissection, thrombus, spasm, or severe residual stenosis at the original target lesion.

B. **ETIOLOGY.** Probably multifactorial; most important mechanism is microvascular spasm.

C. **INCIDENCE.** Varies (0.6-12.2%), depending on clinical setting and definition; more common in vein grafts, thrombus containing lesions, and Rotablator.

D. **CLINICAL MANIFESTATIONS AND PROGNOSIS.** Usually causes chest pain, ST elevation; may result in severe hemodynamic compromise; 10-fold higher risk of death, MI.

E. **PROPHYLAXIS.** Not known; several regimens with adenosine, calcium antagonists, and other vasodilators are under study. Some use "cocktail" of heparin, NTG, verapamil (or adenosine) in

Rotablator flush solution.

F. **MANAGEMENT.** Optimal treatment is unknown; may vary with clinical scenario.
    1. **Reverse Superimposed Spasm.** NTG may reverse superimposed epicardial spasm; probably no value as sole therapy.
    2. **Exclude Coronary Dissection.** Important to exclude; treatment of dissection is more straight forward than that of no-reflow.
    3. **Administer Intracoronary Calcium Antagonists.** Most important treatment for slow-flow or no-reflow; effective in 65-95% of cases; intracoronary verapamil (100-200 mcg bolus) or diltiazem (0.5-2.5 mg bolus) are effective.
    4. **Treat Distal Embolization.** Consider lytic drugs for macroembolization and distal vessel cutoff.
    5. **Clear Microvascular Plugging.** Rapid, forceful injections may clear microvascular plugging.
    6. **Increase Coronary Perfusion Pressure.** Important to maintain adequate perfusion pressure (IABP for hypotension; CPS for hemodynamic collapse).
    7. **Coronary Artery Bypass Surgery.** No value.
    8. **Triage to ICU.** Important to monitor patients for CPK rise.
    9. **Other Approaches.** Papeverine, adenosine have been used in some cases (very little experience).

22   PERFORATION

A. **INCIDENCE AND CLASSIFICATION.** PTCA (0.1%); other non-balloon devices (0.5-3.0%); types of perforation include free perforation, contained perforation, and other unclassified perforations.

B. **MECHANISMS AND RISK FACTORS.** Perforation may be secondary to guidewire, PTCA, devices that ablate or remove tissue. Oversized devices in angulated lesions or tapering vessels are important risk factors.

C. **OUTCOME.** Significant patient morbidity, even with successful treatment. Death (0-9%); MI (4-26%); emergency CABG (24-36%); blood transfusion (34%).

D. **PREVENTION**
    1. **Guidewire Positioning.** Important to maintain free movement of tip of guidewire; avoid placing guidewire in small branches; always verify distal wire position before inflation or device deployment.
    2. **Device Sizing.** Balloon/artery ratio ~ 1 for PTCA; for high risk lesions, use undersized devices such as Rotablator, ELCA (device/artery ratio 0.5-0.6); use adjunctive PTCA rather than larger devices.
    3. **Other Device Considerations.** Avoid DCA for spiral, extensive dissections; avoid hi-pressure balloon inflations outside stents; use balloon/artery ratio ~ 1.

E. MANAGEMENT

1. **Nonoperative Management of Coronary Perforation.** Crucial to identify the perforation and support the patient hemodynamically with pressors, CPS, etc.

    a. **Prolonged Balloon Inflation.** Initial step in virtually all perforations; balloon/artery ratio ~ 1, inflation at 2-6 atm for at least 10 minutes; use perfusion balloon if necessary; May avoid surgery in 60-70%. Stent-vein allografts are "experimental".

    b. **Pericardiocentesis.** Mandatory for rapid accumulation of pericardial effusion, particularly if associated with hemodynamic collapse.

    c. **Reversal of Anticoagulation.** Strongly considered in patients with ongoing perforation despite prolonged balloon inflations, or with free perforation due to lasers or atherectomy.

    d. **Monitoring Following Successful Nonoperative Management.** All patients should be monitored in CCU; pericardial drainage for ~ 24 hours; frequent, serial echo.

2. **Operative Management.** Indicated for large perforations associated with severe ischemia, persistent perforation despite nonoperative measures, or hemodynamic collapse not immediately responsive to pericardiocentesis; required in 30-40% of perforations.

23 EMERGENCY BYPASS SURGERY

A. INTRODUCTION

1. **Levels of Surgical Backup.** Two different levels for surgical support for PTCA include "stand-by" arrangements (a surgical team and operating room are open and available in the event of failed PTCA) and "back-up" arrangements (emergency surgery is performed in the next available operating room).

2. **Surgical Consultation Before PTCA.** Detailed assessment of high risk patients is necessary, particularly for patients with severe LV dysfunction, prior CABG, lack of suitable conduits, severe comorbid medical conditions, etc.

B. INCIDENCE.

Contemporary PTCA is complicated by emergency CABG in 1-2% of procedures (CABG performed within 24 hours of intervention).

C. INDICATIONS FOR EMERGENCY CABG

1. **Important Considerations.** Age of the patient, mental status, conduit availability, history of previous CABG, and use of thrombolytic agents within 6 hours are important.

2. **Indications for Emergency Cardiac Surgery.** Acute coronary occlusion accounts for 70% of emergency CABG after failed PTCA; other indications include suboptimal angioplasty result with refractory ischemia, coronary artery perforation with tamponade, left main injury, and retained angioplasty hardware.

D. CONTRAINDICATIONS TO EMERGENCY SURGERY.

Contraindications are based on patient

life expectancy and cardiopulmonary reserve. Factors that preclude surgery include irreversible cerebral injury, metastatic carcinoma, AIDS, end-stage pulmonary disease, no suitable conduits, and age >80 with cardiogenic shock.

E. **PREPARATION FOR EMERGENCY SURGERY.** Before referring a patient for emergency CABG, it is important to restore adequate oxygen delivery and maintain distal coronary blood flow with perfusion catheters and coronary vasodilators, if possible,

F. **SURGICAL TECHNIQUES**
   1. **Conduit Selection.** Vein grafts may be used for hemodynamically unstable patients; the IMA is preferred for stable patients
   2. **Myocardial Protection.** Blood cardioplegia is important, using antegrade (from the aortic root) and retrograde (from the coronary sinus) techniques. Warm induction cardioplegia is useful for patients in shock.
   3. **Coronary Arterial Repair and Revascularization.** Long-patch angioplasty with saphenous veins is recommended for long spiral dissections or distal perforations. If stents have been implanted, we usually attempt to remove them.
   4. **Special Considerations.** Primary attention is given to the acutely ischemic myocardium; once this territory is grafted, other vessels > 1.5mm with diameter stenosis are grafted.
   5. **Operative Adjuncts.** Inotropic agents, pressors, and intra-aortic balloon pumps are useful in select patients, to sustain myocardial function. Occasionally, single or biventricular support devices are needed.

G. **RESULTS**
   1. **Morbidity.** Operative mortality is 5.7-12.5%, but nearly 40% for patients in shock and nearly 100% for octogenarians in shock.
   2. **Morbidity.** Perioperative MI occurs in 28-63% of patients, characterized by ECG changes and enzyme elevation; LV function usually improves post-operatively. Nonoliguric renal failure and prolonged mechanical ventilation occur in 5-10% of patients.

24   RESTENOSIS

A. **DEFINITION OF RESTENOSIS.** Recurrent symptoms after PTCA may be due to progressive disease in untreated vessels or to restenosis of the original target lesion.
   1. **Angiographic Restenosis.**
      a. **Dichotomous Events** (Restenosis is either present or absent). The most common definition is diameter stenosis > 50% at follow-up; restenosis occurs in 30-50% of patients. Other definitions identify different patients with restenosis.
      b. **Continuous Outcomes** (Restenosis is a continuum; it occurs to some extent in all patients).

Restenosis is the net result of multiple factors, including acute gain and late loss (elastic recoil, intimal hyperplasia, remodeling).

2. **Clinical Restenosis.** Contemporary definitions of restenosis rely on outcomes which reflect hard clinical endpoints, including death, myocardial inflation, and repeat target-lesion revascularization (CABG, rePTCA).

B. **MECHANISMS OF RESTENOSIS.** Restenosis is complex; these mechanisms are not mutually exclusive.

1. **Elastic Recoil.** Simple "stretching" of the arterial wall during balloon inflation, followed by recoil of the vessel to its original dimensions. May be eliminated by stenting.

2. **Intimal hyperplasia.** Manifestation of "healing" after vessel injury, characterized by proliferation of modified vascular smooth muscle cells. Common after all devices; cannot yet be modified by devices or drugs.

3. **Arterial Remodeling.** Changes in the vessel wall leading to vessel expansion or vessel contraction, which can enlarge or constrict the lumen, respectively. Common after DCA and PTCA.

C. **TIME COURSE OF RESTENOSIS.** Most common within 6-months. After stenting, in-stent minimal lumen diameter may improve between 6-months and 3-years after implantation.

D. **PREDICTORS OF RESTENOSIS**

1. **Geometric Factors.** Post-procedure lumen diameter is a strong predictor of restenosis. Some devices (ELCA, Rotablator, DCA) may be associated with greater loss of lumen diameter.

2. **Biological Factors.** Diabetes and the presence of activated smooth muscle cells are important risk factors. Hypercholesterolemia is a risk factor for atherosclerosis, but not restenosis. The impact of LAD location, unstable angina, gender, and smoking is controversial.

3. **Prior Restenosis.** Restenotic lesions have a higher restenosis rate than de novo lesions, but may reflect preselection for other geometric and biologic determinants.

E. **PREVENTION OF RESTENOSIS**

1. **Pharmacological Interventions.** Only calcium channel antagonists, fish oil, and c7E3 (plaque stabilization or "passivation") may decrease clinical restenosis.

2. **Mechanical Interventions.** Stents are associated with a 30% reduction in restenosis compared to PTCA (for de novo lesions in native vessels $\geq$ 3 mm). Restenosis rates after DCA and PTCA are similar (native vessels and vein grafts). ELCA and Rotablator are associated with higher restenosis rates than PTCA. Other randomized trials (optimal atherectomy, optimal stenting) are in progress.

F. **DETECTION OF RESTENOSIS**

1. **Patient's Symptoms.** Absence of symptoms is a good predictor of absence of restenosis; recurrent symptoms are not good predictors of restenosis.

2. **Functional Testing.** Routine serial functional testing in asymptomatic patients is not recommended; functional testing is useful in patients with recurrent chest pain. False positive results are frequent within 6 weeks of intervention. The value of exercise scintigraphy, exercise

echo, and dobutamine echo are similar.

G. **MANAGEMENT OF RESTENOSIS.** Intervention for restenotic lesions is safer than de novo lesions; recurrent restenosis rates are 30-50%. Factors such as patient characteristics, myocardium at risk, lesion morphology, coexisting coronary artery disease, and LV function are important considerations in guiding therapy.

H. **RECOMMENDATIONS.** Optimize the initial result by appropriate device selection and use pharmacologic and other therapies to reduce the progression of atherosclerosis at other sites.

I. **FUTURE DIRECTIONS.** Advances in molecular biology and new pharmacologic agents may have a dramatic impact on restenosis.

25 MEDICAL & PERIPHERAL COMPLICATIONS

RENAL INSUFFICIENCY

A. **ETIOLOGY.** Potential causes of renal insufficiency post intervention include pre-renal (volume depletion, low cardiac output) renal (dye induced or ischemic), or post renal (obstruction) failure..

B. **PREVENTION.** Hydration with or without loop diuretics, mannitol or dopamine are commonly used for prevention of contrast induced renal failure in high risk patients; randomized data supporting their use are limited.

C. **MANAGEMENT.** Management of renal insufficiency includes ruling out obstruction or bleeding and, maintaining adequate hydration and urine output with fluids, diuretics and renal dose dopamine.

CONTRAST REACTIONS

A. **TYPES OF CONTRAST AGENTS**
   1. **Ionic, High osmolar agents** have an osmolarity 5-8 times higher than blood.
   2. **Low osmolar agents** may be either ionic or nonionic, and are half the osmotic load of high-osmolar agents.

B. **ADVERSE DYE REACTIONS**
   1. **Hemodynamic effects:** Transient hypotension and impaired contractility are due to hyperosmolarity of contrast.
   2. **Electrophysiologic effects:** ECG changes, ventricular and bradyarrhythmias are due to high osmolarity and calcium chelating properties.

3. **Minor reactions:** Nausea, urticaria, itching, heat sensation, and vomiting occur more frequently with high osmolar agents.

4. **Allergic reactions:** Observed more frequently with high osmolar contrast.

5. **Thrombosis:** More common with nonionic agents; these agents should be avoided if possible when interventions are performed in unstable angina or MI patients.

6. **Nephrotoxicity:** Not influenced by the type of contrast agents, but high osmolar agents may cause volume overload.

7. **Cost:** High osmolar agents are inexpensive eg, 15-20 times less than high osmolar agents.

C. **RECOMMENDATIONS.** Nonionic contrast should be avoided if possible in patients with unstable ischemic syndromes; high osmolar agents should be used unless allergic, hemodynamic, arrhythmic or volume overload concerns are present.

D. **PREVENTION**

1. **Identify patients at risk** by obtaining a history of prior contrast reactions, severe hay fever, asthma, or other allergies.

2. **Pharmacologic prophylaxis** should be performed with steroids (Prednisone 40 mg q6°, starting 12-18 hrs before procedure), diphenhydramine (50 mg just before procedure); low osmolar contrast is recommended.

E. **TREATMENT**

1. **Minor contrast reactions** (nausea, urticaria, minor bradycardia) usually require no treatment.

2. **Moderate reactions** (urticaria and angioedema) may be treated with IV diphenhydramine, steroids.

3. **Severe reactions** (anaphylaxis - bronchospasm, laryngeal edema and/or profound hypotension) may occur with a single contrast injection and require IV epinephrine (1-5cc of 1:10,000 dilution IV every 2-5 min), steroids, diphenhydramine, bronchodilators, and possible intubation.

PERIPHERAL VASCULAR COMPLICATIONS

A. **AV FISTULA.** May occur in 0.1-1.5% of interventional cases. Diagnosis should be confirmed with color flow Doppler in patients with a continuous bruit. Management usually requires surgical repair, but ultrasound guided compression is used in some cases.

B. **PSEUDOANEURYSM.** May occur due to a low femoral puncture, impaired clotting or inadequate compression following sheath removal. Diagnosis should be confirmed by ultrasound or angiography in any patient with a large hematoma. Management includes observation if small (< 3 cm) or ultrasound guided compression for larger pseudoaneurysms (surgical correction if unsuccessful).

C. **THROMBOTIC OCCLUSION.** Occurs more frequently with the brachial approach, and is recognized by severe pain or numbness, cool extremity and absence of a distal pulse. Management requires thrombectomy or surgical repair.

D. **ARTERIAL PERFORATION.** Infrequent; when wire induced, can usually be managed conservatively. More severe perforation may require surgical repair.

E. **DISSECTION.** Infrequent; can be managed conservatively unless major branches are involved.

F. **RETROPERITONEAL HEMORRHAGE.** Due to a high femoral arterial puncture; manifested by abdominal pain or an asymptomatic drop in hemoglobin. Treatment requires cessation of anticoagulants, removal of sheaths and prolonged compression. Surgical repair is rarely necessary.

G. **ATHEROEMBOLIZATION.** Can result in stroke, renal failure, livedo reticularis, blue toe syndrome or acute arterial ischemia. Management is usually conservative.

H. **BLEEDING COMPLICATIONS.** Related to baseline patient characteristics, sheath size, thrombolytics, glycoprotein IIb/IIIa receptor antagonists, prolonged heparin or coumadin.

I. **VASCULAR CLOSURE DEVICES.** Collagen plugs, percutaneous suture and compression devices are promising techniques to reduce access site bleeding complications.

INFECTION
A. **CLINICAL MANIFESTATIONS.** Infections may manifest as fever, rigors, lethargy, or erythema at the access site.

B. **ETIOLOGY AND TREATMENT.** The most common cause of post procedure sepsis is Staph aureus; management includes blood and catheter cultures, line removal and empiric IV vancomycin until cultures are available.

NEUROLOGIC COMPLICATIONS. Incidence of neurologic events is 0.07% for diagnostic procedures, 0.1-0.5% for interventional procedures; due to emboli (atheroma, air, thrombus), intracranial bleeding, or cerebral hypoperfusion. Management includes reversal of potential drug, metabolic or hemodynamic causes; consideration of reversal of heparin with protamine (if bleeding is suspected); and obtaining a CT scan.

26 CORONARY STENTS

A. **STENT DESIGNS**
1. **Self-Expanding Stents.** The original WallStent is being replaced by a second-generation New WallStent; advantages include less shortening and less thrombogenicity compared to earlier

designs.

2.   **Balloon-Expandable Stents.** Two stainless steel stents are approved by the FDA: The Gianturco-Roubin stent (GRS) and the Palmar-Schatz stent (PSS). Other stainless steel (MultiLink stent, MicroStent) and tantalum (Wiktor stent, Cordis stent) stents are under investigation. The Strecker stent (tantalum) was withdrawn from the market and will be replaced by the Nir stent (stainless steel).

B.   STENT CHARACTERISTICS

1.   **Biocompatibility.** Resistance to thrombosis and corrosion.

2   **Flexibility.** Of extreme practical importance for the coronary circulation. The PSS is the least flexible; the Microstent is the most flexible.

3.   **Visibility.** Important for proper deployment. The radiopacity of tantalum is superior to stainless steel.

4.   **Reliable Expansion.** Balloon-expandable stents provide more reliable expansion than self-expanding stents.

5.   **Stent Surface Area.** 7-20% for most stents; higher surface area results in better coverage of lesion but more thrombogenicity.

C.   TECHNIQUE OF STENT PLACEMENT

1.   **Self-Expanding Stents.** Predilation is required. The stent is delivered by retracting the constraining sheath. PTCA is recommended to smoothe the stent surface after deployment.

2.   **Balloon-Expandable Stents.** Predilation is required. The stent is delivered by inflating the stent delivery balloon; optimal results are achieved by high-pressure balloons after deployment. The PSS and MultiLink-Stents have special delivery sheaths which must be retracted before stent deployment.

3.   **Radial Artery Technique.** May improve patient comfort and reduce bleeding and vascular complications compared to femoral technique.

D.   INDICATION FOR STENTS

1.   **Definite Indications.** FDA approved; based on compelling observational data and randomized trials: Reversal of abrupt closure (GRS), prevention of restenosis (PSS).

2.   **Probable Indications.** Based on compelling observational data; randomized trials are in progress and FDA approval is likely in the near future: Saphenous vein grafts (nondegenerated).

3.   **Possible Indications.** Stents are commonly used, but data are lacking: Bifurcation lesions (technically challenging; only used by experienced operators); ostial lesions; restenotic lesions; small vessels (< 3 mm); chronic total occlusions; and diffuse disease.

4.   **Contraindications.** Lesions with gross thrombus may be considered for stenting after thrombus removal (TEC, angiojet) or dissolution (lytic therapy, anticoagulation).

E.   SPECIFIC CLINICAL SITUATIONS

1.   **Acute MI.** Stents should not be withheld after failed PTCA because of fear of stent thrombosis. Prospective studies of planned stenting in acute MI are in progress.

2. **Unstable angina.** Immediate results, complications, and late outcome after stenting are similar to stable angina.

3. **Single Patent Vessel.** Stents can provide reliable revascularization if patient is not a candidate for CABG, target lesion is suitable for stenting, and distal run-off is good. Optimal stenting is important.

4. **Unprotected Left Main.** Approach is similar to single patent vessel.

5. **Sealing Perforations and Pseudoaneurysms.** Stent-vein allografts have been used in selected patients; technically challenging.

6. **Women.** Vascular complications are increased in women; restenosis and late outcome are similar to men.

F. **ADJUNCTIVE THERAPY.** Medical regimens are largely empiric; randomized trials in progress.

1. **Conventional Anticoagulation Regimen.** Includes aspirin, dipyridamole, low-molecular weight Dextran, heparin, and Warfarin; stent thrombosis (2-3%); bleeding and vascular complications (10-25%); length of hospital stay (5-7 days).

2. **Low-Intensity Anticoagulation Regimen.** Involve "optimal" stent technique and antiplatelet agents (aspirin, Ticlopidine) without prolonged heparin infusion or Warfarin. Low-molecular weight heparin is probably of no additional benefit.

3. **Intravascular Ultrasound (IVUS).** May be useful for guiding "optimal" stent technique. Optimal IVUS criteria include stent coverage (stent cross-sectional area > 80% of reference-vessel cross-sectional area); apposition (gap between stent and vessel wall < 0.1 mm); and symmetry (stent minor axis/stent major axis > 0.7). However, routine need for IVUS has not been confirmed.

4. **Thrombolytic Therapy.** May be useful in degenerated vein grafts and for adjunctive treatment of stent thrombosis.

5. **Vasodilators.** Widely used, but not of proven value.

6. **Antibiotics.** Not routinely recommended; should be used for prophylaxis before invasive procedures associated with transient bacteremia.

7. **Other medications.** Studies of platelet IIb/IIIa inhibitors are planned or in progress.

8. **Angioscopy.** Useful in thrombotic lesions.

9. **Doppler Flow.** Stenting results in normalization of coronary flow reserve. Doppler may be useful for identifying angiographically-inapparent residual disease or dissection which impairs flow reserve after successful PTCA.

10. **Atherectomy.** DCA (ostial lesions), Rotablator (ostial lesions, calcified lesions), and TEC (thrombotic lesions) may be useful adjuncts to stenting.

G. **COMPLICATIONS**

1. **Stent Thrombosis.** Acute (< 1%); Subacute (0.4-4.7%); WallStent (15-24%); Wiktor (12%); after failed PTCA (0-32%). Predictors of stent thrombosis include unstented distal disease or dissection, stent diameter < 3 mm, filling defects inside stent, and need for multiple stents. Treatment includes immediate revascularization by PTCA, adjunctive lytic therapy, and correction of underlying causes, if possible.

2. **Ischemic Complications.** Usually arise as a consequence of abrupt closure after failed PTCA or

stent thrombosis; MI (2-26%), CABG (0-16%), death (0-10%). Overall ischemic complications: Stents for failed PTCA (28%), elective stents (0-6.9%).

3. **Bleeding and Vascular Injury.** Overall bleeding and vascular complications: Conventional anticoagulation (7.3-13.5%); low intensity regimen (1-2.5%). Risk factors include age > 70, female gender, and multiple interventions during the same hospitalization.

4. **Stent Embolization.** Rare with coronary stents (< 1%).

5. **Sidebranch Occlusion.** Occurs with similar frequency after stenting or PTCA. Sidebranches can be retrieved with low-profile balloons through PSS and GRS.

6. **Perforation.** Rare complication. May be related to oversized balloons, high pressure inflations, contained perforation after other devices (before stent deployment), or unrecognized subintimal passage of guidewire when stents are used for abrupt closure.

H. OTHER ISSUES

1. **Cost.** Stents are more expensive than PTCA. If length of stay and bleeding/vascular complications can be reduced by low-intensity regimens without increasing stent thrombosis, stents will be cost-effective because of their favorable impact or restenosis.

2. **Future Directions.** Biodegradable stents, drug-delivery stents, coated stents, radio-active stents, and stent-grafts may increase the utilization of stents in the future.

27

ROTABLATOR

A . **DESCRIPTION** The Rotablator system consists of the Rotablator burr, flexible drive shaft, and a main console. Burr rotational speed is controlled by a compressed air turbine, and speed is monitored by a fiberoptic tachometer on the main console.

B. **PHYSICAL PRINCIPLES AND DESIGN CHARACTERISTICS.** Rotablator operation is based on two physical principles: Differential cutting is the ability to selectively remove tissue based on differences in tissue composition and elasticity; inelastic, calcified tissue is selectively ablated by Rotablator. Orthogonal displacement of friction refers to the eliminination of longitudinal friction at usual rotational speeds of operation.

C. **IMPACT OF HIGH-SPEED ROTATIONAL ABLATION.** The mechanism of Rotablator atherectomy is ablation of inelastic plaque. Unlike other atherectomy devices, tissue is not removed; microembolization of plaque and other debris is well tolerated when particles are small. Larger particles may be generated during forceful advancement of the burr, excessive burr deceleration, or low platform speeds. With proper use, Rotablator is highly efficient at plaque ablation; lumen diameter usually exceeds 90% of burr diameter. Unfortunately, equipment costs for Rotablator are 20-50% more than PTCA.

D. ROTABLATOR PROCEDURE

1. **Preprocedural Assessment.** The general approach is similar to PTCA. Special considerations include the prophylactic insertion of temporary pacemakers (target lesions in the RCA or dominant LCX), and maintenance of adequate hydration to offset-vasodilator induced hypotension.

2. **Adjunctive Medication.** Aspirin is manadatory and calcium channel blockers are strongly recommended. Large doses of intracoronary NTG are frequently used to attenuate spsam. Some operators use a cocktail of NTG, verapamil, and heparin in the Rotablator flush solution; ACT should be maintained > 300 seconds.

3. **Rotablator Technique.** Guiding catheter selection is crucial; coaxial alignment is the most important consideration to prevent "guidewire bias" and inadvertent dissection or perforation. The ideal burr/artery ratio is unknown, but most operators complete the procedure with a final burr/artery ratio of 0.75-0.80. It is important to achieve the proper platform speed before advancing the burr across the target lesion; gentle, slow burr advancement and continuous monitoring of the rotational speed will enhance results and safety.

E. RESULTS

1. **Results.** Procedural success (73-96%); Adjunctive PTCA (42-100%). Lumen dimensions may improve after 24 hours due to release of elastic recoil and spasm.

2. **Complications.** Angiographic complications: Dissection (10-13%), abrupt closure (1.8-11.2%), slow-flow (1.2-7.6%), perforation (0-1.5%), severe spasm (1.6-6.6%). Clinical complications are similar to PTCA: Death (0-2.3%), Q-wave MI (0-4.8%), emergency CABG (0-2.8%). There may be a higher incidence of non-W-wave MI after Rotablator (2.8-8.8%) than after PTCA.

3. **Restenosis.** To date, Rotablator has had no impact on restenosis rates (37-62%) compared to conventional PTCA. The need for target lesion revascularization was higher for Rotablator than PTCA (ERBAC Trial). Further studies are in progress.

4. **Impact of Plaque Composition on Results.** Rotablator can ablate both soft and calcified plaque. However, its main value compared to PTCA is for calcified lesions.

5. **Impact of Lesion Morphology on Results.** Rotablator provides greater lumen enlargement than PTCA for complex lesions, ostial lesions, and undilatable lesions. The value of Rotablator for long lesions is uncertain; there may be a higher incidence of non-Q-wave MI. Rotablator is not recommended for severely angulated or thrombotic lesions.

F. CLINICAL TRIALS.

Three large multicenter trials are in progress: STRATAS (to compare the strategies of aggressive debulking with and without adjunctive PTCA); DART (to compare Rotablator and PTCA for simple lesions); and CARAT (to compare small [burr/artery ratio < 0.7] and big [burr/artery ratio > 0.7] burrs). Other studies of Rotablator as an adjunct to stenting are planned.

G. SUMMARY.

Rotablator may have certain "niche" applications for undilatable, calcified, and ostial lesions. The issues about restenosis are unsettled; available studies suggest no benefit.

28 DIRECTIONAL CORONARY ATHERECTOMY (DCA)

A. DESCRIPTION. Simpson Coronary AtheroCath. Percutaneous over-the-wire cutting and retrieval system; excised atheroma is removed from the patient.

B. DCA EQUIPMENT

1. **Guiding Catheters.** New line of 9.5-10F guides have replaced older 11F guides; new configurations for the RCA and vein grafts.

2. **AtheroCath Designs**
   - **First Generation.** *SCA-1;* only available as 7F Graft cutter with Surlyn balloon.
   - **Second Generation.** *SCA-EX;* better torque and nosecone design compared to SCA-1; PET balloon replaced Surlyn balloon; short-window (5mm) devices available.
   - **Third Generation.** *SCA-GTO;* best support and torque control; not available in short window or 7F Graft devices.

3. **Ancillary Equipment.** Motor-drive unit, 0.014-inch guidewires, and large bore rotating hemostatic valve (ID ≥ 0.094-inch).

C. DCA TECHNIQUE

1. **Preparation of the AtheroCath.** GTO device requires triple negative aspiration prep.

2. **Guiding Catheter Manipulation.** Most important principle is coaxial alignment; over-rotating and deep-seating must be avoided.

3. **AtheroCath Deployment.** Gentle advancement and continuous rotation are necessary, orient cutter toward angiographically evident plaque.

4. **Adjunctive Medical Therapy.** Similar to PTCA; ASA, Heparin (ACT > 300 sec); ReoPro useful for high risk patients.

5. **Adjunctive Devices.** Rotablator useful for calcified ostial lesions; IVUS may be useful for assessing depth, extent of calcification and for guiding optimal atherectomy.

6. **Optimal Atherectomy.** Selection of appropriate device size; cut towards angiographically apparent plaque; larger cutter or PTCA for residual stenosis > 15%; can be accomplished with or without IVUS.

D. MECHANISM OF LUMEN ENLARGEMENT. IVUS suggests tissue removal accounts for ≥ 75% of lumen enlargement.

E. PROCEDURAL RESULTS

1. **Immediate Angiographic Results.** DCA success (83-99%); final diameter stenosis (5-29%); adjunctive PTCA is recommended for optimal atherectomy.

2. **Angiographic Complications.** Overall, similar to PTCA.
   a. **Dissection/Abrupt Closure.** Nonocclusive dissections (20%); severe dissection/abrupt closure

(0-7%) (similar to PTCA); may be due to guide, device, or wires. Treatment includes PTCA, stents, CABG. Nearly half of abrupt closures do not occur at the treatment site.

    b. Thrombosis. Accounts for ≥ 50% of abrupt closures after DCA; treatment includes PTCA, lytics, CABG.

    c. Distal Embolization and No-Reflow. 0-13.4%; more common in vein grafts. Treatment includes disruption of embolus (distal embolization) or calcium antagonists (no-reflow).

    d. Vasospasm. < 2%; readily responds to nitrates or low-pressure PTCA.

    e. Perforation. < 1%; not related to resection of media or adventitia; treatment is identical to perforation of any cause.

    f. Sidebranch Occlusion. Overall incidence (0.7-7.7%); 37% sidebranch occlusion if ostium has disease; treatment is PTCA or DCA of branch.

3. Clinical Complications. Most occur as a consequence of severe angiographic complications (especially abrupt closure).

    a. Major Clinical Complications. 0-10%; due to severe dissection, perforation, guiding catheters, device-related injury and adjunctive PTCA.

    b. Non-Q-Wave MI. May be a higher incidence of non-Q-MI (3-12.5%) after DCA than PTCA; risk of non-Q MI is decreased by ReoPro. Clinical significance of asymptomatic enzyme rise is controversial.

    c. Vascular Injury. Transfusion or vascular repair (1-5%); similar to PTCA.

4. Restenosis and Late Outcome. Randomized studies show no difference in restenosis rates between DCA and PTCA in native vessels or vein graft. Optimal atherectomy trials are in progress; may be able to achieve restenosis rates similar to stents.

5. Correlates of Outcome

    a. Angiographic Results. Lesion calcification is the most important correlate of adverse results; other factors include length > 10 mm, angulation, proximal tortuosity; better results with eccentric and ulcerated lesions.

    b. Complications. Associated with operator inexperience, de novo lesions, and lesion angulation.

    c. Restenosis. Randomized studies suggest post-procedure lumen diameter is strongest predictor; other important determinants are vessel size, diabetes, LAD location, and unstable angina.

F. SPECIAL CONSIDERATIONS

1. Deep Tissue Resection. > 60%; probably no relationship to restenosis, pseudoaneurysm formation, or ectasia.

2. Unstable Angina. Immediate results are excellent (comparable to stable angina); 2-year event-free survival may be lower than stable angina.

3. Acute MI. Overall procedural success (92-93%); may be higher incidence of angiographic and clinical complications.

4. Elderly. Higher incidence of major complications, procedural failure, and blood transfusion.

G. LESION-SPECIFIC APPLICATIONS

1. Ostial Lesions. Procedural success (86-87%); major complications (< 1%); high restenosis rates

(48% de novo, 61% restenotic); DCA not suited as sole therapy for heavy calcification or vessel diameter < 3 mm.

2. **Bifurcation Lesions.** Procedural success (97-100%), major complications (0-3%); transient sidebranch occlusion (37%, salvaged by PTCA or DCA).

3. **Thrombus-Containing Lesions.** DCA not suitable for large thrombus burden; small thrombus burden is ok; adjunctive lytics and/or prolonged (48 hr) heparin may be useful.

4. **Saphenous Vein Grafts.** DCA is suitable for focal lesions; immediate results, complications, and restenosis are similar to PTCA.

5. **Left Main Disease.** Procedural success (88%); emergency CABG (4.5%).

6. **Suboptimal PTCA.** DCA is suitable for focal dissection, elastic recoil, and small thrombus burden; procedural success (63-92%), major complication (0-12.5%). DCA contraindicated in long, spiral dissections.

7. **Restenotic Lesions.** Procedural success (94-98%); similar results compared to PTCA, stents.

8. **Stent Restenosis.** Uncertain risk of excision of stent struts or coils; no advantage over PTCA.

H. **TISSUE ANALYSIS.** DCA provides only opportunity for sampling atherosclerosis from living patients.

29 TRANSLUMINAL EXTRACTION CATHETER (TEC) ATHERECTOMY

A. **DESCRIPTION.** TEC is an over-the-wire cutting and aspiration system with a conical cutting head and stainless steel blades, for cutting and removal of atheroma and thrombus.

B. **EQUIPMENT**
   1. **Cutters.** TEC cutters are available from 5.5-7.5F (1.8-2.5 mm).
   2. **Guiding Catheters.** Special 10F tungsten-braided catheters are available; 9F guides may be used with TEC cutters ≤ 6.5F.

C. **TECHNIQUE**
   1. **Guiding Catheter Manipulation.** Deep-seating and over-rotation should be avoided.
   2. **Hemostatic Valve.** A special rotating hemostatic valve connects the guide to the motor drive unit; special care must be used to eliminate air from the valve.
   3. **Guidewires.** A special 300-cm stainless steel TEC guidewire has a 0.021-inch ball-tip; less steerable than conventional PTCA guidewires.
   4. **Cutter Deployment.** Recommended cutter/artery ratio ~ 0.5-0.7; cutter activation in lesion should be avoided. Ensure that pressurized flush is flowing during TEC.

5. **Adjunctive Medical Treatment.** Similar to PTCA; intracoronary verapamil useful for no-reflow.
6. **Adjunctive Intervention.** Adjunctive PTCA, DCA, or stenting is virtually always required; angioscopy may be useful in vein grafts.

D. **MECHANISM OF ACTION.** Minimal if any plaque removal; partial or complete thrombus extraction; dissection is frequent.

E. **RESULTS**
1. **Native Coronary Arteries.**
   a. **Immediate Results.** Procedural success (84-94%), adjunctive PTCA (79-84%); elastic recoil (30%); final diameter stenosis after TEC (~ 60%), adjunctive PTCA (~ 36%).
   b. **Clinical Complications.** Death (1.4-2.3%); MI (0.6-3.4%); CABG (2.6-3.4%).
   c. **Angiographic Complications.** Abrupt closure (8-11%); dissection (39%); perforation (0.7-2.2%); distal embolization (0.5-1.6%); sidebranch occlusion (2.7%).
   d. **Follow-up.** Angiographic restenosis (56-61%); clinical restenosis (29%).
2. **Saphenous Vein Grafts.**
   a. **Immediate Results.** Procedural success (82-92%); adjunctive PTCA (74-95%).
   b. **Clinical Complications.** Death (0-10.3%); MI (0.7-3.7%); CABG (0.2%).
   c. **Angiographic Complications.** Distal embolization (2-17%); no-reflow (8.8%); abrupt closure (2-5%).
   d. **Follow-up.** Angiographic restenosis (64-69%); late total occlusion (29%).

F. **SPECIAL CONSIDERATIONS.**
1. **Acute Ischemic Syndromes.** May have role for acute MI and after failed thrombolysis; multicenter trial in progress (TOPIT).
2. **Thrombus.** TEC is effective at removing thrombus; nevertheless, procedural success is lower and complications are higher if thrombus is present.
3. **Saphenous Vein Bypass Grafts.** May be an adjunct to stenting in thrombotic vein grafts.
4. **Ostial Lesions.** TEC and adjunctive PTCA result in 22% incremental increase in lumen diameter compared to PTCA alone.
5. **Contraindications.** Heavy calcification, severe angulation, marked eccentricity, and bifurcation lesions should not be treated with TEC.

G. **FUTURE DIRECTIONS.** Expandable cutter heads, improved cutting and aspiration are expected.

30 EXCIMER LASER CORONARY ANGIOPLASTY (ELCA)

A. BACKGROUND. Lasers (Light Amplification by Stimulated Emission of Radiation) ablate tissue by photochemical, localized thermal, and mechanical effects.

B. EQUIPMENT

1. **Laser Unit.** AIS and Spectranetics have merged, now operating under the Spectranetics name. The laser unit has a warm-up time of only 5 minutes.
2. **Laser Catheters.** Contemporary laser catheters are flexible, allow rapid exchange, and achieve greater ablation area. Specialized catheters include a directional laser and a laser guidewire.

C. CLINICAL RESULTS

1. **Observational Studies.** The ELCA Registry reported procedural success in 90%, independent of lesion morphology.
2. **Non-randomized Comparative Studies.** Case controlled series demonstrate lower procedural success, more complications, and higher restenosis rates after ELCA compared to PTCA.
3. **Randomized Trials.** The Dutch AMRO study demonstrated similar angiographic results and complications, but a trend toward higher restenosis rate after ELCA. The German ERBAC study reported higher rates of acute complications and restenosis after ELCA.
4. **Laser Wire for Total Occlusions.** This appears to be a promising technology for refractory total occlusions; however, the incidence of wire perforation was 21%.
5. **Complications.** Dissection and/or perforation occur more commonly with large catheters, higher energies, long lesions, sidebranches, experienced operators, and when blood or contrast enter the ablation field.
6. **New Techniques to Improve Results.** The saline infusion technique has improved angiographic results; the impact on restenosis is unknown.

D. RECOMMENDATIONS AND CASE SELECTION. ELCA is well-suited for long lesions, total occlusions, and ostial lesions. ELCA can be used for in-stent restenosis, but comparative data to PTCA are lacking.

E. TECHNICAL DETAILS

1. **Catheter Selection.** The laser catheter diameter should be less than two-thirds the reference vessel diameter.
2. **The ELCA Procedure.** It is important to use a coaxial guiding catheter, an extra-support guidewire, energy densities between 40 - 60 mJ/mm^2, and the saline infusion technique to minimize acoustic effects and dissection.
3. **Trouble-Shooting.** Never apply additional laser energy once dissection has occurred. If the 1.4 mm catheter does not cross a rigid lesion on a straight segment of the artery, the energy density may be increased to 60 mJ/mm^2, or the frequency increased to 30 Hz. If this is

unsuccessful, the laser procedure should be abandoned.

31 INTRAVASCULAR ULTRASOUND (IVUS)

A. LIMITATIONS OF ANGIOGRAPHY

1. **Stenosis severity.** IVUS is superior to angiography for identifying atherosclerosis and stenosis severity. Angiographically "normal" vessels frequently have significant disease by IVUS.

2. **Post-Intervention Assessment.** IVUS is superior to angiography for assessing the post-interventional "hazy" or "suboptimal" result.

B. IVUS EQUIPMENT. IVUS consists of two principal components: An imaging catheter and an imaging console to reconstruct the image.

1. **Mechanical Devices.** Most widely used imaging catheters; external motor and drive shaft rotates a single transducer at the catheter tip. Main advantage is image quality.

2. **Electronic Devices.** Annular array of 32-64 elements at distal catheter tip; main advantages are flexibility, trackability, and absence of imaging artifacts.

C. IMAGE INTERPRETATION

1. **Normal Lumen Features.** Blood appears as finely-textured specular echoes; permits identification of true lumen. May not be visible in severe lesions.

2. **Normal Wall Anatomy.** Some vessels have 3 distinct layers (internal elastic lamina, media, adventitia); other vessels have 1 distinct layer (internal elastic lamina is inapparent).

3. **Plaque Composition and Distribution.** IVUS can readily distinguish soft, fibrous, and calcified plaque as well as eccentric vs. concentric stenoses. It is less useful for identifying thrombus.

D. ADVANTAGES OF IVUS. Superior to other modalities for precise quantitative analysis of vessel dimensions, plaque characterization, and evaluation of dissection.

E. DISADVANTAGES OF IVUS. Imaging artifacts (non-uniform rotational distortion, ring-down artifact), geometric distortion, inability to distinguish tissue with similar acoustic properties (e.g., soft plaque and thrombus), and cost.

F. TECHNIQUE. IVUS can be performed with standard PTCA guiding catheters ($\geq$ 7F) and 0.014-inch guidewires. Monorail designs with a protective sheath are most widely used. Serious complication are rare.

G. DIAGNOSTIC APPLICATIONS OF IVUS

1. **Angiographically Unrecognized Disease.** IVUS can detect atherosclerosis at sites which appear normal by angiography.

2. **Lesions of Uncertain Severity.** IVUS provides precise quantitative assessment, independent of lesion location.

3. **Cardiac Allograft Vasculoplasty.** Many centers perform routine IVUS to detect allograft atherosclerosis.

H. INTERVENTIONAL APPLICATION OF IVUS

1. **Characterize Plaque for Device Selection.** Plaque distribution (eccentric vs. concentric) and composition (soft, fibrous, calcified, mixed) have implications for device selection (e.g., DCA for highly eccentric plaque, Rotablator for heavily calcified lesions).

2. **Mechanism of Lumen Enlargement.** IVUS can identify plaque removal (DCA), ablation (Rotablator), dissection (PTCA, ELCA), vessel stretching (PTCA), and elimination of elastic recoil (stents).

3. **Precise Quantitative Measurements.** IVUS can identify "normal" vessel size and assist in device selection and sizing.

4. **Guidance of Directional Atherectomy.** IVUS can be used to achieve "optimal" atherectomy results; however, the absolute need for IVUS has not been established, since "optimal" results can also be achieved without IVUS.

5. **Coronary Stent Deployment.** IVUS criteria for "optimal" stenting include excellent stent apposition (< 0.1 mm between vessel wall and strent strut), cross-sectional area (CSA) index > 0. 8 (ratio of stent minimal CSA to reference vessel CSA), and symmetry index > 0.7 (ratio of minor to major stent diameter).

6. **Characterize Dissection After Intervention.** IVUS is useful for identifying the depth, extent, and length of dissection; and may be useful for stent deployment in complex dissections.

I. COMPARISON OF IVUS, ANGIOSCOPY, AND DOPPLER FLOW

1. IVUS is useful in the assessment of lumen dimensions, plaque characterization, and evaluation of suboptimal results after intervention.

2. Angioscopy is most for differentiating thrombus from dissection and residual plaque.

3. Doppler flow is useful for determining the physiologic significance of stenoses before and after intervention.

J. NEW INTRAVASCULAR IMAGING DEVICES.
Future advances include IVUS guidewires and combined IVUS-revascularization devices (PTCA, DCA).

32

ANGIOSCOPY

A. INDICATIONS

1. **Guiding Saphenous Vein Graft Interventions.** Angioscopy is superior to angiography for identification of thrombus; may be useful for guiding interventions in vein grafts and selecting

vessels for prolonged UK infusion.

2. **Evaluation of Suboptimal Results.** Can readily distinguish clot from dissection; may have implications for device selection.

3. **Post-Interventional Assessment.** Can be used to evaluate residual filling defects, and to distinguish clot, dissection, residual plaque.

4. **Assessment of Borderline Lesions.** Less useful than IVUS or Doppler flow.

5. **Identification of Culprit Lesions.** In multivessel disease, angioscopy may identify thrombus and the "culprit" lesion.

6. **Predicting Outcome After Intervention.** Controversial role

B. **LIMITATIONS OF ANGIOSCOPY.** Provides qualitative, not quantitative, information; not useful for ostial lesions or origin lesions of LAD or LCx.

C. **COMPLICATIONS.** Dissection (2.8%), abrupt closure (1%); in degenerated vein grafts, angioscopy may induce transient or sustained no-reflow (50%); transient ischemia occurs when cuff inflation exceeds 60 seconds.

33 DOPPLER BLOOD FLOW

A. **INTRODUCTION.** Coronary blood flow is determined by coronary vascular resistance, which is autoregulated by the microvasculature. Coronary blood flow may also be affected by stenosis in the epicardial vessels. Resting flow is impaired when diameter stenosis > 85%; hyperemic flow is impaired when diameter stenosis > 50%. Coronary blood flow velocity and hyperemic coronary flow reserve (CFR) can be measured by Doppler technique.

B. **APPROACH TO DOPPLER BLOOD FLOW**
1. **Doppler Systems.** Most widely used system is the Doppler FloWire.
2. **Coronary Blood Flow Data.** Instantaneous peak velocities are used to measure average peak velocity (APV) and diastolic/systolic velocity ratio (DSVR). CFR is the ratio of basal APV/hyperemic APV. A full understanding of the limitations of these measurements is crucial.

C. **CLINICAL APPLICATIONS.** Provides complementary information to angiography, IVUS, and angioscopy.
1. **Clinical Applications.** Useful for assessment of borderline lesions; diagnosis of Syndrome X; evaluation of transplant arteriopathy; bypass graft patency; and functional recovery after MI.
2. **Interventional Applications.** Useful for assessment of suboptimal results after intervention; predicting complications; monitoring Urokinase infusions for chronic occlusions; assessment of no-reflow; and studying dynamic turbulence.

34 ADJUNCTIVE PHARMACOTHERAPY

ANALGESIA AND SEDATION. Premedication is used to ease anxiety and discomfort; popular combinations include narcotics and short-acting benzodiazepines. Local anesthesia with warm xylocaine may further reduce discomfort.

CONTRAST REACTIONS

A. **PROPHYLAXIS AGAINST CONTRAST REACTIONS.** Prophylactic medical therapy is recommended for all patients with a previous contrast-induced urticaria, bronchospasm, or anaphylaxis; treatment should be instituted at least 12 hours prior to the procedure. Standard prophylaxis includes a corticosteroid (prednisone, solumedrol, or hydrocortisone) and H-1 blocker (benadryl); H-2 blockers (cimetidine, ranitidine) are considered optional. For emergency PTCA, intravenous prophylaxis is required immediately prior to angiography, and low-osmolar contrast agents are recommended.

B **TREATMENT OF CONTRAST REACTIONS**
   1. **Minor reactions.** Nausea, flushing may occur within minutes of exposure. No specific treatment is required, but cool compresses, benadryl, or atropine may improve patient comfort.
   2. **Moderate reactions.** Persistent nausea and vomiting, anaphylactoid reactions (urticaria, angioedema), or severe vasovagal reactions (bradycardia with hypotension) may occur within minutes to hours of exposure. Treatment is usually required, including IV fluids, H-1 blockers (Benadryl), antiemetics (Compazine), and atropine. Anaphylactoid reactions should be treated with intravenous steroids (solumedrol or hydrocortisone) and epinephrine (0.1-0.5cc of 1:1000 epinephrine SQ), if necessary.
   3. **Severe reactions.** Anaphylaxis (bronchospasm, laryngeal edema, and/or profound hypotension) is a life-threatening medical emergency, which may occur within seconds of exposure to even small amounts of contrast. Immediate treatment includes epinephrine (1-5cc of 1:10,000 epinephrine IV), intravenous steroids (solumedrol or hydrocortisone), and benadryl. Supported ventilation and inhaled (albuterol) or intravenous (theophylline) bronchodilators may be indicated. Patients frequently require prolonged infusions of epinephrine or neosynephrine to support the circulation.

PREVENTION OF ABRUPT CLOSURE
A. **ANTIPLATELET THERAPY**
   1. **Aspirin.** Reduces the risk of abrupt closure by 50-75% when given at least 24 hours before PTCA. The optimal dose is unknown, although most operators use 325 mg daily.
   2. **Ticlopidine.** More potent platelet inhibitor than aspirin, but should be administered for at least 3 days prior to PTCA to achieve platelet inhibition. Usual dose is 250 mg BID, but 500 mg BID for 1-2 days may expedite the onset of antiplatelet action. May be useful in patients with

aspirin-allergy. Neutropenia may occur in 1-2% of patients after 4 weeks of therapy; usually reversible after discontinuation of drug. May also be associated with elevated transaminases. Clopidogrel is a more potent analogue with potentially fewer side effects.

3. **Dipyridamole.** No benefit compared to aspirin alone.

4. **IIb/IIIa Receptor Antagonists.** Multiple agents are under investigation (ReoPro, Integrelin, Xemlofiban, Tirofiban); ReoPro is FDA-approved for use in high-risk interventions with PTCA or DCA (EPIC Trial). Patients receiving bolus and infusion of ReoPro have fewer major ischemic complications and 6-month cardiac events. ReoPro also reduces major ischemic complications in elective PTCA patients (EPILOG Trial). Further studies of "rescue ReoPro" are under evaluation. Integrelin has not yet shown clinical benefit (IMPACT Trial), but further studies are in progress.

B. ANTITHROMBOTIC AGENTS

1. **Heparin.** Always employed during PTCA. Heparin-effect is estimated by ACT, but different techniques achieve different ACT results. The ideal ACT is unknown, but most operators aim for an ACT of approximately 300 seconds. The dose of postprocedural heparin after successful intervention is unknown; further studies are in progress. Elective PTCA patients with good angiographic results probably do not require any additional heparin after the procedure.

2. **Low Molecular Weight Heparin.** No clear advantage over unfractionated heparin; further studies are in progress.

3. **Hirudin and Derivatives.** Hirudin and hirulog are as effective as heparin during PTCA; both reduce ischemic complications and bleeding, but not restenosis. Hirulog has no apparent advantage over hirudin.

4. **Other Antithrombin Agents.** Argatroban, tissue-factor pathway inhibitor (TFPI), and other antithrombin peptides are under evaluation.

C. FIBRINOLYTICS.
Routine use of lytic agents is not justified; intracoronary urokinase has a detrimental effect in unstable angina patients (TAUSA Trial). Lytic infusions should be considered for definite thrombus (confirmed by angioscopy) and for chronic total occlusions that cannot be crossed by a guidewire.

D. DEXTRAN.
No benefit during percutaneous intervention.

PREVENTING ISCHEMIA DURING ANGIOPLASTY

A. NITROGLYCERIN.
Commonly used during PTCA to attenuate spasm; does not prevent or delay onset of ischemia during balloon inflations. Should be used with caution in patients with hypovolemia or hypotension.

B. BETA-BLOCKERS.
Clearly useful for intraprocedural hypertension. May delay the onset and severity of chest pain during balloon inflations, but clear benefit has not been demonstrated.

C. CALCIUM CHANNEL ANTAGONISTS.
Clearly useful for reversing many cases of no-reflow;

routine use is common but not clearly indicated.

TREATMENT OF PERIPROCEDURAL HYPOTENSION. Severe and persistent hypotension increases the risk of abrupt closure after PTCA; the etiology of hypotension must be sought and immediately corrected. If hypotension does not immediately respond to simple measures such as IV fluids or atropine, the systemic circulation should be supported by drugs or other support devices.

35   LOCAL DRUG DELIVERY

A   **OVERVIEW.** Local drug delivery has theoretical applications in restenosis, thrombosis, and promoting neovascularization. Local delivery of high drug concentrations may limit side effects associated with systemic administration.

B.   **MECHANISMS OF INTRAMURAL DRUG DELIVERY.** Passive diffusion: simple diffusion mediated by a concentration or electrochemical gradient; Active bulk transfer: direct introduction by hydrostatic pressure; Facilitated diffusion: delivery by a substrate-carrier complex.

C.   **PHARMACOKINETIC CONSIDERATIONS.** The most important factor is the intramural residence time; some agents may be quickly washed away by the coronary circulation.

D.   **CATHETER-BASED LOCAL DRUG DELIVERY TECHNIQUES**
  1. **The Double-Balloon Catheter.** Standard angioplasty balloon shaft with two latex balloons; drug infusion between the balloons bathes the arterial wall; drug delivery by passive diffusion or applied hydrostatic pressure. Advantage: easy, safe; Disadvantage: need for prolonged dwell times.
  2. **The Wolinsky Perforated Balloon Catheter.** Triple-lumen balloon with 28 holes in longitudinal rows; delivery by bulk transfer through the pores. Advantage: easy; Disadvantage: may injure the vessel wall from barotrauma or high-velocity jets.
  3. **The Microporous Balloon Catheter.** Variation of the perforated balloon.
  4. **The Transport Catheter.** Triple lumen catheter with dual balloons, 36-48 infusion holes. Preliminary trials in progress.
  5. **The Hydrogel-Coated Balloon.** Standard PE balloon coated with a hydrogel polymer, which absorbs water; hydrogel compression during balloon inflation results in pressure diffusion from the polymer to the vessel wall. Clinical trials are in progress. Advantage: homogenous delivery, useful as an angioplasty balloon; Disadvantage: Rapid washoff of drug, low drug concentrations.
  6. **The Dispatch Catheter.** Spiral inflation coil wrapped around a urethane sheath; the spiral coil forms an internal lumen during inflation, which permits antegrade blood flow. Drug is delivered passively through the coils and into the vessel wall. Clinical trials are in progress. Advantage: prolonged delivery times, allows passive perfusion of distal vessel during drug delivery; Disadvantage: ischemia of sidebranches, cannot be used as an angioplasty balloon.

7. **The Channel Balloon.** Standard PET balloon on a triple lumen shaft; 18 longitudinal channels serve as conduits for drug delivery. Advantage: low pressure, atraumatic drug delivery; can function as an angioplasty balloon; Disadvantage: nonhomogenous drug delivery, ischemia during balloon inflation.

8. **The Infusasleeve.** Multilumen catheter tracks over a standard angioplasty balloon; drug infusion occurs directly over the angioplasty balloon during inflations. Clinical trials in progress.

9. **The Iontophoresis Catheter.** Local delivery by electrochemical gradient. Can achieve higher drug concentrations than passive drug delivery.

E. DRUG DELIVERY CATHETERS APPROVED FOR CLINICAL USE

1. **Medical-Legal Implications.** The Dispatch catheter and Infusasleeve are FDA-approved for intraluminal, not intramural, drug delivery. The Hydrogel-coated balloon is approved as angioplasty balloon.

2. **The Hydrogel-Coated Balloon.** Urokinase-coated balloons are being studied for thrombus-containing lesions.

3. **The Dispatch Catheter.** Currently under evaluation for delivery of Urokinase and/or heparin.

4. **The Infusasleeve.** Several studies are planned.

F. CONCLUSIONS.
Several issues need to be resolved: Which drug, what concentration, how long? Local drug delivery appears promising for treatment of thrombus and restenosis.

36 PERIPHERAL AND VISCERAL INTERVENTION

A. PATHOPHYSIOLOGY.
Similar to coronary atherosclerosis; it is useful to consider peripheral vascular disease in 3 anatomic zones: The inflow tract (Zone 1), the outflow tract (Zone 2), and the run-off bed (Zone 3).

B. DIAGNOSIS AND PATIENT EVALUATION

1. **Lower Extremity.** The quality of pulses will help localize the site of obstruction, but is unreliable for estimating disease severity. Objective data are provided by the ankle-brachial index and duplex ultrasound.

2. **Carotid Artery.** Duplex ultrasound is useful for evaluation of carotid atherosclerosis.

3. **Renal and Mesenteric Arteries.** Duplex ultrasound is useful for evaluation of the renal arteries, celiac axis, and superior mesenteric artery.

4. **Subclavian Artery.** Duplex ultrasound is useful for evaluation of subclavian stenosis. A systolic blood pressure difference ≥ 20 mmHg between both arms suggests significant stenosis.

C. PERCUTANEOUS ANGIOPLASTY TECHNIQUES

1. **Adjunctive Medication.** Aspirin recommended for all patients; sublingual nifedipine and intra-arterial nitroglycerin are useful for minimizing vasospasm in the renal and infrapopliteal circulation.

2. **Vascular Access.** Arterial access should be achieved as close as possible to the target lesion. Retrograde femoral (ipsilateral and contralateral approaches), antegrade femoral, axillary, and brachial approaches are useful for specific anatomic situations.

3. **Crossing the Lesion.** Baseline angiography may be performed with diagnostic catheters or guiding catheters. Multiple guidewires are available for different types of lesions.

4. **Balloon Catheter Selection.** A variety of balloon catheters are available. The balloon may be positioned using anatomic landmarks or guiding catheter techniques.

5. **Special Considerations for Renal Artery Angioplasty.** Long-acting antihypertensive therapy should be replaced by short-acting alternatives; vascular surgery back-up is recommended.

D. **RESULTS OF PTA.** There is no universally accepted definition of success; various definitions include angiographic success (residual stenosis < 15-20%), hemodynamic success (residual pressure gradient = 0 mmHg at rest), or clinical success (using clinical endpoints).

1. **Renal Artery PTA.** Angiographic success (79-96%); 6-year patency (70-93%). Better results for fibromuscular dysplasia than atherosclerotic stenosis.

2. **Aortoiliac PTA.** Aorta: Success (83-100%), 5-year patency (70-92%); Iliac artery: Success (73-100%), 5-year patency (32-92%).

3. **Iliofemoral PTA.** Success (90-95%); 3-year patency (75-80%). Worse outcome for total iliac occlusions and lesion length > 10 cm.

4. **Femoropopliteal PTA.** Success (85%); 3-year patency (60%). Long-term success is most influenced by distal run-off.

5. **Infrapopliteal PTA.** Success (95%); 1-year patency (75-80%); coronary angioplasty balloons and guidewires may be useful.

6. **Cerebral PTA.** Success (76-83%); death (3%); stroke (10%).

E. **COMPLICATIONS OF PTA.** Overall incidence (5-10%); emergency surgery (3%); death (0.1-0.5%).

F. **NEW DIRECTIONS IN PERCUTANEOUS VASCULAR INTERVENTIONS**

1. **Intravascular Stents.** The only FDA-approved stent is the Palmaz stent; the WallStent is under clinical evaluation. Procedural success (> 95%), 5-year patency (93%); stenting for carotid artery disease is under investigation (success > 90%).

2. **Peripheral Intra-Arterial thrombolysis (PIAT).** Useful for acute claudication or limb-threatening ischemia due to thromboembolic occlusion; prolonged Urokinase infusions are widely used. Success (60-95%); 2-year patency (80%).

3. **Atherectomy.** Success (80%); 6-month patency (40%); 2-year patency (15%). Overall results are inferior to PTA.

4. **Laser Ablation Techniques.** Rarely used; results are inferior to PTA

37 BALLOON VALVULOPLASTY

PERCUTANEOUS BALLOON MITRAL VALVULOPLASTY (PBMV)

A. MECHANISM OF MITRAL VALVULOPLASTY. Separation of fused commissures; fracture of calcified nodules.

B. PREPROCEDURAL EVALUATION. 2-D echo, TEE to generate echo score, exclude LA clot, assess MR.

C. TECHNIQUE

1. **Antegrade Transvenous Approach (Inoue Technique; Single or Double-Balloon Technique).** All require antegrade transseptal left heart catheterization.
   a. **Technique of transseptal left heart catheterization.** Standard technique of transseptal catheterization using Brochenbrough needle, sklylet, and Mullins sheath and dilator.
   b. **Inoue Technique.** Special "dumbbell" balloon configuration to permit optimal position across mitral value; variable dilating diameters can be achieved with one balloon.
   c. **Single or Double-Balloon Technique.** More difficult to position balloons than Inoue technique; double balloons generally preferred to achieve ideal results.

2. **Retrograde Transarterial Approach.** Requires retrograde left heart catheterization; special catheters must be used to cross mitral valve retrograde.

D. RESULTS

1. **Hemodynamic Results.** 50-70% decrease in transmitral gradient; 50-100% increase in mitral valve area; larger valve areas with double balloon technique; also effective after prior surgical commissurotomy or during pregnancy.

2. **Complications.** Death (0-1.6%); embolic events (0-6.5%); severe MR (0.9-3%); left-right shunt (20%).

3. **Longterm Results.** Restenosis at 5 years (7-24%); predictors of adverse outcome include echo score > 8, high LVEDP, high NYHA class.

4. **Predictors of Early Outcome.** Echo score > 8, advanced age, calcification, AF are associated with less successful outcome.

5. **Comparison of Difference Techniques and Surgical Commissurotomy.** Overall, similar results with single and double balloons; Inoue; and retrograde arterial techniques. Slightly larger valve areas with double balloons. PBMV and surgical commissurotomy achieve similar results, but less restenosis after PBMV.

PERCUTANEOUS BALLOON AORTIC VALVULOPLASTY (PBAV). Not an accepted alternative to aortic valve replacement because of poor longterm outcome.

A. MECHANISM OF AORTIC VALVULOPLASTY. Fracture of calcified nodules, separation of fused commissures (rheumatic etiology), and simple stretching of valve leaflets.

B. **PREPROCEDURAL EVALUATION.**   2-D echo, cardiac catheterization and coronary angiography.

C. **TECHNIQUE.** Immediate and longterm results for all techniques are similar.
    1. **Retrograde Arterial Approach.** Most common; brachial or femoral route; easier to perform than antegrade approach.
    2. **Antegrade Transvenous Approach.** Requires transseptal left heart cath; more difficult than retrograde approach.
    3. **Single vs. Multiple balloon techniques.** Simplest approach is retrograde with single balloon.

D. **RESULTS**
    1. **Hemodynamic Results.** 50-70% decrease in aortic valve gradient and 40-60% increase in valve area.
    2. **Complications.** Death (2.6-10.4%); stroke (0.4-4.6%); perforation (0-1.8%); myocardial infarction (0.3-1.6%); severe AR (0-1.6%); vascular injury (7.5-27%).
    3. **Longterm Results.** Poor 1-3 year outcome. Death (30-60%); AVR (7-27%); repeat PBAV (4-22%).
    4. **Predictors of Late Outcome.** Most important predictors of late outcome are related to baseline LV function, not valve area. LV and aortic systolic pressure, PCW, and percent reduction in gradient.
    5. **Comparison of Balloon Valvuloplasty and Aortic Valve Replacement.** No prospective randomized studies; 2-year event free survival: PBAV (6.5%) and AVR (78%).

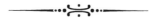

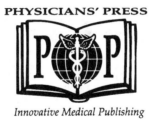

PHYSICIANS' PRESS

Innovative Medical Publishing

Other Interventional Cardiology Publications from Physicians' Press
– 1996 –

- Tough Calls in Interventional Cardiology

- Manual of Interventional Cardiology Slide Series

- Manual of Interventional Cardiology Device Guide

- Rotablator Guidebook

To Order or Receive Information:
Phone: (810) 645-6443 • Fax: (810) 642-4949
CALL FOR PRICING

The Most Unique Atlas in Cardiology!

How Do You Stack Up Against the Experts?

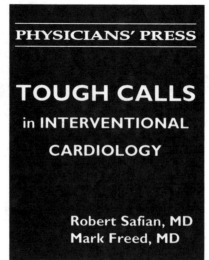

PHYSICIANS' PRESS

TOUGH CALLS in INTERVENTIONAL CARDIOLOGY

Robert Safian, MD
Mark Freed, MD

Here's Your Chance to Get 40 Second Opinions!

The Questions: *In 1996 –*

How do the experts use new devices or perform PTCA if new devices are not available? *Calcified lesions, intracoronary thrombus, degenerated vein grafts…*

How do the experts manage complications? *Dissection, acute closure, no-reflow, perforation, retained hardware…*

How do the experts manage unstable angina? Acute MI? Multivessel disease?

How are the experts using adjunctive pharmacotherapy? Intravascular ultrasound? Doppler? Angioscopy?

What techniques do the experts use to optimize stenting, PTCA, atherectomy and laser?

The Experts: *40 Experts from 10 Countries*

USA: *Spencer King III, MD; William O'Neill, MD; Gary Roubin, MD; Marty Leon, MD; Eric Topol, MD and many more...*

International: *Antonio Colombo, MD (Italy); Nicolas Reifart, MD (Germany); Patrick Serruys, MD (Netherlands); Masakiyo Nobuyoshi, MD (Japan); Ulrich Sigwart, MD (England) and more...*

The Format:

A 55-year old man presents with unstable angina and a thrombus-containing lesion in the mid-RCA.

Q: Would you mechanically intervene now or treat the patient medically for 24-48 hours first?

Q: What is your device (or device combination) of choice in this setting? What adjunctive pharmacotherapy would you use?

Q: Would you stent this lesion for a suboptimal result?

Dr. Baim:
Dr. Topol:
Dr. Serruys:
Editorial Perspective:

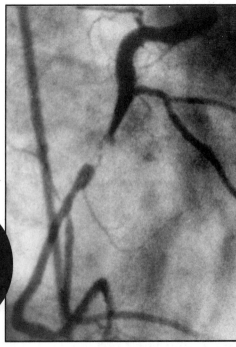

More Than 200 Cases In All!

The Bottom Line:

Tough Calls in Interventional Cardiology allows the reader to appreciate areas of **Consensus & Controversy** among the experts, and is the most unique and practical instructional atlas available.

DUE OUT MARCH 1996

To Order or Receive Information:
Phone: (810) 645-6443 • Fax: (810) 642-4949
CALL FOR PRICING

The New **Manual of Interventional Cardiology**
Full-Color Slide Series

Special Emphasis on Stents

STENT DESIGN

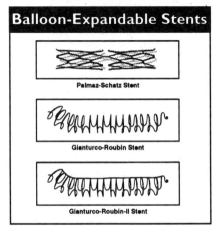

Balloon-Expandable Stents

Palmaz-Schatz Stent

Gianturco-Roubin Stent

Gianturco-Roubin-II Stent

1996 TRIAL RESULTS

Benestent-I Trial: 1 Year Follow-up

516 Patients with stable angina & a de novo coronary lesion randomized to Palmaz-Schatz stent or PTCA.

	Stent (%)	PTCA (%)	*P*
Death	1.2	0.8	NS
MI	5.0	4.2	NS
CABG	6.9	5.1	NS
Repeat PTCA	10	21	0.001
Combined Endpoint	23	32	0.004

CCL: Benefit of elective stenting of native coronaries is maintained at 1 year.

JACC 1996: 2-7: 255

LESION-SPECIFIC TECHNIQUES

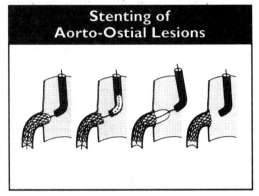

Stenting of Aorto-Ostial Lesions

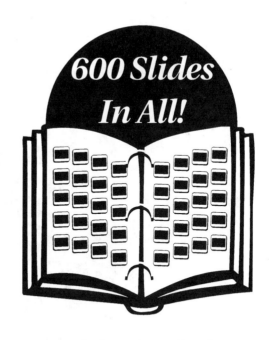

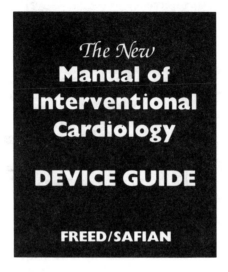

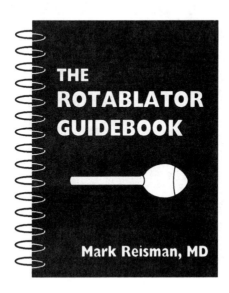